MATHEMATICS FOR NEUROSCIENTISTS

ELSEVIER *science & technology books*

Companion Web Site:

http://www.elsevierdirect.com/companions/9780123748829

Mathematics for Neuroscientists by Fabrizio Gabbiani and Steven J. Cox

Resources:

- All figures from the book available
- MATLAB® codes and exercises for each chapter of the book

Related titles

MATLAB® for Neuroscientists: An Introduction to Scientific Computing in MATLAB, P. Wallisch, M. Lusignan, M. Benayoun, T.I. Baker, A.S. Dickey, N.G. Hatzopoulos. 2009, Academic Press, ISBN: 978-0-12-374551-4

Signal Processing for Neuroscientists: An Introduction to the Analysis of Physiological Signals, W. van Drongelen. 2007, Academic Press, ISBN: 978-0-12-370867-0

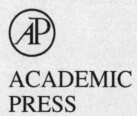

ACADEMIC PRESS

MATHEMATICS
FOR
NEUROSCIENTISTS

Fabrizio Gabbiani

Steven J. Cox

AMSTERDAM • BOSTON • HEIDELBERG • LONDON
NEW YORK • OXFORD • PARIS • SAN DIEGO
SAN FRANCISCO • SINGAPORE • SYDNEY • TOKYO

Academic Press is an imprint of Elsevier
The book's associated website is available at:
www.elsevierdirect.com/companions/9780123748829

Academic Press is an imprint of Elsevier
32 Jamestown Road, London NW1 7BY, UK
30 Corporate Drive, Suite 400, Burlington, MA 01803, USA
525 B Street, Suite 1800, San Diego, CA 92101-4495, USA

First edition 2010

British Library Cataloguing-in-Publication Data
A catalogue record for this book is available from the British Library.

Library of Congress Cataloging-in-Publication Data
A catalog record for this book is available from the Library of Congress.

ISBN: 978-0-12-374882-9

For MATLAB® and Simulink® product information, please contact:
The MathWorks, Inc.
3 Apple Hill Drive
Natick, MA, 01760-2098 USA
Tel: 508-647-7000
Fax: 508-647-7001
E-mail: info@mathworks.com
Web: www.mathworks.com

For information on all Academic Press publications
visit our website at *www.elsevierdirect.com*

Typeset by: diacriTech, India

Printed and bound in United States of America
10 11 12 13   10 9 8 7 6 5 4 3 2 1

Short Contents

1   Introduction   1

2   The Passive Isopotential Cell   9

3   Differential Equations   21

4   The Active Isopotential Cell   33

5   The Quasi-Active Isopotential Cell   49

6   The Passive Cable   67

7   Fourier Series and Transforms   87

8   The Passive Dendritic Tree   103

9   The Active Dendritic Tree   119

10   Reduced Single Neuron Models   143

11   Probability and Random Variables   155

12   Synaptic Transmission and Quantal Release   175

13   Neuronal Calcium Signaling*   193

14   The Singular Value Decomposition and Applications*   223

15   Quantification of Spike Train Variability   237

16   Stochastic Processes   251

17   Membrane Noise*   267

18   Power and Cross Spectra   279

19   Natural Light Signals and Phototransduction   291

20   Firing Rate Codes and Early Vision   299

21   Models of Simple and Complex Cells   311

22   Stochastic Estimation Theory   327

23   Reverse-Correlation and Spike Train Decoding   335

24   Signal Detection Theory   343

25   Relating Neuronal Responses and Psychophysics   355

26   Population Codes*   367

27   Neuronal Networks   381

28   Solutions to Selected Exercises   409

References   473

Index   483

Full Contents

Preface   xi

1. Introduction   1

1.1   How to Use This book   2
1.2   Brain Facts Brief   2
1.3   Mathematical Preliminaries   4
1.4   Units   7
1.5   Sources   8

2. The Passive Isopotential Cell   9

2.1   Introduction   9
2.2   The Nernst Potential   11
2.3   Membrane Conductance   12
2.4   Membrane Capacitance and Current Balance   12
2.5   Synaptic Conductance   14
2.6   Summary and Sources   15
2.7   Exercises   16

3. Differential Equations   21

3.1   Exact Solution   21
3.2   Moment Methods*   23
3.3   The Laplace Transform*   25
3.4   Numerical Methods   27
3.5   Synaptic Input   28
3.6   Summary and Sources   29
3.7   Exercises   29

4. The Active Isopotential Cell   33

4.1   The Delayed Rectifier Potassium Channel   34
4.2   The Sodium Channel   36
4.3   The Hodgkin–Huxley Equations   37
4.4   The Transient Potassium Channel*   40
4.5   Summary and Sources   43
4.6   Exercises   43

5. The Quasi-Active Isopotential Cell   49

5.1   The Quasi-Active Model   49
5.2   Numerical Methods   51
5.3   Exact Solution via Eigenvector Expansion   54
5.4   A Persistent Sodium Current*   58

5.5   A Nonspecific Cation Current that is Activated by Hyperpolarization*   59
5.6   Summary and Sources   60
5.7   Exercises   61

6. The Passive Cable   67

6.1   The Discrete Passive Cable Equation   67
6.2   Exact Solution via Eigenvector Expansion   69
6.3   Numerical Methods   71
6.4   The Passive Cable Equation   73
6.5   Synaptic Input   78
6.6   Summary and Sources   81
6.7   Exercises   82

7. Fourier Series and Transforms   87

7.1   Fourier Series   87
7.2   The Discrete Fourier Transform   89
7.3   The Continuous Fourier Transform   94
7.4   Reconciling the Discrete and Continuous Fourier Transforms   95
7.5   Summary and Sources   98
7.6   Exercises   98

8. The Passive Dendritic Tree   103

8.1   The Discrete Passive Tree   103
8.2   Eigenvector Expansion   105
8.3   Numerical Methods   107
8.4   The Passive Dendrite Equation   110
8.5   The Equivalent Cylinder*   111
8.6   Branched Eigenfunctions*   113
8.7   Summary and Sources   115
8.8   Exercises   115

9. The Active Dendritic Tree   119

9.1   The Active Uniform Cable   120
9.2   On the Interaction of Active Uniform Cables*   122
9.3   The Active Nonuniform Cable   125
9.4   The Quasi-Active Cable*   130
9.5   The Active Dendritic Tree   134
9.6   Summary and Sources   136
9.7   Exercises   136

10. Reduced Single Neuron Models   143

10.1   The Leaky Integrate-and-Fire Neuron   143
10.2   Bursting Neurons   146
10.3   Simplified Models of Bursting Neurons   147
10.4   Summary and Sources   152
10.5   Exercises   153

11. Probability and Random Variables   155

11.1   Events and Random Variables   155
11.2   Binomial Random Variables   157
11.3   Poisson Random Variables   159
11.4   Gaussian Random Variables   159
11.5   Cumulative Distribution Functions   160
11.6   Conditional Probabilities*   161
11.7   Sum of Independent Random Variables*   162
11.8   Transformation of Random Variables*   163
11.9   Random Vectors*   164
11.10 Exponential and Gamma Distributed Random
       Variables   167
11.11 The Homogeneous Poisson Process   168
11.12 Summary and Sources   170
11.13 Exercises   170

12. Synaptic Transmission and Quantal Release   175

12.1   Basic Synaptic Structure and Physiology   175
12.2   Discovery of Quantal Release   177
12.3   Compound Poisson Model of Synaptic Release   178
12.4   Comparison with Experimental Data   180
12.5   Quantal Analysis at Central Synapses   181
12.6   Facilitation, Potentiation, and Depression of
       Synaptic Transmission   183
12.7   Models of Short-Term Synaptic Plasticity   186
12.8   Summary and Sources   189
12.9   Exercises   190

13. Neuronal Calcium Signaling*   193

13.1   Voltage-Gated Calcium Channels   195
13.2   Diffusion, Buffering, and Extraction of Cytosolic
       Calcium   198
13.3   Calcium Release from the ER   201
13.4   Calcium in Spines   209
13.5   Presynaptic Calcium and Transmitter Release   213
13.6   Summary and Sources   217
13.7   Exercises   217

14. The Singular Value Decomposition
       and Applications*   223

14.1   The Singular Value Decomposition   223
14.2   Principal Component Analysis and Spike Sorting   226
14.3   Synaptic Plasticity and Principal Components   228
14.4   Neuronal Model Reduction via Balanced
       Truncation   230

14.5   Summary and Sources   233
14.6   Exercises   233

15. Quantification of Spike Train Variability   237

15.1   Interspike Interval Histograms and Coefficient of
       Variation   238
15.2   Refractory Period   239
15.3   Spike Count Distribution and Fano Factor   240
15.4   Renewal Processes   240
15.5   Return Maps and Empirical Correlation Coefficient   243
15.6   Summary and Sources   245
15.7   Exercises   246

16. Stochastic Processes   251

16.1   Definition and General Properties   251
16.2   Gaussian Processes   252
16.3   Point Processes   254
16.4   The Inhomogeneous Poisson Process   257
16.5   Spectral Analysis   259
16.6   Summary and Sources   262
16.7   Exercises   262

17. Membrane Noise*   267

17.1   Two-State Channel Model   267
17.2   Multistate Channel Models   270
17.3   The Ornstein–Uhlenbeck Process   271
17.4   Synaptic Noise   272
17.5   Summary and Sources   275
17.6   Exercises   275

18. Power and Cross Spectra   279

18.1   Cross Correlation and Coherence   279
18.2   Estimator Bias and Variance   280
18.3   Numerical Estimate of the Power Spectrum*   282
18.4   Summary and Sources   286
18.5   Exercises   286

19. Natural Light Signals and Phototransduction   291

19.1   Wavelength and Intensity   291
19.2   Spatial Properties of Natural Light Signals   293
19.3   Temporal Properties of Natural Light Signals   293
19.4   A Model of Phototransduction   294
19.5   Summary and Sources   297
19.6   Exercises   298

20. Firing Rate Codes and Early Vision   299

20.1   Definition of Mean Instantaneous Firing Rate   299
20.2   Visual System and Visual Stimuli   300
20.3   Spatial Receptive Field of Retinal
       Ganglion Cells   301
20.4   Characterization of Receptive Field Structure   303
20.5   Spatio-Temporal Receptive Fields   306

20.6 Static Nonlinearities* 308
20.7 Summary and Sources 308
20.8 Exercises 309

21. Models of Simple and Complex Cells 311

21.1 Simple Cell Models 311
21.2 Nonseparable Receptive Fields 318
21.3 Receptive Fields of Complex Cells 320
21.4 Motion-Energy Model 321
21.5 Hubel–Wiesel Model 321
21.6 Multiscale Representation of Visual
      Information 322
21.7 Summary and Sources 323
21.8 Exercises 323

22. Stochastic Estimation Theory 327

22.1 Minimum Mean Square Error Estimation 327
22.2 Estimation of Gaussian Signals* 329
22.3 Linear Nonlinear (LN) Models* 331
22.4 Summary and Sources 332
22.5 Exercises 332

23. Reverse-Correlation and Spike
     Train Decoding 335

23.1 Reverse-Correlation 335
23.2 Stimulus Reconstruction 338
23.3 Summary and Sources 340
23.4 Exercises 340

24. Signal Detection Theory 343

24.1 Testing Hypotheses 343
24.2 Ideal Decision Rules 346
24.3 ROC Curves* 348
24.4 Multidimensional Gaussian Signals* 348
24.5 Fisher Linear Discriminant* 351
24.6 Summary and Sources 354
24.7 Exercises 354

25. Relating Neuronal Responses
     and Psychophysics 355

25.1 Single Photon Detection 355
25.2 Signal Detection Theory and Psychophysics 359
25.3 Motion Detection 361
25.4 Summary and Sources 363
25.5 Exercises 364

26. Population Codes* 367

26.1 Cartesian Coordinate Systems 367
26.2 Overcomplete Representations 369
26.3 Frames 370

26.4 Maximum Likelihood 372
26.5 Estimation Error and the Cramer–Rao Bound* 374
26.6 Population Coding in the Superior Colliculus 375
26.7 Summary and Sources 376
26.8 Exercises 378

27. Neuronal Networks 381

27.1 Hopfield Networks 382
27.2 Leaky Integrate-and-Fire Networks 383
27.3 Leaky Integrate-and-Fire Networks with Plastic
      Synapses 389
27.4 Hodgkin–Huxley Based Networks 392
27.5 Hodgkin–Huxley Based Networks with Plastic
      Synapses 397
27.6 Rate Based Networks 398
27.7 Brain Maps and Self-Organizing Maps 401
27.8 Summary and Sources 403
27.9 Exercises 404

28. Solutions to Selected Exercises 409

28.1   Chapter 2 409
28.2   Chapter 3 411
28.3   Chapter 4 413
28.4   Chapter 5 414
28.5   Chapter 6 416
28.6   Chapter 7 419
28.7   Chapter 8 421
28.8   Chapter 9 422
28.9   Chapter 10 422
28.10 Chapter 11 423
28.11 Chapter 12 428
28.12 Chapter 13 430
28.13 Chapter 14 431
28.14 Chapter 15 433
28.15 Chapter 16 436
28.16 Chapter 17 442
28.17 Chapter 18 445
28.18 Chapter 19 452
28.19 Chapter 20 453
28.20 Chapter 21 453
28.21 Chapter 22 455
28.22 Chapter 23 458
28.23 Chapter 24 459
28.24 Chapter 25 464
28.25 Chapter 26 466
28.26 Chapter 27 470

References 473
Index 483

A companion website for this book can be found at:

www.elsevierdirect.com/companions/9780123748829

Preface

This text sprung from a course we have taught jointly over the last 8 years at Rice University to students from Rice and Baylor College of Medicine. The goal of our course, and this text, is to develop mathematical methods that are most relevant to neuroscience, in a fashion that deepens the student's knowledge of each.

Regarding the mathematics, this means working in concrete incremental steps that enable the student to parse and extend the MATLAB code provided for each of the 232 computational examples and exercises. Regarding the neuroscience, this means establishing basic models of stimuli and molecular, cellular, and circuit level phenomena prior to their systematic elaboration and integration. The degree to which we have succeeded in this goal is, in large measure, due to the perspicacity of our many devoted students.

We have also benefited from Houston's rich neuroscience climate and happily acknowledge the leadership of Jack Byrne, Mike Friedlander, Marty Golubitsky, and Kathy Matthews in promoting dialog between mathematics and neuroscience. This dialog has been sustained by our close collaboration with fellow members of the Gulf Coast Consortium for Theoretical and Computational Neuroscience. In particular, we thank Mark Embree, Kreso Josic, Weiji Ma, Peter Saggau, and Harel Shouval for detailed feedback on a number of our chapters. It is also a pleasure to acknowledge comments received from Maurice Chacron, Stephen Coombes, Greg DeAngelis, Brent Doiron, Hans van Hateren, Leonard Maler, Victor Matveev, and Ralf Wessel and his group.

Our deepest thanks go to our wives, Sibylle and Laura, for nurturing the early stages of our work and for accepting our near single mindedness during our final year of writing.

We also thank Colin Cox for an early animation that catalyzed a good fraction of our course and Simon Cox for coordinating our code and figures at a time when they appeared to be taking on a life of their own.

1

Introduction

OUTLINE

1.1	How to Use this Book	2	1.4 Units 7
1.2	Brain Facts Brief	2	1.5 Sources 8
1.3	Mathematical Preliminaries	4	

Faced with the seemingly limitless qualities of the brain, Neuroscience has eschewed provincialism and instead pursued a broad tack that openly draws on insights from biology, physics, chemistry, psychology, and mathematics in its construction of technologies and theories with which to probe and understand the brain. These technologies and theories, in turn, continue to attract scientists and mathematicians to questions of Neuroscience. As a result, we may trace over one hundred years of fruitful interplay between Neuroscience and mathematics. This text aims to prepare the advanced undergraduate or beginning graduate student to take an active part in this dialogue via the application of existing, or the creation of new, mathematics in the interest of a deeper understanding of the brain. Requiring no more than one year of Calculus, and no prior exposure to Neuroscience, we prepare the student by

1. introducing mathematical and computational tools in precisely the contexts that first established their importance for Neuroscience and

2. developing these tools in concrete incremental steps within a common computational environment.

As such, the text may also serve to introduce Neuroscience to readers with a mathematical and/or computational background.

Regarding (1), we introduce ordinary differential equations via the work of Hodgkin and Huxley (1952) on action potentials in the squid giant axon, partial differential equations through the work of Rall on cable theory (see Segev et al. (1994)), probability theory following the analysis of Fatt and Katz (1952) on synaptic transmission, dynamical systems theory in the context of Fitzhugh's (1955) investigation of action potential threshold, and linear algebra in the context of the work of Hodgkin and Huxley (1952) on subthreshold oscillations and the compartmental modeling of Hines (1984) on dendritic trees. In addition, we apply Fourier transforms to describe neuronal receptive fields following Enroth-Cugell and Robson's (1966) work on retinal ganglion cells and its subsequent extension to Hubel and Wiesel's (1962) characterization of cat cortical neurons. We also introduce and motivate statistical decision methods starting with the historical photon detection experiments of Hecht et al. (1942).

Regarding (2), we develop, test, and integrate models of channels, receptors, membranes, cells, circuits and sensory stimuli by working from the simple to the complex within the MATLAB computing environment. Assuming no prior exposure to MATLAB, we develop and implement numerical methods for solving algebraic and differential equations, for computing Fourier transforms, and for generating and analyzing random signals. Through an associated web site we provide the student with MATLAB code for 144 computational figures in the text and we provide the instructor with MATLAB code for 98 computational exercises. The exercises range from routine reinforcement of concepts developed in the text to significant extensions that guide the reader to the research literature. Our reference to exercises both in the text and across the exercises serve to establish them as an integral component of this book.

Concerning the mathematical models considered in the text, we cite the realization of Schrödinger (1961) that "we cannot ask for more than just adequate pictures capable of synthesizing in a comprehensible way all observed facts and giving a reasonable expectation on new ones we are out for." Furthermore, lest "adequate" serve as an invitation to loose or vague modeling, Schrödinger warns that "without an absolutely precise model, thinking itself becomes imprecise, and the consequences derived from the model become ambiguous."

As we enter the 21st century, one of the biggest challenges facing Neuroscience is to integrate knowledge and to craft theories that span multiple scales, both in space from the nanometer neighborhood of an ion channel to the meter that action potentials must travel down the sciatic nerve, and in time from the fraction of a millisecond it takes to release neurotransmitter to the hours it takes to prune or grow synaptic contacts between cells. We hope that this text, by providing an integrated treatment of experimental and mathematical tools within a single computational framework, will prepare our readers to meet this challenge.

1.1 HOW TO USE THIS BOOK

The book is largely self-contained and as such is suited for both self-study and reference use. The chapters need not be read in numerical order. To facilitate a selection for reading, we have sketched in Figure 1.1 the main dependencies between the chapters. The four core chapters that underlie much of the book are Chapters 2–4 and 11. For the reader with limited prior training in mathematics it is in these chapters that we develop, by hand calculation, MATLAB simulation and a thorough suite of exercises, the mathematical maturity required to appreciate the chapters to come. Many of the basic chapters also contain more advanced subsections, indicated by an asterisk, *, which can be skipped on a first reading. Detailed solutions are provided for most exercises, either at the end of the book or through the associated web site. We mark with a dagger, †, each exercise whose solution is not included in this text.

Over the past eight years, we have used a subset of the book's material for a one semester introductory course on Mathematical Neuroscience to an audience comprised of Science and Engineering undergraduate and graduate students from Rice University and Neuroscience graduate students from Baylor College of Medicine. We first cover Chapters 2–5, which set and solve the Hodgkin–Huxley equations for isopotential cells and, via the eigenvector expansion of the cell's subthreshold response, introduce the key concepts of linear algebra needed to tackle the multicompartment cell in Chapters 6 and 8–9. We then open Chapter 11, introduce probabilistic methods and apply them to synaptic transmission, in Chapter 12, and spike train variability, in Chapter 15. We conclude this overview of single neuron properties by covering Chapter 10 on reduced single neuron models. We transition to Systems Neuroscience via the Fourier transform of Chapter 7 and its application to visual neurons in Chapters 20 and 21. Finally, we connect neural response to behavior via the material of Chapters 24 and 25. An alternative possibility is to conclude with Chapters 22 and 23, after an informal introduction to stochastic processes, and power and cross spectra in Chapters 16 and 18.

We have also used the following chapters for advanced courses: 13, 14, 16–19, and 26. Chapter 13 provides a comprehensive coverage of calcium dynamics within single neurons at an advanced level. Similarly, Chapter 14 introduces the singular value decomposition, a mathematical tool that has important applications both in spike sorting and in model reduction. Chapters 16 and 18 introduce stochastic processes and methods of spectral analysis. These results can be applied at the microscopic level to describe single channel gating properties, Chapter 17, and at the macroscopic level to describe the statistical properties of natural scenes and their impact on visual processing, Chapter 19. Finally the chapters on population codes and networks, Chapters 26 and 27, address the coding and dynamical properties of neuronal ensembles.

To ease the reading of the text, we have relegated all references to the **Summary and Sources** section located at the end of each chapter. These reference lists are offered as pointers to the literature and are not intended to be exhaustive.

1.2 BRAIN FACTS BRIEF

The brain is the central component of the nervous system and is incredibly varied across animals. In vertebrates, it is composed of three main subdivisions: the forebrain, the midbrain, and the hindbrain. In mammals and particularly in humans, the cerebral cortex of the forebrain is highly expanded. The human brain is thought to contain on the order of 100 billion (10^{11}) nerve cells, or neurons. Each neuron "typically" receives 10,000 inputs (synapses, §2.1) from other neurons, but this number varies widely across neuron types. For example: granule cells of the cerebellum, the most abundant neurons in the brain, receive on average four inputs while Purkinje cells, the output neurons of the cerebellar cortex, receive on the order of 100,000. In the mouse cerebral cortex, the number of neurons per cubic millimeter has been estimated at 10^5, while there are approximately 7×10^8 synapses and 4 km of cable (axons, §2.1) in the same volume. Brain size (weight) typically scales with body size, thus the human brain is far from the largest. At another extreme, the brain of the honey bee is estimated to contain less than a million (10^6) neurons within a single cubic millimeter. Yet the honey bee can learn a variety of complex tasks, not unlike those learned by a macaque monkey for instance. Although it is often difficult to draw comparisons across widely different species, the basic principles underlying information processing as they are discussed in this book appear to be universal, in spite of obvious differences in implementation. The electrical properties of cells (Chapter 2), the generation and propagation of signals along axons (Chapters 4 and 9), and the detection of visual motion (Chapters 21 and 25) or population codes (Chapter 26), for instance, are observed to follow very similar principles across very distantly related species.

Information about the environment reaches the brain through five common senses: vision, touch, hearing, smell, and taste. In addition, some animals are able to sense electric fields through specialized electroreceptors. These include many species of fish and monotremes (egg-laying mammals) like the platypus. Most sensory information is gathered from the environment passively, but some species are able to emit signals and register their perturbation by the environment and thus possess active sensory systems. This includes bats that emit sounds at specific frequencies and hear the echoes bouncing off objects in the environment, a phenomenon called echolocation. In addition some species of fish, termed weakly electric, possess an electric organ allowing them to generate an electric field around their body and sense its distortion by the environment, a phenomenon called electrolocation.

Ultimately, the brain controls the locomotor output of the organism. This is typically a complex process, involving both commands issued to the muscles to execute movements, feedback from sensors reporting the actual state of the musculature and skeletal elements, and inputs from the senses to monitor progress towards a goal. So efficient is this process that even the tiny brain of a fly is, for instance, able to process information sufficiently fast to allow for highly acrobatic flight behaviors, executed in less than 100 ms from sensory transduction to motor output.

To study the brain, different biological systems have proven useful for different purposes. For example, slices of the rat hippocampus, a structure involved in learning and memory as well as navigation, are particularly adequate for electrophysiological recordings of pyramidal neurons and a detailed characterization of their subcellular properties, because their cell bodies are tightly packed in a layer that is easy to visualize. The fruit fly *Drosophila melanogaster* and the worm *Caenorhabditis elegans* (whose nervous system comprises exactly 302 neurons) are good models to investigate the relation between simple behaviors and genetics, as their genomes are sequenced and many tools are available to selectively switch on and off genes in specific brain structures or neurons. One approach that has been particularly successful to study information processing in the brain is "neuro-ethological," based on the study of natural behaviors

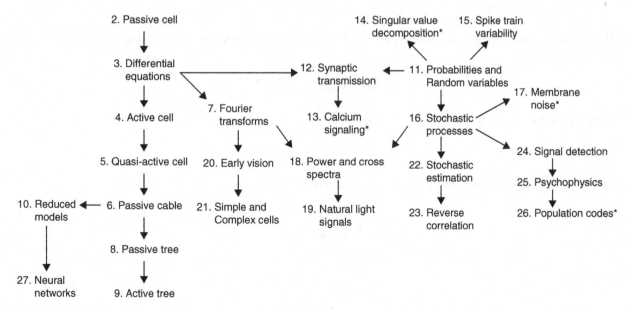

FIGURE 1.1 Chapter dependencies. Each arrow points to a chapter that depends significantly on the content of the current chapter. The asterisk is used to denote chapters that cover advanced material.

(ethology) in relation to the brain structures involved in their execution. Besides the already mentioned weakly electric fish and bats, classical examples, among many others, include song learning in zebrafinches, the neural control of flight in flies, sound localization in barn owls, and escape behaviors in a variety of species, such as locust, goldfish, or flies.

1.3 MATHEMATICAL PRELIMINARIES

MATLAB. Native MATLAB functions are in typewriter font, e.g., `svd`. Our contributed code, available on the book's web site, has a trailing `.m`, e.g., `bepswI.m`.

Numbers. The counting numbers, $\{0,1,2,\ldots\}$, are denoted by $\mathbb{N}$, while the reals are denoted by $\mathbb{R}$ and the complex numbers by $\mathbb{C}$. Each complex number, $z \in \mathbb{C}$, may be decomposed into its real and imaginary components. We will write

$$z = x + iy, \quad \text{where} \quad x = \Re(z), \quad y = \Im(z), \quad \text{and} \quad i \equiv \sqrt{-1}.$$

Here x and y are each real and $\equiv$ signifies that one side is defined by the other. We denote the complex conjugate and magnitude of z by

$$z^* \equiv x - iy \quad \text{and} \quad |z| \equiv \sqrt{x^2 + y^2},$$

respectively.

Sets. Sets are delimited by curly brackets, $\{\}$. For example the set of odd numbers between 4 and 10 is $\{5,7,9\}$.

Intervals. For $a,b \in \mathbb{R}$ with $a < b$ the open interval (a,b) is the set of numbers x such that $a < x < b$. The closed interval $[a,b]$ is the set of numbers x such that $a \leq x \leq b$. The semiclosed (or semiopen) intervals $[a,b)$ and $(a,b]$ are the set of numbers x such that $a \leq x < b$ and $a < x \leq b$, respectively.

Vectors and matrices. Given n real or complex numbers, $x_1, x_2, \ldots, x_n$, we denote their arrangement into a vector, or column, via bold lower case letters,

$$\mathbf{x} = \begin{pmatrix} x_1 \\ x_2 \\ \vdots \\ x_n \end{pmatrix}. \tag{1.1}$$

The collections of all real and complex vectors with n components are denoted $\mathbb{R}^n$ and $\mathbb{C}^n$, respectively. The transpose of a vector, $\mathbf{x}$, is the row,

$$\mathbf{x}^T = (x_1 \ x_2 \ \cdots \ x_n),$$

and the conjugate transpose of a vector, $\mathbf{z} \in \mathbb{C}^n$, is the row

$$\mathbf{z}^H = (z_1^* \ z_2^* \ \cdots \ z_n^*).$$

We next define the inner, or scalar, or "dot," product for $\mathbf{x}$ and $\mathbf{y}$ in $\mathbb{C}^n$,

$$\mathbf{x}^H \mathbf{y} \equiv \sum_{j=1}^{n} x_j^* y_j,$$

and note that as

$$\mathbf{z}^H \mathbf{z} = \sum_{i=1}^{n} |z_i|^2 \geq 0$$

it makes sense to define the **norm**

$$\|\mathbf{z}\| \equiv \sqrt{\mathbf{z}^H \mathbf{z}}.$$

To gain practice with these definitions you may wish to confirm that

$$\|(\mathbf{y}^H\mathbf{y})\mathbf{x} - (\mathbf{y}^H\mathbf{x})\mathbf{y}\|^2 = \|\mathbf{y}\|^2(\|\mathbf{y}\|^2\|\mathbf{x}\|^2 - |\mathbf{x}^H\mathbf{y}|^2).$$

As the left hand side is nonnegative the right hand side reveals the important **Schwarz inequality**

$$|\mathbf{x}^H\mathbf{y}| \leq \|\mathbf{x}\|\|\mathbf{y}\|. \tag{1.2}$$

We will transform vectors in $\mathbb{C}^n$ to vectors in $\mathbb{C}^m$ via multiplication by $m \times n$ matrices, $\mathbf{A} \in \mathbb{C}^{m \times n}$, of the form

$$\mathbf{A} = \begin{pmatrix} A_{11} & A_{12} & \cdots & A_{1n} \\ A_{21} & A_{22} & \cdots & A_{2n} \\ \vdots & \vdots & \ddots & \vdots \\ A_{m1} & A_{m2} & \cdots & A_{mn} \end{pmatrix}$$

where each $A_{ij} \in \mathbb{C}$. Thus, $\mathbf{y} = \mathbf{A}\mathbf{x}$ means that $y_i = \sum_{j=1}^{n} A_{ij}x_j$ for $i = 1, \ldots m$. We will consistently denote matrices by bold upper case letters. Given $\mathbf{A} \in \mathbb{C}^{m \times n}$ and $\mathbf{B} \in \mathbb{C}^{n \times p}$ we define their product $\mathbf{C} \in \mathbb{C}^{m \times p}$ via

$$\mathbf{C} = \mathbf{A}\mathbf{B} \quad \text{where} \quad C_{jk} = \sum_{l=1}^{n} A_{jl}B_{lk}.$$

If we reflect $\mathbf{A}$ about its diagonal we arrive at its transpose, $\mathbf{A}^T \in \mathbb{C}^{n \times m}$, where $(\mathbf{A}^T)_{ij} = A_{ji}$. The associated conjugate transpose is denoted $\mathbf{A}^H$, where $(\mathbf{A}^H)_{ij} = A_{ji}^*$. We will often require the conjugate transpose of the product $\mathbf{A}\mathbf{B}$, and so record

$$(\mathbf{A}\mathbf{B})_{jk}^H = \sum_{l=1}^{n} A_{kl}^* B_{lj}^* = (\mathbf{B}^H\mathbf{A}^H)_{jk}, \quad \text{i.e.,} \quad (\mathbf{A}\mathbf{B})^H = \mathbf{B}^H\mathbf{A}^H. \tag{1.3}$$

Similarly, $(\mathbf{A}\mathbf{B})^T = \mathbf{B}^T\mathbf{A}^T$.

The identity matrix, denoted $\mathbf{I}$, is the square matrix of zeros off the diagonal, and ones on the diagonal,

$$\mathbf{I} \equiv \begin{pmatrix} 1 & 0 & \cdots & 0 \\ 0 & \ddots & \ddots & \vdots \\ \vdots & \ddots & 1 & 0 \\ 0 & \cdots & 0 & 1 \end{pmatrix}.$$

We often use the Kronecker delta

$$\delta_{jk} \equiv \begin{cases} 1, & \text{if } j = k \\ 0, & \text{otherwise} \end{cases} \tag{1.4}$$

to denote the elements of $\mathbf{I}$. A matrix $\mathbf{B} \in \mathbb{C}^{n \times n}$ is said to be invertible if there exists a matrix $\mathbf{B}^{-1} \in \mathbb{C}^{n \times n}$ such that

$$\mathbf{B}\mathbf{B}^{-1} = \mathbf{B}^{-1}\mathbf{B} = \mathbf{I}. \tag{1.5}$$

In this case $\mathbf{B}^{-1}$ is called the inverse of $\mathbf{B}$.

Functions. We will make frequent use of the characteristic function

$$\mathbb{1}_{(a,b)}(x) \equiv \begin{cases} 1, & \text{if} \quad a < x < b \\ 0, & \text{otherwise} \end{cases} \tag{1.6}$$

of the interval, (a,b). In the common case that (a,b) is the set of nonnegative reals we will simply write $\mathbb{1}(x)$ and refer to it as the **Heaviside function**.

We will often need to differentiate the running integral,

$$F(x) = \int_0^x f(y)\mathrm{d}y.$$

To see that

$$F'(x) = f(x) \tag{1.7}$$

when f is continuous at x, note that the mean value theorem establishes the second equality in

$$\frac{F(x+h) - F(x)}{h} = \frac{1}{h}\int_x^{x+h} f(y)\mathrm{d}y = f(x_h) \tag{1.8}$$

for some $x_h \in (x, x+h)$. As $h \to 0$ the left hand side approaches $F'(x)$ while on the right $x_h \to x$ and so, by continuity, $f(x_h) \to f(x)$.

We will often need to sample, or discretize, scalar valued functions, $f : \mathbb{R} \to \mathbb{R}$, of time and/or space. For example, if time is divided into increments of size $\mathrm{d}t$ then we will denote the samples of $f(t)$ by superscripted letters in the "typewriter" font

$$\mathtt{f}^j \equiv f((j-1)\mathrm{d}t), \quad j = 1, 2, 3, \ldots.$$

Similarly, we will denote the samples of a vector valued function, $\mathbf{f} : \mathbb{R} \to \mathbb{R}^n$, by superscripted letters in the bold typewriter font

$$\mathbf{f}^j \equiv \mathbf{f}((j-1)\mathrm{d}t), \quad j = 1, 2, 3, \ldots.$$

The elements of $\mathbf{f}^j$ are samples of the elements of $\mathbf{f}$. We express this in symbols as $\mathtt{f}_m^j = f_m((j-1)\mathrm{d}t)$. Where the superscript, j, may interfere with exponents we will be careful to make the distinction.

Random variables. In chapters dealing with random variables, we will try whenever possible to use upper case letters for a random variable and lower case letters for a specific value of the same random variable. We denote the expectation or mean of a random variable X by $E[X]$. The variance is the expectation of the squared deviation of X from the mean: $E[(X - E[X])^2]$. A Gaussian or normal random variable of mean μ and variance σ^2 is denoted by $\mathcal{N}(\mu, \sigma^2)$. An estimator of, e.g., the mean m_X of a random variable X is denoted by $\breve{m}_X$.

Fourier transforms. The Fourier transform of a function $f(t)$ of time, t, is denoted by $\hat{f}(\omega)$:

$$\hat{f}(\omega) \equiv \int_{-\infty}^{\infty} f(t)\mathrm{e}^{-2\pi i\omega t}\,\mathrm{d}t.$$

The variable ω is the ordinary frequency. If t has units of seconds (s) then ω has units of $1/\mathrm{s} = \mathrm{Hz}$ (Hertz). The convolution of two functions f and g is denoted by $f \star g$:

$$(f \star g)(t) \equiv \int_{-\infty}^{\infty} f(t_1)g(t - t_1)\,\mathrm{d}t_1. \tag{1.9}$$

Landau symbols. Let ε be a small real number. For a function $f(\varepsilon)$, we write

$$f(\varepsilon) = O(\varepsilon) \quad (\varepsilon \to 0)$$

when there exists a constant $C > 0$ such that for ε sufficiently small,

$$|f(\varepsilon)| \leq C|\varepsilon| \quad \text{equivalently} \quad \lim_{\varepsilon \to 0} |f(\varepsilon)/\varepsilon| \leq C.$$

Intuitively, this means that $f(\varepsilon)$ decays no slower than ε as ε tends to zero. The notation extends naturally to other functions of ε; e.g., $f(x+\varepsilon) = f(x) + O(\varepsilon^2)$ means that for ε sufficiently small,

$$|f(x+\varepsilon) - f(x)| \leq C|\varepsilon^2|.$$

Similarly, $f(\varepsilon) = o(\varepsilon)$ for $\varepsilon \to 0$ means that

$$\lim_{\varepsilon \to 0} f(\varepsilon)/\varepsilon = 0.$$

Intuitively, this means that the function f decays faster than ε as ε tends to zero.

1.4 UNITS

All units are based on the Système International (SI). The main ones used in this book and their prefixes are briefly summarized here.

The **length** of subcellular components, such as the length of the synaptic cleft, are expressed in nanometers ($1 \text{ nm} = 10^{-9}$ m), while cellular components are expressed in micrometers ($1 \ \mu\text{m} = 10^{-6}$ m) and centimeters ($1 \text{ cm} = 10^{-2}$ m).

An **angle** denotes the length of a circular arc divided by its radius, r. The radius is also the distance of the arc to the point of observation. Equivalently, an angle denotes the length of the arc projected on the corresponding unit circle. Angles are dimensionless since they are the ratio of two distances, but they are often assigned "units" of radians (rad), with the angle subtended by a full circle from its center equal to 2π (since the circumference of a circle is $2\pi r$). One degree (deg) is equal to $2\pi/360$ rad or $360 \text{ deg} = 2\pi$ rad. A **solid angle** denotes the area of a spherical cap, divided by its squared radius, or equivalently the area projected on the corresponding unit sphere. Solid angles are measured in steradians (sr) with the solid angle subtended by the full sphere from its center equal to 4π (since the area of a sphere is $4\pi r^2$).

Temperature is in degrees Kelvin (K), with $0 \text{ K} = -273.15 \text{ °C}$ (degrees centigrade).

Mass is measured in kilograms (kg) with $1 \text{ kg} = 1000$ g (grams) being approximately equal to the mass of one liter (one cubic decimeter, 1 dm^3) of pure water.

The **amount** of a substance is measured in moles, with one mole corresponding to 6.0221415×10^{23} (Avogadro's number) atoms or molecules of pure substance. One mole of substance, in grams, is given by the atomic (or molecular) weight of the substance under consideration; e.g., one mole of sodium is equal to 22.99 g, as may be determined from the periodic table of elements.

Concentration of a solute in a solution, is measured in mole/liter and is abbreviated by M: $1 \text{ M} = 1$ mole/liter. In the context of this book, we will typically consider ions like Na^+, K^+, or Cl^- dissolved in water and denote their concentration by enclosing them in square brackets, e.g., $[Na^+]$.

Time is measured in second (s) or millisecond ($1 \text{ ms} = 10^{-3}$ s) and its inverse, **frequency**, in Hertz ($1 \text{ Hz} = 1 \text{ s}^{-1}$).

Current is measured in micro-, nano-, or picoampere ($1 \text{ pA} = 10^{-12}$ A). One ampere (A) corresponds approximately to the flow of 6.242×10^{18} protons at a given point per second.

The corresponding **charge**, Q, passing at that point in one second is one coulomb (C). In other words, $1 \text{ A} = 1 \text{ C/s}$. By definition, *positive* current corresponds to the flow of positive charge in a given direction and thus a negatively charged particle will flow in the opposite direction. When considering the current flowing across the membrane of a cell, we define by convention positive current as the flow of positive charge *outwards*. Therefore the flow of positive charge *inwards* corresponds to a negative current. The elementary charge of the proton and electron are $\pm 1.602 \times 10^{-19}$ C, respectively. We will often consider current densities, i.e., currents per unit area.

In the SI system, force (mass times acceleration) is measured in newton (N) and work (force times distance) or energy in joule ($1 \text{ J} = 1 \text{ N m}$). Since the electrical (Coulomb's) force is proportional to charge, electrical potential energy is measured in joule/coulomb or **volt** ($1 V = 1 J/C$). We will use most often the unit of millivolt (mV) to measure electrical potential energy differences, e.g., between the inside and outside of a single neuron.

Resistance to current flow in a conductor is measured in ohm (Ω) according to Ohm's law: $R = V/I$, where V is the electrical potential difference and I the current. In other words, 1Ω is the resistance of a conductor that passes a current of 1 A under an electrical potential difference of 1 V. Neurophysiologists often restate Ohm's law in term of conductance: $I = gV$, where $g = 1/R$. The unit of conductance is the siemens ($1 S = 1 \Omega^{-1}$). We will most often deal with megaohm ($1 M\Omega = 10^6 \Omega$) and mS or μS.

Capacitance is the ability to store charge under a given electrical potential difference. For example, given two conducting plates separated by an insulator and maintained at a fixed potential difference V, the stored charge per plate will be proportional to V, i.e., $C = Q/V$, where the capacitance, C, is measured in farad (F), with $1 F = 1 C/V$. We will mainly deal with the microfarad, μF, but also with the femtofarad in Chapter 13 ($1 fF = 10^{-15} F$).

The **luminous intensity** measures the integrated light power emitted by a point source per unit solid angle, weighted by the varying sensitivity of the human eye to light wavelength. It is measured in candela (cd). The precise definition of the candela is given in §19.1.

1.5 SOURCES

For a history of the interplay between Neuroscience and Mathematics see the chapter by Rall in Schwartz (1990). An elementary introduction to brain anatomy is contained in Squire et al. (2008, Chapter 2). Anatomical figures on the mouse brain are taken from Braitenberg and Schüz (1998). A good reference on neuron numbers is Williams and Herrup (1988). The facts on honey bees are taken from Menzel and Giurfa (2001). The following web page also has an extensive list of data on the human and other brains, including references to the original literature: http://faculty.washington.edu/chudler/facts.html. For an overview of neural information processing, see Gabbiani and Midtgaard (2001) and for classical case studies in neuroethology, see Carew (2000) and Heiligenberg (1991). North and Greenspan (2007) offers a broad overview of invertebrate neurobiology, including chapters on *C. elegans* and *D. melanogaster*. The web page "Constants, Units and Uncertainty" from the Physics Laboratory of the National Institute of Standards and Technology (http://physics.nist.gov/cuu) or the web site of the Bureau International des Poids et Mesures (http://www.bipm.org) contain further information on the units used in this book.

A companion website for this book can be found at: *www.elsevierdirect.com/companions/9780123748829.*

2

The Passive Isopotential Cell

OUTLINE

2.1	Introduction	9	2.5	Synaptic Conductance	14
2.2	The Nernst Potential	11	2.6	Summary and Sources	15
2.3	Membrane Conductance	12	2.7	Exercises	16
2.4	Membrane Capacitance and Current Balance	12			

2.1 INTRODUCTION

Modern neuroscience can be traced back to the work of Camillo Golgi, an Italian physician and scientist who invented, in the late 1890s, a method for staining neural tissue. As the Golgi stain only "took" to a small and well-separated population of cells it permitted, for the first time, one to see the trees for the forest. The Spanish neuroanatomist Santiago Ramón y Cajal took quick advantage of the Golgi method to systematically describe the different types of neurons contained in the brain of many animal species. By demonstrating that neurons, though widely varying in shape, nonetheless share common structural components, from which function may be inferred, Ramón y Cajal can be said to have founded modern neuroscience. With reference to Figure 2.1, Ramón y Cajal identified the cell body, or soma, that contains the cell nucleus, the axon that carries electrical impulses to downstream neurons, and the dendrites, where a neuron typically receives inputs from other, upstream neurons through electrical or chemical synapses. Pyramidal neurons, such as that illustrated in Figure 2.1, are the most prevalent neuron type in the mammalian cortex and are characterized by the presence of a single apical dendrite, usually with a larger diameter than the other basal dendrites, that extends towards the brain's surface.

The neuron interacts with its extracellular environment by controlling the flow of ions that pass through pumps, exchangers, and channels that perforate the lipid bilayer that comprises the cell membrane. In Figure 2.2 we offer a schematic of a cross section of a simplified spherical cell and a magnified segment of membrane depicting such a pump, exchanger, or channel.

The pumps and exchangers are constantly at work to maintain a significant imbalance between the intracellular and extracellular concentrations of the principal anion, Cl^- (chloride), and cations, Na^+ (sodium), K^+ (potassium), and Ca^{2+} (calcium). In particular, at rest,

$$[K^+]_{in} \gg [K^+]_{out}, \qquad (2.1)$$

i.e., the intracellular concentration of K^+ is significantly greater than its extracellular concentration, while the situation is the opposite

$$[Na^+]_{in} \ll [Na^+]_{out}, \quad [Cl^-]_{in} \ll [Cl^-]_{out}, \quad \text{and} \quad [Ca^{2+}]_{in} \ll [Ca^{2+}]_{out}, \qquad (2.2)$$

Mathematics for Neuroscientists. DOI: 10.1016/B978-0-12-374882-9.00002-2

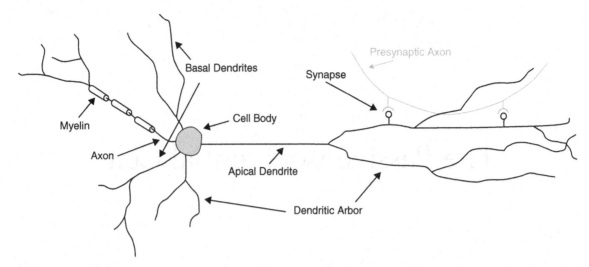

FIGURE 2.1 Schematic illustration of a pyramidal neuron and its main compartments. Input from an action potential in an upstream neuron arrives via the (red) axon and is delivered at synapses that, here, reside on the heads of spines that stud the dendrites. The action potential liberates neurotransmitter from the red axon. Neurotransmitter molecules then bind to channels, in the spine head, that then open and permit ions to flow into the (black) dendrite. These ionic currents are then conducted to the cell body and (black) axon. The initial segment of axon is typically the most "excitable" part of the cell, and hence, if the received currents reach a certain threshold this segment will ignite an action potential that will travel down the axon, to signal downstream neurons, and up into its dendrites, to signal synapses that contributed to its creation. Those axons that communicate with cells outside of their immediate neighborhoods are typically wrapped, with periodic breaks, in layers of insulating fat (myelin) from neighboring glial cells.

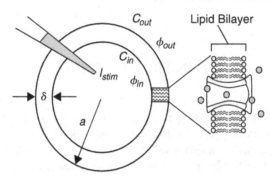

FIGURE 2.2 A cross section of a spherical cell with radius a and membrane thickness δ. The inner and outer concentrations of a particular ion are denoted c_{in} and c_{out} while the inner and outer potentials are denoted ϕ_{in} and ϕ_{out}. Given this simplified geometry we make the further assumption that c_{in} and ϕ_{in} do not vary with position within the cell. This permits us to define a single membrane potential, $V \equiv \phi_{in} - \phi_{out}$, and as such we refer to our cell as **isopotential**. We have also impaled the cell with a sharp, needle-like intracellular electrode ready to deliver the current I_{stim}. The zoom at right depicts the passage of ions through a protein (pump, exchanger, or channel) that spans the membrane.

for the other species. One net effect of this imbalance is to induce a difference in electrical potential across the cell membrane. In particular, we will see that the inside of the cell is typically 70 millivolts (mV) less than the outside. We will refer to this potential difference (in minus out) as the cell's **membrane potential**. These imbalances in concentration and resulting rest potential set the stage for ion channels, the main actors in our neuronal drama.

We have schematized such a channel, and its surrounding lipid bilayer, in the right side of Figure 2.2. These channels are typically ion selective, e.g., we speak of chloride channels and sodium channels, and they are further categorized into passive, active (or voltage-gated), and ligand-gated. **Passive** signifies that the conductance of the channel does not depend on the cell's membrane potential. **Active** signifies that it does, and so we say that the channel is voltage-gated. A ligand-gated channel is one that requires the binding of a helper molecule (the ligand) to open the channel. The ligands we will see first will be molecules of neurotransmitter that have been liberated by an upstream action potential, as discussed in Figure 2.1. We will begin our modeling and analysis of passive and ligand-gated channels in this chapter in preparation for our study of active channels in Chapter 4.

In the sections to follow we will interpret the schematic in Figure 2.2 in terms of an electrical circuit diagram that can then be quantified by a differential equation that may be solved for the membrane potential, $V(t)$, in terms of the stimulus, $I_{stim}(t)$, and the cell's effective electrical properties.

2.2 THE NERNST POTENTIAL

The gradients, Eqs. (2.1) and (2.2), in both concentration and charge trigger associated Fickian and Ohmic fluxes through the membrane. These fluxes have dimensions of mole/(area time). To fix ideas we will consider the flux of a single species, namely chloride. Fick's law states that the flux of matter across a surface is proportional to its concentration gradient, i.e.,

$$J_{Fick}(r) = -D\frac{dc}{dr}(r) \tag{2.3}$$

where r denotes distance from the center of the cell, $c(r)$ denotes concentration (in units of M $\equiv$ mole/liter) of Cl^- at r, and D (area/time) denotes diffusivity. The sign convention in Eq. (2.3) corresponds to positive flux in the direction of *decreasing* concentration. The diffusivity is typically decomposed into $D = \mu kT$ where T is temperature (K), k is Boltzmann's constant (1.381×10^{-23} joule/K), and μ denotes mobility (time/mass). Mobility is a measure of the average drift speed acquired by a Cl^- ion per unit applied external force between collisions with other particles. Its units can be understood by noting that it is proportional to the mean time between collisions (the larger the time, the higher the speed) and inversely proportional to mass (the smaller the mass, the higher the acquired speed).

Ohm's law states that the flux of ions in solution across a surface is proportional to the potential gradient, to the charge density, and to mobility, i.e.,

$$J_{Ohm}(r) = -\mu zec(r)\frac{d\phi}{dr}(r) \tag{2.4}$$

where z denotes the ion's valence ($z = -1$ for Cl^-), e denotes the elementary electronic charge (1.602×10^{-19} C), and so zec is a measure of charge density. The combined or net flux is therefore given by the Nernst-Planck equation

$$J(r) = -\mu kT\frac{dc}{dr}(r) - \mu zec(r)\frac{d\phi}{dr}(r). \tag{2.5}$$

This will now permit us to deduce the resting potential gradient from the resting concentration gradient. At rest we expect the net flux, J, to vanish. As such, we note that Eq. (2.5) takes the form

$$-kT\frac{d}{dr}(\log c(r)) = ze\frac{d\phi}{dr}(r).$$

We next integrate each side through the membrane, i.e., from $r = a - \delta$ to $r = a$ (see Figure 2.2), and arrive at

$$ze(\phi(a-\delta) - \phi(a)) = kT\log(c(a)/c(a-\delta)). \tag{2.6}$$

In terms of in-out notation of Figure 2.2 and $V \equiv \phi_{in} - \phi_{out}$, Eq. (2.6) takes the form

$$V = \frac{kT}{ze}\log\frac{c_{out}}{c_{in}}. \tag{2.7}$$

At room temperature, $T = 27\,°C$, the leading coefficient is $kT/e = 25.8$ mV. If c is indeed pegged to chloride concentration then noting that its valence, z, is -1, and adopting the concentrations

$$c_{in} = [Cl^-]_{in} = 0.04 \text{ M} \quad \text{and} \quad c_{out} = [Cl^-]_{out} = 0.56 \text{ M}$$

associated with the squid giant axon, we find

$$V_{Cl} = -68 \text{ mV} \tag{2.8}$$

for the value of the chloride Nernst potential, i.e., the value of the membrane potential at which the net chloride flux, Eq. (2.5), is zero.

2.3 MEMBRANE CONDUCTANCE

When the transmembrane potential, V, is different from V_{Cl} we expect a flux of ions to cross the membrane and for an associated current to flow. Our goal here is to establish an associated membrane conductance. In fact the membrane is an insulating sheet perforated with a significant number of channels through which chloride ions may pass fairly easily. This conductor/insulator composite presents an effective bulk resistivity (largely independent of V) of

$$\rho_{Cl} = \frac{1}{3} 10^{10} \ \Omega \text{cm}$$

to current flow. Resistivity is the resistance to current flow exerted by the membrane, multiplied by its area, A, and divided by its thickness, δ, or $R_{Cl} = \rho_{Cl}\delta/A$. It is a specific property of the membrane, since we expect its resistance to be proportional to thickness and inversely proportional to area. When scaled by the membrane thickness, e.g., $\delta = 10 \, \text{nm}$, we arrive at the effective membrane conductance (per unit area)

$$g_{Cl} = \frac{1}{\rho_{Cl}\delta} = 0.3 \ \text{mS/cm}^2$$

where S is for siemens, the reciprocal of Ω. Next to V_{Cl}, the membrane conductance takes its place in the simple circuit diagram of Figure 2.3.

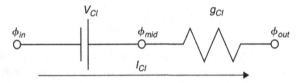

FIGURE 2.3   The equivalent circuit model of the cell's leaky biased membrane. We interpret V_{Cl} as a "battery," or voltage source, that drives or "biases" current flow across the cell's resistive membrane. We have labeled the intermediate potential solely for clarity. The arrow indicates the direction of positive current flow when $V > V_{Cl}$.

We may now use Ohm's law to represent the associated current density. We take potential differences in the direction of the arrow, namely, tail minus head. As such, in accordance with the convention of the previous section,

$$\phi_{in} - \phi_{mid} = V_{Cl}$$

and so Ohm's law reveals

$$I_{Cl} = g_{Cl}(\phi_{mid} - \phi_{out}) = g_{Cl}(\phi_{in} - V_{Cl} - \phi_{out}) = g_{Cl}(V - V_{Cl}), \tag{2.9}$$

in units of $\mu\text{A/cm}^2$. We shall abide by these conventions throughout the remainder of the text. In particular, outward currents are positive and the polarity of the battery is the tail potential minus the head potential.

2.4 MEMBRANE CAPACITANCE AND CURRENT BALANCE

In addition to presenting significant resistance, biological membranes form good dielectrics between their conducting surfaces. The effective dielectric constant is

$$\varepsilon = 10^{-12} \ \text{F/cm}.$$

The dielectric constant is the capacitance of the membrane per unit area multiplied by its thickness ($C = \varepsilon A/\delta$) and is a specific property of the membrane, since capacitance is proportional to area and inversely proportional to thickness. When scaled by the membrane thickness, $\delta = 10 \, \text{nm}$, we arrive at the membrane capacitance (per unit area)

$$C_m = \varepsilon/\delta = 1 \ \mu\text{F/cm}^2.$$

The associated displacement current operates in parallel, see Figure 2.4, with the Ohmic current.

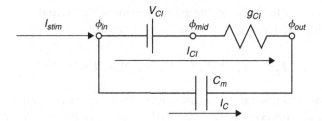

FIGURE 2.4 The equivalent circuit model of the cell's leaky biased and dielectric membrane. The two currents I_C and I_{Cl} will balance the injected current, I_{stim}.

The current density associated with a membrane capacitance is proportional to the rate of change of the potential across the capacitor. That is

$$I_C(t) = C_m \frac{\mathrm{d}}{\mathrm{d}t}(\phi_{in}(t) - \phi_{out}(t)) = C_m \frac{\mathrm{d}V}{\mathrm{d}t}(t). \tag{2.10}$$

Our interest is in tracking how these two membrane currents respond to an injected pulse of current. In order to apply Kirchhoff's Current Law we scale the membrane current densities by membrane surface area, A, and find

$$I_{stim}(t) = AI_C(t) + AI_{Cl}(t). \tag{2.11}$$

On substituting (2.9) and (2.10) this becomes an ordinary differential equation for the membrane potential V. Namely,

$$I_{stim}(t) = AC_m V'(t) + Ag_{Cl}(V(t) - V_{Cl}). \tag{2.12}$$

It is common to divide this equation by Ag_{Cl} and rearrange it to read

$$\tau V'(t) = V_{Cl} - V(t) + I_{stim}(t)/(Ag_{Cl}), \tag{2.13}$$

where

$$\tau \equiv C_m/g_{Cl} \tag{2.14}$$

is known as the **membrane time constant**. As we shall see in the coming chapter, it follows from Eq. (2.13) that in the absence of stimuli $V(t)$ returns to V_{Cl} at the exponential rate $1/\tau$. Given our estimates for C_m and g_{Cl} we find $\tau = 10/3$ ms. We illustrate in Figure 2.5 the computed response of such a cell to a typical current pulse.

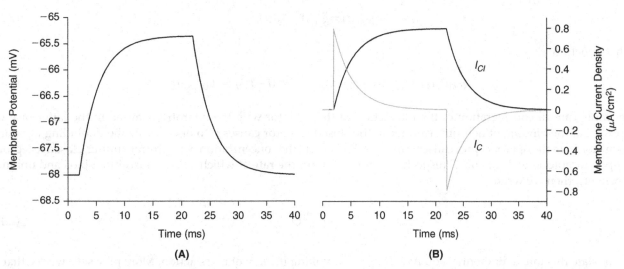

(A) **(B)**

FIGURE 2.5 The solution (A) to (2.12) and the associated membrane currents (B) for a cell of radius 10 μm, with $C_m = 1$ μF/cm^2 and $g_{Cl} = 0.3$ mS/cm^2, subject to a 20 ms, 10 pA current injection. (bepsw1.m)

This model is indeed rich enough to replicate the passive response of actual cells. In coming chapters we shall spend considerable effort developing detailed models of more complicated, active, membrane conductances.

2.5 SYNAPTIC CONDUCTANCE

As ligand-gated channels bind and unbind neurotransmitter, they produce a transient conductance change biased by an associated reversal potential. This is modeled, see Figure 2.6, by adding a third parallel branch to the membrane circuit of Figure 2.4.

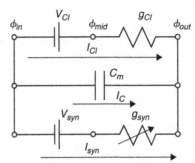

FIGURE 2.6   The circuit diagram for the passive cell with synapse. The arrow through the synaptic conductance is there to indicate that its conductance density varies with time, in a manner that reflects the concentration of available neurotransmitter.

Kirchhoff's Current Law, in the absence of injected current, now reveals that V must satisfy

$$C_m V'(t) + g_{Cl}(V(t) - V_{Cl}) + g_{syn}(t)(V(t) - V_{syn}) = 0. \tag{2.15}$$

The synaptic reversal potential is determined by the equilibrium concentrations of the ions that the associated channel selects. The principal neurotransmitters in the mammalian central nervous system are glutamate and γ-aminobutyric acid, or GABA. The simplest glutamate receptor is the AMPA-type receptor, named after AMPA, or α-amino-3-hydroxyl-5-methyl-4-isoxazole-propionate, which mimics the effect of glutamate on the receptor. The channel associated with the AMPA-type glutamate receptor has a voltage-independent conductance and is selective for Na^+ and K^+. We find $V_{syn}^{ampa} \approx 0\,\text{mV}$. The associated GABA channel is selective for Cl^- and we find $V_{syn}^{gaba} \approx -68\,\text{mV}$. As we will learn in more detail in Chapter 12, the conductance, g_{syn}, is a consequence of the transient dose of neurotransmitter released by the presynaptic terminal in the synaptic cleft (the $\approx 50\,\text{nm}$ gap that separates the presynaptic and postsynaptic cells) and its binding to postsynaptic receptors. Let us denote by $\overline{g}_{syn}$ the peak synaptic conductance. The synaptic conductance is often approximated as either a step function, built from the $\mathbb{1}$ function of Eq. (1.6),

$$g_{syn}(t) = \overline{g}_{syn} \mathbb{1}_{(t_1,t_2)}(t) \tag{2.16}$$

or an α-function

$$g_{syn}(t,t_1) = \overline{g}_{syn}((t-t_1)/\tau_\alpha) \exp(1 - (t-t_1)/\tau_\alpha) \mathbb{1}_{(t_1,\infty)}(t) \tag{2.17}$$

or by more careful consideration of the interaction of the receptor with the neurotransmitter. In the latter case we suppose that the binding of neurotransmitter to the closed receptor causes it to open while the unbinding of neurotransmitter from the open receptor causes it to close. We denote the concentration of neurotransmitter, closed receptors, and open receptors by $\mathcal{T}$, $\mathcal{C}$, and $\mathcal{O}$ respectively. If $k_\pm$ denotes the rate at which neurotransmitter binds and unbinds respectively, then we write

$$\mathcal{T} + \mathcal{C} \underset{k_-}{\overset{k_+}{\rightleftharpoons}} \mathcal{O}, \tag{2.18}$$

and translate this into a differential equation for $\mathcal{O}$ by invoking the law of mass action. More precisely, we see that $\mathcal{O}$ is produced in the forward reaction and consumed in the latter (backward reaction). The law of mass action permits us to equate its rate of production with the product of the forward rate, k_+, and the product of the concentrations of

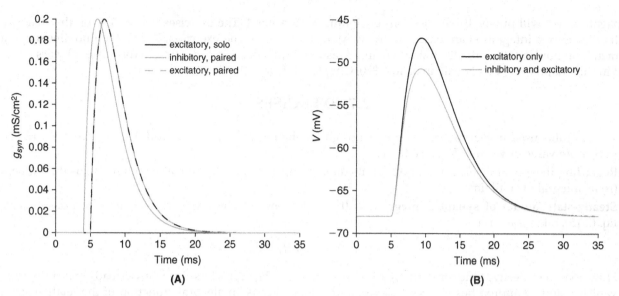

FIGURE 2.7 We first drive the cell with an excitatory α-synapse with $\overline{g}_{syn} = 0.2\,\mathrm{mS/cm^2}$, $\tau_\alpha = 2\,\mathrm{ms}$, $t_1 = 5\,\mathrm{ms}$, and $V_{syn} = 0\,\mathrm{mV}$. The conductance is graphed in black in **A** and its response is graphed in black in **B**. We then precede this with an inhibitory α-synapse with $\overline{g}_{syn} = 0.2\,\mathrm{mS/cm^2}$, $\tau_\alpha = 2\,\mathrm{ms}$, $t_1 = 4\,\mathrm{ms}$, and $V_{syn} = -68\,\mathrm{mV}$. The new conductance is graphed in red in **A** while the additional (original) excitatory conductance is graphed in dashed red in **A**. The response to the pair of inputs is graphed in red in **B**. We see that inhibitory input diminishes the response to the excitatory input by $\approx 20\%$. (trapsyndrive.m)

the two reactants. That is, the rate of production of $\mathcal{O}$ is $k_+ \mathcal{T} \mathcal{C}$. With regard to the reverse reaction we find that the rate of consumption of $\mathcal{O}$ is simply $k_- \mathcal{O}$ and so the number of open receptors obeys the differential equation

$$\mathcal{O}'(t) = k_+ \mathcal{T}(t)\mathcal{C}(t) - k_- \mathcal{O}(t). \tag{2.19}$$

If the total number of receptors is fixed then $\mathcal{O} + \mathcal{C}$ is constant and the fraction of open receptors, $R \equiv \mathcal{O}/(\mathcal{O}+\mathcal{C})$, obeys

$$R'(t) = k_+ \mathcal{T}(t)(1 - R(t)) - k_- R(t). \tag{2.20}$$

The resultant synaptic conductance is then

$$g_{syn}(t) = \overline{g}_{syn} R(t), \tag{2.21}$$

where $\overline{g}_{syn}$ is the product of a single channel conductance and the number of receptors per unit area. We will contrast these three conductances, Eqs. (2.16), (2.17), and (2.21), in the next chapter, once we have acquired a bit more knowledge about differential equations like Eq. (2.15). As a preview, we close in Figure 2.7 with an example of the interaction of excitatory and inhibitory α-synapses.

Figure 2.7 indicates the subtlety associated with the interaction of synaptic inputs. This interaction is nonlinear in the sense that the response to a pair of synapses is not the sum of the individual responses. We will see further illustration of this in the exercises.

2.6 SUMMARY AND SOURCES

We progressed, via the laws of circuit and chemical equilibrium, from a descriptive view of neuronal form and function to a quantitative model of the passive isopotential cell's response to synaptic input. Fundamental neuroscience sourcebooks that provide comprehensive background information on synapses, neurons, and circuits are the texts of Kandel et al. (2008) and Squire et al. (2008). For a thorough account of the membrane electrophysiology of §§2.2–2.5 we recommend Hille (2001). Golgi and Cajal were awarded the 1906 Nobel Prize in Medicine for their work. Nernst received the 1920 Nobel Prize for Chemistry. The press releases announcing the prizes and the Nobel laureate lectures are available at http://nobelprize.org. The giant axon of the squid, mentioned at the end of §2.2, is the setting in which theory and experiment together first gave us a clear picture of action potential generation and propagation. We will pursue these questions beginning in Chapter 4. The exercises below, 3–6, on the steady-state model of synaptic integration are based on the work of Rall (1964). The exercises, 7 and 8, on nonlinear synaptic interaction in nonisopotential cells, follow Vu and Krasne (1992). For an introduction to the basics physics concepts used in this chapter see, e.g., Feynman et al. (1970, Chapters I-43 and II-10).

2.7 EXERCISES

1. The stimulus used in Figure 2.5 is on long enough for the response V to level off. Deduce from Eq. (2.12) the maximum value of V. Hint: $V'(t) = 0$ there.

2. Regarding the g_{syn} of Eq. (2.17), compute (i) its maximum value and the time at which it attains this value, and (ii) its integral over all time.

3. **Steady-state model of synaptic integration.** If g_{syn} is constant show that the synaptic response equation, Eq. (2.15), takes the form

$$\tau_{eff} V'(t) + V(t) = V_{ss}. \tag{2.22}$$

How does this effective time constant, τ_{eff} differ from the τ_m of Eq. (2.14)? As V reaches a steady state its derivative vanishes and so approaches V_{ss}. Set $V_{syn} = 0$, and express V_{ss} as an algebraic function of the relative synaptic strength, $c_e = g_{syn}/g_{Cl}$. Graph it as in Figure 2.8.

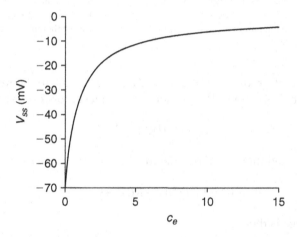

FIGURE 2.8   Steady-state potential associated with steady synaptic input. $V_{Cl} = -68\,\text{mV}$. Excitatory input, Eq. (2.22) with $V_{syn} = 0$. Note the distinctly nonlinear response. (sse.m)

4. The differential equation for the membrane potential of a cell receiving input from two synapses is given by

$$C_m \frac{dV}{dt} + g_{Cl}(V - V_{Cl}) + g_{syn1}(V - V_{syn1}) + g_{syn2}(V - V_{syn2}) = 0. \tag{2.23}$$

Suppose that g_{syn1} and g_{syn2} are constant and write Eq. (2.23) as

$$\tau_{eff,2} \frac{dV}{dt} + V = V_{ss}. \tag{2.24}$$

Express $\tau_{eff,2}$ and V_{ss} as functions of the normalized synaptic conductances, $c_1 = g_{syn1}/g_{Cl}$ and $c_2 = g_{syn2}/g_{Cl}$.

5. With regard to the previous exercise show that if $g_{syn1} = g_{syn2} = g_e$ and $V_{syn1} = V_{syn2} = 0$ then

$$V_{ss} = V_{ss,2e} = \frac{V_{Cl}}{1 + 2c_e} = V_{Cl} - \frac{2c_e}{1 + 2c_e}V_{Cl} \tag{2.25}$$

where $c_e = g_e/g_{Cl}$. Compare, by plotting as in Figure 2.9, this response to that generated (as computed in Exercise 3) by a single excitatory synapse

$$V_{ss,e} = V_{Cl} - \frac{c_e}{1 + c_e}V_{Cl}, \tag{2.26}$$

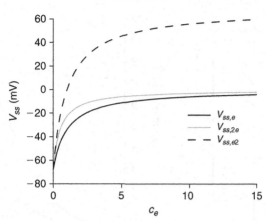

FIGURE 2.9 Steady-state depolarization as a function of normalized conductance for a single, $V_{ss,e}$, and two excitatory, $V_{ss,2e}$, synapses, and the relative sum, $V_{ss,e2}$, of the responses to a single excitatory synapse. Synaptic inputs are said to sum "sublinearly" in the sense that $V_{ss,2e} \leq V_{ss,e2}$. (ss2e.m)

as well as that associated with the sum (relative to V_{Cl}) of the two single excitatory synaptic inputs

$$V_{ss,e2} = V_{Cl} - 2\frac{c_e}{1+c_e}V_{Cl}. \tag{2.27}$$

6. †Let us now investigate the interaction of steady excitatory and inhibitory synaptic currents. The equation for V_{ss} in this case takes the form

$$V_{ss} - V_{Cl} + c_e(V_{ss} - V_e) + c_i(V_{ss} - V_i) = 0, \tag{2.28}$$

where c_e and c_i are the relative excitatory and inhibitory synaptic strengths and V_e and V_i are the respective reversal potentials. Set $V_e = 0$ and $V_i = V_{Cl}$ and solve for V_{ss} as a function of c_e and c_i. Plot, as in Figure 2.10, V_{ss} as a function of c_e for $c_i = 0, 25$, and 50. Show that, for $c_i >> 1 + c_e$, the steady-state membrane potential may be approximated by $V_{ss} \approx V_{Cl} - (c_e/c_i)V_{Cl}$. Thus, in that regime inhibition has a divisive effect on membrane potential.

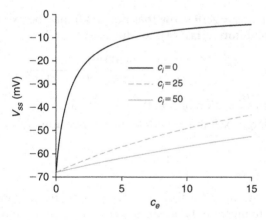

FIGURE 2.10 Steady-state potential associated with steady synaptic input. $V_{Cl} = -68$ mV. Excitatory and inhibitory input, Eq. (2.28). Inhibition has a "linearizing" effect. (ssEI.m)

7. **Illustration of the "veto property" of proximal inhibition**. Consider a two-compartment model representing sites proximal and distal to the spike initiation zone of a neuron. We suppose, as in Figure 2.11A, that the distal compartment receives excitation while the proximal compartment receives inhibition.

(i) Derive the system of coupled differential equations for the membrane potentials

$$V_p \equiv \phi_p - \phi_0 \quad \text{and} \quad V_d \equiv \phi_d - \phi_0.$$

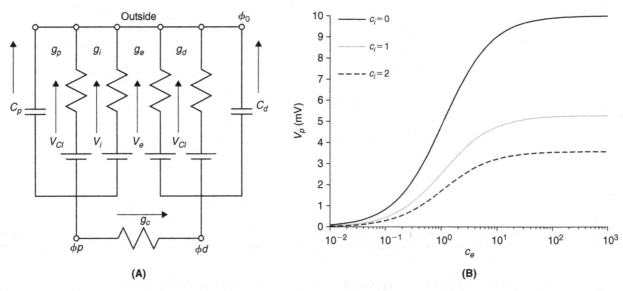

(A)   **(B)**

FIGURE 2.11   **A.** Passive model of a two-compartment cell with proximal conductance, g_p, and capacitance c_p and distal conductance, g_d, and capacitance c_d and a coupling conductance, g_c. An excitatory synapse (g_e, V_e) is located in the distal compartment and an inhibitory one (g_i, V_i) in the proximal compartment. **B.** The relative proximal potential, v_p per Eq. (2.31), as a function of the normalized excitatory conductance at several values of the normalized inhibitory conductance. (`Comp2syn1.m`)

In particular, derive

$$c_p V_p' + g_p(V_p - V_{Cl}) + g_i(V_p - V_i) = g_c(V_d - V_p)$$
$$c_d V_d' + g_d(V_d - V_{Cl}) + g_e(V_d - V_e) = g_c(V_p - V_d). \tag{2.29}$$

(ii) Assume that g_e and g_i are constant and that inhibition is silent ($V_i = V_{Cl}$). Solve for $v_p \equiv V_p - V_{Cl}$, the proximal membrane potential relative to rest at steady state. In particular, confirm that

$$v_p = \frac{g_c g_e v_e}{(g_c + g_p + g_i)(g_c + g_d + g_e) - g_c^2}, \quad \text{where} \quad v_e \equiv V_e - V_{Cl}. \tag{2.30}$$

(iii) With $v_e = 100\,\text{mV}$, $g_p = g_d$, and $g_c = g_p/9$ show that Eq. (2.30) may be expressed in terms of the normalized excitatory, $c_e \equiv g_e/g_d$, and inhibitory, $c_i \equiv g_i/g_d$, conductances as

$$v_p = \frac{(100/9)c_e}{(c_i + 10/9)(c_e + 10/9) - 1/81}. \tag{2.31}$$

Plot v_p, as in Figure 2.11B, as a function of c_e at three values of c_i.

(iv) Show that in the limit of a large excitatory conductance v_p becomes

$$\lim_{g_e \to \infty} v_p = \frac{g_c v_e}{g_c + g_p + g_i}. \tag{2.32}$$

This shows that, no matter how large the distal excitatory input, the proximal inhibitory input can effectively *veto* it: it is always possible to increase the inhibitory conductance, g_i, and overcome the effect of excitation.

8. [†]**Distal inhibition.** Consider the two-compartment circuit of Figure 2.12A where now the distal compartment receives both inhibition and excitation while the proximal compartment is unstimulated. Proceeding as in the previous exercise,

(i) Derive the analogous system of differential equations for V_p and V_d.

(ii) Confirm that the steady-state membrane potential in the proximal compartment satisfies

$$v_p = \frac{g_c g_e v_e}{(g_c + g_p)(g_c + g_d + g_e + g_i) - g_c^2}. \tag{2.33}$$

(iii) Adopting the choices of Exercise 7 show that

$$v_p = \frac{(100/9)c_e}{(10/9)(c_e + c_i + 10/9) - 1/81}$$ (2.34)

and reproduce the graph in Figure 2.12B.

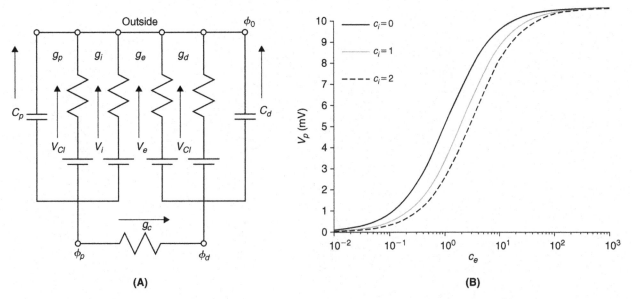

(A) **(B)**

FIGURE 2.12 **A.** Passive model of a two-compartment cell with distal excitatory and inhibitory conductances. **B.** The relative proximal potential, v_p per Eq. (2.34), as a function of the normalized excitatory conductance at several values of the normalized inhibitory conductance. (`Comp2syn2.m`)

(iv) Show that in the limit of a large excitatory conductance Eq. (2.33) becomes

$$\lim_{g_e \to \infty} v_p = \frac{g_c v_e}{g_p + g_c}.$$ (2.35)

The important difference with Eq. (2.32) is that distal inhibition cannot veto excitation. In other words, an increase of excitation can always overcome distal inhibition since the limiting value is independent of g_i.

9. Divide Eq. (2.19) by $\mathcal{O} + \mathcal{C}$ and explain how one arrives at Eq. (2.20).

Differential Equations

O U T L I N E

3.1   Exact Solution   21   3.5   Synaptic Input   28

3.2   Moment Methods*   23   3.6   Summary and Sources   29

3.3   The Laplace Transform*   25   3.7   Exercises   29

3.4   Numerical Methods   27

In constructing a model of the voltage response to a stimulated passive isopotential cell we encountered three linear ordinary differential equations, Eqs. (2.12), (2.15), and (2.20). As we progress from the passive isopotential cell to the active multipotential dendritic tree, these same three equations will continue to determine the background local membrane potential. As preparation for the more complex case, we analyze our three equations in some detail from multiple points of view. In particular we pursue exact analytical integration, approximate numerical integration, as well as solution via the Laplace transform. We also develop one simple consequence of our analysis, namely a method for representing the coefficients in Eq. (2.12) in terms of moments of the solution. Such methods permit the experimentalist to infer their cell's effective electrical properties from measurement of the voltage response to a prescribed current.

3.1 EXACT SOLUTION

To begin, we write Eq. (2.12) as

$$V'(t) + V(t)/\tau = f(t) \qquad V(0) = b, \tag{3.1}$$

where τ is the membrane time constant in Eq. (2.14), $b = V_{Cl}$, and $f(t) = V_{Cl}/\tau + I_{stim}(t)/(AC_m)$. If $\tau = \infty$ then we may simply integrate

$$\int_0^T V'(t)\,dt = \int_0^T f(t)\,dt \quad \text{and find} \quad V(T) = b + \int_0^T f(t)\,dt.$$

When τ is finite we strive to make $V' + V/\tau$ look like a derivative. More precisely, we note that

$$(V(t)e^{t/\tau})' = (V'(t) + V(t)/\tau)e^{t/\tau}$$

and so

$$(V(t)e^{t/\tau})' = e^{t/\tau}f(t) \qquad V(0) = b.$$

Mathematics for Neuroscientists. DOI: 10.1016/B978-0-12-374882-9.00003-4

Now integrate each side from 0 to T and find

$$V(T)e^{T/\tau} - b = \int_0^T e^{t/\tau} f(t)\,dt$$

which, on multiplying through by $e^{-T/\tau}$ gives

$$V(T) = be^{-T/\tau} + \int_0^T e^{(t-T)/\tau} f(t)\,dt$$

$$= V_{Cl}e^{-T/\tau} + \int_0^T e^{(t-T)/\tau}\{I_{stim}(t)/(AC_m) + V_{Cl}/\tau\}\,dt \tag{3.2}$$

$$= V_{Cl} + \frac{1}{AC_m}\int_0^T e^{(t-T)/\tau} I_{stim}(t)\,dt.$$

For simple stimuli we may compute this integral by hand. We consider two examples here and then two more in the exercises.

Square pulse stimulus. With regard to our previous chapter, we choose $t_1 < t_2$ and consider the response to

$$I_{stim}(t) = \frac{Q}{t_2 - t_1}\mathbb{1}_{(t_1,t_2)}(t). \tag{3.3}$$

Here $\mathbb{1}_{(t_1,t_2)}(t)$ is the characteristic function, Eq. (1.6), of the interval (t_1,t_2). Hence I_{stim} is a pulse that begins at t_1, ends at t_2 and delivers a total charge of Q to the cell. Its response is then

$$V(t) = V_{Cl} + \frac{Q\tau}{(t_2 - t_1)AC_m}\begin{cases} 0 & \text{when}\quad t \leq t_1\quad\text{and} \\ 1 - e^{(t_1-t)/\tau} & \text{when}\quad t_1 \leq t \leq t_2 \\ e^{(t_2-t)/\tau} - e^{(t_1-t)/\tau} & \text{when}\quad t_2 \leq t. \end{cases}$$

This is indeed the solution approximated in Figure 2.5.

There is considerable interest in the case of very fast pulses. We achieve this by fixing t_1, evaluating

$$V(t_2) = V_{Cl} + \frac{Q\tau}{(t_2 - t_1)AC_m}(1 - e^{(t_1-t_2)/\tau}),$$

and noting that this approaches

$$V(t_1) = V_{Cl} + \frac{Q}{AC_m}$$

as $t_2 \to t_1$. Using the same reasoning for $t > t_2$, it follows that the full response to this "impulse" is

$$V_{imp}(t) = V_{Cl} + \frac{Q}{AC_m}e^{(t_1-t)/\tau}\mathbb{1}_{(t_1,\infty)}(t). \tag{3.4}$$

As we shall invoke impulsive stimuli throughout the rest of the text it seems wise to develop one or two other essential properties. Let us then consider the integral of the product of I_{stim} and a continuous function, u,

$$\int_0^\infty I_{stim}(t)u(t)\,dt = \frac{Q}{t_2 - t_1}\int_{t_1}^{t_2} u(t)\,dt = Qu(\tilde{t})$$

for some $\tilde{t}$ which, by the mean value theorem, lies between t_1 and t_2. It follows that

$$\int_0^\infty I_{stim}(t)u(t)\,\mathrm{d}t \to Qu(t_1) \quad \text{as} \quad t_2 \to t_1. \tag{3.5}$$

We speak of this limit by saying that I_{stim} converges to the Dirac delta function, centered at t_1, with magnitude Q. The Dirac delta function is defined by the pair of conditions

$$\delta(t) = 0 \text{ when } t \neq 0 \quad \text{and} \quad \int_{-\infty}^\infty \delta(t)u(t)\,\mathrm{d}t = u(0) \tag{3.6}$$

for all functions u that are continuous at 0. The Dirac delta function, centered at t_1, with magnitude Q is then simply $Q\delta(t-t_1)$.

Sinusoidal stimulus. For our next example we compute the response to the sinusoidal input

$$I_{stim}(t) = I_0 \sin(2\pi\omega t).$$

Namely,

$$\begin{aligned}
V(T;\omega) &= V_{Cl} + \frac{I_0}{AC_m}\int_0^T e^{(t-T)/\tau}\sin(2\pi\omega t)\,\mathrm{d}t \\
&= V_{Cl} + \frac{I_0}{AC_m}\frac{2\pi\omega e^{-T/\tau} - 2\pi\omega\cos(2\pi\omega T) + (1/\tau)\sin(2\pi\omega T)}{(2\pi\omega)^2 + 1/\tau^2} \\
&= V_{Cl} + \frac{I_0}{AC_m}\frac{2\pi\omega e^{-T/\tau} + \sqrt{(2\pi\omega)^2 + 1/\tau^2}\sin[2\pi\omega T - \tan^{-1}(2\pi\omega\tau)]}{(2\pi\omega)^2 + 1/\tau^2}.
\end{aligned}$$

For large time, T, after the exponential transient dies away we see that V oscillates about V_{Cl} with amplitude $I_0/(AC_m\sqrt{(2\pi\omega)^2 + 1/\tau^2})$. If we divide this by the strength of the input current we arrive at the so-called input resistance of the cell,

$$R_{in}(\omega) = \frac{1}{AC_m\sqrt{(2\pi\omega)^2 + 1/\tau^2}}. \tag{3.7}$$

We also see that the membrane potential oscillates with a phase lag equal to $\tan^{-1}(2\pi\omega\tau)$ relative to the input current. We plot these results in Figure 3.1.

3.2 MOMENT METHODS*

We derived Eq. (3.2) in order to express the response, V, of the passive isopotential cell, with known parameters A, C_m, g_{Cl}, and V_{Cl}, to the known stimulus I_{stim}. However, in the case where one can measure V for a given I_{stim} we may instead view Eq. (3.2) as a means for determining, or "reverse engineering," the model parameters. We illustrate below that C_m and g_{Cl} may be "read" from simple geometric descriptors (moments) of the stimulus and response. We define the nth moment of the function f to be

$$M_n(f) \equiv \int_0^\infty t^n f(t)\,\mathrm{d}t.$$

The zeroth moment is often called the "strength" of the signal while the ratio of the first to the zeroth is referred to as the "centroid" or "characteristic time," and denoted

$$\tau_c(f) \equiv M_1(f)/M_0(f). \tag{3.8}$$

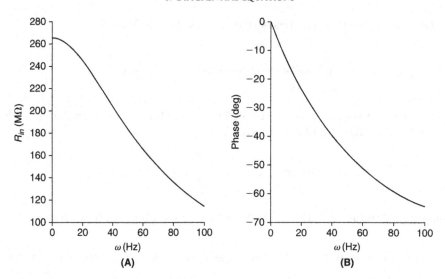

FIGURE 3.1　The input resistance (**A**) and phase lag (**B**) of the membrane potential relative to sinusoidal current injection as a function of frequency. As the response, R_{in}, decreases with frequency we speak of the passive isopotential cell as a **low-pass filter**. (`ffreq.m`)

Regarding moments of the response we find after integrating by parts

$$
\begin{aligned}
M_0(V - V_{Cl}) &= \frac{1}{AC_m} \int_0^\infty \int_0^T e^{(t-T)/\tau} I_{stim}(t)\, dt\, dT \\
&= \frac{1}{AC_m} \int_0^\infty e^{-T/\tau} \int_0^T e^{t/\tau} I_{stim}(t)\, dt\, dT \\
&= \frac{1}{AC_m} \left\{ -\tau e^{-T/\tau} \int_0^T e^{t/\tau} I_{stim}(t)\, dt \Big|_{T=0}^{T=\infty} + \tau \int_0^\infty e^{-t/\tau} I_{stim}(t) e^{t/\tau}\, dt \right\} \\
&= \frac{\tau}{AC_m} \int_0^\infty I_{stim}(t)\, dt = \frac{1}{Ag_{Cl}} M_0(I_{stim})
\end{aligned}
\tag{3.9}
$$

and so one may infer the chloride conductance, g_{Cl}, from the ratio of the strengths of the stimulus and response. That is,

$$
\boxed{Ag_{Cl} = \frac{M_0(I_{stim})}{M_0(V - V_{Cl})}.}
\tag{3.10}
$$

Regarding the next moment, we find

$$
\begin{aligned}
M_1(V - V_{Cl}) &= \frac{1}{AC_m} \int_0^\infty T e^{-T/\tau} \int_0^T e^{t/\tau} I_{stim}(t)\, dt\, dT \\
&= \frac{1}{AC_m} \left\{ -\tau(T+\tau) e^{-T/\tau} \int_0^T e^{t/\tau} I_{stim}(t)\, dt \Big|_{T=0}^{T=\infty} + \tau \int_0^\infty (t+\tau) e^{-t/\tau} I_{stim}(t) e^{t/\tau}\, dt \right\} \\
&= \frac{\tau}{AC_m} \int_0^\infty (t+\tau) I_{stim}(t)\, dt = \frac{M_1(I_{stim}) + \tau M_0(I_{stim})}{Ag_{Cl}}
\end{aligned}
\tag{3.11}
$$

and so τ is simply the lag between the characteristic times of the response and stimulus, i.e.,

$$\boxed{\tau = \tau_c(V - V_{Cl}) - \tau_c(I_{stim}).} \tag{3.12}$$

As above, this gives one an experimental means for estimating τ. For example, the strength of the impulse, $I_{stim}(t) = Q\delta(t - t_1)$ is Q and its characteristic time is t_1. The strength of the relative response, via Eq. (3.4), is $Q/(Ag_{Cl})$ and its characteristic time is $t_1 + \tau$.

3.3 THE LAPLACE TRANSFORM*

The Laplace transform is typically credited with taking dynamical problems into static problems. The Laplace transform of V is

$$\mathcal{L}(V)(s) \equiv \int_0^\infty e^{-st} V(t) \, dt \tag{3.13}$$

where s is a complex variable. We will have occasion to evaluate the Laplace transform of a number of functions, e.g., for constant c

$$\mathcal{L}(c)(s) = \frac{c}{s}, \quad \mathcal{L}(e^{-ct})(s) = \frac{1}{s+c}, \quad \text{and} \quad \mathcal{L}(\sin(ct))(s) = \frac{c}{s^2 + c^2}. \tag{3.14}$$

Regarding its effect on the derivative we find, on integrating by parts, that

$$\mathcal{L}(V') = \int_0^\infty e^{-st} V'(t) \, dt = V(t)e^{-st} \Big|_0^\infty + s \int_0^\infty e^{-st} V(t) \, dt. \tag{3.15}$$

Supposing that V and s are such that $V(t)e^{-st} \to 0$ as $t \to \infty$ we arrive at

$$\mathcal{L}(V') = s\mathcal{L}(V) - V(0). \tag{3.16}$$

It is natural to define $v(t) = V(t) - V_{Cl}$ and write Eq. (2.12) as

$$\tau v'(t) + v(t) = I_{stim}(t)/(Ag_{Cl}). \tag{3.17}$$

If we now take the Laplace transform of each side of Eq. (3.17) we find

$$s\tau \mathcal{L}(v) + \mathcal{L}(v) = \mathcal{L}(I_{stim})/(Ag_{Cl}),$$

and so

$$\mathcal{L}(v) = \frac{1}{1+s\tau} \frac{\mathcal{L}(I_{stim})}{Ag_{Cl}}. \tag{3.18}$$

We have expressed the Laplace transform of the response in terms of the Laplace transform of the stimulus. It remains to invert $\mathcal{L}$ and recover v. This is, in general, a difficult task. It is made easy here by first recognizing that the factor $1/(1+s\tau)$ in Eq. (3.18) is itself the Laplace transform of $\exp(-t/\tau)/\tau$ (recall Eq. (3.14)). Our second and final step in the recovery of v is to associate the product of transforms with convolution. We denote the convolution of two functions, f and g, as in Eq. (1.9), by

$$(f \star g)(t) = \int_0^t f(t-r)g(r) \, dr, \tag{3.19}$$

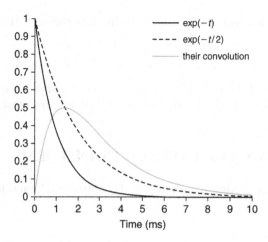

FIGURE 3.2 An illustration of the convolution in Eq. (3.20) with $\tau_1 = 1$ and $\tau_2 = 2$ ms. (`convex.m`)

where f and g are presumed zero for negative arguments. For example, the convolution of two exponentials, see Figure 3.2, is their weighted difference,

$$\exp(-t/\tau_1) \star \exp(-t/\tau_2) = \frac{\tau_1 \tau_2}{\tau_1 - \tau_2}(\exp(-t/\tau_1) - \exp(-t/\tau_2)).$$ (3.20)

On taking the Laplace transform of each side of Eq. (3.19) we find

$$
\begin{aligned}
\mathcal{L}(f \star g) &= \int_0^\infty \int_0^t f(t-r)g(r)\,dr\,e^{-st}\,dt \\
&= \int_0^\infty g(r)e^{-sr} \int_0^\infty f(t-r)e^{-s(t-r)}\,dt\,dr, \quad \text{as } g(r)=0 \text{ for } r<0 \text{ and } f(t-r)=0 \text{ for } r>t \\
&= \int_0^\infty g(r)e^{-sr} \int_0^\infty f(y)e^{-sy}\,dy\,dr, \quad \text{using } y=t-r \text{ and } f(y)=0 \text{ for } y<0 \\
&= \mathcal{L}(f)\mathcal{L}(g).
\end{aligned}
$$ (3.22)

This identity, $\mathcal{L}(f \star g) = \mathcal{L}(f)\mathcal{L}(g)$, is known as the Convolution Theorem. Applying this to Eq. (3.18) we conclude that

$$v(t) = \frac{\exp(-t/\tau) \star I_{stim}(t)}{\tau A g_{Cl}} = \frac{1}{AC_m}\int_0^t e^{(r-t)/\tau}I_{stim}(r)\,dr$$

as in Eq. (3.2).

We next demonstrate that the Laplace transform provides an alternate path to our moment identities, Eqs. (3.10)–(3.12). The connection stems from the identities

$$M_0(f) = \mathcal{L}(f)(0) \quad \text{and} \quad M_1(f) = -\mathcal{L}(f)'(0).$$ (3.23)

The first of these follows from simply setting $s=0$ in Eq. (3.13). The second requires that we first differentiate Eq. (3.13) with respect to s, i.e.,

$$\mathcal{L}(f)'(s) = \frac{d}{ds}\int_0^\infty e^{-st}f(t)\,dt = \int_0^\infty f(t)\frac{d}{ds}e^{-st}\,dt = -\int_0^\infty f(t)te^{-st}\,dt,$$

and then set $s = 0$. From the first identity in Eq. (3.23) we now set $s = 0$ in Eq. (3.18) and find

$$M_0(v) = M_0(I_{stim})/(Ag_{Cl}) \tag{3.24}$$

in agreement with Eq. (3.10). To exploit the second moment identity we differentiate Eq. (3.18) with respect to s and find

$$\mathcal{L}(v)'(s) = \frac{-\tau}{(1+s\tau)^2}\frac{\mathcal{L}(I_{stim})(s)}{Ag_{Cl}} + \frac{1}{1+s\tau}\frac{\mathcal{L}(I_{stim})'(s)}{Ag_{Cl}}. \tag{3.25}$$

Setting $s = 0$ here and then applying Eq. (3.24) brings

$$-M_1(v) = \frac{\tau}{Ag_{Cl}}M_0(I_{stim}) - \frac{1}{Ag_{Cl}}M_1(I_{stim}) = \tau M_0(v) - M_0(v)M_1(I_{stim})/M_0(I_{stim}).$$

On dividing through by $M_0(v)$ we arrive at Eq. (3.12).

3.4 NUMERICAL METHODS

We consider numerical methods with which to systematically approximate the solution of Eq. (3.1). By approximate we mean that we partition time into small intervals of length dt and produce a discrete sequence of voltages, $V^1, V^2, \ldots$ that approximate the true voltage at integer multiples of dt. In other words,

$$V^j \approx V((j-1)dt) \quad j = 1, 2, 3, \ldots \tag{3.26}$$

These V^j will be the solution of a difference approximation to the associated differential equation. We consider three natural means for constructing such difference equations.

The forward Euler scheme. We express Eq. (3.1) as

$$(V^j - V^{j-1})/dt + V^{j-1}/\tau = f^{j-1} \quad j = 1, 2, 3, \ldots$$

and note that the derivative looks beyond (forward) the time point at which the remaining functions are approximated or evaluated. This results in the simple march

$$\boxed{V^j = (1 - dt/\tau)V^{j-1} + dt f^{j-1}} \quad j = 2, 3, \ldots \tag{3.27}$$

starting from $V^1 = b$. We have coded this in MATLAB, see feps.m, with a 1 pA stimulus for 18 ms. This routine asks the user to specify the time step, dt, and the final time, T_{fin}. One naturally asks: does this routine work for every dt and, when it works, how does the answer differ from the exact solution computed in the previous section. To answer the first question we denote $a \equiv 1 - dt/\tau$ and execute the step (3.27) by hand

$$V^2 = aV^1 + dt f^1$$
$$V^3 = aV^2 + dt f^2 = a^2 V^1 + dt(af^1 + f^2)$$
$$V^4 = aV^3 + dt f^3 = a^3 V^1 + dt(a^2 f^1 + af^2 + f^3)$$

until we recognize the pattern

$$V^j = a^{j-1}V^1 + dt \sum_{i=1}^{j-1} a^{j-i-1} f^i.$$

We see that this sequence is bounded so long as $|a| < 1$, i.e., so long as

$$dt < 2\tau. \tag{3.28}$$

What does this mean in practice? Run feps(7,180) and watch the potential grow without bound. When the iterates of a marching scheme take bounded inputs to bounded outputs one calls the scheme **stable**. In our case, forward Euler is stable when dt obeys (3.28).

The backward Euler scheme. We approximate Eq. (3.1) via

$$(\mathsf{v}^j - \mathsf{v}^{j-1})/dt + \mathsf{v}^j/\tau = \mathsf{f}^j \quad j = 2, 3, \ldots$$

and note that the derivative now looks back from where the remaining functions are approximated or evaluated. The resulting marching scheme is

$$\mathsf{v}^j = \frac{\mathsf{v}^{j-1} + dt\,\mathsf{f}^j}{1 + dt/\tau} \tag{3.29}$$

starting from $\mathsf{v}^1 = b$. We shall see that this scheme is stable for every choice of dt. We have coded this in `beps.m` with our same 1 pA stimulus for 18 ms.

The trapezoid scheme. We integrate Eq. (3.1) across one time step,

$$V((j-1)dt) - V((j-2)dt) + (1/\tau) \int\limits_{(j-2)dt}^{(j-1)dt} V(s)\,ds = \int\limits_{(j-2)dt}^{(j-1)dt} f(s)\,ds$$

and approximate each integral via the trapezoid rule, i.e., by the product of the mean of the integrand and the length of the base. This produces

$$\mathsf{v}^j - \mathsf{v}^{j-1} + (1/\tau)(dt/2)(\mathsf{v}^{j-1} + \mathsf{v}^j) = (dt/2)(\mathsf{f}^{j-1} + \mathsf{f}^j)$$

which, upon rearrangement takes the form

$$\mathsf{v}^j = \frac{(2 - dt/\tau)\mathsf{v}^{j-1} + dt(\mathsf{f}^{j-1} + \mathsf{f}^j)}{2 + dt/\tau}. \tag{3.30}$$

This routine is also stable for all dt. In the exercises to come we will find it accurate to order $(dt)^2$ while backward (and forward) Euler are only accurate to order dt.

3.5 SYNAPTIC INPUT

In the case that the cell receives synaptic input rather than current injection we recall Eq. (2.15) and so must instead solve

$$V'(t) + a(t)V(t) = b(t), \quad V(0) = V_{Cl} \tag{3.31}$$

where

$$a(t) = (g_{Cl} + g_{syn}(t))/C_m \quad \text{and} \quad b(t) = (g_{Cl}V_{Cl} + g_{syn}(t)V_{syn})/C_m.$$

This too has an exact solution, for $V' + aV$ is transformed into an exact derivative by multiplication. In particular

$$(V'(t) + a(t)V(t))e^{\int_0^t a(s)\,ds} = (V(t)e^{\int_0^t a(s)\,ds})' = b(t)e^{\int_0^t a(s)\,ds}$$

and so

$$V(t) = V_{Cl}e^{-\int_0^t a(s)\,ds} + \int\limits_0^t b(s)e^{-\int_s^t a(y)\,dy}\,ds. \tag{3.32}$$

Although explicit, this expression is cumbersome for all but the most simple g_{syn}, and so one often resorts to the trapezoid scheme

$$\mathsf{v}^j - \mathsf{v}^{j-1} + (dt/2)(a^j\mathsf{v}^j + a^{j-1}\mathsf{v}^{j-1}) = (dt/2)(b^j + b^{j-1})$$

which leads to the update rule

$$v^j = \frac{(2/dt - a^{j-1})v^{j-1} + b^j + b^{j-1}}{2/dt + a^j}. \tag{3.33}$$

We have coded this in `trapsyn.m` and used it to achieve Figure 2.7 in the previous chapter.

We note that the product term, $a(t)V(t)$, in Eq. (3.31), prohibits the direct application of both the Laplace transform and moment methods to problems with time-varying synaptic conductances.

3.6 SUMMARY AND SOURCES

We have presented three attacks on Eq. (2.12), the linear ordinary differential equation that governs the response of a passive cell to current injection. Each of our methods, exact integration, the Laplace transform, and numerical integration are developed in full in the beautiful introductory text of Redheffer and Port (1992). The Laplace transform is also an effective tool for studying renewal point processes, as we will learn in the exercises of Chapters 11, 15, and 16. Regarding MATLAB programming there is no substitute for practice, for few can learn a language strictly from reading a grammar book. We intend to give the reader considerable practice. For a more systematic introduction to MATLAB in a neuroscience context see Wallisch et al. (2008). To learn more about the mathematics behind the curve-fitting in Exercise 12 see Cheney and Kincaid (2007).

3.7 EXERCISES

1. Find the exact solution to Eq. (3.1) with $I_{stim}(t) = te^{-t}$.

2. †Find the exact solution to Eq. (3.1) with $I_{stim}(t) = e^{-t/\tau_1} - e^{-t/\tau_2}$.

3. Establish the validity of the three transforms in Eq. (3.14).

4. Show that $\mathcal{L}(t)(s) = 1/s^2$ and $\mathcal{L}(t^2)(s) = 2/s^3$. Hint: Use Eq. (3.16).

5. †Generalize the result of Exercise 4 to arbitrary positive integers n:

$$\mathcal{L}(t^n)(s) = \frac{n!}{s^{n+1}}. \tag{3.34}$$

6. Establish the validity of the two basic scaling properties of the Laplace transform.
   (i) If $g(t) = f(t-a)$ and $a > 0$ then $\mathcal{L}(g)(s) = \mathcal{L}(f)(s)e^{-as}$.
   (ii) If $g(t) = f(t/a)$ and $a > 0$ then $\mathcal{L}(g)(s) = a\mathcal{L}(f)(as)$.

7. Show that the Laplace transform of the gamma density distributions, to be studied in Chapters 11, 15, and 16,

$$p_n(t) = \frac{\varrho(\varrho t)^{n-1}}{(n-1)!}\exp(-\varrho t), \quad n = 1,2,\ldots$$

is given by

$$\mathcal{L}(p_n)(s) = \frac{\varrho^n}{(s+\varrho)^n}.$$

Hint: Proceed by *induction*, showing the assertion for $n = 1$ and then showing that $\mathcal{L}(p_{n+1})(s) = (\varrho/(s+\varrho))\mathcal{L}(p_n)(s)$. This last equality may be derived by integrating by parts.

8. †Use Eq. (3.32) when

$$g_{syn}(t) = \frac{\overline{g}_{syn}}{\varepsilon}\mathbb{1}_{(0,\varepsilon)}(t)$$

and evaluate

$$\lim_{\varepsilon \to 0} V(\varepsilon),$$

the response to a conductance "impulse," $g(t) = \overline{g}_{syn}\delta(t)$.

9. Show that the backward Euler and trapezoid schemes are each stable for every positive dt.

10. Let us contrast, by example, the accuracies of the backward Euler and trapezoid schemes. Using V, the exact solution when $I_{stim}(t) = 2(t/\tau)\exp(-t/\tau)/10^5$ μA, we compute the maximum absolute error

$$E(dt) \equiv \max_{1 \leq j \leq T/dt} |V(jdt) - v^j|$$

as a function of the time step, dt, over a time span of $T = 20$ ms. Write a program that evaluates this error for a given dt for both the backward Euler and trapezoid schemes and produces Figure 3.3.

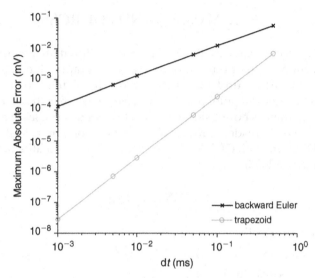

FIGURE 3.3   Contrasting the error in backward Euler and trapezoid approximations. The former decays like dt and the latter like dt^2. (be_vs_trap.m)

11. We will here contrast current injection and synaptic input. The comparison is made easier in terms of $v \equiv V - V_{Cl}$, for v obeys

$$C_m v'(t) + g_{Cl} v(t) + g_{syn}(t) v(t) = g_{syn}(t)E, \quad v(0) = 0,$$

where $E = V_{syn} - V_{Cl}$. Please check that the trapezoid scheme leads to

$$v^j = \frac{(2C_m/dt - g_{Cl} - g_{syn}^{j-1})v^{j-1} + (g_{syn}^j + g_{syn}^{j-1})E}{2C_m/dt + g_{Cl} + g_{syn}^j}.$$

If we denote by w the response, with respect to V_{Cl}, then w obeys

$$C_m w'(t) + g_{Cl} w(t) = g_{syn}(t)E, \quad w(0) = 0,$$

where $E = V_{syn} - V_{Cl}$. Please check that the trapezoid scheme leads to

$$w^j = \frac{(2C_m/dt - g_{Cl})w^{j-1} + (g_{syn}^j + g_{syn}^{j-1})E}{2C_m/dt + g_{Cl}}.$$

The difference here is that in the latter, current approximation, the synaptic conductance acts on the "driving force" E, while in the former, the driving force is $E - v$. In situations where v deviates appreciably from rest, i.e., $v = 0$, we say that the cell experiences a loss of driving force. As a result, we may expect this loss to produce less depolarization than the current approximation.

Confirm this loss of driving force by modifying trapsyn.m to accommodate the square wave conductance

$$g_{syn}(t) = \overline{g}_{syn} \mathbb{1}_{(0,s_p)}(\mathrm{mod}(t, s_T)) \tag{3.35}$$

with amplitude, $\bar{g}_{syn}$ mS/cm^2, pulsewidth, s_p ms, and period, s_T ms. Here mod is the MATLAB function, $\text{mod}(t, s_T) \equiv t - \lfloor t/s_T \rfloor s_T$, where $\lfloor x \rfloor$ is the greatest integer that does not exceed x. Reproduce Figure 3.4.

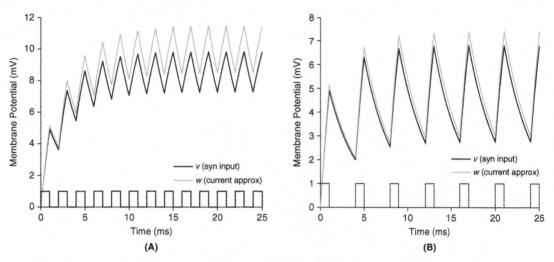

FIGURE 3.4   Response to square wave synaptic input, with amplitude $\bar{g}_{syn} = 0.1$ mS/cm^2 and pulsewidth $s_p = 1$ ms and periods $s_T = 2$ ms at left and $s_T = 4$ ms at right. The square waves are inset and we contrast the true synaptic response, v, and the approximate response, w. In the high frequency case, **A**, the voltage does not have enough time to return to rest before the next input, and hence each input acts on a reduced driving force, and so $v - w$ is much larger in **A** than in **B**. (curvssyn.m)

12. †Please solve the transmitter equation, (2.20), and find

$$R(t) = \frac{\mathcal{T}_0}{\mathcal{T}_0 + K_d} \exp(k_- \min(0, t_2 - t))\{1 - \exp((k_+ \mathcal{T}_0 + k_-)(t_1 - \min(t, t_2)))\} \mathbb{1}_{(t_1, \infty)}(t) \qquad (3.36)$$

where $K_d = k_-/k_+$ is the dissociation constant. As we have stated above, the associated $g_{syn}(t) = G_{syn} R(t)$ is often approximated by an α-function. We accomplish this approximation via lsqcurvefit in MATLAB. In particular, we solve the least-squares problem

$$\min_{\bar{g}_{syn}, \tau_\alpha} \sum_{j=1}^{N_t} |g_{syn}(j dt) - \bar{g}_{syn}(j dt/\tau_\alpha) \exp(1 - j dt/\tau_\alpha)|^2$$

where N_t is the number of time samples. For example, with $\mathcal{T}_0 = 1$ mM, $t_1 = 0$, $t_2 = 4$, $T_{fin} = 20$, $dt = 0.1$ ms, and the AMPA receptor parameters $k_+ = 1.1$ (mM ms)$^{-1}$, $k_- = 0.18$ (ms)$^{-1}$, and $G_{syn} = 100$ mS/cm^2, reproduce Figure 3.5.

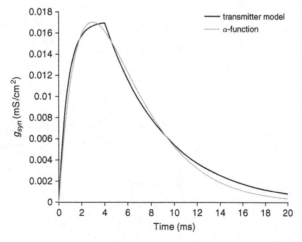

FIGURE 3.5   The best fit of an α-function to the transmitter response, $\bar{g}_{syn} = 0.017$ mS/cm^2 and $\tau_\alpha = 2.943$ ms. (alphafit.m)

The GABA receptor binds so fast that R quickly saturates. To illustrate this, increase k_+ from 1.1 to 5 and run alphafit.m and observe the plateau. Argue that this plateau value is $\mathcal{T}_0/(\mathcal{T}_0 + K_d)$.

The Active Isopotential Cell

OUTLINE

4.1	The Delayed Rectifier Potassium Channel	34		4.4	The Transient Potassium Channel[*]	40
4.2	The Sodium Channel	36		4.5	Summary and Sources	43
4.3	The Hodgkin–Huxley Equations	37		4.6	Exercises	43

The passive model constructed in Chapter 2 provides a fairly accurate prediction of the cell's response to "small" current and/or synaptic input. For inputs of moderate size the passive model, however, fails to capture the characteristic oscillatory overshoot and undershoot, as in Figure 4.1A, while for large inputs it cannot reproduce the cell's characteristic "action potential," see Figure 4.1B.

Following Hodgkin and Huxley, the oscillations and action potential stem from voltage-gated conductances in the cell's plasma membrane that permit the coordinated influx of sodium, Na^+, and the efflux of potassium, K^+. As with chloride, the respective concentration gradients beget associated Nernst potentials, and we are compelled to consider a more complex circuit diagram, Figure 4.2.

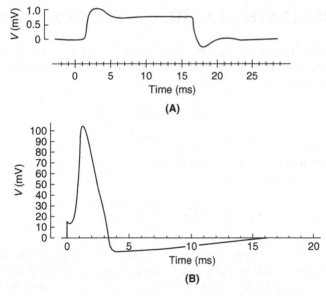

FIGURE 4.1   Voltage response, with respect to rest, of the space-clamped squid giant axon to "moderate" (A) and "large" (B) current stimulus, recorded by Hodgkin and Huxley (1952, Figs. 23 and 13).

Mathematics for Neuroscientists.   DOI: 10.1016/B978-0-12-374882-9.00004-6

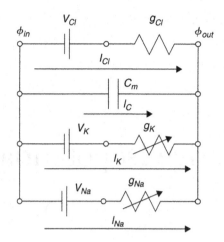

FIGURE 4.2   The equivalent circuit model of the cell's active membrane. We have added two membrane currents to the passive circuit of Figure 2.4. The arrows through the new conductances signify that they are gated by the membrane potential itself.

The Nernst potentials for the two new currents are derived, as in Eq. (2.7), from the respective inner and outer ionic concentrations (in mM),

$$[K^+]_{in} = 400, \quad [K^+]_{out} = 20, \quad [Na^+]_{in} = 50, \quad [Na^+]_{out} = 440. \tag{4.1}$$

These lead, at $T = 27\,°\text{C}$, to

$$V_K = \frac{kT}{ze} \log \frac{[K^+]_{out}}{[K^+]_{in}} \approx -77\,\text{mV} \quad \text{and} \quad V_{Na} = \frac{kT}{ze} \log \frac{[Na^+]_{out}}{[Na^+]_{in}} \approx 56\,\text{mV}. \tag{4.2}$$

Determination of the conductances, g_K and g_{Na}, is considerably more difficult. We take them up in §§4.1 and 4.2 respectively. We integrate these channel models in §4.3 and arrive at the full (space-clamped) system of Hodgkin and Huxley. We then introduce, apply, and study numerical methods for its solution. The channel types expressed in the squid giant axon have now been found to be but two among a vast array of voltage-gated channels. It is remarkable that the formalism developed by Hodgkin and Huxley has survived application to each of these channels. We close this chapter with an application to the transient potassium channel.

4.1 THE DELAYED RECTIFIER POTASSIUM CHANNEL

Hodgkin and Huxley observed that the potassium conductance varied with time and voltage. At a fixed voltage, however, they observed that the conductance grew monotonically in time to a steady level. They therefore postulated a potassium conductance of the form

$$g_K = \bar{g}_K n^p(t; V) \tag{4.3}$$

where $\bar{g}_K$ is the conductance/area of open K^+ channels and $n^p(t; V)$ is the probability that a K^+ channel is open at time t. To say that n approaches a steady (voltage dependent) level, $n_\infty(V(t))$, at the (voltage dependent) rate, $\tau_n(V(t))$, is to ask that

$$n'(t) = \frac{n_\infty(V(t)) - n(t)}{\tau_n(V(t))}. \tag{4.4}$$

Hodgkin and Huxley determined the exponent, $p = 4$, and the functional forms of n_∞ and τ_n via an ingenious combination of theory and experiment. Regarding the latter, they could chemically and electrically rig their (squid giant axon) preparation in such a way that I_K was the only current. This meant doctoring the bath to eliminate other ions, achieving a **space clamp** by inserting a long axial conductor along the axon's interior, and, most importantly, using a **voltage clamp** to simultaneously thwart the capacitive current and so measure the K^+ current over a range of physiological voltages. More precisely, they could hold the membrane at some fixed prestep potential, V_{ps}, and then "activate" the chosen current by stepping to a new holding potential, V_s, and recording the current necessary to maintain this potential. As I_K was the only uninterrupted current their measured current was indeed I_K. If we denote by $\{t_1, t_2, \ldots, t_N\}$ the times at which the current was measured then we can invert Ohm's law and find

$$g_K(t_j; (V_{ps}, V_s)) = I_K(t_j)/(V_s - V_K) \quad j = 1, \ldots, N. \tag{4.5}$$

The simulated voltage clamp and g_K curves presented in Figure 4.13A and B offer, among many other things, an explanation for the adjective "delayed rectifier," as the conductance changes after a delay following a step in potential. In fact, this delay was the main motivation for introducing the exponent p in Eq. (4.3) as Hodgkin and Huxley observed that an exponent $p > 1$ effectively delays the conductance rise.

Next, in order to reconcile the data, Eq. (4.5), with the model, Eq. (4.3), we note that if $V(t) = V_s$ independent of t and $n(0) = n_\infty(V_{ps})$ then Eq. (4.4) implies that

$$n(t; (V_{ps}, V_s)) = n_\infty(V_s) + \exp(-t/\tau_n(V_s))(n_\infty(V_{ps}) - n_\infty(V_s)). \tag{4.6}$$

This led Hodgkin and Huxley to determine $\bar{g}_K$, p, n_∞, and τ_n by minimizing (for fixed p) the sum of the squared differences

$$\sum_{(V_{ps}, V_s)} \sum_{j=1}^{N} |\bar{g}_K(n_\infty(V_s) + \exp(-t_j/\tau_n(V_s))(n_\infty(V_{ps}) - n_\infty(V_s)))^p - g_K(t_j; (V_{ps}, V_s))|^2 \tag{4.7}$$

where the outer sum is over all experimental pairings of V_{ps} and V_s. They then chose the power p that yielded the smallest misfit.

Once the functionals have been determined they are further interpolated by combinations of exponentials. In particular, Hodgkin and Huxley found

$$\bar{g}_K = 36 \text{ mS/cm}^2, \quad \tau_n(V) = \frac{1}{\alpha_n(V) + \beta_n(V)}, \quad \text{and} \quad n_\infty(V) = \alpha_n(V)\tau_n(V) \tag{4.8}$$

where

$$\alpha_n(V) = \frac{0.01(61 + V)}{1 - \exp(-(61 - V)/10)} \quad \text{and} \quad \beta_n(V) = \exp(-(V + 71)/80)/8 \tag{4.9}$$

are illustrated in Figure 4.3.

The expression of n_∞ and τ_n in terms of α_n and β_n permits one to express the gating equation, (4.4), as

$$n'(t) = \alpha_n(V(t))(1 - n(t)) - \beta_n(V(t))n(t). \tag{4.10}$$

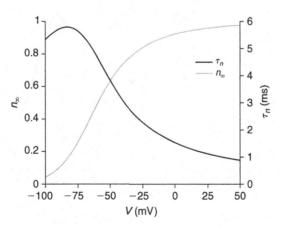

FIGURE 4.3   The gating functions that govern the potassium channel. (hhfuncs.m)

Recalling our work in Chapter 2, in particular Eq. (2.20), we recognize α_n as the rate at which a closed K^+ channel opens and β_n as the rate at which an open K^+ channel closes.

4.2 THE SODIUM CHANNEL

With sodium back in the bath the response is considerably different. Applying the identical voltage clamp procedure, Hodgkin and Huxley discovered that the associated sodium conductance rose quickly and then fell off. They chose to model this via two, independent, voltage-gated processes; m to capture the upstroke or "activation" and h to capture the downstroke or "inactivation." Presuming activation and inactivation to be dependent on voltage and yet independent of one another, the resulting sodium conductance took the form

$$g_{Na} = \bar{g}_{Na} m^{p_m}(t;V) h^{p_h}(t;V) \tag{4.11}$$

where m and h obey, as in Eq. (4.4),

$$m'(t) = \frac{m_\infty(V(t)) - m(t)}{\tau_m(V(t))} \quad \text{and} \quad h'(t) = \frac{h_\infty(V(t)) - h(t)}{\tau_h(V(t))}.$$

As above if the membrane potential is stepped to V_s from a fixed prestep value, V_{ps}, then m and h take the form

$$m(t;(V_{ps},V_s)) = m_\infty(V_s) + \exp(-t/\tau_m(V_s))(m_\infty(V_{ps}) - m_\infty(V_s))$$
$$h(t;(V_{ps},V_s)) = h_\infty(V_s) + \exp(-t/\tau_h(V_s))(h_\infty(V_{ps}) - h_\infty(V_s)).$$

(We will simulate these experiments in Exercise 1 and arrive at Figure 4.13A and C.) For fixed powers, p_m and p_h, we then minimize the full trace

$$\sum_{(V_{ps},V_s)} \sum_{j=1}^{N} |\bar{g}_{Na} m^{p_m}(t;(V_{ps},V_s)) h^{p_h}(t;(V_{ps},V_s)) - g_{Na}(t_j;(V_{ps},V_s))|^2 \tag{4.12}$$

to arrive at the maximal conductance,

$$\bar{g}_{Na} = 120 \text{ mS/cm}^2, \tag{4.13}$$

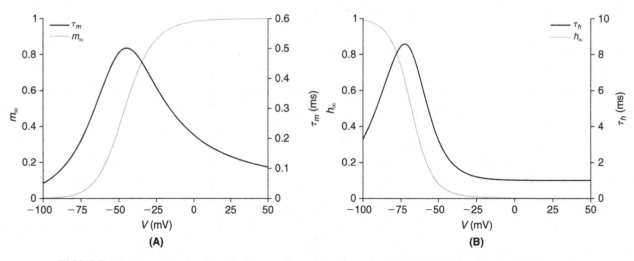

FIGURE 4.4 The gating functions that govern the sodium channel. **A.** Activation. **B.** Inactivation. (hhfuncs.m)

the activation functionals, m_∞ and τ_m, and the inactivation functionals, h_∞ and τ_h. These are illustrated in Figure 4.4 and parametrized in terms of

$$\tau_m(V) = \frac{1}{\alpha_m(V) + \beta_m(V)} \quad \text{and} \quad m_\infty(V) = \alpha_m(V)\tau_m(V)$$

$$\tau_h(V) = \frac{1}{\alpha_h(V) + \beta_h(V)} \quad \text{and} \quad h_\infty(V) = \alpha_h(V)\tau_h(V)$$

where

$$\alpha_m(V) = \frac{0.1(51 + V)}{1 - \exp(-(51 + V)/10)} \quad \text{and} \quad \beta_m(V) = 4\exp(-(V + 71)/18)$$

$$\alpha_h(V) = 0.07\exp(-(V + 71)/20) \quad \text{and} \quad \beta_h(V) = \frac{1}{\exp(-(41 + V)/10) + 1}.$$

(4.14)

4.3 THE HODGKIN–HUXLEY EQUATIONS

Returning to the circuit diagram of Figure 4.2 we apply Kirchhoff's Current Law and arrive at the system of ordinary differential equations

$$C_m V'(t) = -\overline{g}_{Na} m^3 h (V - V_{Na}) - \overline{g}_K n^4 (V - V_K) - g_{Cl}(V - V_{Cl}) + I_{stim}/A$$
$$n'(t) = \alpha_n(V)(1 - n) - \beta_n(V)n$$
$$m'(t) = \alpha_m(V)(1 - m) - \beta_m(V)m$$
$$h'(t) = \alpha_h(V)(1 - h) - \beta_h(V)h$$

(4.15)

and note that, in the absence of stimulus, the membrane sits at a resting potential, V_r. This potential is the value of V for which the steady-state membrane current

$$I_{ss}(V) \equiv \overline{g}_K n_\infty^4(V)(V - V_K) + \overline{g}_{Na} m_\infty^3(V)h_\infty(V)(V - V_{Na}) + g_{Cl}(V - V_{Cl})$$

(4.16)

vanishes. We graph this function in Figure 4.5 and estimate $V_r = -71$ mV. More accurate values may of course be found by solving the nonlinear equation, $I_{ss}(V) = 0$, numerically. We demonstrate below how to use MATLAB's fsolve routine for this task.

Once the rest state is computed we may proceed to solve Eq. (4.15). Recalling the discretization schemes of the previous chapter, we choose a time step, dt, and note that forward Euler would be cheap, not necessarily stable, and

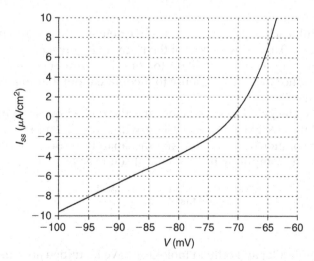

FIGURE 4.5   The steady ionic current of the squid giant axon. (hhfuncs.m)

only accurate to order dt. Backward Euler is stable, but at a great cost, namely we would have to solve a nonlinear system at each advance of dt. The trapezoid rule suffers the same cost but with the advantage of second order accuracy. Fortunately, Hines has discovered a fourth way. By staggering the discretization of the voltage and gating equations he delivers a second order scheme that does not require the solution of any nonlinear equations. In particular, we define

$$V^j \approx V((j-1)dt), \quad n^j \approx n((j-3/2)dt), \quad \text{and} \quad I^j = I((j-3/2)dt) \quad j=1,2,3,\ldots \tag{4.17}$$

and initialize via

$$V^1 = V_r \quad \text{and} \quad n^1 = n_\infty(V_r), \ m^1 = m_\infty(V_r), \ h^1 = h_\infty(V_r).$$

We begin by advancing the gating variables via the trapezoid-like approximation of the n-equation in Eq. (4.15),

$$n^j - n^{j-1} = \alpha_n(V^{j-1})dt - (\alpha_n(V^{j-1}) + \beta_n(V^{j-1}))(n^j + n^{j-1})dt/2.$$

This permits the explicit representation

$$n^j = \frac{(1/dt - (\alpha_n(V^{j-1}) + \beta_n(V^{j-1}))/2)n^{j-1} + \alpha_n(V^{j-1})}{1/dt + (\alpha_n(V^{j-1}) + \beta_n(V^{j-1}))/2} \tag{4.18}$$

or, equivalently

$$n^j = \frac{(2\tau_n(V^{j-1}) - dt)n^{j-1} + 2n_\infty(V^{j-1})dt}{2\tau_n(V^{j-1}) + dt}. \tag{4.19}$$

After updating the remaining gating variables we update the voltage via the half-step backward Euler rule

$$C_m \frac{V^{j-1/2} - V^{j-1}}{dt/2} = -\bar{g}_{Na}(m^j)^3 h^j(V^{j-1/2} - V_{Na}) - \bar{g}_K(n^j)^4(V^{j-1/2} - V_K) - g_{Cl}(V^{j-1/2} - V_{Cl}) + I^j/A. \tag{4.20}$$

This permits the explicit update

$$V^{j-1/2} = \frac{2C_m V^{j-1}/dt + \bar{g}_K(n^j)^4 V_K + \bar{g}_{Na}(m^j)^3 h^j V_{Na} + g_{Cl} V_{Cl} + I^j/A}{2C_m/dt + \bar{g}_K(n^j)^4 + \bar{g}_{Na}(m^j)^3 h^j + g_{Cl}}$$

and finally we advance another half-step via

$$V^j = 2V^{j-1/2} - V^{j-1}. \tag{4.21}$$

We have coded this **staggered Euler scheme** in stEdemo.m. If we deliver a 40 pA current pulse for 2 ms, commencing at $t = 2$ ms, and use a time step $dt = 0.01$ ms, we arrive at the traces in Figure 4.6.

We may discern from the above simulation that 40 pA for 2 ms is sufficient current to elicit an action potential. In Figure 4.7 we use stE.m to reproduce the cell's response to moderate input and to ascertain the precise threshold at which "moderate" becomes "large."

Regarding the accuracy of the staggered Euler scheme, and the related question of how small the time step, dt, must be chosen, we have solved the Hodgkin–Huxley system, with a 40 pA, 2 ms stimulus at $dt = 10^{-k}$ for $k = 1, 2, 3, 4$, and 5. We denote the associated solution by V_k. Absent an exact analytical solution we measure the accuracy of each V_k against our best candidate, V_5, by computing the maximal absolute error

$$E(k) \equiv \max_j \left| V_k^j - V_5^{j \times 10^{5-k}} \right|. \tag{4.22}$$

We plot this error in Figure 4.8.

Since Hodgkin and Huxley, molecular and cellular biologists have identified an incredible variety of voltage-gated ion channels. For example, there are sodium channels that do not inactivate and potassium channels that do.

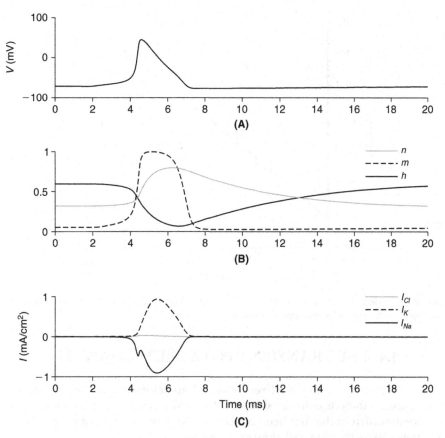

FIGURE 4.6 The action potential (**A**), its gating variables (**B**), and the associated membrane currents (**C**). This computed V agrees quite well with the measured V in Figure 4.1B. Its upstroke is facilitated by m while its downstroke comes thanks to n and h. These variables are fundamental components of the individual ionic currents. stEdemo.m

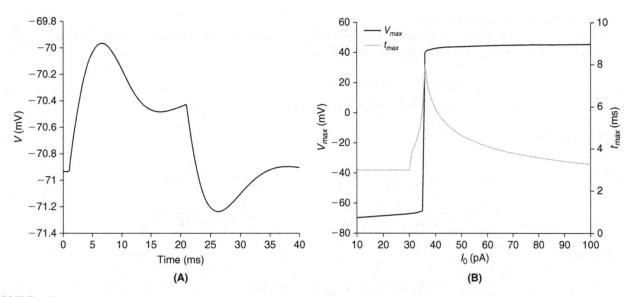

FIGURE 4.7 **A**. The response to a 5 pA, 20 ms current step. This moderate stimulus reproduces the measured oscillatory overshoot and undershoot of Figure 4.1A. (stEdemo2.m) **B**. We fix the current on and off times at 1 and 3 ms and examine the maximum depolarization (black), and the time at which it was achieved (red), as the current amplitude is increased from 10 to 100 pA. The threshold at which the cell fires is approximately 35 pA. At this current the cell however takes 6 ms, after termination of the stimulus, to fire. As the stimulus amplitude is increased, this lag in firing time approaches zero. (stEthresh.m)

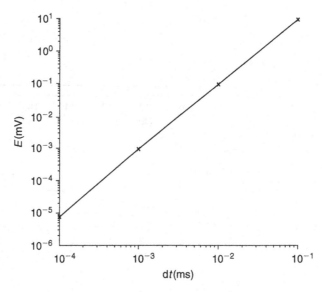

FIGURE 4.8 Illustration of the second order accuracy of the staggered Euler scheme. The error function of Eq. (4.22) decreases by two orders of magnitude when the time step, dt, decreases by one order of magnitude. (stEerr.m)

4.4 THE TRANSIENT POTASSIUM CHANNEL[*]

Channels that activate and then inactivate, at a fixed potential, are referred to as "transient." Even within the family of transient potassium channels there is considerable variation. We here develop a channel model of a transient, or so-called "A-type," potassium current that has been observed in stellate neurons of the cerebellum. We suppose that it has fast (in fact instantaneous) activation and slow inactivation,

$$I_A = \overline{g}_A a_\infty(V) b(V - V_K), \quad \tau_b b' = b_\infty(V) - b, \quad \tau_b = 15 \text{ ms},$$

$$a_\infty(V) = \frac{1}{1 + \exp(-(V + 27)/8.8)}, \quad b_\infty(V) = \frac{1}{1 + \exp((V + 68)/6.6)}. \tag{4.23}$$

We illustrate these functionals in Figure 4.9.

To investigate the shape of the resulting current, and its role in shaping the associated action potential we adopt sodium and delayed rectifier potassium currents of the form

$$I_{Na} = \overline{g}_{Na} m_\infty(V) h(V - V_{Na}), \quad \tau_h(V) h' = h_\infty(V) - h$$

$$I_K = \overline{g}_K n(V - V_K), \quad \tau_n n' = n_\infty(V) - n \tag{4.24}$$

with gating functionals

$$m_\infty(V) = \frac{1}{1 + \exp(-(V + 35)/4)}, \quad n_\infty(V) = m_\infty(V), \quad \tau_n = 0.5,$$

$$h_\infty(V) = \frac{1}{1 + \exp((V + 35)/4)}, \quad \tau_h(V) = \frac{12992}{4\pi(V + 74)^2 + 784} - 0.15, \tag{4.25}$$

and parameters,

$$\overline{g}_{Na} = 30, \overline{g}_K = 7, g_{Cl} = 1, \overline{g}_A = 16 \text{ mS/cm}^2$$

$$V_{Na} = 45, V_K = -90, V_{Cl} = -70 \text{ mV}, \quad C_m = 1.5 \text{ } \mu\text{F/cm}^2. \tag{4.26}$$

Regarding the solution of the system of ordinary differential equations for V, h, n, and b, we advance the gating variables exactly as in Eq. (4.18) but note that the voltage equation offers more difficulty here. In particular, instantaneous

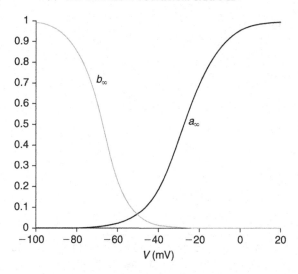

FIGURE 4.9   Activation, a_∞, and inactivation, b_∞, functionals for the A-type potassium channel, Eq. (4.23). (moliA.m)

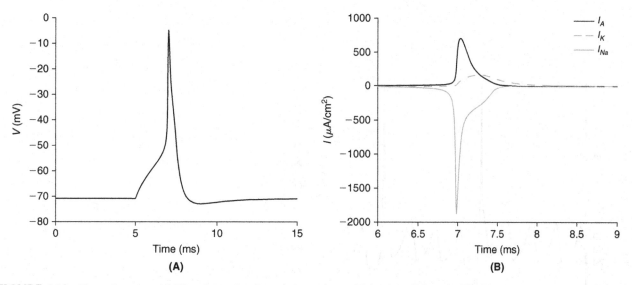

FIGURE 4.10   The action potential (**A**) and associated membrane currents (**B**) for the cell described by Eqs. (4.23)–(4.26). (stmolidemo.m)

activation introduces explicit nonlinearities into the voltage equation. In order to avoid having to solve a nonlinear equation, at each increment of dt, we replace the implicit rule, Eq. (4.20), with the mixed rule

$$C_m \frac{V^j - V^{j-1}}{dt} = -\overline{g}_{Na} m_\infty(V^{j-1}) h^j (V^j - V_{Na}) - \overline{g}_K n^j (V^j - V_K)$$
$$- \overline{g}_A a_\infty(V^{j-1}) b^j (V^j - V_{Na}) - g_{Cl}(V^j - V_{Cl}) + I^j/A, \tag{4.27}$$

and so arrive at

$$V^j = \frac{C_m V^{j-1}/dt + \overline{g}_{Na} m_\infty(V^{j-1}) h^j V_{Na} + \overline{g}_K n^j V_K + \overline{g}_A a_\infty(V^{j-1}) b^j V_{Na} + g_{Cl} V_{Cl} + I^j/A}{C_m/dt + \overline{g}_{Na} m_\infty(V^{j-1}) h^j + \overline{g}_K n^j + \overline{g}_A a_\infty(V^{j-1}) b^j + g_{Cl}}.$$

We have coded this **hybrid Euler scheme** in stmolidemo.m and illustrated its results in Figure 4.10 with a 300 pA, 2 ms, current injection, with d$t = 0.01$ ms.

As may be expected from the use of a mixed update rule, application of this hybrid scheme results in a loss of second order accuracy, see Figure 4.11.

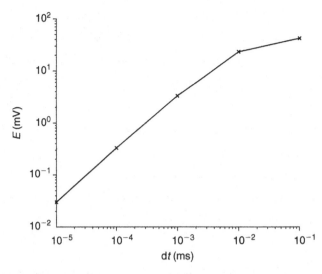

FIGURE 4.11　An illustration of the first order accuracy of the hybrid Euler scheme Eq. (4.27). The error, E, is computed as per Eq. (4.22). (stmolierr.m)

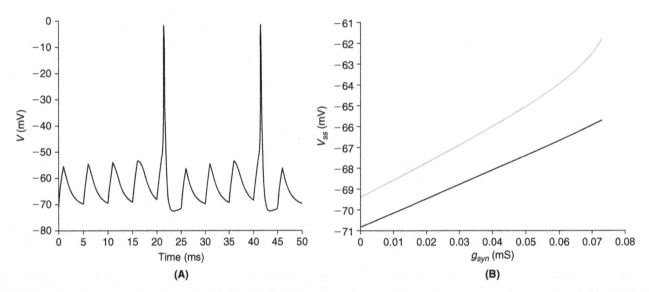

FIGURE 4.12　Response of the cell described by Eqs. (4.23)–(4.26) to synaptic input. **A.** Dynamic response to square wave g_{syn} of amplitude 0.5 mS/cm^2, period 5 ms, and $V_{syn} = 0$. Although an individual pulse is subthreshold, when they arrive at the "right" frequency they eventually fire the cell. (stmolisyn.m) **B.** Steady-state membrane potential response as a function of steady synaptic conductance, with $V_{syn} = 0$, and with (black) and without (red) the A-current. This demonstrates that I_A has a linearizing effect on the cell's membrane potential. Figure 2.10A. (molisynss.m)

If we wish to drive the cell with synaptic input rather than current injection then the I_j/A term in Eq. (4.27) is simply replaced with $-g_{syn}^j(V^j - V_{syn})$. We investigate, in Figure 4.12, the associated response when g_{syn} is the periodic pulse of Eq. (3.35), as well as when g_{syn} is simply constant. For the latter case we return to Exercise 2.3, and ask for the associated steady-state potential, i.e., the solution to

$$(V_{ss} - V_{Cl}) + c_{Na}m_\infty(V_{ss})h_\infty(V_{ss})(V_{ss} - V_{Na})$$
$$+ \{c_A a_\infty(V_{ss})b_\infty(V_{ss}) + c_K n_\infty(V_{ss})\}(V_{ss} - V_K) + c_{syn}(V_{ss} - V_{syn}) = 0 \tag{4.28}$$

where each of the conductances c_{Na}, c_A, c_K, and c_{syn} has been scaled by g_{Cl} so that, in particular, $c_{syn} = g_{syn}/g_{Cl}$.

4.5 SUMMARY AND SOURCES

We have constructed phenomenological models of a sodium channel and two potassium channels. These models permit us to predict the conductance of the channel as a function of the cell's transmembrane potential difference. We combined these channel models in a well-defined system of four (or more) ordinary differential equation, and derived and tested a numerical approximation method that permitted us to discern the threshold, in both amplitude and frequency, at which current injection yielded an action potential. Figure 4.1, as well as most of the first three sections, is drawn from the fundamental work of Hodgkin and Huxley (1952), who were awarded the 1963 Nobel Prize in Medicine. The preparation of a squid giant axon and actual recordings are presented in videos available at www.iac-usnc.org/Methods. This web site contains videos of several other classical electrophysiological preparations. Hille (2001) synthesizes this material, addresses the value of model building, and considers challenges to a number of the assumptions in Hodgkin and Huxley (1952), notably that of independence of the sodium gating variables, m and h. Willms et al. (1999) extend and improve the fitting of voltage clamp data. The lovely staggered Euler scheme of §4.3 is due to Hines (1984). The model of §4.4 with the A-type potassium channel is adapted from Molineux et al. (2005). Exercise 6 is from Fitzhugh (1955). This exercise is a gateway into the very rich world of phase plane analysis of neural models, see, e.g., Izhikevich (2007).

4.6 EXERCISES

1. Let us attempt to simulate the voltage clamp experiments of Hodgkin and Huxley. More precisely, suppose

$$V(t) = \mathbb{1}_{(2,15)}(t)V_c,$$

where V_c is the desired clamp potential, and modify stEdemo.m to solve for the associated gating variables and plot, as in Figure 4.13, V and

$$g_K(t) = \overline{g}_K n^4(t) \quad \text{and} \quad g_{Na}(t) = \overline{g}_{Na} m^3(t)h(t)$$

for a range of clamp potentials.

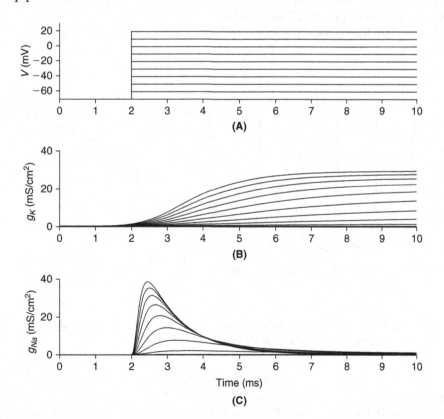

FIGURE 4.13 Simulated voltage clamp experiments of Hodgkin and Huxley. **A.** Command potential. **B.** Potassium conductance. **C.** Sodium conductance. (clamp.m)

2. The next two exercises will help us understand the rate at which our cell may fire. To begin, modify stE.m to deliver 60 pA, 2 ms current pulses at $t_1 = 1$ ms and a variable t_2. Experiment with several values of t_2 and reproduce Figure 4.14.

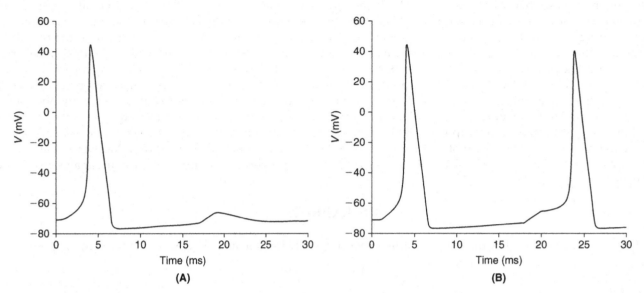

FIGURE 4.14 Illustration of the refractory period observed in the Hodgkin–Huxley model. In **A** the second stimulus is delivered at $t_2 = 17$ ms and produces a slight depolarization. In **B** the second stimulus is delivered at $t_2 = 18$ ms and produces a full action potential. This period, of roughly 17 ms, in which the cell does not spike when subjected to suprathreshold stimulus, is known as the refractory period. (stErefracdrive.m)

3. We notice that for sustained current input our cell enters a regime of periodic firing. For example, if $I_{stim}(t) = 100\mathbb{1}_{(2,\infty)}(t)$ pA we observe the response in Figure 4.15A.

    Modify stE.m to calculate the interspike interval and reproduce the "f/I" curve in Figure 4.15B.

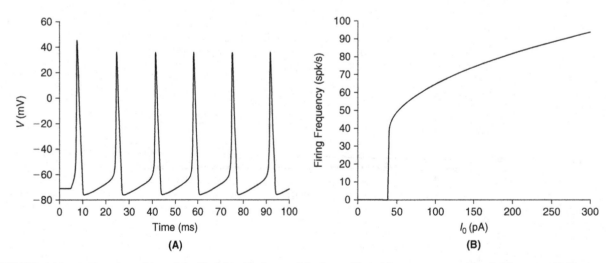

FIGURE 4.15 **A.** Periodic spiking of the Hodgkin–Huxley model when subjected to constant suprathreshold current. **B.** The number of spikes per second as a function of (constant) stimulus amplitude. (stEfreq.m)

4. The f/I curve of the previous exercise exhibits clear thresholds in both amplitude and frequency. We will demonstrate here that addition of the A-current removes the frequency threshold. In particular, show that the cell of §4.4 can fire at arbitrarily low frequencies by modifying stmolidemo.m, in the manner of the previous exercise, and reproduce Figure 4.16.

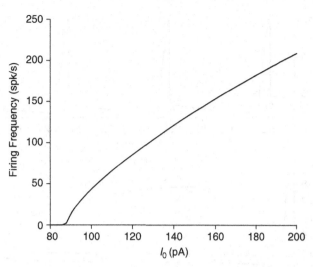

FIGURE 4.16 The number of spikes per second as a function of (constant) stimulus amplitude for the cell of §4.4 with the A-type potassium current. (molifreq.m)

5. One may excite a cell without impaling it, by instead upsetting the balance of extracellular ions. Modify stE.m to deliver a pulse of extracellular potassium ions, of concentration K_{stim}, in the time interval $[t_1, t_2]$, and so reproduce Figure 4.17. This stimulus resets the reversal potential, via (recall Eq. (4.2))

$$[K^+]_{out}(t) = 20 + K_{stim}\mathbb{1}_{(t_1,t_2)}(t), \quad E_K = 25.8\log([K^+]_{out}/400),$$

where $[K^+]_{out} = 20$ and $[K^+]_{in} = 400$ mM are drawn from Eq. (4.1).

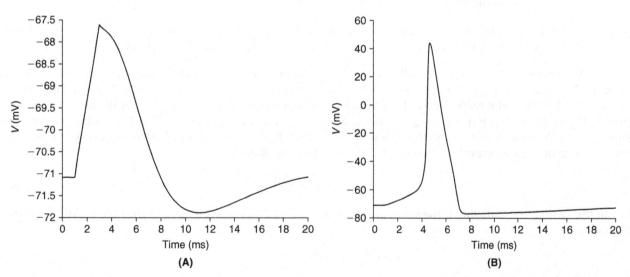

FIGURE 4.17 Depolarization of the Hodgkin–Huxley model by a 2 ms pulse of extracellular potassium ions. A. $K_{stim} = 5$ mM is subthreshold. B. $K_{stim} = 10$ mM elicits a spike. (stEKstimdrive.m)

6. Returning to Figure 4.6 we pursue a pair of simple observations. First, m, the gating variable of sodium activation is so fast that perhaps we can simply presume that it instantaneously reaches its steady-state level, $m_\infty(V(t))$. That is

$$m(t) \approx m_\infty(V(t)).$$

Second, we observe that $n + h$ is fairly flat. In, particular.

$$h(t) \approx 0.87 - n(t). \tag{4.29}$$

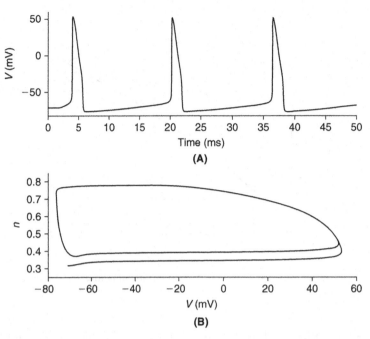

FIGURE 4.18   Response of the FitzHugh model, Eq. (4.30). **A.** Membrane potential as a function of time. **B.** Phase diagram of n and V. (stE2d.m)

With these approximations, the Hodgkin–Huxley system Eq. (4.15) reduces to

$$C_m V'(t) = -\bar{g}_{Na} m_\infty^3(V)(0.87 - n)(V - V_{Na}) - \bar{g}_K n^4(V - V_K) - g_{Cl}(V - V_{Cl}) + I_{stim}/A$$
$$n'(t) = \alpha_n(V)(1 - n) - \beta_n(V)n. \tag{4.30}$$

Modify stE.m to solve this two-variable reduced system and graph its response to $I_{stim} = 50\,\mathbb{1}_{(2,\infty)}(t)$ pA in the "phase plane" as in Figure 4.18. This reduced model is sometimes called the FitzHugh model.

7. One great feature of planar systems, like that of the previous exercise, is that the equations, when interpreted graphically, dictate how the solution must behave. The principal objects are the two nullclines. These are the curves on which V and n respectively, do not change. With reference to Eq. (4.30), the n nullcline is simply those points, (V, n), for which $n'(t) = 0$, i.e., it is the graph of n_∞, namely $(V, n_\infty(V))$. The V nullcline is a bit more complicated. We recognize it as a quartic in n with coefficients that depend on V. We arrive at a very simple quartic if we replace our initial approximation, Eq. (4.29), with the arguably better

$$h(t) = 0.7 - n^2(t). \tag{4.31}$$

For in this case, the V nullcline is the set of points $(V, n_1(V, I_{stim}))$ where $n_1(V, I_{stim})$ is the lone positive root of the biquadratic

$$a(V)n^4 + b(V)n^2 + c(V) + I_{stim}/A, \tag{4.32}$$

for constant I_{stim}.

i. Please write out $a(V)$, $b(V)$, and $c(V)$ and argue that Eq. (4.32) indeed has only one root

$$n_1(V, I_{stim}) = \sqrt{\frac{-b(V) - \sqrt{b^2(V) - 4a(V)(c(V) + I_{stim}/A)}}{2a(V)}} \tag{4.33}$$

for each V for which $V_K < V < V_{Na}$.

ii. Graph, as in Figure 4.19A the n nullcline and V nullcline for $I_{stim} = 0$, 10, and 20 pA. Argue that these curves constrain the resulting dynamics by explaining why the solution, $(V(t), n(t))$ can only cross the n nullcline when moving horizontally and that it can only cross the V nullcline when moving vertically.

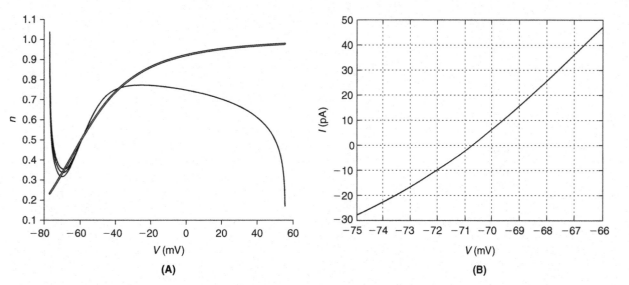

FIGURE 4.19 **A.** The n nullcline (red) and V nullclines (black) for $I_{stim} = 0$, 10, and 20 pA. The three V nullclines coincide outside of the interval $-75 < V < -55$ mV. In this interval, increasing I_{stim} serves to "lift" the V nullcline and so produce more depolarized rest states. **B.** The $I - V$ rest curve associated with Eq. (4.34). (fhpp.m)

iii. Next argue that the system is at rest only where its two nullclines cross. Argue that this occurs when V and I_{stim} satisfy

$$I_{stim} = -A(a(V)n_\infty^4(V) + b(V)n_\infty^2(V) + c(V)),$$ (4.34)

and graph this as in Figure 4.19B.

iv. Now address, as in Figure 4.20, the stability of a pair of rest states by incrementing I_{stim} by 1 pA at the 2 ms mark.

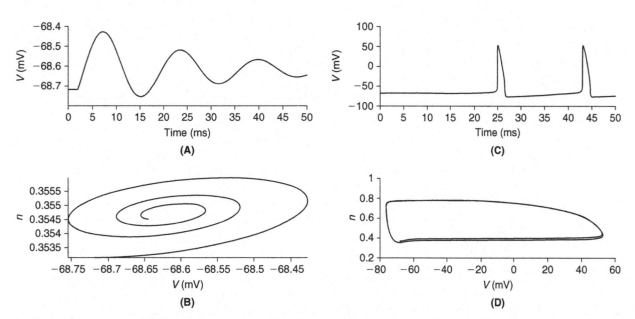

FIGURE 4.20 Voltage traces and phase planes of the modified FitzHugh system for $I_{stim} = 20 + 1_{(2,\infty)}(t)$ pA (**A, B**) and $I_{stim} = 30 + 1_{(2,\infty)}(t)$ pA (**C, D**). In the former case the incremental current brought us to a nearby rest state, while in the latter the same increment produced a large excursion and eventual periodic spiking. The mathematics developed in the next chapter will permit us to take a closer look at this threshold. (fhpp.m)

5

The Quasi-Active Isopotential Cell

OUTLINE

5.1	The Quasi-Active Model	49	5.5	A Nonspecific Cation Current that is Activated by Hyperpolarization*	59
5.2	Numerical Methods	51			
5.3	Exact Solution via Eigenvector Expansion	54	5.6	Summary and Sources	60
5.4	A Persistent Sodium Current*	58	5.7	Exercises	61

The passive model is a severe reduction of the active cell. In this chapter we establish a middle ground by linearizing the full Hodgkin–Huxley system, Eq. (4.15), about its rest state. This will help both determine the stability of the rest state and to predict the response to subthreshold stimuli. In addition, the resulting four-dimensional linear system of ordinary differential equations is amenable to careful mathematical and computational analysis. In particular, we introduce and compute determinants, eigenvalues, eigenvectors, the matrix exponential, and the LU factorization and apply these methods to two new channels, responsible for the persistent sodium current, I_{NaP}, and the hyperpolarization activated nonspecific cation current, I_h.

5.1 THE QUASI-ACTIVE MODEL

The full set of Hodgkin–Huxley equations, Eq. (4.15), is often said to model the "active" or "excitable" cell. With regard to this active system we suppose that ε is small and that our current stimulus is $I_{stim} = \varepsilon \tilde{I}(t)$. We note that at rest, $V = V_r$ where $I_{ss}(V_r) = 0$ (recall Eq. (4.16)), and

$$m(0) = m_\infty(V_r) \equiv \overline{m}, \quad h(0) = h_\infty(V_r) \equiv \overline{h}, \quad \text{and} \quad n(0) = n_\infty(V_r) \equiv \overline{n}.$$

In response to I_{stim} it seems natural to assume that

$$
\begin{aligned}
V(t) &= V_r + \varepsilon \tilde{V}(t) + O(\varepsilon^2) \\
m(t) &= \overline{m} + \varepsilon \tilde{m}(t) + O(\varepsilon^2) \\
h(t) &= \overline{h} + \varepsilon \tilde{h}(t) + O(\varepsilon^2) \\
n(t) &= \overline{n} + \varepsilon \tilde{n}(t) + O(\varepsilon^2)
\end{aligned}
\tag{5.1}
$$

and to attempt to solve for the unknown "first order" or "quasi-active" variables, $\tilde{V}, \tilde{m}, \tilde{h},$ and $\tilde{n}$. Here $O(\varepsilon^2)$ signifies terms of size ε^2. On substituting Eq. (5.1) into the Hodgkin–Huxley equations, (4.15), and identifying terms of order ε we will arrive at a consistent **linear** system of ordinary differential equations for the quasi-active variables. In particular, we note that each gating equation takes the form

$$\tau_m(V_r + \varepsilon \tilde{V} + O(\varepsilon^2)) \frac{d}{dt}(\overline{m} + \varepsilon \tilde{m} + O(\varepsilon^2)) = m_\infty(V_r + \varepsilon \tilde{V} + O(\varepsilon^2)) - (\overline{m} + \varepsilon \tilde{m} + O(\varepsilon^2)).$$

Mathematics for Neuroscientists. DOI: 10.1016/B978-0-12-374882-9.00005-8

Applying the time derivative on the left and developing τ_m and m_∞ in Taylor series about V_r we find

$$\left(\tau_m(V_r) + \varepsilon \frac{d\tau_m}{dV}(V_r)\tilde{V}\right)\varepsilon\frac{d\tilde{m}}{dt} = \left(m_\infty(V_r) + \varepsilon\frac{dm_\infty}{dV}(V_r)\tilde{V}\right) - (\overline{m} + \varepsilon\tilde{m}) + O(\varepsilon^2).$$

Identifying terms of order ε then yields

$$\tau_m(V_r)\frac{d\tilde{m}}{dt}(t) = \frac{dm_\infty}{dV}(V_r)\tilde{V}(t) - \tilde{m}(t).$$

Equations with identical structure govern the evolution of $\tilde{n}$ and $\tilde{h}$. Regarding current balance, we note that the potassium contribution is

$$n^4(V - V_K) = (\overline{n} + \varepsilon\tilde{n} + O(\varepsilon^2))^4(V_r + \varepsilon\tilde{V} + O(\varepsilon^2) - V_K)$$
$$= \overline{n}^4(V_r - V_K) + \{\overline{n}^4\tilde{V} + 4\overline{n}^3\tilde{n}(V_r - V_K)\}\varepsilon + O(\varepsilon^2),$$

while the sodium term contributes

$$m^3h(V - V_{Na}) = (\overline{m} + \varepsilon\tilde{m} + O(\varepsilon^2))^3(\overline{h} + \varepsilon\tilde{h} + O(\varepsilon^2))(V_r + \varepsilon\tilde{V} + O(\varepsilon^2) - V_{Na})$$
$$= \overline{m}^3\overline{h}(V_r - V_{Na}) + \{\overline{m}^3\overline{h}\tilde{V} + (3\overline{m}^2\overline{h}\tilde{m} + \overline{m}^3\tilde{h})(V_r - V_{Na})\}\varepsilon + O(\varepsilon^2).$$

Combining these forms we arrive at the so-called quasi-active model

$$C_m\tilde{V}' = -\overline{g}_{Na}\{\overline{m}^3\overline{h}\tilde{V} + (3\tilde{m}\overline{m}^2\overline{h} + \overline{m}^3\tilde{h})v_{Na}\} - \overline{g}_K\{\overline{n}^4\tilde{V} + 4\tilde{n}\overline{n}^3v_K\} - g_{Cl}\tilde{V} + \tilde{I}/A$$

$$\tilde{m}' = \frac{(dm_\infty(V_r)/dV)\tilde{V} - \tilde{m}}{\tau_m(V_r)}$$

$$\tilde{h}' = \frac{(dh_\infty(V_r)/dV)\tilde{V} - \tilde{h}}{\tau_h(V_r)} \qquad\qquad (5.2)$$

$$\tilde{n}' = \frac{(dn_\infty(V_r)/dV)\tilde{V} - \tilde{n}}{\tau_n(V_r)}$$

where

$$v_{Na} \equiv V_r - V_{Na} \quad\text{and}\quad v_K \equiv V_r - V_K.$$

Although simpler than the full Hodgkin–Huxley system, Eq. (4.15), the behavior of this system is not immediately apparent. To begin, we express Eq. (5.2) as the linear system

$$\boxed{\mathbf{y}'(t) = \mathbf{B}\mathbf{y}(t) + \mathbf{f}(t), \quad\text{where}\quad \mathbf{y} = (\tilde{m}\ \tilde{h}\ \tilde{n}\ \tilde{V})^T} \qquad\qquad (5.3)$$

where $\mathbf{f} = (0\ 0\ 0\ \tilde{I}/A)^T$, and $\mathbf{B}$ is the matrix

$$\mathbf{B} = \begin{pmatrix} -1/\overline{\tau}_m & 0 & 0 & \overline{m}'_\infty/\overline{\tau}_m \\ 0 & -1/\overline{\tau}_h & 0 & \overline{h}'_\infty/\overline{\tau}_h \\ 0 & 0 & -1/\overline{\tau}_n & \overline{n}'_\infty/\overline{\tau}_n \\ -3\overline{m}^2\overline{h}v_{Na}/\tau_{Na} & -\overline{m}^3 v_{Na}/\tau_{Na} & -4\overline{n}^3 v_K/\tau_K & -\overline{m}^3\overline{h}/\tau_{Na} - \overline{n}^4/\tau_K - 1/\tau_{Cl} \end{pmatrix} \qquad (5.4)$$

with

$$\overline{m}'_\infty \equiv dm_\infty(V_r)/dV, \quad \overline{\tau}_m \equiv \tau_m(V_r), \quad \tau_{Na} = C_m/\overline{g}_{Na}, \quad \tau_K = C_m/\overline{g}_K, \quad \text{and} \quad \tau_{Cl} = C_m/g_{Cl}.$$

Given expressions for m_∞, n_∞, and h_∞ we invoke the symbolic toolbox in MATLAB to compute the requisite derivatives in Eq. (5.4). We implement this in `hhsym.m` and, using the functions and parameters of §4.3, arrive at

$$\mathbf{B} = \begin{pmatrix} -4.2097 & 0 & 0 & 0.0265 \\ 0 & -0.1175 & 0 & -0.0041 \\ 0 & 0 & -0.1833 & 0.0028 \\ 77.2344 & 2.3133 & -28.2822 & -0.6822 \end{pmatrix}. \tag{5.5}$$

If, rather than direct current injection, we instead wish to consider subthreshold synaptic input over a steady background conductance, i.e.,

$$g_{syn}(t) = g_{ss} + \varepsilon \tilde{g}_{syn}(t)$$

then we must develop

$$I_{syn}(t) = g_{syn}(t)(V(t) - V_{syn}) = (g_{ss} + \varepsilon \tilde{g}_{syn}(t))(V_r + \varepsilon \tilde{V}) = g_{ss}(V_r - V_{syn}) + \varepsilon(g_{ss}\tilde{V} + \tilde{g}_{syn}(V_r - V_{syn})) + O(\varepsilon^2).$$

This then subtracts an additional g_{ss}/C_m from B_{44} in Eq. (5.4) and causes $\mathbf{f}$ to take the form

$$\mathbf{f}(t) = (0 \ 0 \ 0 \ \tilde{g}_{syn}(t)(V_r - V_{syn}))^T. \tag{5.6}$$

We now consider the two standard means by which Eq. (5.3) is solved.

5.2 NUMERICAL METHODS

With $\mathbf{B}$ in hand, we set $\mathbf{f}^j = \mathbf{f}((j-1)dt)$ and construct a marching scheme for $\mathbf{y}^j \approx \mathbf{y}((j-1)dt)$. We note, in particular, that $\mathbf{y}^1 = \mathbf{y}(0) = 0$ as $\mathbf{y}$ measures perturbation from rest. The trapezoid scheme applied to Eq. (5.3) requires

$$\mathbf{y}^j - \mathbf{y}^{j-1} = \mathbf{B}(\mathbf{y}^j + \mathbf{y}^{j-1})dt/2 + (\mathbf{f}^j + \mathbf{f}^{j-1})dt/2$$

and so yields the update procedure

$$\boxed{((2/dt)\mathbf{I} - \mathbf{B})\mathbf{y}^j = ((2/dt)\mathbf{I} + \mathbf{B})\mathbf{y}^{j-1} + \mathbf{f}^j + \mathbf{f}^{j-1}} \tag{5.7}$$

where $\mathbf{I}$ is the 4-by-4 identity matrix (ones on the diagonal, zeros elsewhere). Eq. (5.7) requires us to solve four simultaneous linear equations at each step. We pause to develop the standard approach to the solution of such systems.

Gaussian Elimination is a simple procedure for decoupling simultaneous linear equations. It succeeds by replacing rows with linear combinations of rows. For example, taking up the $\mathbf{B}$ of Eq. (5.5), if $dt = 0.1$ then

$$\mathbf{A} \equiv (2/dt)\mathbf{I} - \mathbf{B} = \begin{pmatrix} 24.2097 & 0 & 0 & -0.0265 \\ 0 & 20.1175 & 0 & 0.0041 \\ 0 & 0 & 20.1833 & -0.0028 \\ -77.2344 & -2.3133 & 28.2822 & 20.6822 \end{pmatrix}$$

and we may view Eq. (5.7) as an instance of $\mathbf{A}\mathbf{y} = \mathbf{b}$. The elimination procedure of Gauss is best viewed as sequential transformation by very simple "row mixers." For example, the matrix that multiplies row 1 by $a \equiv -A_{41}/A_{11}$ and then adds that to row 4 is

$$\mathbf{E}_1 \equiv \begin{pmatrix} 1 & 0 & 0 & 0 \\ 0 & 1 & 0 & 0 \\ 0 & 0 & 1 & 0 \\ a & 0 & 0 & 1 \end{pmatrix}.$$

On applying it to both sides of $\mathbf{A}\mathbf{y} = \mathbf{b}$ we find $\mathbf{E}_1\mathbf{A}\mathbf{y} = \mathbf{E}_1\mathbf{b}$ where

$$\mathbf{E}_1\mathbf{A} = \begin{pmatrix} 24.2097 & 0 & 0 & -0.0265 \\ 0 & 20.1175 & 0 & 0.0041 \\ 0 & 0 & 20.1833 & -0.0028 \\ 0 & -2.3133 & 28.2822 & 20.5978 \end{pmatrix}$$

indeed has eliminated one of $\mathbf{A}$'s nonzeros. If we continue in this vein to eliminate the remaining two nonzeros below the diagonal, via $\mathbf{E}_2$ and $\mathbf{E}_3$, then we arrive at the "upper triangular" matrix

$$\mathbf{U} = \mathbf{E}_3\mathbf{E}_2\mathbf{E}_1\mathbf{A} = \begin{pmatrix} 24.2097 & 0 & 0 & -0.0265 \\ 0 & 20.1175 & 0 & 0.0041 \\ 0 & 0 & 20.1833 & -0.0028 \\ 0 & 0 & 0 & 20.6022 \end{pmatrix}. \tag{5.8}$$

In general, it is possible that elimination in columns 1 through j may inadvertently eliminate the diagonal element of the subsequent column. In this case we exchange row $j+1$ with a later row that possesses a nonzero in its $(j+1)$st column. For example, if

$$\mathbf{B} = \begin{pmatrix} 2 & 2 & 2 \\ 1 & 4 & 0 \\ 0 & 5 & 3 \end{pmatrix}$$

then elimination in column one brings

$$\mathbf{E}_1\mathbf{B} = \begin{pmatrix} 2 & 2 & 2 \\ 0 & 0 & -4 \\ 0 & 5 & 3 \end{pmatrix}.$$

Rather than eliminating the 5 in column 2 we simply exchange rows 2 and 3 and find

$$\mathbf{U} = \mathbf{P}_2\mathbf{E}_1\mathbf{B} = \begin{pmatrix} 2 & 2 & 2 \\ 0 & 5 & 3 \\ 0 & 0 & -4 \end{pmatrix} \quad \text{where} \quad \mathbf{P}_2 = \begin{pmatrix} 1 & 0 & 0 \\ 0 & 0 & 1 \\ 0 & 1 & 0 \end{pmatrix} \tag{5.9}$$

is the elementary permutation matrix obtained by exchanging the corresponding rows of the identity matrix.

The diagonal elements of $\mathbf{U}$ are referred to as the **pivots** of $\mathbf{A}$. If each of these pivots is nonzero then we say that $\mathbf{A}$ is **invertible** and note that we may solve $\mathbf{U}\mathbf{y} = \mathbf{E}_3\mathbf{E}_2\mathbf{E}_1\mathbf{b}$ by elementary back substitution. For this latter system is "uncoupled" in the sense that the last equation has but one unknown and solving for it leaves the previous equation with but one unknown, and so on. MATLAB accomplishes this reduction to $\mathbf{U}$ and subsequent back substitution with its "backslash" command, i.e., the solution, $\mathbf{y}$, to $\mathbf{A}\mathbf{y} = \mathbf{b}$ is computed via $\mathbf{y} = \mathbf{A}\backslash\mathbf{b}$. This is algebraically equivalent to $\mathbf{y} = \mathbf{A}^{-1}\mathbf{b}$ where $\mathbf{A}^{-1}$ is the inverse of $\mathbf{A}$. The inverse however is typically expensive to compute and rarely worth the effort, though see Exercises 2–3 for nice examples and a general approach.

We have invoked the MATLAB backslash in our implementation of Eq. (5.7), and illustrate our findings in Figure 5.1 for current injections of increasing magnitude.

We quantify the quasi-active model's ability to capture the frequency response of the active cell by contrasting, in Figure 5.2, the active and quasi-active responses to

$$I_{stim}(t) = I_0 \sin(2\pi\omega t) \tag{5.10}$$

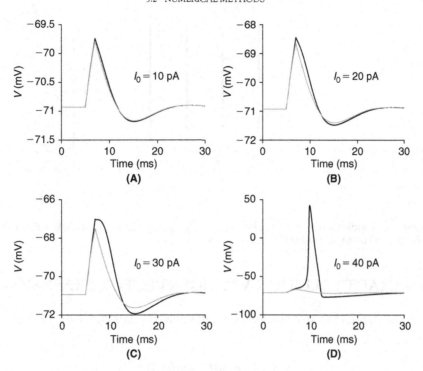

FIGURE 5.1 The full (black) and quasi-active (red) response to step current injection at four different levels (**A–D**). On recalling Figure 4.1 we see that the quasi-active model accurately reproduces the oscillatory components in the response to small to moderate stimulus. (stEqa.m)

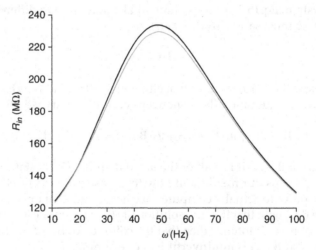

FIGURE 5.2 Input resistance, Eq. (5.11), as a function of frequency, given the stimuli Eq. (5.10) with $I_0 = 1$ pA, for the full (black) and quasi-active (red) models. We see that the low-pass nature of the passive cell, as depicted in Figure 3.1A, has shifted to a band-pass filter with resonant peak near 45 Hz. (stEqafreq.m)

over a wide range of ω values. We quantify the active response in terms of the input resistance

$$R_{in} \equiv \frac{1}{I_0} \max_{t > T} |V(t) - V_r| \tag{5.11}$$

where T is chosen to suppress the transient term. For the quasi-active response we simply replace $V(t) - V_r$ with $\tilde{V}$.

We see that the quasi-active model does an excellent job of capturing the band-pass feature of the active cell. To further illustrate this we next contrast, in Figure 5.3, the active response to input trains at three distinct frequencies.

The resonance exhibited in Figure 5.3 is reminiscent of that seen in Figure 4.12. Although these are active phenomena, the quasi-active model properly identifies the resonant frequency. To better appreciate this feature of the quasi-active approach we now turn to exact methods.

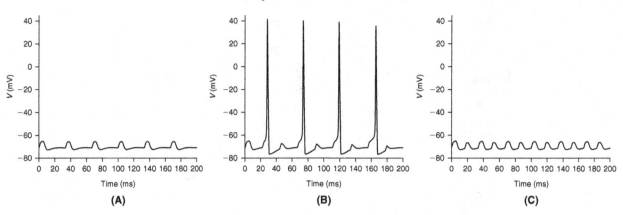

FIGURE 5.3   Active response to periodic train of current pulses, $I_{stim}(t) = I_0 \mathbf{1}_{(0,w)}(\mathrm{mod}(t, 1/f))$, where $I_0 = 35$ pA, the pulsewidth is $w = 2$ ms, and the frequency is $f = 30$ Hz (**A**), 45 Hz (**B**), and 60 Hz (**C**). (stEperdrive.m)

5.3 EXACT SOLUTION VIA EIGENVECTOR EXPANSION

Recalling the exact solution, Eq. (3.2), to a single linear differential equation, we may ask if

$$\mathbf{y}(t) = \int_0^t \exp((t-s)z)\mathbf{f}(s)\,\mathrm{d}s \tag{5.12}$$

solves, for some scalar z, our system, Eq. (5.3), of four differential equations. On differentiating each side of Eq. (5.12) we find $\mathbf{y}'(t) = \mathbf{f}(t) + z\mathbf{y}(t)$ and so z must satisfy $\mathbf{B}\mathbf{y}(t) = z\mathbf{y}(t)$, or

$$(\mathbf{B} - z\mathbf{I})\mathbf{y}(t) = 0, \tag{5.13}$$

where $\mathbf{I}$ is the identity matrix. Now Eq. (5.13) requires that either $\mathbf{y}(t) = 0$ or that $\mathbf{B} - z\mathbf{I}$ annihilates a nonzero vector. As the former is not the case then $\mathbf{B} - z\mathbf{I}$ must annihilate a nonzero vector. In that case, $(\mathbf{B} - z\mathbf{I})\mathbf{y} = 0$ is often expressed as

$$y_1(\mathbf{B} - z\mathbf{I})_1 + y_2(\mathbf{B} - z\mathbf{I})_2 + y_3(\mathbf{B} - z\mathbf{I})_3 + y_4(\mathbf{B} - z\mathbf{I})_4 = 0 \tag{5.14}$$

where $(\mathbf{B} - z\mathbf{I})_j$ is the jth column of $\mathbf{B} - z\mathbf{I}$. If not all of the $y_j = 0$ then Eq. (5.14) states that the columns of $\mathbf{B} - z\mathbf{I}$ are **linearly dependent**. This then gives us our first hint at how to choose z – namely, choose it to create dependencies among the columns of $\mathbf{B} - z\mathbf{I}$. In order to actually compute z we next argue that one may instead create dependencies among the *rows* of $\mathbf{B} - z\mathbf{I}$. To see this, note that if in the solution of $(\mathbf{B} - z\mathbf{I})\mathbf{y} = 0$ via Gaussian Elimination each pivot is nonzero then $\mathbf{y} = 0$ is the only solution. It follows then that the columns of $\mathbf{B} - z\mathbf{I}$ are linearly dependent if $\mathbf{B} - z\mathbf{I}$ has a zero pivot. In this case we say that $\mathbf{B} - z\mathbf{I}$ is **noninvertible**. For example, if

$$\mathbf{B} = \begin{pmatrix} B_{11} & B_{12} \\ B_{21} & B_{22} \end{pmatrix} \quad \text{then} \quad \mathbf{B} - z\mathbf{I} = \begin{pmatrix} B_{11} - z & B_{12} \\ B_{21} & B_{22} - z \end{pmatrix}$$

and so, if $B_{21} = 0$ then the pivots are $B_{11} - z$ and $B_{22} - z$ and so $z = B_{11}$ and $z = B_{22}$ render the columns of $\mathbf{B} - z\mathbf{I}$ linearly dependent. If $B_{21} \neq 0$ then one step of Gaussian Elimination produces

$$\begin{pmatrix} B_{11} - z & B_{12} \\ 0 & B_{22} - z - B_{12}\frac{B_{21}}{B_{11} - z} \end{pmatrix}$$

and so the zero pivot condition reveals that z must obey

$$B_{22} - z - B_{12}\frac{B_{21}}{B_{11} - z} = 0,$$

i.e., z must be a root of the quadratic,

$$(B_{11} - z)(B_{22} - z) - B_{12}B_{21} = 0. \tag{5.15}$$

While for **B** three dimensional

$$\mathbf{B} - z\mathbf{I} = \begin{pmatrix} B_{11} - z & B_{12} & B_{13} \\ B_{21} & B_{22} - z & B_{23} \\ B_{31} & B_{32} & B_{33} - z \end{pmatrix}$$

and so if $B_{21} = B_{31} = 0$ then $z = B_{11}$ produces a zero pivot. If both are nonzero then Gaussian Elimination in the first column yields

$$\begin{pmatrix} B_{11} - z & B_{12} & B_{13} \\ 0 & B_{22} - z - B_{21}B_{12}/(B_{11} - z) & B_{23} - B_{21}B_{13}/(B_{11} - z) \\ 0 & B_{32} - B_{31}B_{12}/(B_{11} - z) & B_{33} - z - B_{31}B_{13}/(B_{11} - z) \end{pmatrix}.$$

Elimination of the (3,2) element yields the (3,3) element of the form

$$B_{33} - z - \frac{B_{31}B_{13}}{B_{11} - z} - \frac{(B_{32} - B_{31}B_{12})(B_{23} - B_{21}B_{13}/(B_{11} - z))}{B_{22} - z - B_{21}B_{12}}.$$

This vanishes when z is a root of the cubic

$$((B_{33} - z)(B_{11} - z) - B_{31}B_{13})(B_{22} - B_{21}B_{12} - z) - (B_{32} - B_{31}B_{12})(B_{23}(B_{11} - z) - B_{31}B_{12}) = 0 \tag{5.16}$$

In general, if **B** is N-by-N then the Nth pivot in Gaussian Elimination of $(\mathbf{B} - z\mathbf{I})$ will vanish when z is the root of an associated Nth order polynomial. By the Fundamental Theorem of Algebra this polynomial has N complex (possibly coincident) roots, $\{z_n\}_{n=1}^{N}$. We call these roots the **eigenvalues** of **B**. The German prefix may be translated as "self" for the eigenvalues depend solely on **B** itself.

We are now half way to unraveling the consequences of our hopeful guess, Eq. (5.12). The fact that there is more than one z that renders the columns of $(\mathbf{B} - z\mathbf{I})$ dependent suggests that Eq. (5.12) is too naive. The resolution comes from making these dependencies explicit, i.e., by solving

$$(\mathbf{B} - z_j\mathbf{I})\mathbf{w}_j = 0 \tag{5.17}$$

for the nontrivial **eigenvectors**, $\mathbf{w}_j$. As $\mathbf{B}\mathbf{w}_j = z_j\mathbf{w}_j$ we call $\mathbf{w}_j$ the **eigenvector** of **B** associated with z_j. These are typically determined by Gaussian Elimination. For small matrices this is easier done than said. For example, if

$$\mathbf{B} = \begin{pmatrix} 1 & 3 \\ 0 & 2 \end{pmatrix} \quad \text{then the eigenvalues are} \quad z_1 = 1 \quad \text{and} \quad z_2 = 2$$

and $\mathbf{w}_1$ must solve $(\mathbf{B} - z_1\mathbf{I})\mathbf{w}_1 = 0$, i.e.,

$$\begin{pmatrix} 0 & 3 \\ 0 & 1 \end{pmatrix} \begin{pmatrix} w_{11} \\ w_{12} \end{pmatrix} = \begin{pmatrix} 0 \\ 0 \end{pmatrix} \quad \text{and so} \quad \mathbf{w}_1 = \begin{pmatrix} 1 \\ 0 \end{pmatrix},$$

while $\mathbf{w}_2$ must solve $(\mathbf{B} - z_2\mathbf{I})\mathbf{w}_2 = 0$, i.e.,

$$\begin{pmatrix} -1 & 3 \\ 0 & 0 \end{pmatrix} \begin{pmatrix} w_{21} \\ w_{22} \end{pmatrix} = \begin{pmatrix} 0 \\ 0 \end{pmatrix} \quad \text{and so} \quad \mathbf{w}_2 = \begin{pmatrix} 3 \\ 1 \end{pmatrix}.$$

Although we have made concrete choices of $\mathbf{w}_1$ and $\mathbf{w}_2$ please note that each may be multiplied by any nonzero scalar and still remain an eigenvector. We observe that $\mathbf{w}_1$ is independent of $\mathbf{w}_2$, i.e., neither is a multiple of the other. This notion is generalized to larger sets of vectors, each with N components via

Definition. The collection of vectors $\{\mathbf{u}_1, \mathbf{u}_2, \ldots \mathbf{u}_m\} \subset \mathbb{R}^N$ is said to be **linearly independent** if the only solution, $\mathbf{a}$, to $a_1\mathbf{u}_1 + a_2\mathbf{u}_2 + \cdots + a_m\mathbf{u}_m = 0$ is $\mathbf{a} = 0$.

It follows that if the N columns of an N-by-N matrix $\mathbf{U}$ are linearly independent then $\mathbf{U}$ is invertible. Hence given any $\mathbf{b} \in \mathbb{R}^N$ there exists a unique $\mathbf{c} \in \mathbb{R}^N$ such that $\mathbf{U}\mathbf{c} = \mathbf{b}$. These notions, coupled with the Theorem below, will help us "expand" both the stimulus, $\mathbf{f}$, and response, $\mathbf{y}$, in terms of the eigenvectors of $\mathbf{B}$.

Theorem 1. If an N-by-N matrix has N distinct eigenvalues then its N associated eigenvectors are linearly independent.

To see whether this criterion applies to our quasi-active cell we call on MATLAB to compute the associated eigenpairs of eigenvalues and eigenvectors. The command [W,Z]=eig(B) delivers the four eigenvectors as the columns of $\mathbf{W}$ and the four eigenvalues as the associated diagonal entries of $\mathbf{Z}$. In this case, the eigenvalues are

$$z_1 = -4.72, \quad z_2 = -0.12, \quad z_3 = -0.18 + 0.28i, \quad \text{and} \quad z_4 = -0.18 - 0.28i \tag{5.18}$$

where $i = \sqrt{-1}$. It follows from Theorem 1 that the associated eigenvectors are linearly independent, and hence, for each t, there is a unique solution $\mathbf{c}(t)$ to

$$\mathbf{W}\mathbf{c}(t) = \mathbf{f}(t). \tag{5.19}$$

In components, this takes the form of an eigenvector expansion of the stimulus,

$$\sum_{j=1}^{N} c_j(t)\mathbf{w}_j = \mathbf{f}(t).$$

We next attempt a similar expansion of the response

$$\mathbf{y}(t) = \sum_{j=1}^{N} a_j(t)\mathbf{w}_j. \tag{5.20}$$

To determine the coefficients a_j we equate

$$\mathbf{y}'(t) = \sum_{j=1}^{N} a_j'(t)\mathbf{w}_j$$

and

$$\mathbf{B}\mathbf{y}(t) + \mathbf{f}(t) = \mathbf{B}\sum_{j=1}^{N} a_j(t)\mathbf{w}_j + \sum_{j=1}^{N} c_j(t)\mathbf{w}_j = \sum_{j=1}^{N} (z_j a_j(t) + c_j(t))\mathbf{w}_j,$$

and so find that the a_j must obey the familiar initial value problem

$$a_j'(t) = z_j a_j(t) + c_j(t), \qquad a_j(0) = 0.$$

We solved this equation in §3.1 and found

$$a_j(t) = \int_0^t \exp((t-s)z_j)c_j(s)\,\mathrm{d}s.$$

Returning to Eq. (5.20) we find

$$\boxed{\mathbf{y}(t) = \sum_{j=1}^{N} \mathbf{w}_j \int_0^t \exp((t-s)z_j)c_j(s)\,\mathrm{d}s.} \tag{5.21}$$

where $\mathbf{c}$ satisfies Eq. (5.19).

Resonance*. As each of the z_k in Eq. (5.18) has negative real part we see that $\mathbf{y}$ in Eq. (5.21) decays to zero exponentially. For those nonreal eigenvalues we will now show that there will be oscillatory terms "near" the frequency

$$\omega_k = \frac{1000}{2\pi}\Im z_k. \tag{5.22}$$

The significance of "near" will be made precise in Eq. (5.26) below. The factor 2π in Eq. (5.22) converts from circular to temporal frequency (see, e.g., Eq. (5.10)) and the factor 1000 from kHz to Hz, since each τ in Eq. (5.4) is measured in ms. Note, using z_3 from Eq. (5.18), that $\omega_3 = 44.1$ Hz, is close to the resonant frequency identified in Figure 5.2.

To better understand this connection between eigenvalues and resonance we now take a close look at both the structure of the eigenvectors and the nature of the characteristic polynomial. The arrowhead structure of $\mathbf{B}$ in Eq. (5.4) permits us to deduce that solutions of the eigenproblem $\mathbf{Bw} = z\mathbf{w}$ take the form

$$\mathbf{w} = \begin{pmatrix} \overline{m}'_\infty/(1+z\overline{\tau}_m) \\ \overline{h}'_\infty/(1+z\overline{\tau}_h) \\ \overline{n}'_\infty/(1+z\overline{\tau}_n) \\ 1 \end{pmatrix} \tag{5.23}$$

where the eigenvalues, z, are roots of the quartic polynomial

$$\begin{aligned}
P(z) &= (z+\gamma)(1+z\overline{\tau}_m)(1+z\overline{\tau}_h)(1+z\overline{\tau}_n) + 3\overline{m}^2\overline{h}v_{Na}\overline{m}'_\infty(1+z\overline{\tau}_h)(1+z\overline{\tau}_n)/\tau_{Na} \\
&\quad + \overline{m}^3 v_{Na}\overline{h}'_\infty(1+z\overline{\tau}_m)(1+z\overline{\tau}_n)/\tau_{Na} + 4\overline{n}^3 v_K\overline{n}'_\infty(1+z\overline{\tau}_m)(1+z\overline{\tau}_h)/\tau_K
\end{aligned} \tag{5.24}$$

and $\gamma = \overline{m}^3\overline{h}/\tau_{Na} + \overline{n}^4/\tau_K + 1/\tau_{Cl}$. It then follows from Eq. (5.21) that

$$\tilde{V}(t) = \sum_{j=1}^{4} \int_0^t \exp((t-s)z_j)c_j(s)\,ds. \tag{5.25}$$

Moreover, when $\mathbf{f} = (0\ 0\ 0\ \tilde{I}/A)^T$ then Exercise 9 reveals that $\mathbf{c} = \mathbf{W}\backslash\mathbf{f}$ has components

$$c_j(t) = \frac{\tilde{I}(t)}{A}\frac{(1+z_j\overline{\tau}_m)(1+z_j\overline{\tau}_h)(1+z_j\overline{\tau}_n)}{\overline{\tau}_m\overline{\tau}_h\overline{\tau}_n\prod_{k\neq j}(z_j-z_k)}. \tag{5.26}$$

We now suppose, as in Eq. (5.18), z_1 and z_2 to be real, $z_3 = z_{3,r} + iz_{3,i}$, and $z_4 = z_3^*$ and we show how $z_{3,i}$ leads to resonance. If $\tilde{I}(t) = \sin(2\pi\omega t)$ and $j = 1$ or 2 then

$$\int_0^t \exp((t-s)z_j)\sin(2\pi\omega s)\,ds = \frac{\exp(z_j t) + \sqrt{(2\pi\omega)^2+z_j^2}\sin(2\pi\omega t + \arctan(2\pi\omega/z_j))}{(2\pi\omega)^2+z_j^2}$$

and so the associated gain is the familiar (recall Eq. (3.7)) low-pass function $1/\sqrt{(2\pi\omega)^2+z_j^2}$. We next write $c_3(t) = (c_{3,r} + ic_{3,i})\sin(2\pi\omega t)$, note that $c_4 = c_3^*$ and so

$$\int_0^t \{\exp((t-s)z_3)c_3(s) + \exp((t-s)z_4)c_4(s)\}\,ds$$

$$= 2\int_0^t \exp((t-s)z_{3,r})\{c_{3,r}\cos((t-s)z_{3,i}) - c_{3,i}\sin((t-s)z_{3,i})\}\sin(2\pi\omega s)\,ds$$

$$= 2\sqrt{\frac{(z_{3,r}c_{3,r}+z_{3,i}c_{3,i})^2+c_{3,r}^2(2\pi\omega)^2}{(z_{3,r}^2+(z_{3,i}+2\pi\omega)^2)(z_{3,r}^2+(z_{3,i}-2\pi\omega)^2)}}\sin(2\pi\omega t+\theta)+\exp(z_{3,r}t)\phi(t)$$

where θ is a phase shift and ϕ, as the coefficient of an evanescent term, need not concern us here. The associated gain

$$G_{34}(\omega) \equiv \sqrt{\frac{(z_{3,r}c_{3,r}+z_{3,i}c_{3,i})^2+c_{3,r}^2(2\pi\omega)^2}{(z_{3,r}^2+(z_{3,i}+2\pi\omega)^2)(z_{3,r}^2+(z_{3,i}-2\pi\omega)^2)}} \tag{5.27}$$

indeed peaks at $\omega = z_{3,i}/(2\pi)$ when the associated real part, $z_{3,r}$, vanishes. When $z_{3,r} \neq 0$ the associated peak in G_{34} shifts and broadens, precisely as in Figure 5.2.

The matrix exponential*. We close this section by noting that Eq. (5.21) is often written much more compactly as

$$\mathbf{y}(t) = \int_0^t \exp((t-s)\mathbf{B})\mathbf{f}(s)\,ds \tag{5.28}$$

where $\exp(t\mathbf{B})$, the matrix exponential of $t\mathbf{B}$, is built from the eigendecomposition of $\mathbf{B}$. In particular, Eq. (5.17) may be written in matrix fashion as $\mathbf{BW} = \mathbf{WZ}$. As the columns of $\mathbf{W}$ are linearly independent it follows that $\mathbf{W}$ is invertible, and so multiplication of $\mathbf{BW} = \mathbf{WZ}$ by $\mathbf{W}^{-1}$ from the left brings the representation

$$\mathbf{B} = \mathbf{WZW}^{-1}. \tag{5.29}$$

Now if Taylor's theorem is to hold in the matrix case we may expect that

$$\exp(t\mathbf{B}) = \mathbf{I} + t\mathbf{B} + (t\mathbf{B})^2/2 + (t\mathbf{B})^3/3! + \cdots \tag{5.30}$$

These powers are made easy by Eq. (5.29). In particular,

$$\mathbf{B}^2 = \mathbf{BB} = \mathbf{WZW}^{-1}\mathbf{WZW}^{-1} = \mathbf{WZ}^2\mathbf{W}^{-1}$$

where $\mathbf{Z}^2$ is simply the diagonal matrix comprised of the squares of the eigenvalues. In a similar fashion we find $\mathbf{B}^k = \mathbf{WZ}^k\mathbf{W}^{-1}$ and so

$$\exp(t\mathbf{B}) = \mathbf{W}\exp(t\mathbf{Z})\mathbf{W}^{-1} \tag{5.31}$$

where $\exp(t\mathbf{Z})$ is the diagonal matrix comprised of $\exp(tz_j)$ as j runs from 1 to 4. On substituting (5.31) into (5.28) we find

$$\mathbf{y}(t) = \int_0^t \mathbf{W}\exp((t-s)\mathbf{Z})\mathbf{W}^{-1}\mathbf{f}(s)\,ds = \int_0^t \mathbf{W}\exp((t-s)\mathbf{Z})\mathbf{c}(s)\,ds = \sum_{j=1}^4 \mathbf{w}_j \int_0^t \exp((t-s)z_j)c_j(s)\,ds$$

which indeed is nothing other than Eq. (5.21). Finally, we observe that these integrals are well behaved, for the real part of each of the z_j, recall Eq. (5.18), is negative. As this dictates that small perturbations from the rest state, V_r, will vanish over time we say that V_r is a **stable** rest point.

5.4 A PERSISTENT SODIUM CURRENT*

The methods we have developed so far apply readily to a vast array of active models. In this and the next section we will construct and study active and quasi-active models of the Hodgkin–Huxley system augmented by two important currents.

The first of these is a fast activating and noninactivating sodium current. It is therefore referred to as a persistent sodium current. As a concrete example, we study

$$I_{NaP} = \overline{g}_{NaP}p_\infty(V)(V - V_{Na}), \quad p_\infty(V) = \frac{1}{1 + \exp(-(V+49)/5)}. \tag{5.32}$$

We contrast p_∞ and m_∞, the steady-state activation functional of the transient sodium current, in Figure 5.5A. We now add I_{NaP} to the Hodgkin–Huxley system and ask how this changes the cell's rest potential, resonant frequency, and action potential. We do this by computing the rest potential and the eigenvalues of the augmented quasi-active system over a range of channel conductances. Its effect on the latter is felt through the addition of $(\overline{p}'_\infty v_{Na} + \overline{p}_\infty)/\tau_{NaP}$ to B_{44} in Eq. (5.4). We illustrate our findings in Figure 5.4.

We next illustrate, in Figure 5.5, the recruitment of this current during a spike.

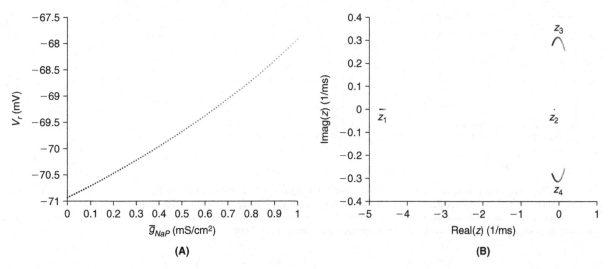

FIGURE 5.4   Rest potential (**A**) and spectrum (**B**) of the Hodgkin–Huxley system, Eq. (4.15), with a persistent sodium current, Eq. (5.32), as a function of $\overline{g}_{NaP}$. In both we indicate increasing values of $\overline{g}_{NaP}$ by moving from black to red. In **A** we see that I_{NaP} is active at rest and that it serves to depolarize the cell. In **B** the depolarizing effect of increasing $\overline{g}_{NaP}$ is seen by the rightward shift of the eigenvalues of the associated **B** matrix. The complex pair in fact enters the right half plane as $\overline{g}_{NaP}$ exceeds 0.5. We note that the active cell lacks a stable rest state in this case. (NaPtrack.m)

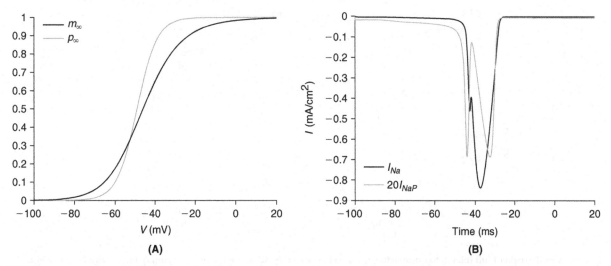

FIGURE 5.5   **A**. The activation functionals for both I_{Na} and I_{NaP}. **B**. The transient and persistent sodium currents associated with an action potential sparked by a 40 pA, 2 ms current injection, with $\overline{g}_{NaP} = 0.4$ mS/cm^2. We note that I_{NaP} is active at rest and is recruited much earlier than I_{Na}. (INaP.m)

5.5 A NONSPECIFIC CATION CURRENT THAT IS ACTIVATED BY HYPERPOLARIZATION*

We consider a fascinating channel that passes both sodium and potassium, has a reversal potential well above rest and so acts to depolarize the cell, but is gated in a fashion that permits activation only upon hyperpolarization. The associated current is denoted I_h, and we here study the concrete form

$$I_h = \overline{g}_h q^2(t)(V - V_h), \qquad \tau_q(V(t))q'(t) = q_\infty(V(t)) - q(t)$$

$$q_\infty(V) = \frac{1}{1 + \exp((V + 69)/7.1)}$$

$$\tau_q(V) = \frac{1000}{\exp((V + 66.4)/9.3) + \exp(-(V + 81.6)/13)} \text{ ms}, \qquad V_h = -40 \text{ mV}.$$

(5.33)

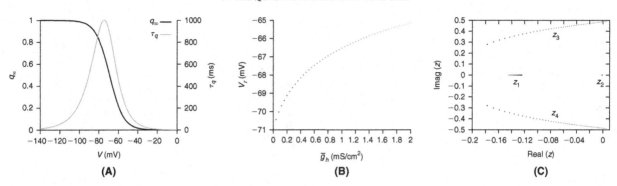

FIGURE 5.6   **A.** The h-current gating functionals. **B.** Rest potential. **C.** Quasi-active spectrum of the Hodgkin–Huxley system Eq. (4.15) plus the h-current of Eq. (5.33), as a function of $\overline{g}_h$. In **B** we observe that I_h, like I_{NaP}, is active at rest and that it serves to depolarize the cell. In **C** the transition from black to red denotes increasing values of $\overline{g}_h$. Like I_{NaP}, as we increase its conductance the nonreal eigenvalues move right and with increasing (absolute) imaginary part and eventually cross the imaginary axis. (`htrack.m`)

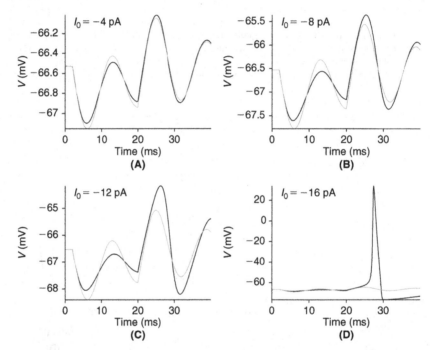

FIGURE 5.7   Comparison of full (black) to quasi-active (red) response of the Hodgkin–Huxley system Eq. (4.15) with an h-current, Eq. (5.33), to increasing amounts of hyperpolarization. In each case we used $\overline{g}_h = 1$ mS/cm^2 and delivered the current stimulus for 18 ms. In **A** and **B** we observe, as expected, the quasi-active response to track the full, active, response to small to moderate stimulus. The overshoot and action potential exhibited in **C** and **D** following sustained hyperpolarization, or inhibition, is known as "postinhibitory rebound." (`stEqah.m`)

In Figure 5.6 we illustrate its gating functionals and track its effect on the Hodgkin–Huxley system as $\overline{g}_h$ is increased. We note that the associated quasi-active system is now five dimensional.

We next contrast, in Figure 5.7, the response of the quasi-active and active cells, with I_h, to single hyperpolarizing current pulses.

5.6 SUMMARY AND SOURCES

We have linearized the Hodgkin–Huxley system about its rest state and arrived at a linear system of ordinary differential equations for the so-called quasi-active response. Their numerical solution led us to a system of algebraic equations, which we solved via Gaussian Elimination, while their exact solution was represented in terms of eigenvalues and eigenvectors of the underlying matrix. We found the nonreal eigenvalue with the largest real part to be an excellent predictor of the active cell's resonant frequency. The determinant serves as a natural link between Gaussian Elimination and eigenvalues. We develop its properties in a sequence of exercises.

The quasi-active model appears already in Hodgkin and Huxley (1952). Our mix of linear algebra and systems of differential equations is well supported by Redheffer and Port (1992). For more on persistent sodium currents, currents activated by hyperpolarization, and their interaction with other currents that are "active" near rest, see Desjardins et al. (2003). We will consider their role in the bursting of thalamic relay neurons in Chapter 10. Newton's method for root finding, Exercise 1, and the LU matrix factorization, Exercise 2, are both discussed at length by Cheney and Kincaid (2007). Exercise 11 is based on Morris and Lecar (1981).

5.7 EXERCISES

1. The derivatives required to specify the quasi-active model can be used to accelerate the computation of the rest potential. We recall that V_r is the value of V for which the steady-state function

$$I_{ss}(V) \equiv \bar{g}_K n_\infty^4(V)(V - V_K) + \bar{g}_{Na} m_\infty^3(V) h_\infty(V)(V - V_{Na}) + g_{Cl}(V - V_{Cl}) \qquad (5.34)$$

vanishes. Given a guess, V_j, we may follow Newton in improving this guess by writing the Taylor approximation of I_{ss} at the better guess, V_{j+1},

$$I_{ss}(V_{j+1}) = I_{ss}(V_j) + \frac{dI_{ss}}{dV}(V_j)(V_{j+1} - V_j) + O((V_{j+1} - V_j)^2).$$

On setting the left hand side to zero and ignoring the second order terms we arrive at the explicit expression

$$V_{j+1} = V_j - I_{ss}(V_j)/(dI_{ss}(V_j)/dV) \qquad (5.35)$$

for the improved guess. Newton's method is little more than repeated application of Eq. (5.35) until $|I_{ss}(V_j)|$ is sufficiently small. MATLAB has implemented a variant of this scheme in its fsolve routine. In its default mode fsolve presumes that the user has not provided any derivative information and so resorts to brute force finite difference approximation. We offer in getVrJac.m an example of the computation of I_{ss}, for a reduced cell, with specification of dI_{ss}/dV. Modify (and test) this code by adding in the Hodgkin–Huxley sodium current.

2. Recalling Eq. (5.8) (i) please find $\mathbf{E}_2$ and $\mathbf{E}_3$. (ii) Show that

$$\mathbf{E}_1^{-1} = \begin{pmatrix} 1 & 0 & 0 & 0 \\ 0 & 1 & 0 & 0 \\ 0 & 0 & 1 & 0 \\ -a & 0 & 0 & 1 \end{pmatrix}$$

and find $\mathbf{E}_2^{-1}$ and $\mathbf{E}_3^{-1}$. (iii) Working, at the algebraic level, show that $\mathbf{U} = \mathbf{E}_3 \mathbf{E}_2 \mathbf{E}_1 \mathbf{A}$ may be written $\mathbf{E}_1^{-1} \mathbf{E}_2^{-1} \mathbf{E}_3^{-1} \mathbf{U} = \mathbf{A}$. (iv) Argue, in general, that the product of two lower triangular matrices, each with ones on their diagonal, is itself lower triangular with ones on its diagonal. (v) Conclude that $\mathbf{A} = \mathbf{LU}$ where $\mathbf{L}$ is lower triangular, with ones its diagonal, and $\mathbf{U}$ is upper triangular. (vi) In general we may need to intersperse our elimination matrices with elementary permutation matrices, e.g., $\mathbf{U} = \mathbf{E}_2 \mathbf{P}_2 \mathbf{E}_1 \mathbf{P}_1 \mathbf{A}$, where $\mathbf{P}_j$ exchanges row j and $\mathbf{E}_j$ conducts elimination in column j. Argue that $\mathbf{F}_1 \equiv \mathbf{P}_2 \mathbf{E}_1 \mathbf{P}_2$ is lower triangular, define $\mathbf{P} \equiv \mathbf{P}_1 \mathbf{P}_2$, and conclude that $\mathbf{A}$ enjoys the factorization $\mathbf{A} = \mathbf{PLU}$. What is $\mathbf{L}$? MATLAB achieves this "LU factorization" via the command [L,U,P] = lu(A).

3. [†]We have used Gaussian Elimination in a top-down fashion to arrive at a lower triangular system. If we then follow this with a bottom-up sweep we arrive at a method, deemed Gauss–Jordan, for assembling the inverse of a matrix. To illustrate this we begin in the 2-by-2 case and augment our $\mathbf{B}$ matrix with the identity,

$$\begin{pmatrix} B_{11} & B_{12} & 1 & 0 \\ B_{21} & B_{22} & 0 & 1 \end{pmatrix}.$$

The process of transforming $\mathbf{B}$ to $\mathbf{I}$ on the left will simultaneously transform $\mathbf{I}$ to $\mathbf{B}^{-1}$ on the right. Elimination in the (2,1) slot produces

$$\begin{pmatrix} B_{11} & B_{12} & 1 & 0 \\ 0 & B_{22} - B_{12}B_{21}/B_{11} & -B_{21}/B_{11} & 1 \end{pmatrix}. \qquad (5.36)$$

Dividing the first row by B_{11} and the second row by $B_{22} - B_{12}B_{21}/B_{11}$ yields

$$\begin{pmatrix} 1 & B_{12}/B_{11} & 1/B_{11} & 0 \\ 0 & 1 & -B_{21}/(B_{22}B_{11} - B_{21}B_{12}) & 1/(B_{22} - B_{12}B_{21}/B_{11}) \end{pmatrix}. \tag{5.37}$$

Finally, elimination in the (1,2) slot yields

$$\begin{pmatrix} 1 & 0 & 1/B_{11} + (B_{12}/B_{11})B_{21}/(B_{22}B_{11} - B_{21}B_{12}) & B_{12}/(B_{22}B_{11} - B_{21}B_{12}) \\ 0 & 1 & -B_{21}/(B_{22}B_{11} - B_{21}B_{12}) & 1/(B_{22} - B_{12}B_{21}/B_{11}) \end{pmatrix}. \tag{5.38}$$

(i) Show that the matrix on the right is

$$\mathbf{B}^{-1} = \frac{1}{B_{22}B_{11} - B_{21}B_{12}} \begin{pmatrix} B_{22} & -B_{12} \\ -B_{21} & B_{11} \end{pmatrix} \tag{5.39}$$

and confirm that indeed $\mathbf{B}^{-1}\mathbf{B} = \mathbf{B}\mathbf{B}^{-1} = \mathbf{I}$.

(ii) Given

$$\mathbf{B} = \begin{pmatrix} -2 & 1 \\ 1 & -2 \end{pmatrix} \tag{5.40}$$

compute $\mathbf{B}^{-1}$ via Eq. (5.39).

(iii) We may also interpret the Gauss–Jordan method as a sequence of elementary transformations. In particular, explain how Eq. (5.36) obeys $\mathbf{E}_1\mathbf{B} = \mathbf{U}$, how Eq. (5.37) is then $\mathbf{M}_2\mathbf{M}_1\mathbf{E}_1\mathbf{B} = \mathbf{M}_2\mathbf{M}_1\mathbf{U}$ and finally how Eq. (5.38) is then $\mathbf{E}_2\mathbf{M}_2\mathbf{M}_1\mathbf{E}_1\mathbf{B} = \mathbf{E}_2\mathbf{M}_2\mathbf{M}_1\mathbf{U} = \mathbf{I}$. Reversing the process, please explain how

$$\mathbf{B} = \mathbf{E}_1^{-1}\mathbf{M}_1^{-1}\mathbf{M}_2^{-1}\mathbf{E}_2^{-1}, \tag{5.41}$$

by producing each of the $\mathbf{E}_j$, $\mathbf{M}_j$ and their inverses. These $\mathbf{M}_j$ may be called elementary row multipliers. We offer

$$\mathbf{M}_1 = \begin{pmatrix} 1/B_{11} & 0 \\ 0 & 1 \end{pmatrix} \quad \text{and} \quad \mathbf{M}_1^{-1} = \begin{pmatrix} B_{11} & 0 \\ 0 & 1 \end{pmatrix}. \tag{5.42}$$

4. [†]Show that if $\mathbf{B}$ is invertible then so too is its transpose and that the inverse of its transpose is the transpose of its inverse, i.e., $(\mathbf{B}^T)^{-1} = (\mathbf{B}^{-1})^T$. We typically denote this common value by $\mathbf{B}^{-T}$.

5. [†]Suppose that $\mathbf{P} \in \mathbb{R}^{n \times n}$ is an elementary permutation matrix obtained by exchanging two rows of the identity matrix.

(i) Argue that $\mathbf{PP} = \mathbf{I}$.
(ii) Prove that $z = 1$ and $z = -1$ are the only eigenvalues of $\mathbf{P}$ and that to $z = 1$ are associated $n - 1$ eigenvectors and to $z = -1$ is associated 1 eigenvector.

6. Compute, by hand, the eigenvalues and eigenvectors of the $\mathbf{B}$ in Eq. (5.40). To witness the action of $\mathbf{B}$, and the role played by its eigenvalues and eigenvectors, please reproduce Figure 5.8.

Argue that the area of the ellipse in (A) is 3π and that the area of the parallelogram in (B) is 3. In each case our matrix scaled the area of the original shape by factor of 3 and in each case we see that $\mathbf{B}$ stretched its subject by z_1 in eigendirection $\mathbf{w}_1$ and by z_2 in eigendirection $\mathbf{w}_2$. This fact is a consequence of the general statement that each matrix $\mathbf{B} \in \mathbb{R}^{n \times n}$ scales the n-dimensional volume of its subject by $|\det \mathbf{B}|$ where det is short for "determinant" and is the product of the eigenvalues of $\mathbf{B}$, i.e.,

$$\det \mathbf{B} \equiv \prod_{j=1}^{n} z_j. \tag{5.43}$$

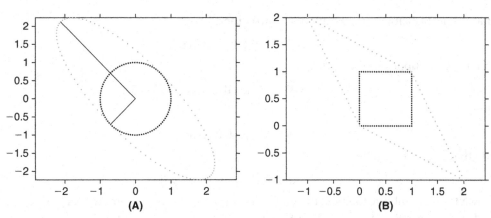

FIGURE 5.8 The unit circle and unit square (black dots) and their images under the matrix $\mathbf{B}$ (red dots). In (A) we have also plotted scaled unit eigenvectors $z_j\mathbf{w}_j$ for $j = 1$ and 2. (distort.m)

Please confirm that in the general 2-by-2 case, if

$$\mathbf{B} = \begin{pmatrix} B_{11} & B_{12} \\ B_{21} & B_{22} \end{pmatrix} \tag{5.44}$$

then $\det \mathbf{B} = z_1 z_2 = B_{11}B_{22} - B_{12}B_{21}$. In addition, check that the matrix trace, $\mathrm{tr}\mathbf{B} \equiv B_{11} + B_{22}$, obeys $\mathrm{tr}\mathbf{B} = z_1 + z_2$.

7. (i) †Argue that if z_j is an eigenvalue of $\mathbf{B}$ then $z_j - z$ is an eigenvalue of $\mathbf{B} - z\mathbf{I}$. Use this to deduce from Eq. (5.43) that the eigenvalues of $\mathbf{B}$ are the roots of the characteristic polynomial

$$\det(\mathbf{B} - z\mathbf{I}) = \prod_{j=1}^{n} (z_j - z). \tag{5.45}$$

(ii) If one had a definition of det that was independent of eigenvalues then one could use Eq. (5.45) to compute the eigenvalues. We offer the telescoping definition

$$\det(\mathbf{B}) \equiv \sum_{j=1}^{n} B_{ij}(-1)^{i+j} \det(\mathbf{B}_{\neg i, \neg j}) \tag{5.46}$$

where i is at the user's discretion, $\{\neg i, \neg j\}$ indicates the removal of row i and column j, and the determinant of a scalar is that scalar. The term $(-1)^{i+j}\det(\mathbf{B}_{\neg i, \neg j})$ is often called a cofactor of $\mathbf{B}$, in which case Eq. (5.46) is referred to as the "cofactor expansion of $\det \mathbf{B}$ along row i." Please confirm that this agrees with the previous exercise for the 2-by-2 $\mathbf{B}$ of Eq. (5.44) and that, if $\mathbf{B}$ is 3-by-3, that expansion along row 1

$$\det \mathbf{B} = B_{11}\det\begin{pmatrix} B_{22} & B_{23} \\ B_{32} & B_{33} \end{pmatrix} - B_{12}\det\begin{pmatrix} B_{21} & B_{23} \\ B_{31} & B_{33} \end{pmatrix} + B_{13}\det\begin{pmatrix} B_{21} & B_{22} \\ B_{31} & B_{32} \end{pmatrix}$$
$$= B_{11}\{B_{22}B_{33} - B_{23}B_{31}\} - B_{12}\{B_{21}B_{33} - B_{23}B_{31}\} + B_{13}\{B_{21}B_{32} - B_{23}B_{31}\},$$

indeed agrees with the expansion along row 2.

8. (i) †Deduce from Eq. (5.46) that if $\mathbf{B}$ is triangular then

$$\det \mathbf{B} = \prod_{j=1}^{n} B_{jj}. \tag{5.47}$$

(ii) Show that if $\mathbf{P}$ is an elementary permutation matrix then

$$\det(\mathbf{PB}) = -\det(\mathbf{B}) = \det(\mathbf{P})\det(\mathbf{B}). \tag{5.48}$$

(iii) Show that if $\mathbf{E}$ is an elementary elimination matrix then

$$\det(\mathbf{EB}) = \det(\mathbf{B}) = \det(\mathbf{E})\det(\mathbf{B}). \tag{5.49}$$

(iv) Show that if $\mathbf{M}$ multiplies row k by m then

$$\det(\mathbf{MB}) = m\det(\mathbf{B}) = \det(\mathbf{M})\det(\mathbf{B}). \tag{5.50}$$

(v) Show that

$$\det(\mathbf{AB}) = \det(\mathbf{A})\det(\mathbf{B}). \tag{5.51}$$

(vi) Conclude that if $\mathbf{C}$ is invertible

$$\det(\mathbf{C}^{-1}) = \det(\mathbf{C})^{-1} \neq 0.$$

9. Assemble, in MATLAB's symbolic toolbox, the matrix $\mathbf{W} = (\mathbf{w}_1 \; \mathbf{w}_2 \; \mathbf{w}_3 \; \mathbf{w}_4)$ where $\mathbf{w}_k$ is Eq. (5.23) with $z = z_k$. With $\mathbf{f} = (0 \; 0 \; 0 \; \tilde{I}/A)^T$ now solve $\mathbf{Wc} = \mathbf{f}$ for $\mathbf{c}$ and confirm Eq. (5.26).

10. We will now use our quasi-active analysis to determine the so-called threshold current, I_θ, i.e., the greatest value of I_{stim} at which the cell does not spike. We computed this empirically in Figure 4.7B. We will now derive it analytically for the reduced model of Exercise 4.7 by calculating the value of I_{stim} at which the eigenvalues of the quasi-active system cross into the right half plane.

    Derive the quasi-active counterpart to the reduced system of Exercise 4.7. Note that rest is determined by Eq. (4.34) and show that the quasi-active matrix, Eq. (5.4), is

$$\mathbf{B} = \begin{pmatrix} -\alpha_n(V) - \beta_n(V) & (1-n)\alpha_n'(V) - n\beta_n'(V) \\ 4a(V)n^3 + 2b(V)n & a'(V)n^4 + b'(V)n^2 + c'(V) \end{pmatrix}.$$

The eigenvalues of $\mathbf{B}$ cross into the right half plane when $\mathrm{tr}\mathbf{B} = 0$, i.e., when V is a root of

$$S(V) \equiv a'(V)n^4 + b'(V)n^2 + c'(V) - \alpha_n(V) - \beta_n(V). \tag{5.52}$$

Graph S as in Figure 5.9, and show that it has a root at $V_\theta \approx -68.23$ mV. Now return with this voltage to the $I - V$ rest curve, Figure 4.19B and conclude that the threshold for spiking in the modified FitzHugh system is $I_\theta \approx 23.925$ pA.

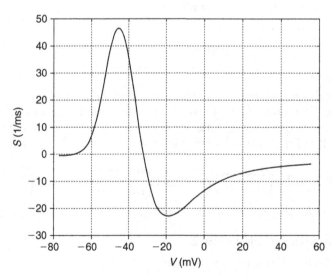

FIGURE 5.9 The S curve, Eq. (5.52), associated with the modified FitzHugh system. As the trace of the quasi-active matrix, its roots are the potentials at which the eigenvalues are a conjugate pair of imaginary numbers.

11. Derive the quasi-active counterpart to the system of Morris and Lecar

$$C_m V'(t) = -\overline{g}_{Ca} m_\infty(V)(V - V_{Ca}) - \overline{g}_K w(V - V_K) - g_L(V - V_L) + I_{stim}/A$$
$$w'(t) = (w_\infty(V) - w)/\tau_w(V)$$

where

$$C_m = 10 \ \mu F/cm^2, \ \bar{g}_{Ca} = 44, \ \bar{g}_K = 80, \ g_L = 20 \ mS/cm^2,$$
$$V_{Ca} = 100, \ V_K = -70, \ V_L = -50 \ mV,$$

and the gating functional are

$$m_\infty(V) = \frac{1 + \tanh((V+1)/15))}{2}, \quad w_\infty(V) = \frac{1 + \tanh(V/30))}{2}, \quad \text{and} \quad \tau_w(V) = \frac{2}{\cosh(V/60)}.$$

Compute the rest potential, V_r, the associated 2×2 matrix $\mathbf{B}$, and its eigenvalues. Is V_r stable?

12. †Prove Theorem 1 by assembling these parts. (i) Show that if $z_1 \neq z_2$ then $\mathbf{w}_1$ is not a multiple of $\mathbf{w}_2$.
    (ii) Show that if z_1, z_2, and z_3 are distinct then $\{\mathbf{w}_1, \mathbf{w}_2, \mathbf{w}_3\}$ is a linearly independent set. Hint: Show that if this set were dependent then we would violate (i).
    Generalize (ii) to sets with more than three vectors.

13. We now attack the quasi-active system, Eq. (5.2), with the Laplace transform.

    (i) Take the Laplace transform of each gating equation in Eq. (5.2) and solve the transformed gating variable in terms of the transformed potential. In particular, show that

    $$\mathcal{L}\tilde{m} = \frac{\overline{m}'_\infty}{1 + s\overline{\tau}_m} \mathcal{L}\tilde{V}. \tag{5.53}$$

    (ii) Transform the potential equation in Eq. (5.2) and substitute your results from part (i) to arrive at the input conductance

    $$G_{in}(s) \equiv \frac{\mathcal{L}\tilde{I}}{A\mathcal{L}\tilde{V}} = sC_m + g_{Cl} + \bar{g}_{Na}\left\{ \overline{m}^3\overline{h} - \left(\frac{3\overline{m}^2\overline{h}\overline{m}'_\infty}{1 + s\overline{\tau}_m} + \frac{\overline{m}^3\overline{h}'_\infty}{1 + s\overline{\tau}_h} \right)v_{Na} \right\} + \bar{g}_K\left\{ \overline{n}^4 - \frac{4\overline{n}^3 v_K \overline{n}'_\infty}{1 + s\overline{\tau}_n} \right\}.$$

    (iii) As in §3.3 we view this equation as an opportunity to reverse engineer the quasi-active parameter set $\{C_m, g_{Cl}, \bar{g}_{Na}, \bar{g}_K\}$ from moments of the stimulus, $\tilde{I}$ and response, $\tilde{V}$. With that in mind, please confirm

    $$G_{in}(0) = g_{Cl} + \bar{g}_{Na}(\overline{m}^3\overline{h} - (3\overline{m}^2\overline{h}\overline{m}'_\infty + \overline{m}^3\overline{h}'_\infty)v_{Na}) + \bar{g}_K(\overline{n}^4 - 4\overline{n}^3 v_K \overline{n}'_\infty)$$
    $$G'_{in}(0) = C_m + \bar{g}_{Na}(3\overline{m}^2\overline{h}\overline{m}'_\infty\overline{\tau}_m + \overline{m}^3\overline{h}'_\infty\overline{\tau}_h)v_{Na} + \bar{g}_K 4\overline{n}^3 v_K \overline{n}'_\infty \overline{\tau}_n$$
    $$G''_{in}(0) = -2\bar{g}_{Na}(3\overline{m}^2\overline{h}\overline{m}'_\infty\overline{\tau}_m^2 + \overline{m}^3\overline{h}'_\infty\overline{\tau}_h^2)v_{Na} - 2\bar{g}_K 4\overline{n}^3 v_K \overline{n}'_\infty \overline{\tau}_n^2$$
    $$G'''_{in}(0) = 6\bar{g}_{Na}(3\overline{m}^2\overline{h}\overline{m}'_\infty\overline{\tau}_m^3 + \overline{m}^3\overline{h}'_\infty\overline{\tau}_h^3)v_{Na} + 6\bar{g}_K 4\overline{n}^3 v_K \overline{n}'_\infty \overline{\tau}_n^3. \tag{5.54}$$

    This "exposes" the desired parameter set. To establish the moment connection please confirm, arguing as in Eq. (3.23), that

    $$AG_{in}(0) = \frac{M_0(\tilde{I})}{M_0(\tilde{V})}$$
    $$AG'_{in}(0) = \frac{M_1(\tilde{V})AG_{in}(0) - M_1(\tilde{I})}{M_0(\tilde{V})}$$
    $$AG''_{in}(0) = \frac{M_2(\tilde{I}) + 2M_1(\tilde{V})AG'_{in}(0) - M_2(\tilde{V})AG_{in}(0)}{M_0(\tilde{V})}$$
    $$AG'''_{in}(0) = \frac{3M_1(\tilde{V})AG''_{in}(0) - 3M_2(\tilde{V})AG'_{in}(0) + M_3(\tilde{V})AG_{in}(0) - M_3(\tilde{I})}{M_0(\tilde{V})}. \tag{5.55}$$

    (iv) With Eq. (5.55) we recognize Eq. (5.54) as four linear equations in the four unknowns, $\{C_m, g_{Cl}, \bar{g}_{Na}, \bar{g}_K\}$. Write a program that takes the response computed by stEqa.m, computes the moments used in Eq. (5.55) and solves the resulting linear system for $\{C_m, g_{Cl}, \bar{g}_{Na}, \bar{g}_K\}$. How well does this approach tolerate added noise in the response and stimulus?

The Passive Cable

OUTLINE

6.1	The Discrete Passive Cable Equation	67	6.5	Synaptic Input		78
6.2	Exact Solution via Eigenvector Expansion	69	6.6	Summary and Sources		81
6.3	Numerical Methods	71	6.7	Exercises		82
6.4	The Passive Cable Equation	73				

Up to this point we have assumed that membrane potential varies in time but not in space. No cell fits this hypothesis exactly and very few cells even fit it approximately, for most neurons resemble dendritic trees or bushes with tens or hundreds of fine thin branches. As each branch resembles, both geometrically and electrically, Lord Kelvin's RC model of the transatlantic telegraph cable, the mathematical study of dendritic branches has come to be called "cable theory." The electrical analogy to Kelvin, however, only holds in the subthreshold, in fact passive, regime, for Kelvin's cables possessed nothing like our ion channels. In this chapter, our first step into space is softened by the fact that we limit ourselves to uniform, unbranched, passive cables. This permits us to develop analytical and numerical methods with minimal distraction. We will then argue in Chapters 8 and 9 that these survive the extension to active dendritic trees.

We proceed by first deriving the discrete, or compartmental, passive cable equation. We construct its exact (via an eigenvector expansion) and approximate (via the trapezoid rule) solution to current injection. As the compartment size shrinks, and the number of compartments grows, we arrive at the passive cable equation. Methods for studying partial differential equations of this form have been under continuous development for over 150 years. We construct and analyze its exact solution (via an eigenfunction expansion) to current injection in a manner that permits us to reconcile the discrete and continuous formulations. In the final section we consider synaptic input onto a spine appended to the cable.

6.1 THE DISCRETE PASSIVE CABLE EQUATION

We consider a cable of length ℓ and radius a. We choose an integer N and divide the cable into N compartments each of length $dx = \ell/N$ and surface area $2\pi a\, dx$ and cross-sectional area πa^2. We suppose that each compartment is isopotential but permit this potential to vary from compartment to compartment, see Figure 6.1. The only new object here is the coupling resistance between compartments. We express it in terms of R_a in Ωcm, the resistivity of the cytoplasm. The circuit elements are then

$$C = (2\pi a\, dx)C_m, \quad G = (2\pi a\, dx)g_{Cl}, \quad \text{and} \quad R = dx R_a/(\pi a^2).$$

Current balance at the first node in Figure 6.1 now reads

$$I_{stim} = I_1 + I_2 + I_3 = C(\phi_1 - \phi_0)' + G((\phi_1 - V_{Cl}) - \phi_0) + (\phi_1 - \phi_2)/R$$

Mathematics for Neuroscientists. DOI: 10.1016/B978-0-12-374882-9.00006-X

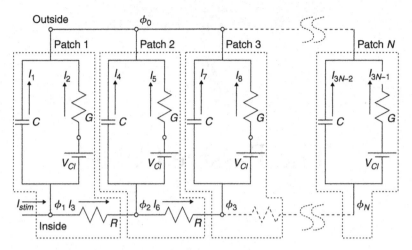

FIGURE 6.1   The compartmentalization of a simple cable.

which, in terms of the relative transmembrane potential

$$v_n \equiv \phi_n - \phi_0 - V_{Cl}, \quad n = 1, \dots, N$$

reads

$$I_{stim} = Cv'_1 + Gv_1 + (v_1 - v_2)/R. \tag{6.1}$$

On recalling the time constant, $\tau = C/G$, and defining the "space constant"

$$\lambda \equiv \sqrt{\frac{a}{2R_a g_{Cl}}} \tag{6.2}$$

division of Eq. (6.1) by G produces

$$\tau v'_1 + v_1 - \lambda^2 (v_2 - v_1)/dx^2 = I_{stim}/G. \tag{6.3}$$

Current balance at the second node requires $I_4 + I_5 = I_3 - I_6$, that is

$$Cv'_2 + Gv_2 = (v_1 - v_2)/R - (v_2 - v_3)/R \tag{6.4}$$

or, on division by G,

$$\tau v'_2 + v_2 - \lambda^2 (v_1 - 2v_2 + v_3)/dx^2 = 0.$$

Similarly, at the nth compartment,

$$Cv'_n + Gv_n = (v_{n+1} - 2v_n + v_{n-1})/R$$

or

$$\tau v'_n + v_n - \lambda^2 (v_{n+1} - 2v_n + v_{n-1})/dx^2 = 0. \tag{6.5}$$

Current balance at the final compartment reads $I_{3N-2} + I_{3N-1} = I_{3N-3}$, that is

$$Cv'_N + Gv_N = (v_{N-1} - v_N)/R$$

or

$$\tau v'_N + v_N - \lambda^2 (v_{N-1} - v_N)/dx^2 = 0. \tag{6.6}$$

Collecting the potentials in the column vector

$$\mathbf{v}(t) = (v_1 \ v_2 \ \dots \ v_N)^T$$

we may express the above as

$$\mathbf{v}'(t) = \mathbf{B}\mathbf{v}(t) + \mathbf{f}(t) \tag{6.7}$$

where

$$\mathbf{B} = (\lambda^2 \mathbf{S} - \mathbf{I})/\tau, \tag{6.8}$$

$\mathbf{S}$ is the second difference matrix

$$\mathbf{S} = \frac{1}{dx^2} \begin{pmatrix} -1 & 1 & 0 & 0 & \cdots & 0 \\ 1 & -2 & 1 & 0 & \cdots & 0 \\ \cdot & \cdot & \cdot & \cdot & \cdot & \cdot \\ 0 & \cdots & 0 & 1 & -2 & 1 \\ 0 & \cdots & 0 & 0 & 1 & -1 \end{pmatrix} \tag{6.9}$$

and the forcing term is

$$\mathbf{f} = \frac{I_{stim}(t)}{(2\pi a \ dx)C_m} \mathbf{e}_k \quad \text{where} \quad \mathbf{e}_k \equiv (0 \ 0 \ \dots \ 0 \ 1 \ 0 \ \dots \ 0)^T, \tag{6.10}$$

is associated with current injection into compartment k. Our illustration, Figure 6.1, uses $k=1$ but we will be interested in the general case. We also presume that each compartment starts from rest, i.e.,

$$\mathbf{v}(0) = 0. \tag{6.11}$$

As in the previous chapter, we solve Eq. (6.7) both exactly, via eigenvectors of $\mathbf{B}$, and approximately, via Euler's method.

6.2 EXACT SOLUTION VIA EIGENVECTOR EXPANSION

The second difference matrix, $\mathbf{S}$, is symmetric, i.e., obeys $\mathbf{S} = \mathbf{S}^T$, and negative semidefinite, i.e., obeys $\mathbf{u}^T \mathbf{S} \mathbf{u} \leq 0$ for every $\mathbf{u} \in \mathbb{R}^N$. As such, its eigenvalues are real and nonpositive (Exercises 1–3). It is also noninvertible and so 0 is an eigenvalue. We may therefore order the eigenvalues as

$$0 = \theta_0 \geq \theta_1 \geq \cdots \geq \theta_{N-1}$$

and denote the corresponding eigenvectors by

$$\mathbf{q}_0, \ \mathbf{q}_1, \ \dots, \ \mathbf{q}_{N-1}.$$

Together they obey

$$\mathbf{S}\mathbf{q}_n = \theta_n \mathbf{q}_n \tag{6.12}$$

and we note that regardless of whether or not these eigenvalues are distinct (they are) every N-by-N symmetric matrix has an orthonormal basis of N eigenvectors (Exercise 4). That is, the $\mathbf{q}_n$ obey

$$\mathbf{q}_m^T \mathbf{q}_n = \delta_{mn}, \tag{6.13}$$

where δ_{mn} is the Kronecker delta of Eq. (1.4). As **B** (recall Eq. (6.8)) is simply an affine function of **S** it follows that its eigenvalues are

$$z_n = (\lambda^2 \theta_n - 1)/\tau, \tag{6.14}$$

and that its eigenvectors remain $\mathbf{q}_n$ (Exercise 5). Recalling Eq. (5.18) it remains to solve $\mathbf{Q}\mathbf{c}(t) = \mathbf{f}(t)$ where

$$\mathbf{Q} = (\mathbf{q}_0 \ \mathbf{q}_1 \ \cdots \ \mathbf{q}_{N-1}) \tag{6.15}$$

is the N-by-N matrix composed of the orthonormal eigenvectors of **S**. Now by orthonormality we note (Exercise 6) that $\mathbf{Q}^{-1} = \mathbf{Q}^T$ and so, recalling the **f** of Eq. (6.10),

$$\mathbf{c}(t) = \frac{I_{stim}(t)}{2\pi a \, dx C_m} \mathbf{Q}^T \mathbf{e}_k = \frac{I_{stim}(t)}{2\pi a \, dx C_m} (q_{0,k} \ q_{1,k} \ \cdots \ q_{N-1,k})^T.$$

We see that $\mathbf{Q}^T \mathbf{e}_k$ is comprised of the kth component of each of the eigenvectors. Now, following the lead of Eq. (5.21), we conclude that

$$\boxed{\mathbf{v}(t) = \frac{N}{2\pi a \ell C_m} \sum_{n=0}^{N-1} \mathbf{q}_n q_{n,k} \int_0^t I_{stim}(s) \exp((t-s)z_n) \, ds.} \tag{6.16}$$

Although cumbersome in appearance, this expression is the sum of elementary objects that should be familiar from our isopotential work back in Chapter 3. More precisely, Eq. (6.16) states that $\mathbf{v}(t)$ is a weighted sum of convolutions, $I_{stim} \star \exp(tz_n)$, that differ from the isopotential case, Eq. (3.2), only in the sense that the membrane time constant, τ, has been replaced with $-1/z_n$. This difference in fact permits us to interpret the N eigenvalues, z_n, as a sequence of decay rates for the N-compartment cable. These rates, however, are not specific to individual compartments but instead to individual eigenvectors, $\mathbf{q}_n$, for these (together with the signature, $q_{n,k}$, of the stimulus location) serve as the weights for the individual convolutions. We will soon derive exact expressions for the z_n and $\mathbf{q}_n$. For now, we invoke eig in MATLAB and illustrate in Figure 6.2 the first few eigenvectors as "functions" of cable length.

As a concrete application of Eq. (6.16) let us consider the cable

$$\ell = 1 \text{ mm}, \quad a = 1 \ \mu\text{m}, \quad C_m = 1 \ \mu\text{F/cm}^2, \quad g_{Cl} = 1/15 \text{ mS/cm}^2, \quad R_a = 0.3 \text{ k}\Omega\text{cm} \tag{6.17}$$

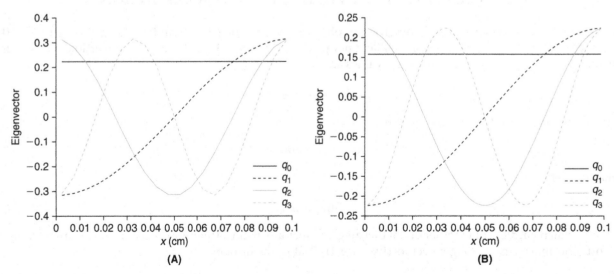

FIGURE 6.2   The first four eigenvectors of **S** for $N = 20$ (**A**) and $N = 40$ (**B**) on a cable of length $\ell = 0.1$ cm. These eigenvectors appear to approximate (scalar multiples of) 1, $\cos(x/\ell)$, $\cos(2x/\ell)$, and $\cos(3x/\ell)$ while the associated eigenvalues of **S** are very close to integer multiples of $(\pi/\ell)^2$. (evecS.m)

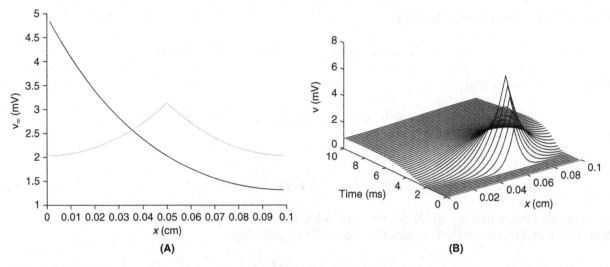

FIGURE 6.3 **A**. The steady-state solution, Eq. (6.18), for the cable parameters in Eq. (6.17) and $I_0 = 1$ nA and $N = 41$ and stimulus at compartments $k = 1$, black, and $k = 21$, red. (steady.m) **B**. Dynamic response, Eq. (6.20), of the same cable to the stimulus of Eq. (6.19), $I_0 = 10$ nA, $t_1 = 1$, and $t_2 = 2$ ms at $x = 0.06$ cm, with $N = 100$. (eigcab.m)

and suppose that $I_{stim}(t)$ takes the constant value I_0. In this case, Eq. (6.16) reduces to

$$\mathbf{v}(t) = \frac{I_0 N}{2\pi a \ell C_m} \sum_{n=0}^{N-1} \frac{\mathbf{q}_n q_{n,k}}{z_n} (e^{z_n t} - 1)$$

which, as $t \to \infty$, converges to

$$\mathbf{v}_\infty = \frac{-I_0 N}{2\pi a \ell C_m} \sum_{n=0}^{N-1} \frac{\mathbf{q}_n q_{n,k}}{z_n} \tag{6.18}$$

as illustrated in Figure 6.3A. As a second example, if we inject the pulse

$$I_{stim}(t) = I_0 \mathbb{1}_{(t_1, t_2)}(t) \tag{6.19}$$

at compartment k then Eq. (6.16) takes the form

$$\mathbf{v}(t) = \frac{-I_0 N}{2\pi a \ell C_m} \sum_{n=0}^{N-1} \frac{\mathbf{q}_n q_{n,k}}{z_n} (e^{\max(t-t_2,0)z_n} - e^{\max(t-t_1,0)z_n}) \tag{6.20}$$

as presented in Figure 6.3B. We will establish below that the attenuation in the steady response away from the site of stimulation is of the form $\exp(-x/\lambda)$. In other words, the response drops by factor of $1/e$ within one space constant, λ, from the stimulus. Note that $\lambda = 0.05$ cm for the cable specified in Eq. (6.17).

6.3 NUMERICAL METHODS

We formulate three straightforward marching schemes for the

$$\text{stimulus} \quad \mathbf{f}^j = \mathbf{f}((j-1)dt) \quad \text{and response} \quad \mathbf{v}^j \approx \mathbf{v}((j-1)dt)$$

associated with the discrete cable equation, Eq. (6.7). The forward Euler scheme reads

$$(\mathbf{v}^j - \mathbf{v}^{j-1})/dt = \mathbf{B}\mathbf{v}^{j-1} + \mathbf{f}^{j-1}, \quad \text{i.e.,} \quad \mathbf{v}^j = (\mathbf{I} + dt\mathbf{B})\mathbf{v}^{j-1} + dt\mathbf{f}^{j-1} \tag{6.21}$$

while the backward Euler scheme requires

$$(v^j - v^{j-1})/dt = \mathbf{B}v^j + f^j, \quad \text{i.e.,} \quad (\mathbf{I} - dt\mathbf{B})v^j = v^{j-1} + dt f^j \tag{6.22}$$

and the trapezoid scheme that

$$v^j - v^{j-1} = \mathbf{B}(v^j + v^{j-1})dt/2 + (f^j + f^{j-1})dt/2$$

or

$$(\mathbf{I} - (dt/2)\mathbf{B})v^j = (\mathbf{I} + (dt/2)\mathbf{B})v^{j-1} + (dt/2)(f^j + f^{j-1}). \tag{6.23}$$

At first sight it appears that Eq. (6.23) requires one additional (over backward Euler) matrix-vector product per iteration. To see that this is not the case note that Eq. (6.23) is equivalent to

$$\text{set} \quad \mathbf{r}^2 = (dt/2)(f^2 + f^1)$$

and for $j = 2, 3, \ldots,$

$$\text{solve } (\mathbf{I} - (dt/2)\mathbf{B})v^j = \mathbf{r}^j \quad \text{and set } \mathbf{r}^{j+1} = 2v^j - \mathbf{r}^j + (dt/2)(f^{j+1} + f^j). \tag{6.24}$$

Regarding implementation, we note that both Eq. (6.22) and Eq. (6.24) require the solution of a linear system of equations at each step in time. As the matrix in each case **does not** depend on j we may decompose it, once and for all, into lower and upper triangular factors. This provides significant acceleration of the associated time marching scheme. MATLAB constructs these factors (recall Exercise 4.2) via [L,U]=lu(speye(N)-(dt/2)**B**) and so the solution of Eq. (6.24) is reduced to two triangular solves, $v^j = \mathbf{U}\backslash(\mathbf{L}\backslash\mathbf{r}^j)$. We have coded this in trapcab.m and illustrate it in Figure 6.4 in the case of dual injection

$$\mathbf{I}_{stim}(t) = I_0\{\mathbf{e}_{c_1}\mathbb{1}_{(t_{1,1},t_{2,1})} + \mathbf{e}_{c_2}\mathbb{1}_{(t_{1,2},t_{2,2})}\} \tag{6.25}$$

at compartments c_1 and c_2. These compartment indices are computed from the specified cable length, ℓ, space-step, dx, and stimulation locations x_1 and x_2 via $c_i = \text{round}(x_i/dx)$.

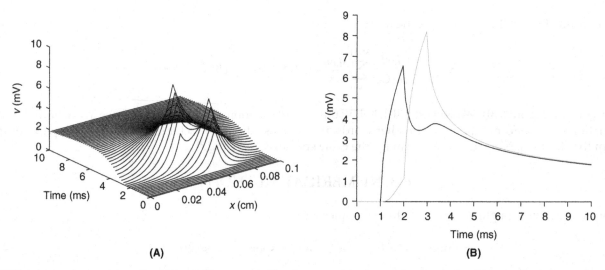

(A)   **(B)**

FIGURE 6.4   Response of the cable of Eq. (6.17), as revealed by the trapezoid scheme ($dx = 1\ \mu$m, $dt = 0.05$ ms), Eq. (6.24), to the double stimulation in Eq. (6.25), $I_0 = 100$ pA, $x_1 = 0.06$ cm, $t_{1,1} = 1$, $t_{2,1} = 2$ ms, and $x_2 = 0.04$, $t_{1,2} = 3$, $t_{2,2} = 4$. The proximity of the two stimuli, in both space and time, leads to significant boosting of the latter response. **A.** The full space-time response. **B.** The response in time at the early site, x_1 (black), and the late site, x_2, (red). (trapcab.m)

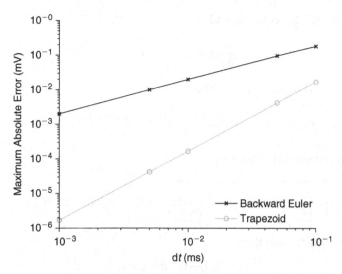

FIGURE 6.5 Illustration of the fact that backward Euler is accurate to $O(dt)$ while trapezoid is accurate to $O(dt^2)$. $N = 100$. (cndrive.m, cnpfib.m)

We next compare the accuracy of the trapezoid and backward Euler schemes, under the assumption that

$$\mathbf{f}(t) = \frac{e^{-t} - e^{-2t}}{10C_m 2\pi a}\mathbf{q}_1.$$

In this case, the exact solution, recall Eq. (6.16), is

$$\mathbf{v}^{(ex)}(t) = \frac{e^{z_1 t} - e^{-t}(z_1 + 2) + e^{-2t}(z_1 + 1)}{10C_m 2a\pi(z_1 + 1)(z_1 + 2)}\mathbf{q}_1$$

and so, with sc denoting either the backward Euler or trapezoid scheme, we compute the maximum absolute error by

$$E(dt, sc) \equiv \max_j \max_n |\mathbf{v}_n^j(sc) - \mathbf{v}_n^{(ex)}((j-1)dt)|$$

and illustrate our findings in Figure 6.5.

6.4 THE PASSIVE CABLE EQUATION

We have examined the role of the time step dt in our resolution of the voltage response of the discrete passive cable. We now investigate the role of the space step, dx. To begin, we let the number, N, of compartments approach ∞. As $dx = \ell/N$ this limit is equivalent to $dx \to 0$. In this limit we will pass from a spatially discrete set of potentials, $\mathbf{v}(t) = (v_1(t)\, v_2(t) \cdots v_N(t))^T$, to a continuous set of potentials, $v(x, t)$, $0 \le x \le \ell$. For small dx we expect $v((n - 1/2)dx, t)$ to be the potential at the center of the nth compartment, i.e., $v_n(t)$. To begin, we will suppose that current is injected into the first compartment. Discrete current balance at the left end, Eq. (6.1), in terms of our approximation $v((n - 1/2)dx, t) \approx v_n(t)$, takes the form

$$C_m(2\pi a dx)\frac{\partial v}{\partial t}(dx/2, t) + g_{Cl}(2\pi a dx)v(dx/2, t) - \frac{\pi a^2}{R_a}\frac{v(3dx/2, t) - v(dx/2, t)}{dx} = I_{stim}(t). \tag{6.26}$$

As dx approaches zero this takes the form

$$\frac{\partial v}{\partial x}(0, t) = -\frac{R_a}{\pi a^2}I_{stim}(t), \qquad 0 < t. \tag{6.27}$$

By identical reasoning at the cable's far end, we find

$$\frac{\partial v}{\partial x}(\ell, t) = 0, \qquad 0 < t. \tag{6.28}$$

Now at an interior point, x, we deduce from Eq. (6.5) that

$$\tau \frac{\partial v}{\partial t}(x, t) + v(x, t) - \lambda^2 \frac{v(x + \mathrm{d}x, t) - 2v(x, t) + v(x - \mathrm{d}x, t)}{\mathrm{d}x^2} = 0 \tag{6.29}$$

which, as $\mathrm{d}x$ approaches zero becomes (Exercise 10)

$$\boxed{\tau \frac{\partial v}{\partial t}(x, t) + v(x, t) - \lambda^2 \frac{\partial^2 v}{\partial x^2}(x, t) = 0,} \quad 0 < x < \ell, \quad 0 < t. \tag{6.30}$$

Finally, if the entire cable is initially at rest then

$$v(x, 0) = 0 \quad 0 < x < \ell. \tag{6.31}$$

The cable equation, (6.30), together with its boundary conditions, Eqs. (6.27) and (6.28), and initial condition, Eq. (6.31), is an instance of a well-studied class of partial differential equations.

The steady-state solution to end-point stimulus. To begin, we suppose a constant current stimulus, $I_{stim}(t) = I_0$, and search for the steady-state solution $v_\infty(x) \equiv v(x, t \to \infty)$. In this limit we may ignore the time derivative in the cable equation, (6.30), and so find that v_∞ must obey the ordinary differential equation

$$\lambda^2 v_\infty''(x) = v_\infty(x), \tag{6.32}$$

subject to the boundary conditions,

$$v_\infty'(0) = -\frac{R_a}{\pi a^2} I_0, \quad v_\infty'(\ell) = 0. \tag{6.33}$$

In Exercise 11 the reader will construct the solution

$$v_\infty(x) = \frac{I_0 R_a \lambda \cosh((\ell - x)/\lambda)}{\pi a^2 \sinh(\ell/\lambda)} \tag{6.34}$$

and contrast it to the discrete steady state, Eq. (6.18), computed in the previous section. This function takes its maximum value at the site, $x = 0$, of stimulation, and so it is natural to define the associated input resistance

$$R_{in}(0) \equiv \frac{v_\infty(0)}{I_0} = \frac{R_a \lambda \cosh(\ell/\lambda)}{\pi a^2 \sinh(\ell/\lambda)}. \tag{6.35}$$

We note that this decreases with cable length ℓ.

The transient solution to end-point stimulus. We now return to the full cable equation and derive an eigenrepresentation of v reminiscent of Eq. (6.16). The basic idea is to **separate variables**, i.e., to suppose that v may be written as a product of univariate functions of space and time. Note that if we substitute the guess

$$v(x, t) = q(x)p(t) \tag{6.36}$$

into the cable equation, Eq. (6.30), we find

$$\tau q(x)p'(t) + q(x)p(t) = \lambda^2 q''(x)p(t).$$

If we now divide this through by qp we arrive at

$$\tau p'(t)/p(t) + 1 = \lambda^2 q''(x)/q(x).$$

Now note that the function on the right depends solely on x while that on the left depends solely on t. Taking then an x derivative of each side we find that $q''(x)/q(x)$ must be constant. We write this constant as ϑ and so arrive at

$$q''(x) = \vartheta q(x), \quad 0 < x < \ell. \tag{6.37}$$

This eigenvalue problem will be the infinite dimensional analog of the matrix eigenvalue problem, Eq. (6.12), once we prescribe the domain of permissible q. More precisely, it remains to translate the top and bottom rows of $\mathbf{S}$ into boundary conditions on Eq. (6.37). Recalling Eq. (6.28) it seems "natural" to prescribe $q'(\ell) = 0$. At the near end, where I_{stim} is applied, the correct prescription is less obvious. If q is, however, to be an eigenfunction of $\mathrm{d}^2/\mathrm{d}x^2$ we expect it to be independent of the stimulus. An indication of the "right" way forward can be glimpsed from Figure 6.2. The "cosinesque" functions indeed suggest the prescription $q'(0) = 0$. Appending

$$q'(0) = q'(\ell) = 0 \tag{6.38}$$

to Eq. (6.37) we arrive, via Exercise 12, at the eigenvalues and eigenfunctions

$$\vartheta_0 = 0, \quad q_0(x) = 1/\sqrt{\ell},$$
$$\vartheta_n = -n^2\pi^2/\ell^2, \quad q_n(x) = \sqrt{2/\ell}\cos(n\pi x/\ell), \ n = 1, 2, \ldots \tag{6.39}$$

We note that these q_n are orthonormal in the sense that

$$\int_0^\ell q_n(x)q_m(x) = \delta_{mn}. \tag{6.40}$$

Finding many q we modify our naive guess, Eq. (6.36), to

$$v(x, t) = \sum_{n=0}^{\infty} q_n(x)p_n(t) \tag{6.41}$$

and proceed to determine the p_n. First, thanks to orthonormality, we may multiply each side of Eq. (6.41) by an eigenfunction, integrate, and arrive at

$$p_n(t) = \int_0^\ell q_n(x)v(x, t)\,\mathrm{d}x. \tag{6.42}$$

We now use the cable equation to derive an ordinary differential equation for each of the p_n.

$$\tau p_n'(t) = \tau \int_0^\ell q_n(x)\frac{\partial v}{\partial t}(x, t)\,\mathrm{d}x = \int_0^\ell q_n(x)\left(\lambda^2\frac{\partial^2 v}{\partial x^2}(x, t) - v(x, t)\right)$$

$$\tag{6.43}$$

$$= \lambda^2 \int_0^\ell q_n(x)\frac{\partial^2 v}{\partial x^2}(x, t)\,\mathrm{d}x - p_n(t).$$

We unravel the remaining integral by twice integrating by parts. Namely,

$$\int_0^\ell q_n(x)\frac{\partial^2 v}{\partial x^2}(x, t)\,\mathrm{d}x = q_n(x)\frac{\partial v}{\partial x}(x, t)\Big|_{x=0}^\ell - \int_0^\ell q_n'(x)\frac{\partial v}{\partial x}(x, t)\,\mathrm{d}x$$

$$= -q_n(0)\frac{\partial v}{\partial x}(0, t) - \int_0^\ell q_n'(x)\frac{\partial v}{\partial x}(x, t)\,\mathrm{d}x$$

$$= -q_n(0)\frac{\partial v}{\partial x}(0, t) - q_n'(x)v(x, t)\Big|_{x=0}^\ell + \int_0^\ell q_n''(x)v(x, t)\,\mathrm{d}x$$

$$= q_n(0)R_a I_{stim}(t)/(\pi a^2) + \vartheta_n p_n(t).$$

It follows that each $p_n(t)$ obeys the initial value problem

$$\tau p'_n(t) + (1 - \lambda^2 \vartheta_n) p_n(t) = \lambda^2 q_n(0) R_a I_{stim}(t)/(\pi a^2), \quad p_n(0) = 0. \tag{6.44}$$

We note that the time-varying stimulus now appears as a driving term in the time-varying component of v. This equation is exactly the one we derived back in Chapter 2 for the isopotential cell. Recalling Eq. (3.2), we find

$$p_n(t) = \frac{q_n(0)}{2\pi a C_m} \int_0^t I_{stim}(s) \exp((t-s)\zeta_n) \, ds$$

where

$$\zeta_n = (\lambda^2 \vartheta_n - 1)/\tau$$

and so, returning to Eq. (6.41), we conclude that

$$v(x,t) = \sum_{n=0}^{\infty} \frac{q_n(0)q_n(x)}{C_m 2a\pi} \int_0^t I_{stim}(s) \exp((t-s)\zeta_n) \, ds. \tag{6.45}$$

This is identical in structure to the solution, Eq. (6.16), of the discrete passive cable. We will investigate in Exercise 13 the sense in which this sum converges.

The transient solution to interior-point stimulus. In the case that we deliver the stimulus at $x = x_s$ the discrete current balance there takes the form

$$(2\pi a \, dx)\left(C_m \frac{\partial v}{\partial t}(x_s,t) + g_{Cl} v(x_s,t)\right) - \frac{\pi a^2}{R_a} \frac{v(x_s+dx,t) - 2v(x_s,t) + v(x_s-dx,t)}{dx} = I_{stim}(t),$$

or, after division by $2\pi a \, dx$,

$$\tau \frac{\partial v}{\partial t}(x_s,t) + v(x_s,t) - \lambda^2 \frac{v(x_s+dx,t) - 2v(x_s,t) + v(x_s-dx,t)}{dx^2} = \frac{I_{stim}(t)}{2\pi a \, dx g_{Cl}}.$$

As we pass to the limit we see that the spatial "footprint" of the injection is of length dx and magnitude $1/dx$. Recalling our work in Chapter 3, in particular Eq. (3.6), we see that this footprint converges to the delta function centered at x_s. It follows that our cable equation now takes the form

$$\tau \frac{\partial v}{\partial t}(x,t) + v(x,t) - \lambda^2 \frac{\partial^2 v}{\partial x^2}(x,t) = I_{stim}(t)\delta(x-x_s)/(2\pi a g_{Cl}) \tag{6.46}$$

and that *both* ends are now sealed, i.e.,

$$\frac{\partial v}{\partial x}(0,t) = \frac{\partial v}{\partial x}(\ell,t) = 0.$$

To solve Eq. (6.46) we retrace each of the steps in our previous derivation and find that Eq. (6.45) retains its form but shifts its attention from $q_n(0)$ to $q_n(x_s)$. That is, the solution to Eq. (6.46) is

$$v(x,t) = \sum_{n=0}^{\infty} \frac{q_n(x_s)q_n(x)}{C_m 2a\pi} \int_0^t I_{stim}(s) \exp((t-s)\zeta_n) \, ds, \tag{6.47}$$

where q_n and ζ_n are exactly as above.

The steady-state solution given interior-point current injection. If I_{stim} is held constant at I_0 then the potential will approach the solution of the steady-state equation

$$v_\infty(x) - \lambda^2 v_\infty''(x) = I_0 \delta(x - x_s)/(2\pi a g_{Cl}), \tag{6.48}$$

subject to $v_\infty'(0) = v_\infty'(\ell) = 0$. Arguing as in Exercise 11 we find that v_∞ is proportional to $\cosh(x/\lambda)$ for $x < x_s$ and proportional to $\cosh((\ell-x)/\lambda)$ for $x > x_s$. The ambiguity is resolved by enforcing continuity of v_∞ and current balance at x_s. The latter follows from integrating Eq. (6.48) in a vanishingly small interval about x_s. More precisely,

$$-\lambda^2(v_\infty'(x_s^+) - v_\infty'(x_s^-)) = I_0/(2\pi a g_{Cl}).$$

These observations lead us to

$$v_\infty(x) = \frac{I_0}{2\pi a \lambda g_{Cl}} \frac{1}{\sinh(x_s/\lambda) + \cosh(x_s/\lambda)\tanh((\ell-x_s)/\lambda)} \begin{cases} \cosh(x/\lambda) & \text{if } 0 \leq x \leq x_s \\ \frac{\cosh(x_s/\lambda)\cosh((\ell-x)/\lambda)}{\cosh((\ell-x_s)/\lambda)} & \text{if } x_s \leq x \leq \ell. \end{cases}$$

This attains its maximum at x_s, the site of stimulation, and so the associated input resistance takes the form

$$R_{in}(x_s) \equiv \frac{v_\infty(x_s)}{I_0} = \frac{1}{2\pi a \lambda g_{Cl}} \frac{1}{\tanh(x_s/\lambda) + \tanh((\ell-x_s)/\lambda)}. \tag{6.49}$$

We graph this in Figure 6.6 for the cable at hand.

Reconciling the discrete and the continuous. Given the eigenfunctions, Eq. (6.39), of the cable we might guess that the jth component of the nth eigenvector of the discrete cable (neglecting the normalization constant) is the value that the nth eigenfunction takes at the center of the jth compartment. That is,

$$q_{n,j} = q_n((j-1/2)dx) = \cos(n\pi(j-1/2)/N). \tag{6.50}$$

This indeed agrees with the eigenvectors of Figure 6.2 and, on substituting Eq. (6.50) into Eq. (6.12) we indeed find equality so long as the associated compartmental eigenvalues obey

$$\theta_n = -4(N/\ell)^2 \sin^2(n\pi/(2N)). \tag{6.51}$$

This is welcome news in that we now have exact knowledge of every term in the solution, Eq. (6.16), to the discrete cable equation. In addition, by contrasting θ_n and ϑ_n we see that the eigenvalues of the discrete cable accurately capture only the lowest $N/3$ of the true eigenvalues, as illustrated in Figure 6.7.

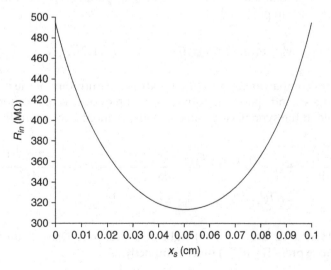

FIGURE 6.6   The input resistance, R_{in}, Eq. (6.49), as a function of stimulus site, x_s, for the cable described by Eq. (6.17). We see a marked increase in R_{in} as the stimulus moves away from the center and toward a sealed end. (Rinxs.m)

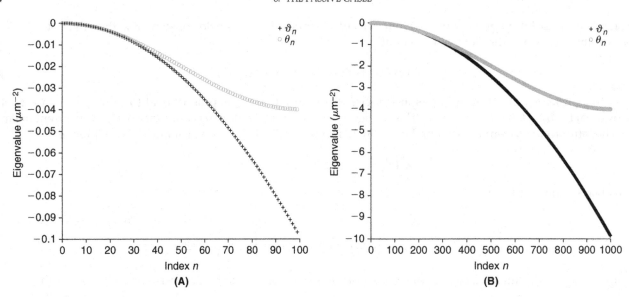

FIGURE 6.7　The eigenvalues of the discrete, θ_n, and continuous, ϑ_n, cable of length $\ell = 1$ mm for $N = 100$ and $dx = 10$ μm (A) and $N = 1000$ and $dx = 1$ μm (B). (thvsvth.m)

6.5 SYNAPTIC INPUT

If rather than current injection we instead have synaptic input, with conductance g_{syn} (in units of mS) and reversal potential V_{syn} (in mV), at x_s then the cable equation, Eq. (6.46), takes the form

$$\tau \frac{\partial v}{\partial t}(x,t) + v(x,t) - \lambda^2 \frac{\partial^2 v}{\partial x^2}(x,t) + c_{syn}(t)(v(x,t) - v_{syn})\delta(x - x_s) = 0 \tag{6.52}$$

where

$$v_{syn} \equiv V_{syn} - V_{Cl} \quad \text{and} \quad c_{syn}(t) \equiv \frac{g_{syn}(t)}{2\pi a g_{Cl}}.$$

The time dependence of g_{syn} here defeats the separation of variables that led to our clean representations in Eqs. (6.45) and (6.47). We turn therefore to approximate means. We choose a spatial step, dx, and a time step, dt, and build a consistent linear system for the discrete potentials

$$v_n^j \approx v((n - 1/2)dx, (j - 1)dt), \quad n = 1, 2, \ldots, N \tag{6.53}$$

where $N = \ell/dx$ is the number of compartments and $(n - 1/2)dx$ is the midpoint of the nth compartment. With regard to Eq. (6.52) we approximate the second space derivative via action of our second difference matrix, $\mathbf{S}$, and the time derivative by the trapezoid rule. If the synapse is located at compartment k then our discrete system takes the form

$$2\tau \frac{v_n^j - v_n^{j-1}}{dt} + v_n^j + v_n^{j-1} - \lambda^2 \frac{v_{n+1}^j - 2v_n^j + v_{n-1}^j}{dx^2} - \lambda^2 \frac{v_{n+1}^{j-1} - 2v_n^{j-1} + v_{n-1}^{j-1}}{dx^2}$$
$$+ (c^j v_n^j + c^{j-1} v_n^{j-1})\delta_{nk} = (c^j + c^{j-1})v_{syn}\delta_{nk} \tag{6.54}$$

where $c^j = c_{syn}((j-1)dt)/dx$. Here $1/dx$ denotes the height of the discrete Dirac delta associated with the synaptic footprint at compartment k. We express Eq. (6.54) more compactly as

$$((2\tau/dt)\mathbf{I} - \mathbf{B} + c^j \mathbf{e}_k \mathbf{e}_k^T)v^j = ((2\tau/dt)\mathbf{I} + \mathbf{B} - c^{j-1}\mathbf{e}_k \mathbf{e}_k^T)v^{j-1} + (c^j + c^{j-1})v_{syn}\mathbf{e}_k \tag{6.55}$$

where $\mathbf{B} = \lambda^2\mathbf{S} - \mathbf{I}$ and $\mathbf{v}^j = (v_1^j \ v_2^j \ \cdots \ v_N^j)^T$. We solve Eq. (6.55) by setting $\mathbf{v}^1 = 0$ and then

$$\mathbf{r}^j \equiv \begin{cases} (c^1 + c^2)v_{syn}\mathbf{e}_k & \text{if } j = 2, \\ 2(2\tau/dt)\mathbf{v}^{j-1} - \mathbf{r}^{j-1} + (c^j + c^{j-1})v_{syn}\mathbf{e}_k & \text{if } j > 2, \end{cases} \quad \text{and} \quad ((2\tau/dt)\mathbf{I} - \mathbf{B} + c^j\mathbf{e}_k\mathbf{e}_k^T)\mathbf{v}^j = \mathbf{r}^j.$$

We note that this procedure generalizes easily to the polysynaptic case

$$\tau\frac{\partial v}{\partial t}(x,t) + v(x,t) - \lambda^2\frac{\partial^2 v}{\partial x^2}(x,t) = \sum_{m=1}^{M} c_{syn,m}(t)(v_{syn,m} - v(x,t))\delta(x - x_{s,m}) \tag{6.56}$$

where $c_{syn,m}(t)$ is the normalized conductance change associated with a synapse at $x_{s,m}$ with relative reversal potential $v_{syn,m}$. We have coded its solution in `trapcabsyn.m` and illustrate its use in Figure 6.8.

On cortical pyramidal cells and several other neuron types, the vast majority of excitatory synaptic contacts are made not onto the soma or dendrites but onto the heads of small spines, as illustrated in Figure 6.9. We suppose that the spine head is isopotential, with transmembrane potential W, and we describe the spine geometry in terms of ℓ_{sn}, the spine neck length, a_{sn}, the spine neck radius, and A_{sh}, the surface area of the spine head. We adopt the typical values

$$\ell_{sn} = 1 \ \mu\text{m}, \quad a_{sn} = 0.1 \ \mu\text{m}, \quad A_{sh} = 1 \ \mu\text{m}^2. \tag{6.57}$$

The spine neck presents an axial resistance while the spine head sports both a membrane capacitance and conductance and a synapse. In particular,

$$R_{sn} = \ell_{sn}R_a/(\pi a_{sn}^2), \quad G_{sh} = g_{Cl}A_{sh}, \quad \text{and} \quad g_{syn} = \overline{g}_{syn}(t)\rho_{syn}A_{sh}$$

where $\overline{g}_{syn}$ is in mS and ρ_{syn} is the number of conductances per unit area. With $w \equiv W - V_{Cl}$ and

$$c_{syn}(t) = g_{syn}(t)/G_{sh}, \quad \text{and} \quad \gamma_1 = 1/(R_{sn}G_{sh}) \quad \text{and} \quad \gamma_2 = 1/(R_{sn}2\pi a g_{Cl})$$

current balance at the spine head reads

$$\tau w'(t) + w(t) + c_{syn}(t)(w(t) - v_{syn}) = \gamma_1(v(x_s,t) - w(t)) \tag{6.58}$$

while the associated cable equation reads

$$\tau\frac{\partial v}{\partial t}(x,t) + v(x,t) - \lambda^2\frac{\partial^2 v}{\partial x^2}(x,t) = \gamma_2(w(t) - v(x,t))\delta(x - x_s). \tag{6.59}$$

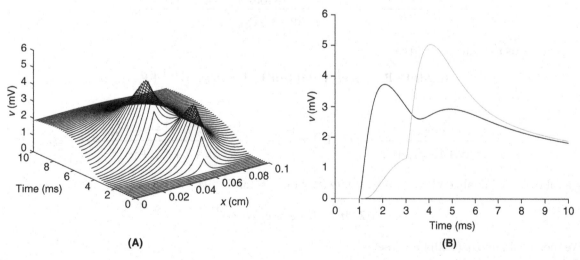

(A) (B)

FIGURE 6.8 Response to α-function synaptic input with $\overline{g}_{syn} = 100$ nS, $\tau_\alpha = 1/2$ ms at $x = 0.06$ cm at $t_1 = 1$ ms and $x = 0.04$ at $t_1 = 3$. (`trapcabsyn.m`)

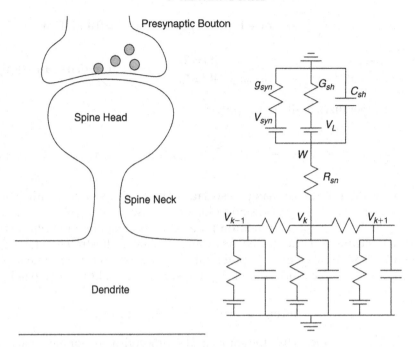

FIGURE 6.9 A schematic of synaptic contact onto the head of a spine emanating from compartment k of our discrete cable, and its associated circuit diagram. The red circles are synaptic vesicles. Depolarization of the presynaptic bouton causes one or more of these vesicles to fuse with the plasma membrane and deliver their payload of neurotransmitter to the synaptic cleft. Upon diffusion across the cleft the neurotransmitter then gates ion channels on the spine head.

To solve this coupled cable/spine system we first apply the trapezoid rule to the spine equation, Eq. (6.58), finding

$$w^j = \frac{(2\tau/dt - 1 - c_{syn}^{j-1} - \gamma_1)w^{j-1} + v_{syn}(c_{syn}^{j-1} + c_{syn}^j) + (v_k^{j-1} + v_k^j)\gamma_1}{2\tau/dt + 1 + c_{syn}^j + \gamma_1} \tag{6.60}$$

and then apply the trapezoid rule to the cable equation, Eq. (6.59), bringing

$$((2/dt)\mathbf{I} - \mathbf{B} + \gamma_2 \mathbf{e}_k \mathbf{e}_k^T)\mathbf{v}^j = ((2/dt)\mathbf{I} + \mathbf{B} - \gamma_2 \mathbf{e}_k \mathbf{e}_k^T)\mathbf{v}^{j-1} + \gamma_2(w^j + w^{j-1})\mathbf{e}_k. \tag{6.61}$$

The latter suggests that we compile

$$w^j + w^{j-1} = \frac{(4\tau/dt + c_{syn}^j - c_{syn}^{j-1})w^{j-1} + v_{syn}(c_{syn}^{j-1} + c_{syn}^j) + (v_k^{j-1} + v_k^j)\gamma_1}{2\tau/dt + 1 + c_{syn}^j + \gamma_1}.$$

This now permits us to write Eq. (6.61) as

$$((2/dt)\mathbf{I} - \mathbf{B} + \xi^j \mathbf{e}_k \mathbf{e}_k^T)\mathbf{v}^j = ((2/dt)\mathbf{I} + \mathbf{B} - \xi^j \mathbf{e}_k \mathbf{e}_k^T)\mathbf{v}^{j-1} + \mathbf{f}^j \tag{6.62}$$

where

$$\xi^j = \gamma_2 - \frac{\gamma_1 \gamma_2}{2\tau/dt + 1 + c_{syn}^j + \gamma_1} \quad \text{and} \quad \mathbf{f}^j = \gamma_2 \frac{(4\tau/dt + c_{syn}^j - c_{syn}^{j-1})w^{j-1} + v_{syn}(c_{syn}^{j-1} + c_{syn}^j)}{2\tau/dt + 1 + c_{syn}^j + \gamma_1}\mathbf{e}_k.$$

Arguing as above, we initialize $\mathbf{v}^1 = w^1 = 0$, evaluate $\mathbf{f}^2$, set $\mathbf{r}^2 = \mathbf{f}^2$, and solve

$$((2/dt)\mathbf{I} - \mathbf{B} + \xi^2 \mathbf{e}_k \mathbf{e}_k^T)\mathbf{v}^2 = \mathbf{f}^2$$

for $\mathbf{v}^2$. We then evaluate Eq. (6.60) for w^2, set

$$\mathbf{r}^j \equiv ((4/dt)\mathbf{I} + (\xi^{j-1} - \xi^j)\mathbf{e}_k \mathbf{e}_k^T)\mathbf{v}^{j-1} - \mathbf{r}^{j-1} + \mathbf{f}^j, \quad j = 3, 4, \ldots$$

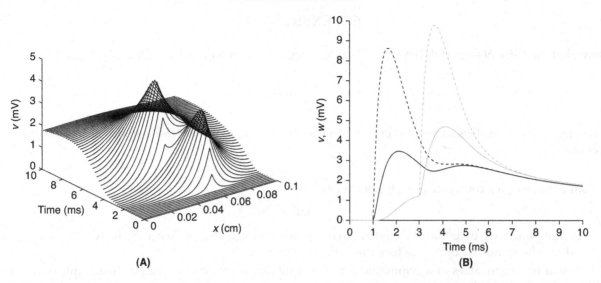

(A)   **(B)**

FIGURE 6.10   Response of the passive cable to two α-function synaptic inputs at spines with $\overline{g}_{syn} = 100$ nS, $\tau_\alpha = 1/2$ ms at $x = 0.06$ cm at $t_1 = 1$ ms and $x = 0.04$ cm at $t_1 = 3$ ms. **A.** The full space-time response. **B.** The time response at the early site, $x = 0.06$ cm (black), and the late site, $x = 0.04$ cm, (red). The solid curves depict the cable potential, $v(x_s, t)$, at that site while the dashed depict spine head potential, $w(t)$. The spine increases the input resistance at x_s and so amplifies w over v. This may have important consequences for active channels in the spine head. (trapcabspine.m)

and solve

$$((2/dt)\mathbf{I} - \mathbf{B} + \xi^j \mathbf{e}_k \mathbf{e}_k^T)\mathbf{v}^j = \mathbf{r}^j \quad j = 3, 4, \ldots$$

Finally, we solve Eq. (6.60) for w^j and repeat. We have coded this in trapcabspine.m and illustrate it in Figure 6.10.

6.6 SUMMARY AND SOURCES

We derived the discrete passive cable equation and expressed its solution, when driven by current injected at a single compartment, in terms of the eigenvalues and eigenvectors of the associated second difference matrix. The expression is simply a weighted sum of convolutions familiar from our single compartment work – where the weights are eigenvectors and the constituents of the convolutions are the current stimulus and exponentials with decay rates parametrized by the eigenvalues. This representation persists as the number of compartments grows. In fact, it is the limiting case that permits exact, closed form, solution. In the case that input is delivered through changes in conductance rather than direct current injection our analytical techniques become unwieldy and we return to the trapezoid rule to build a time marching approximation scheme. This scheme permitted us to explore the interaction of synaptic input onto distinct spines.

Dendritic Cable Theory was developed by Wilfrid Rall, see Rall and Agmon-Snir (1998) for a modern survey and Segev et al. (1994) for the original papers. We have argued that the eigenvectors of the second difference matrix, **S**, and eigenfunctions of the second order differential operator, ∂_{xx}, permit us to represent the response of the cable to current stimuli. We will see in Exercise 16, that these eigenvectors, and values, also permit us to analyze the performance of the associated approximation schemes. The separation of space and time variables executed in §6.4 was pioneered by Fourier, Sturm, and Liouville. We will hear more from Fourier in Chapter 7. Redheffer and Port (1992) provides an excellent introduction to Sturm–Liouville theory. The cable equation is an instance of the well-studied heat, or diffusion, equation. As such, there exist a number of alternate approaches, e.g., Green's functions, that have been exploited by neuroscientists. We recommend Strauss (2007) for the mathematics and Tuckwell (1988) for the applications. The spine model of §6.5 is drawn from Baer and Rinzel (1991). For a rigorous presentation of the perturbation argument invoked in Exercise 4 to prove that **every** symmetric matrix in $\mathbb{R}^{N \times N}$ has N orthonormal eigenvectors, see §17.3 in Redheffer and Port (1992). For a deeper look at the Cholesky decomposition of Exercise 5 see Golub and van Loan (1996). The Weierstrass M-test for uniform convergence, Eq. (6.74), is proven in Redheffer and Port (1992). The determination of the cable parameters in Exercise 9 from moments of the end potential and current is drawn from Cox (1998). The summation identities, Eqs. (6.66), (6.69), and (6.72) are consequences of the Residue theorem, see Spiegel et al. (2009).

6.7 EXERCISES

1. Show that the N-by-N second difference matrix, S, is negative semidefinite by confirming the identity

$$\mathbf{u}^T \mathbf{S} \mathbf{u} = -\sum_{j=1}^{N-1} (u_j - u_{j+1})^2 / \mathrm{d}x^2.$$

2. Prove that the eigenvalues of a real symmetric matrix are real by following these steps. Suppose $\mathbf{A} = \mathbf{A}^T$ is real and that

$$\mathbf{A}\mathbf{u} = z\mathbf{u}. \tag{6.63}$$

   (i) Take the complex conjugate of each side and arrive at

$$\mathbf{A}\mathbf{u}^* = z^* \mathbf{u}^*. \tag{6.64}$$

   (ii) Multiply Eq. (6.63) by $\mathbf{u}^H \equiv (\mathbf{u}^*)^T$ and Eq. (6.64) by $\mathbf{u}^T$, and take the difference of the two resulting products and use the symmetry of $\mathbf{A}$ to reduce this difference to $0 = z - z^*$.

3. [†]Prove that the eigenvalues of a symmetric negative semidefinite matrix are nonpositive. Hint: Write $\mathbf{A}\mathbf{u} = z\mathbf{u}$ and multiply each side by $\mathbf{u}^T$.

4. [*](i) Prove that the eigenvectors, associated with distinct eigenvalues, of a symmetric matrix are orthogonal to one another by following these steps. Write $\mathbf{A}\mathbf{u}_1 = z_1 \mathbf{u}_1$ and $\mathbf{A}\mathbf{u}_2 = z_2 \mathbf{u}_2$ and suppose that $z_1 \neq z_2$. Now as above, multiply the former by $\mathbf{u}_2^T$ and the latter by $\mathbf{u}_1^T$, take the difference of the products and conclude that $0 = (z_1 - z_2)\mathbf{u}_1^T \mathbf{u}_2$.

   (ii) In the case that $\mathbf{A}$ does not possess distinct eigenvalues we note $\mathbf{A}$ must be very close to a symmetric matrix that does possess distinct eigenvalues. For example, the double eigenvalue of the 2×2 identity matrix stems from the degenerate characteristic polynomial $(1 - z)^2$ and is easily split by perturbing $\mathbf{I}$ to

$$\mathbf{I}_\varepsilon \equiv \begin{pmatrix} 1 & \varepsilon \\ \varepsilon & 1 \end{pmatrix}.$$

   Compute, by hand, its eigenvalues and eigenvectors and show that they converge, as $\varepsilon \to 0$, to the eigenvalue, and two orthogonal eigenvectors, of the 2×2 identity matrix.

5. [†]Given $\mathbf{A}\mathbf{u} = z\mathbf{u}$ and two constants, α and β, show that $\mathbf{u}$ is also an eigenvector of $\alpha \mathbf{I} + \beta \mathbf{A}$ and that $\alpha + \beta z$ is the associated eigenvalue. If $\mathbf{A}$ is also invertible explain how the eigenvalues and eigenvectors of $\mathbf{A}^{-1}$ may be determined by those of $\mathbf{A}$.

6. Use Eq. (6.13) to show that the $\mathbf{Q}$ defined in Eq. (6.15) indeed obeys $\mathbf{Q}^T = \mathbf{Q}^{-1}$.

7. If $\mathbf{A}$ is symmetric and positive definite then its LU factorization, recall Exercise 5.2, simplifies to $\mathbf{A} = \mathbf{L}\mathbf{L}^T$ where $\mathbf{L}$ is lower triangular, but not necessarily with ones on its diagonal. $\mathbf{A} = \mathbf{L}\mathbf{L}^T$ is known as the Cholesky factorization.

   (i) Show that any $\mathbf{A}$ may be written $\mathbf{A} = \mathbf{L}\mathbf{D}\mathbf{U}$ where $\mathbf{L}$ is lower triangular, $\mathbf{D}$ is diagonal, $\mathbf{U}$ is upper triangular, and both $\mathbf{L}$ and $\mathbf{U}$ have ones on their diagonal.

   (ii) If $\mathbf{A} = \mathbf{A}^T$ show that $\mathbf{L}\mathbf{D}\mathbf{U} = \mathbf{U}^T \mathbf{D} \mathbf{L}^T$ and then $\mathbf{L}^{-1}\mathbf{U}^T \mathbf{D} = \mathbf{D}\mathbf{U}\mathbf{L}^{-T}$.

   (iii) Observe, in this last equation, that the left is lower triangular while the right is upper triangular and so conclude that each side is diagonal. Given ones on the diagonals of $\mathbf{L}$ and $\mathbf{U}$ establish in fact that $\mathbf{L}^{-1}\mathbf{U}^T \mathbf{D} = \mathbf{D}$ and conclude that $\mathbf{U} = \mathbf{L}^T$ and $\mathbf{A} = \mathbf{L}\mathbf{D}\mathbf{L}^T$.

   (iv) If, in addition, $\mathbf{A}$ is positive definite conclude that each element of $\mathbf{D}$ is positive and so $\mathbf{D} = \mathbf{D}^{1/2}\mathbf{D}^{1/2}$ and $\mathbf{A} = (\mathbf{L}\mathbf{D}^{1/2})(\mathbf{L}\mathbf{D}^{1/2})^T$.

8. [†]Suppose that $\mathbf{A} \in \mathbb{R}^{n \times n}$ is symmetric and positive definite. If λ_1 and λ_n are its largest and smallest eigenvalues, respectively, then show that

$$\lambda_n \mathbf{x}^T \mathbf{x} \leq \mathbf{x}^T \mathbf{A} \mathbf{x} \leq \lambda_1 \mathbf{x}^T \mathbf{x} \quad \forall \, \mathbf{x} \in \mathbb{R}^n.$$

9. We now generalize the moment calculations of §3.2 to the cable.

   (i) First deduce from Eq. (6.45) that

$$M_0(v(0, \cdot)) = \frac{M_0(I_{stim})}{2\pi a C_m} \sum_{n=0}^{\infty} \frac{q_n^2(0)}{\zeta_n}. \tag{6.65}$$

Next define $L \equiv \ell/\lambda$ and use

$$\sum_{n=1}^{\infty} \frac{1}{c^2+n^2} = \frac{\pi}{2c}\coth(\pi c) - \frac{1}{2c^2} \tag{6.66}$$

to deduce that

$$\sum_{n=0}^{\infty} \frac{q_n^2(0)}{\zeta_n} = \frac{\tau}{\ell} + \frac{2\tau}{\ell}\sum_{n=1}^{\infty} \frac{1}{1+n^2\pi^2/L^2} = \frac{\tau}{\lambda}\coth(L)$$

and so conclude that

$$\boxed{\frac{M_0(v(0,\cdot))}{M_0(I_{stim})} = \frac{\coth(L)}{2\pi a\lambda g_{Cl}}.} \tag{6.67}$$

(ii) Deduce from Eq. (6.45) that

$$M_1(v(0,\cdot)) = \frac{M_1(I_{stim})}{2\pi aC_m}\sum_{n=0}^{\infty}\frac{q_n^2(0)}{\zeta_n} + \frac{M_0(I_{stim})}{2\pi aC_m}\sum_{n=0}^{\infty}\frac{q_n^2(0)}{\zeta_n^2} \tag{6.68}$$

and use

$$\sum_{n=1}^{\infty}\frac{1}{(c^2+n^2)^2} = \frac{\pi^2c+\pi\cosh(\pi c)\sinh(\pi c)}{4c^3\sinh^2(\pi c)} - \frac{1}{2c^4} \tag{6.69}$$

to evaluate

$$\sum_{n=0}^{\infty}\frac{q_n^2(0)}{\zeta_n^2} = \frac{\tau^2}{\ell}\left\{1+2\frac{L^4}{\pi^4}\sum_{n=1}^{\infty}\frac{1}{((L/\pi)^2+n^2)^2}\right\} = \frac{\tau^2}{\lambda}\frac{L+\cosh(L)\sinh(L)}{2\sinh^2(L)}$$

and so arrive at

$$\boxed{\frac{M_1(v(0,\cdot))}{M_0(v(0,\cdot))} - \frac{M_1(I_{stim})}{M_0(I_{stim})} = \frac{\tau}{2}\left(1+\frac{2L}{\sinh(2L)}\right).} \tag{6.70}$$

(iii) Finally, deduce from Eq. (6.45) that

$$M_2(v(0,\cdot)) = \frac{M_2(I_{stim})}{2\pi aC_m}\sum_{n=0}^{\infty}\frac{q_n^2(0)}{\zeta_n} + \frac{M_1(I_{stim})}{\pi aC_m}\sum_{n=0}^{\infty}\frac{q_n^2(0)}{\zeta_n^2} + \frac{M_0(I_{stim})}{\pi aC_m}\sum_{n=0}^{\infty}\frac{q_n^2(0)}{\zeta_n^3} \tag{6.71}$$

and use

$$\sum_{n=1}^{\infty}\frac{1}{(c^2+n^2)^3} = \frac{3\pi^2c+2\pi^3c^2\coth(\pi c)+(3/2)\sinh(2\pi c)}{16c^5\sinh^2(\pi c)} - \frac{1}{2c^6} \tag{6.72}$$

to evaluate

$$\sum_{n=0}^{\infty}\frac{q_n^2(0)}{\zeta_n^3} = \frac{\tau^3}{\lambda}\frac{3L+2L^2\coth(L)+(3/2)\sinh(2L)}{8\sinh^2(L)}.$$

Use this expression together with Eqs. (6.67) and (6.70) to write a single equation for L, namely

$$F(L) = \frac{M_2(v_0)/M_0(v_0) - M_2(I)/M_0(I) - 2\tau_c(I)(\tau_c(v_0)-\tau_c(I))}{(\tau_c(v_0)-\tau_c(I))^2}$$

where

$$F(L) \equiv \frac{\sinh^2(2L)}{(\sinh(2L)+2L)^2} \frac{3L\tanh(L)+2L^2+3\sinh^2(L)}{\sinh^2(L)}.$$

It follows that the first three moments of the stimulus and response uniquely determine L if their combination above strikes F where it is monotone. Over what interval is F monotone?

10. †Develop both $f(x+dx)$ and $f(x-dx)$ in Taylor series about x. Add these two series and conclude that

$$\frac{f(x+dx)-2f(x)+f(x-dx)}{dx^2} \to f''(x) \quad \text{as} \quad dx \to 0.$$

This justifies our passage from Eqs. (6.29) to (6.30).

11. To solve the steady-state cable equation, Eq. (6.32), we attempt the educated (linear equations are solved by exponentials) guess $v_\infty(x)=e^{\alpha x}$.
   (i) Insert this guess into Eq. (6.32), find that $\alpha=\pm 1/\lambda$, and deduce that $v_\infty(x)=c_1 e^{x/\lambda}+c_2 e^{-x/\lambda}$.
   (ii) Determine the values of the two constants c_1 and c_2 from the boundary conditions, Eq. (6.33).
   (iii) Confirm that your answer agrees with Eq. (6.34) where

$$\sinh(x) = \frac{e^x - e^{-x}}{2} \quad \text{and} \quad \cosh(x) = \frac{e^x + e^{-x}}{2}.$$

   Plot Eq. (6.34) and compare with Figure 6.3.

12. †We approach the eigenvalue problem, Eq. (6.37), via the same tack as that of the previous exercise.
   (i) Attempt $q(x)=\exp(\alpha x)$ and show that $q(x)=c_1\exp(\sqrt{\vartheta}x)+c_2\exp(-\sqrt{\vartheta}x)$.
   (ii) Show that $q'(0)=0$ translates into $c_1=c_2$ while $q'(\ell)=0$ requires that $\exp(2\sqrt{\vartheta}\ell)=1$. Argue that this requires $2\sqrt{\vartheta}\ell=i2\pi n$ for $n=0,1,2,\ldots$ and conclude that $\vartheta=-(n\pi/\ell)^2$.

13. Regarding the convergence of the infinite sum in Eq. (6.45), suppose that $I_{stim}^{max}=\max\{|I_{stim}(s)|;0\leq s\leq\infty\}$ and show that

$$\left|\int_0^t I_{stim}(s)\exp((t-s)\zeta_n)\,ds\right| \leq I_{stim}^{max}\int_0^t \exp((t-s)\zeta_n)\,ds \leq \frac{\tau I_{stim}^{max}}{1+(n\pi(\lambda/\ell))^2}. \tag{6.73}$$

Deduce from Eq. (6.66) that this sequence is summable. Finally, invoke the

Weierstrass M-Test. If each $v_n(x,t)$ obeys $\max\{|v_n(x,t)|:x\in[0,\ell],0\leq t\}\leq M_n$ and M_n is summable then there exists a function $v(x,t)$ such that given any $\varepsilon>0$ there exists an index N such that

$$\max_{x\in[0,\ell],0\leq t}\left|v(x,t)-\sum_{n=1}^m v_n(x,t)\right| \leq \varepsilon \tag{6.74}$$

whenever $m\geq N$.

In particular, use the Weierstrass M-test to conclude that the sum in Eq. (6.45) indeed converges. In this case we say that the sum of the v_n converges uniformly to v. As each v_n is continuous it then follows that so too is v, and although integrals of the v_n will sum to integrals of v the same cannot be said for derivatives. To see this, differentiate each side of Eq. (6.45) with respect x and then set $x=0$.

14. We now show that our analytical methods are general enough to accommodate an arbitrary spatio-temporal current stimulus, I ($\mu A/cm$). In particular, solve

$$\tau\frac{\partial v}{\partial t}(x,t)+v(x,t)-\lambda^2\frac{\partial^2 v}{\partial x^2}(x,t)=I(x,t)/(2\pi ag_{Cl}), \tag{6.75}$$

subject to $v_x(0,t)=v_x(\ell,t)=v(x,0)=0$ by mimicking our separation of variables argument. First show that p_n obeys

$$\tau p_n'(t)+(1+\lambda^2\vartheta_n)p_n(t)=I_n(t)/(2\pi ag_{Cl}), \quad p_n(0)=0, \tag{6.76}$$

where

$$I_n(t) = \int\limits_0^\ell I(x,t) q_n(x) \, dx. \tag{6.77}$$

You should then arrive at

$$v(x,t) = \sum_{n=0}^\infty \frac{q_n(x)}{C_m 2a\pi} \int\limits_0^t I_n(s) \exp((t-s)\zeta_n) \, ds. \tag{6.78}$$

Please show that if

$$I(x,t) = -\sqrt{2/\ell} \cos(\pi x/\ell)(e^{-t} - e^{-2t})/500 \tag{6.79}$$

then v is simply

$$v(x,t) = -\frac{\sqrt{2/\ell} \cos(\pi x/\ell)}{C_m 2a\pi} \frac{e^{-t}(\zeta_1 - 2) + e^{-2t}(1 - \zeta_1) + e^{-\zeta_1 t}}{500(\zeta_1 - 1)(\zeta_1 - 2)}. \tag{6.80}$$

Use `meshgrid` and `mesh` to illustrate this solution as in Figure 6.11.

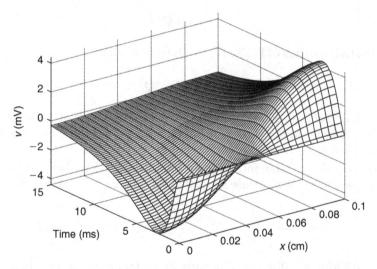

FIGURE 6.11   The graph of the v in Eq. (6.80) using passive parameters defined in Eq. Eq. (6.17). (pfibexact.m)

15. We show that our moment methods allow us to ascertain the location of synaptic input from indirect measurements. In particular, we suppose that v obeys Eq. (6.52) with sealed ends and that we have recorded both end potentials, $v(0,t)$ and $v(\ell,t)$.

(i) Define the left and right moments

$$M_L(x) \equiv \int\limits_0^\infty v(x,t) \, dt, \quad 0 \le x \le x_s \quad \text{and} \quad M_R(x) \equiv \int\limits_0^\infty v(x,t) \, dt, \quad x_s \le x \le \ell$$

and use Eq. (6.52) to conclude that $\lambda^2 M_L''(x) = M_L(x)$ and $\lambda^2 M_R''(x) = M_R(x)$.

(ii) Using known information about M_L at $x = 0$ and M_R at $x = \ell$ show that

$$M_L(x) = M_0(v(0,\cdot)) \cosh(x/\lambda) \quad \text{and}$$
$$M_R(x) = M_0(v(\ell,\cdot)) \cosh((\ell - x)/\lambda).$$

(iii) Explain why $M_L(x_s) = M_R(x_s)$ and use this to derive the following equation for x_s,

$$\sigma(x_s) \equiv \frac{\cosh((\ell - x_s)/\lambda)}{\cosh(x_s/\lambda)} = \frac{M_0(v(0, \cdot))}{M_0(v(\ell, \cdot))}. \tag{6.81}$$

Demonstrate that σ is a monotone function of x_s and hence that the end moments uniquely determine the site of synaptic input.

16. Let us investigate the stability of the unforced (i.e., without current or synaptic inputs) forward Euler scheme

$$v^j = (I + dtB)v^{j-1}.$$

As above, it follows that $v^j = (I - dtB)^{j-1}v^1$ and so we look for a condition on dt that will guarantee that $(I - dtB)^{j-1}$ remains bounded. We label this forward Euler matrix

$$F \equiv I + dtB = I + (dt/\tau)(\lambda^2 S - I)$$

and deduce from Exercise 5 that $Fq_n = \gamma_n q_n$ where the q_n are the eigenvectors of S and

$$\gamma_n = 1 + (dt/\tau)(\lambda^2 \theta_n - 1).$$

Show that if $\Gamma = \text{diag}(\gamma)$ then $FQ = Q\Gamma$ and moreover that

$$F = Q\Gamma Q^T. \tag{6.82}$$

We are now prepared to study powers of F. Use Eq. (6.82) to show that

$$F^{j-1} = Q\Gamma^{j-1}Q^T$$

and note that to raise a diagonal matrix to a power is simply to raise each of its elements to that power. Argue then that forward Euler is stable so long as $|\gamma_{N-1}|$, the magnitude of the largest eigenvalue of F, is less than 1. Use Eq. (6.51) to derive an explicit stability bound for dt.

17. [†]Few cables are uniform in shape. Most branches taper with distance from their cell body. In the compartmental case, if the radius of compartment n is a_n please show that the current balance, Eq. (6.5), takes the form

$$\frac{a_{n-1}^2 v_{n-1} - (a_{n-1}^2 + a_n^2)v_n + a_n^2 v_{n+1}}{2R_a dx^2} = a_n(C_m v'_n + g_{Cl}v_n). \tag{6.83}$$

Next show, that as $dx \to 0$ and $n \to \infty$ this takes the form of the tapered cable equation

$$\frac{\partial}{\partial x}\left(a^2(x)\frac{\partial v}{\partial x}(x,t)\right) = 2R_a a(x)\{C_m \frac{\partial v}{\partial t}(x,t) + g_{Cl}v(x,t)\}. \tag{6.84}$$

7

Fourier Series and Transforms

O U T L I N E

7.1 Fourier Series	87	7.4 Reconciling the Discrete and Continuous
7.2 The Discrete Fourier Transform	89	Fourier Transforms 95
7.3 The Continuous Fourier Transform	94	7.5 Summary and Sources 98
		7.6 Exercises 98

The series expansion and integral transform named after Joseph Fourier are powerful techniques for decomposing complex signals into simpler, and often biologically salient, components. These components are typically sine waves oscillating at a fixed frequency. We observed in §§5.2–5.5 that ion channels tune neurons to respond best to input delivered at a specific resonant frequency. The cochlea of the vertebrate inner ear in fact distributes its key receptors, called hair cells, such that their resonant frequencies increase steadily with distance from the auditory canal. In this way the cochlea generates a tonotopic map by decomposing the pressure wave arriving at the ear into its individual frequency components. We take a closer look at such hair cells in Exercise 13.3 and, in Chapters 20 and 21, study a number of cells in the visual pathway that are tuned to specific temporal and/or spatial frequencies of visual stimuli. In this chapter we present the mathematical and computational aspects of the Fourier analysis of signals, with particular emphasis on its role in convolution and its application to the cable equation.

7.1 FOURIER SERIES

The eigenfunctions of the passive sealed cable are cosine functions and the exact solution, Eq. (6.45), is an example of a Fourier cosine series. The cosines were "chosen" (as opposed to sines) by our sealed end conditions. In general, we will expand functions into combinations of both sines and cosines and so find it most convenient to begin with the complex exponentials

$$e^{2\pi i n x} = \cos(2\pi n x) + i \sin(2\pi n x). \tag{7.1}$$

For integers m and n these functions enjoy the orthogonality relation

$$\int_{-1/2}^{1/2} e^{2\pi i n x} e^{-2\pi i m x} \, dx = \int_{-1/2}^{1/2} e^{2\pi i (n-m)x} \, dx = \delta_{mn}, \tag{7.2}$$

Mathematics for Neuroscientists. DOI: 10.1016/B978-0-12-374882-9.00007-1

where δ_{mn} is the Kronecker delta of Eq. (1.4). For a function f with period 1, we develop it in a Fourier series

$$f(x) = \sum_{n=-\infty}^{\infty} \hat{f}_n e^{2\pi i n x} \tag{7.3}$$

and note that multiplication of each side by $e^{-2\pi i m x}$ followed by integration, thanks to Eq. (7.2), allows us to express the Fourier coefficients

$$\hat{f}_m = \int_{-1/2}^{1/2} f(x) e^{-2\pi i m x} \, dx. \tag{7.4}$$

For example, if $f(x) = \mathbb{1}_{(-a,a)}(x)$ is the characteristic function (recall Eq. (1.6)) of the interval $(-a,a)$ and $a = 1/(2\pi)$ then Eq. (7.4) yields

$$\hat{f}_m = \frac{\sin(m)}{m\pi} \quad \text{and so} \quad f(x) = \frac{1}{\pi} + 2\sum_{n=1}^{\infty} \frac{\sin(n)}{n\pi} \cos(2\pi n x). \tag{7.5}$$

As this step narrows and grows in height, i.e., as $a \to 0$ and $f(x) = \mathbb{1}_{(-a,a)}(x)/(2a)$, we arrive at the Dirac delta function $f(x) = \delta(x)$ of Eq. (3.6). In this case Eq. (7.4) reveals

$$\hat{f}_m = 1 \quad \text{and so} \quad \delta(x) = 1 + 2\sum_{n=1}^{\infty} \cos(2\pi n x). \tag{7.6}$$

It is natural to ask in what sense, and at what rate, these series expansions approach their limits. We truncate both sums at the Nth term and plot the results in Figure 7.1.

The partial sum in the expansion of the Dirac delta is in fact amenable to hand calculation. In particular, we will establish in Exercise 1 that

$$1 + 2\sum_{n=1}^{N} \cos(2\pi n x) = \frac{\sin((N+1/2)2\pi x)}{\sin(\pi x)} \tag{7.7}$$

and so find Eq. (7.6) equivalent to

$$\lim_{N\to\infty} \frac{\sin((N+1/2)2\pi x)}{\sin(\pi x)} = \delta(x). \tag{7.8}$$

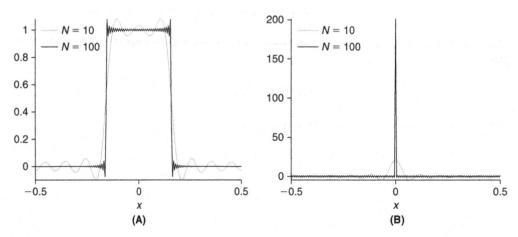

FIGURE 7.1   Fourier series representations of the step (**A**) and the Dirac delta function (**B**) upon truncation of Eq. (7.5) and Eq. (7.6) at the levels indicated in the respective legends. (`fourierex2.m`)

We next examine the interaction of two Fourier expansions. In particular, if

$$f(x) = \sum_{n=-\infty}^{\infty} \hat{f}_n e^{2\pi i n x} \quad \text{and} \quad g(x) = \sum_{n=-\infty}^{\infty} \hat{g}_n e^{2\pi i n x}$$

then we arrive, on exchanging the order of integration and summation, at the so-called reciprocity formula,

$$\int_{-1/2}^{1/2} f(x)g(x)\,dx = \int_{-1/2}^{1/2} f(x) \sum_{n=-\infty}^{\infty} \hat{g}_n e^{2\pi i n x}\,dx = \sum_{n=-\infty}^{\infty} \hat{g}_n \int_{-1/2}^{1/2} f(x)e^{2\pi i n x}\,dx = \sum_{n=-\infty}^{\infty} \hat{g}_n \hat{f}_{-n}. \tag{7.9}$$

From this formula we will derive, in Exercises 2 and 3, two very important special cases, namely Parseval's identity,

$$\boxed{\int_{-1/2}^{1/2} |f(x)|^2\,dx = \sum_{n=-\infty}^{\infty} |\hat{f}_n|^2} \tag{7.10}$$

and the Convolution Theorem

$$\boxed{(f \star g)(y) \equiv \int_{-1/2}^{1/2} f(x)g(y-x)\,dx = \sum_{n=-\infty}^{\infty} \hat{f}_n \hat{g}_n e^{2\pi i n y}.} \tag{7.11}$$

Parseval's identity is often interpreted as conservation of energy or information between the original and Fourier representation of f, while the Convolution Theorem reveals that the Fourier coefficients of the convolution of two functions, f and g, are simply the products of the Fourier coefficients of f and g.

7.2 THE DISCRETE FOURIER TRANSFORM

If we truncate the sum, as well as discretize our interval, in the Fourier expansion, Eq. (7.3), we arrive at the discrete Fourier transform. Let us first, however, permit more general intervals and periods. To be precise, we suppose a signal u to have period T, i.e., $u(t+T) = u(t)$ for each t and that we have sampled the signal at an even number, N, of equally spaced instants in time. In particular, $dt \equiv T/N$, $t_m = m\,dt$, and $u_m \equiv u(t_m)$. We now attempt to develop u in a discrete Fourier series of the form

$$u(t_m) = \frac{1}{N} \sum_{n=0}^{N-1} c_n \exp(2\pi i n t_m/T). \tag{7.12}$$

On defining

$$w \equiv \exp(2\pi i/N)$$

and using the relation $m = t_m T/N$, we note that Eq. (7.12) takes the very simple form,

$$\frac{1}{N} \sum_{n=0}^{N-1} w^{mn} c_n = u_m. \tag{7.13}$$

This in turn may be written as the matrix equation

$$\frac{1}{N} \mathbf{Fc} = \mathbf{u} \tag{7.14}$$

where, noting that $w^N = 1$,

$$\mathbf{F} = \begin{pmatrix} 1 & 1 & 1 & \cdot & 1 \\ 1 & w & w^2 & \cdot & w^{N-1} \\ 1 & w^2 & w^4 & \cdot & w^{2(N-1)} \\ \cdot & \cdot & \cdot & & \cdot \\ 1 & w^{N-1} & w^{2(N-1)} & \cdot & w^{(N-1)^2} \end{pmatrix}. \tag{7.15}$$

We now exploit this very special structure of $\mathbf{F}$ and arrive at an elegant solution to Eq. (7.14). To begin we examine the jk element of $\mathbf{F}^H\mathbf{F}$, i.e., row j of $\mathbf{F}^H$ (the conjugate transpose of $\mathbf{F}$) times column k of $\mathbf{F}$,

$$(\mathbf{F}^H\mathbf{F})_{jk} = 1 \cdot 1 + (w^*)^{j-1}w^{k-1} + (w^*)^{2(j-1)}w^{2(k-1)} + \cdots + (w^*)^{(N-1)(j-1)}w^{(N-1)(k-1)}.$$

If $j = k$ then $(w^*)^{m(j-1)}w^{m(k-1)} = \exp(-2\pi i m(j-1))\exp(2\pi i m(j-1)) = 1$ for each m and $(\mathbf{F}^H\mathbf{F})_{jj} = N$. If $j \neq k$ we let $z = (w^*)^{(j-1)}w^{(k-1)}$ and find the finite geometric series

$$(\mathbf{F}^H\mathbf{F})_{jk} = 1 + z + z^2 + \cdots + z^{N-1} = \frac{1-z^N}{1-z} = 0, \tag{7.16}$$

where the final equality stems from $z^N = 1$. Gathering the above computations, we have shown that

$$\mathbf{F}^H\mathbf{F} = N\mathbf{I} \quad \text{and so} \quad \mathbf{F}^{-1} = \frac{1}{N}\mathbf{F}^H \quad \text{and} \quad \mathbf{c} = \mathbf{F}^H\mathbf{u} \tag{7.17}$$

is the solution to Eq. (7.14). We speak of $\mathbf{c}$ as the discrete Fourier transform of $\mathbf{u}$, and to make the connection clear we often write $\hat{\mathbf{u}}$ for $\mathbf{c}$. With this convention, the latter equation in (7.17) may be expressed in component form as

$$\hat{u}_m = c_m = \sum_{n=0}^{N-1} (w^*)^{mn}u_n = \sum_{n=0}^{N-1} e^{-2\pi i mn/N}u_n = \sum_{n=0}^{N-1} e^{-2\pi i \omega_m t_n}u(t_n) \tag{7.18}$$

where $\omega_m = m/T$ is the associated discrete frequency. The best implementations of Eq. (7.18) take still further advantage of the gorgeous structure of the Fourier matrix, $\mathbf{F}$, and assume that N is a power of 2, i.e., $N = 2^M$. The resulting algorithm is known as the fast Fourier transform, or fft in MATLAB. The choice, however, of whether to place the dimension, N, in the forward or inverse transform, is implementation dependent. Our Eq. (7.18) matches the definition uhat = fft(u) in MATLAB. We illustrate the computation of the fast Fourier transform with a small data set in Figure 7.2.

We observe from Figure 7.2B, and then confirm using Eq. (7.18), that

$$\hat{u}_{N/2+j} = \hat{u}_{N/2-j}^*, \quad j = 1, 2, \ldots, N/2 - 1, \tag{7.19}$$

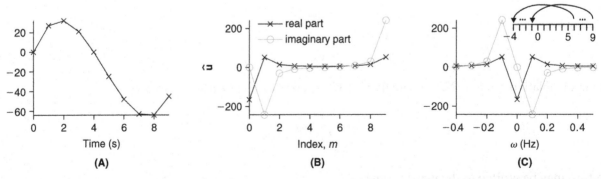

FIGURE 7.2   **A.** $N = 10$ samples of $u(t) = t(4-t)(10-t)$ on the interval $[0, T = 10]$. **B.** The real and imaginary components of its discrete Fourier transform, as a function of the index, m. **C.** As in **B** but now with zero frequency centered by circshift. The numerical index in **B** is now replaced by true frequency, $\omega_m = m/T$ where $m = -N/2 + 1 : N/2$. The inset illustrates how indices corresponding to frequencies above the Nyquist frequency, $1/2$, are wrapped around. (fftexcoarse2.m)

since u is real (Exercise 13). More generally, Eq. (7.18) implies that the discrete Fourier transform is periodic, $\hat{u}_{-j} = \hat{u}_{N-j}$, $j = 1, \ldots, N/2 + 1$. For graphical purposes the latter half of the frequency content is typically wrapped around to the "front" of the vector. This is done via `fftshift` or `circshift` in MATLAB, which center the discrete Fourier transform around zero frequency and so permit a monotonic ordering of the true frequency

$$\omega_m = m/T, \quad m = -N/2 + 1, \ldots, -1, 0, 1, \ldots, N/2 - 1, N/2.$$

These considerations should also explain the common practice of only presenting the real and imaginary parts of $\hat{u}_0$ through $\hat{u}_{N/2}$. The example in Figure 7.2 also suggests that we should be careful to choose enough sample points to properly capture the full frequency content of the data. More precisely, if the signal possesses oscillations up to a frequency of ω_{max}, then one needs at least two samples in each interval of length $1/\omega_{max}$. In other words, we require $N \geq 2\omega_{max}T$ samples in the full interval $[0, T]$. The number $2\omega_{max}$ is known as the Nyquist rate. We offer a concrete example in Figure 7.3.

We next note that it follows immediately from Eq. (7.17) that one may recover $\mathbf{u}$ from its discrete Fourier transform via

$$\mathbf{u} = \frac{1}{N}\mathbf{F}\hat{\mathbf{u}}. \tag{7.20}$$

We therefore refer to application by $(1/N)\mathbf{F}$ as the inverse discrete Fourier transform. In MATLAB this is achieved by the `ifft` function. We next consider a common application of this transform pair.

The band-pass filter. We suppose that our signal has been corrupted by noise in a known frequency band. We mask this band and so clean our dirty signal via the sequence of transformations

$$\mathbf{u}_{clean} = \mathbf{FMF}^{-1}\mathbf{u}_{dirty}$$

where $\mathbf{M}$ is the "mask" matrix. In the simplest case $\mathbf{M}$ is the identity matrix with ones masked by zeros if their indices jibe with unwanted frequencies. In the low-pass case we specify a cut-off frequency, ω_{cut}, and then simply zero out

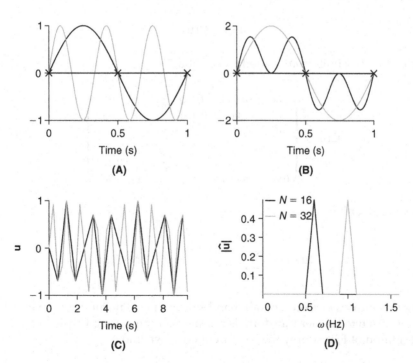

FIGURE 7.3 Illustration of the aliasing phenomenon. **A.** If $f(t) = \sin(2\pi t)$ (black) is sampled at intervals $dt = 0.5$ s (black crosses), it is indistinguishable from $g(t) = \sin(2\pi(3t))$ (red line). **B.** Similarly $f(t) + g(t)$ (black) is indistinguishable from $2f(t)$ at the same sampling points. **C, D.** Sampling $u(t) = \sin(2\pi t)$ on either side of the Nyquist rate. Here $\omega_{max} = 1$ and $T = 10$ and so we need 20 samples to reliably capture its frequency content. Sampling u with 16 or 32 samples (**C**) and magnitude of the respective discrete Fourier transforms (**D**). We recognize the black peak, associated with the undersampled signal, as an "alias" of the red, oversampled signal. (`aliascombined.m`)

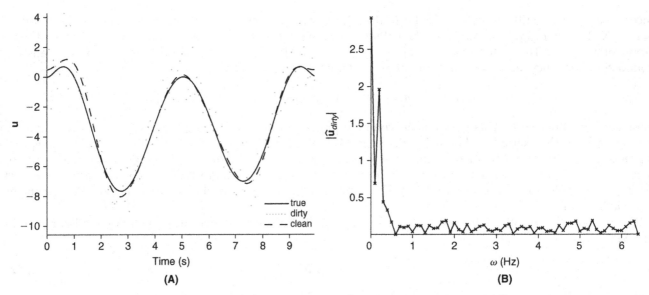

FIGURE 7.4   Low-pass filtering of $u_{dirty}(t) = u_{true}(t) + v(t)$ where $u_{true} = t^2(1-t)(5-t)(5.1-t)(9-t)(10-t)^2/3000$ and the noise, v, is drawn from the standard normal distribution. **A.** The true, dirty, and cleaned signals with $N = 128$ samples and a cut-off frequency $\omega_{cut} = 0.5$ Hz. **B.** The frequency content of the dirty signal. (fftexfine.m)

the elements of $\hat{\mathbf{u}}_{dirty}$ associated with frequencies in excess of ω_{cut}. A discrete frequency version of this is spelled out in fftexfine.m and illustrated in Figure 7.4.

Discrete convolution. We have seen in §3.3 and §7.1 that both the Laplace transform and Fourier series turned convolutions into products. We now develop the discrete analog. As the convolution of two functions is the integral of a shifted product we define the convolution of two vectors $\mathbf{u}$ and $\mathbf{v}$ to be

$$\mathbf{u} \star \mathbf{v} \equiv \mathbf{C(u)v}$$

where $\mathbf{C(u)}$ is the **circulant** matrix built from shifted copies of $\mathbf{u}$, i.e.,

$$\mathbf{C(u)} = \begin{pmatrix} u_0 & u_{N-1} & u_{N-2} & \cdot & \cdot & u_1 \\ u_1 & u_0 & u_{N-1} & \cdot & \cdot & u_2 \\ u_2 & u_1 & u_0 & \cdot & \cdot & \cdot \\ \cdot & \cdot & \cdot & \cdot & \cdot & \cdot \\ \cdot & \cdot & \cdot & \cdot & \cdot & u_{N-1} \\ u_{N-1} & u_{N-2} & \cdot & \cdot & u_1 & u_0 \end{pmatrix}. \tag{7.21}$$

The components of $\mathbf{u} \star \mathbf{v}$ are given by

$$(\mathbf{u} \star \mathbf{v})_l = \sum_{k=0}^{N-1} u_{l-k} v_k, \quad l = 0, \ldots, N-1,$$

with the understanding that indices $l - k$ on the right hand side are periodic modulo N, i.e., $-1 \to N-1$, $-2 \to N-2$, etc. The connection to the discrete Fourier transform is revealed on computing $\mathbf{C(u)F}$. Let us take this one column at a time. As $\mathbf{F}_{:,1}$, the first column of $\mathbf{F}$, is simply the column of ones, we find

$$\mathbf{C(u)F}_{:,1} = \mathbf{F}_{:,1} \sum_{n=0}^{N-1} u_n = \mathbf{F}_{:,1} \hat{u}_0.$$

The second column requires more care,

$$\mathbf{C}(\mathbf{u})\mathbf{F}_{:,2} = \begin{pmatrix} u_0 + wu_{N-1} + w^2 u_{N-2} + \cdots + w^{N-1} u_1 \\ u_1 + wu_0 + w^2 u_{N-1} + \cdots + w^{N-1} u_2 \\ u_2 + wu_1 + w^2 u_0 + \cdots + w^{N-1} u_3 \\ \cdots \\ u_{N-1} + wu_{N-2} + w^2 u_{N-3} + \cdots + w^{N-1} u_0 \end{pmatrix}. \tag{7.22}$$

Each of these rows on the right hand side of Eq. (7.22) resemble scrambled version of $\hat{u}_1$. To unscramble we need only (see Exercise 7)

$$ww^* = 1 \quad \text{and} \quad w^{N-j} = (w^*)^j. \tag{7.23}$$

In particular, this permits us to recognize the first row in Eq. (7.22) as

$$u_0 + (w^*)^{N-1} u_{N-1} + (w^*)^{N-2} u_{N-2} + \cdots + w^* u_1 = \hat{u}_1.$$

In the second row of Eq. (7.22) we find u_0 scaled by w and so we factor

$$w(w^* u_1 + u_0 + w^* w^2 u_{N-1} + \cdots + w^* w^{N-1} u_2) = w(w^* u_1 + u_0 + (w^*)^{N-1} u_{N-1} + \cdots + (w^*)^2 u_2) = w\hat{u}_1.$$

In the third row in Eq. (7.22) we find u_0 scaled by w^2 and so we find $w^2 (\mathbf{C}(\mathbf{u})\mathbf{F}_{:,2})_3 = w^2 \hat{u}_1$. This pattern continues and so

$$\mathbf{C}(\mathbf{u})\mathbf{F}_{:,2} = \mathbf{F}_{:,2}\hat{u}_1.$$

As subsequent columns of $\mathbf{F}$ are simply powers of its second column we find

$$\mathbf{C}(\mathbf{u})\mathbf{F}_{:,n} = \mathbf{F}_{:,n}\hat{u}_{n-1}. \tag{7.24}$$

That is, the nth column of $\mathbf{F}$ is an eigenvector of $\mathbf{C}(\mathbf{u})$ and its associated eigenvalue is $\hat{u}_{n-1}$. We may collect these into

$$\mathbf{C}(\mathbf{u})\mathbf{F} = \mathbf{F}\,\text{diag}\,(\hat{\mathbf{u}}).$$

Multiplying on the right by $\mathbf{F}^{-1}$ reveals $\mathbf{C}(\mathbf{u}) = \mathbf{F}\,\text{diag}\,(\hat{\mathbf{u}})\mathbf{F}^{-1}$ and so

$$\widehat{\mathbf{u} \star \mathbf{v}} = \mathbf{F}^{-1}\mathbf{C}(\mathbf{u})\mathbf{v} = \text{diag}\,(\hat{\mathbf{u}})\mathbf{F}^{-1}\mathbf{v} = \hat{\mathbf{u}}\hat{\mathbf{v}}$$

where the final product is elementwise. This is the discrete Convolution Theorem. As a simple application of these ideas let us consider the "autaptic" cable.

The discrete cable of length ℓ and N compartments that loops back on itself produces the circulant second difference matrix, of the form Eq. (7.21),

$$\mathbf{S}^o = \frac{1}{\mathrm{d}x^2} \begin{pmatrix} -2 & 1 & 0 & \cdot & 0 & 1 \\ 1 & -2 & 1 & 0 & \cdot & 0 \\ 0 & 1 & -2 & 1 & \cdot & 0 \\ \cdot & \cdot & \cdot & \cdot & \cdot & \cdot \\ 0 & \cdot & 0 & 1 & -2 & 1 \\ 1 & 0 & \cdot & 0 & 1 & -2 \end{pmatrix}$$

where $dx = \ell/N$. It follows from Eq. (7.24) that the eigenvalues of $\mathbf{S}^o$ are simply the discrete Fourier transform of the first column of $\mathbf{S}^o$. That is

$$
\begin{aligned}
\theta_n^o &= \frac{-2 + \exp(-2\pi i n dx/\ell) + \exp(-2\pi i n (N-1)dx/\ell)}{dx^2} \\
&= \frac{\exp(-2\pi i n/N) + \exp(2\pi i n/N) - 2}{dx^2} \\
&= -4(N/\ell)^2 \sin^2(n\pi/N), \quad n = 0,1,\ldots,N-1.
\end{aligned}
$$

The bulk of these are double eigenvalues, for $\theta_n^o = \theta_{N-n}^o$ when $n = 1,2,\ldots,N/2-1$. In addition, for such n we note that $\theta_n^o < \theta_n$ where θ_n (recall Eq. (6.51)) is the nth eigenvalue of the sealed cable. As a result, the same stimulus delivered to both the sealed and autaptic cables (of the same length, radii and space, and time constants) will decay faster in the latter than the former.

7.3 THE CONTINUOUS FOURIER TRANSFORM

Given the expansion, Eq. (7.3), of a 2π-periodic function in terms of an infinite sum of oscillating exponentials, it seems natural to attempt to represent a general, nonperiodic, function, u, in the form

$$
u(t) = \int_{-\infty}^{\infty} \hat{u}(\xi) e^{2\pi i \xi t} \, d\xi \tag{7.25}
$$

for some function $\hat{u}$. To uncover this $\hat{u}$ we multiply each side by $\exp(-2\pi i \omega t)$ and integrate in t over the finite interval $[-T, T]$. This brings

$$
\begin{aligned}
\int_{-T}^{T} e^{-2\pi i \omega t} u(t) \, dt &= \int_{-T}^{T} \int_{-\infty}^{\infty} \hat{u}(\xi) e^{2\pi i (\xi - \omega) t} \, d\xi \, dt \\
&= \int_{-\infty}^{\infty} \hat{u}(\xi) \int_{-T}^{T} e^{2\pi i (\xi - \omega) t} \, dt \, d\xi \\
&= \int_{-\infty}^{\infty} \hat{u}(\xi) \frac{\sin(2\pi T(\xi - \omega))}{\pi(\xi - \omega)} \, d\xi.
\end{aligned}
$$

It remains to let $T \to \infty$. Here we note that

$$
\lim_{T \to \infty} \frac{\sin(2\pi T(\xi - \omega))}{\pi(\xi - \omega)} \to \delta(\xi - \omega)
$$

in the same sense as Eq. (7.8). Recalling the fundamental properties of the delta function, Eq. (3.6), we find

$$
\hat{u}(\omega) = \int_{-\infty}^{\infty} e^{-2\pi i \omega t} u(t) \, dt \tag{7.26}
$$

and we speak of $\hat{u}$ as the Fourier transform of u. It follows that the inverse Fourier transform is given by Eq. (7.25). Note that the choice of the sign in the exponential $\exp(-2\pi i \omega t)$ is arbitrary, as is the inclusion of the factor 2π in the exponent. Our definition allows a simple transition from continuous to discrete transforms, as explained in the next section. Regarding examples, we note that the Fourier transform of the constant function was implicitly computed above. To make it explicit, $u(t) = a$ has the Fourier transform

$$
a \int_{-\infty}^{\infty} e^{-2\pi i \omega t} \, dt = a \lim_{T \to \infty} \int_{-T}^{T} e^{-2\pi i \omega t} \, dt = a \lim_{T \to \infty} \frac{\sin(2\pi \omega T)}{\pi \omega} = a\delta(\omega). \tag{7.27}
$$

If instead u is the scaled pulse

$$u(t) = \frac{\mathbb{1}_{(-a,a)}(t)}{2a}, \quad \text{then} \quad \hat{u}(\omega) = \frac{1}{2a}\int_{-a}^{a} e^{-2\pi i\omega t}\,dt = \frac{\sin(2\pi\omega a)}{2\pi\omega a}.$$

In the limit as $a \to 0$ this reveals

$$u(t) = \delta(t) \quad \text{and} \quad \hat{u}(\omega) = 1.$$

From here one may argue, precisely as in §3.3, that the Fourier transform, like the Laplace transform, is well suited to differentiation and convolution. Namely, the Fourier transform of the derivative of a function is simply $2\pi i\omega$ times the Fourier transform of that function,

$$\widehat{u'}(\omega) = 2\pi i\omega\hat{u}(\omega), \tag{7.28}$$

and the Fourier transform of a convolution of two functions is the product of their Fourier transforms,

$$\widehat{u \star v} = \hat{u}\hat{v}. \tag{7.29}$$

7.4 RECONCILING THE DISCRETE AND CONTINUOUS FOURIER TRANSFORMS

We now derive a numerical estimate of the continuous Fourier transform of a function $g(t)$ defined over $\mathbb{R}$, based on the results from the previous sections. The first step is to select an interval $[-T/2, T/2]$ over which the function will be discretized. If g is different from zero only over a finite interval $[a, b]$, then any choice of $T/2 > \max(|a|, |b|)$ will do. Otherwise, the value of T needs to be sufficiently large to include a "representative" sample of g, and its selection may require some experimentation. The next step is to select a discretization step h so as to define the discrete samples

$$g_j = g(-T/2 + t_j), \qquad t_j = jh, \, j = 0, \ldots, N-1.$$

The step h determines the Nyquist frequency $\omega_{Nyquist} = 1/(2h)$ above which frequencies will be folded over to lower ones, as explained in §7.2. Therefore, h needs to be small enough that the frequency components of g above $\omega_{Nyquist}$ are negligible. When a continuous waveform like the membrane potential of a neuron is recorded experimentally, this is achieved by low-pass filtering to zero any component above the Nyquist frequency before sampling. Note that the Nyquist frequency is half the sampling frequency $\omega_s = 1/h$. The sampling step in the frequency domain is given by $d\omega = 1/(Nh)$ and the frequency samples by $\omega_k = kd\omega$, $k = 0, \ldots, N-1$. As explained in §7.2, frequencies above the Nyquist frequency correspond to negative frequencies greater than $-\omega_{Nyquist}$ through the correspondence $\hat{g}_{-j} = \hat{g}_{N-j}$ for $j = 1, \ldots, (N/2) - 1$.

We now apply the trapezoid rule to the continuous definition of $\hat{g}(\omega_k)$

$$\hat{g}(\omega_k) = \int_{-\infty}^{\infty} g(t)e^{-2\pi i\omega_k t}\,dt \approx \int_{-T/2}^{T/2} g(t)e^{-2\pi i\omega_k t}\,dt$$

$$\approx e^{2\pi i\omega_k T/2}\sum_{j=0}^{N-1} g_j e^{-2\pi i\omega_k t_j}(t_{j+1} - t_j) = e^{\pi ik}h\sum_{j=0}^{N-1} g_j e^{-2\pi kj/N}.$$

Thus, we see that the continuous Fourier transform $\hat{g}(\omega_k)$ is approximated by the discrete transform $\hat{g}_k$ via $\hat{g}(\omega_k) \approx he^{\pi ik}\hat{g}_k$. The phase factor $e^{\pi ik}$ stems from our choice of the time origin at $-T/2$, and would equal one if our time origin was $T = 0$. As an application of the mixing of discrete and continuous Fourier transforms we finish the work begun in Exercise 6.15.

*Recovery of a synaptic conductance from end potentials.** Recall that with respect to the passive sealed cable with synaptic input at x_s, i.e.,

$$\lambda^2 v_{xx} = \tau v_t + v + c_{syn}(t)\delta(x - x_s)(v - v_{syn}),$$ (7.30)

we showed that x_s may be determined by knowledge of the "strength" of the associated end potentials,

$$v(0,t) \equiv v_0(t) \quad \text{and} \quad v(\ell,t) \equiv v_1(t).$$

We will now use the Fourier transforms of v_0 and v_1 to determine the time course, $c_{syn}(t)$, of the normalized synaptic conductance. To begin, we integrate Eq. (7.30) over a vanishingly small interval about x_s, use the fundamental properties, Eq. (3.6), of the Dirac delta function, and arrive at the representation

$$c_{syn}(t) = \lambda^2 \frac{v_x(x_s^+,t) - v_x(x_s^-,t)}{v(x_s,t) - v_{syn}}$$ (7.31)

of the unknown time course. We now use the Fourier transform to propagate the known end potentials inward to the known synaptic location and so arrive at the quantities on the right side of Eq. (7.31). As in Exercise 6.15 we start from the left and note that v satisfies

$$\lambda^2 v_{xx} = \tau v_t + v, \quad 0 < x < x_s, \quad v(0,t) = v_0(t), \ v_x(0,t) = 0.$$

On taking the Fourier transform of each side we find that

$$\hat{v}(x,\omega) = \int_0^\infty v(x,t)\exp(-2\pi i t\omega)\,dt,$$

obeys the ordinary differential equation

$$\lambda^2 \hat{v}_{xx}(x,\omega) = (2\pi i \tau\omega + 1)\hat{v}(x,\omega) \quad 0 < x < x_s, \quad \hat{v}(0,\omega) = \hat{v}_0(\omega), \quad \hat{v}_x(0,\omega) = 0.$$ (7.32)

We have used the derivative rule, Eq. (7.28), for differentiation in t and the fact that differentiation in x may pass untouched through integration in t. We next set $\mu(\omega) \equiv \sqrt{1 + 2\pi i \tau\omega}/\lambda$ and argue, as in Exercise 6.11, that $\hat{v}$ has the exact solution

$$\hat{v}(x,\omega) = \hat{v}_0(\omega)\cosh(x\mu(\omega)), \quad 0 < x < x_s.$$ (7.33)

We may now differentiate this in x and arrive at (the Fourier transform) of the necessary flux

$$\hat{v}_x(x,\omega) = \hat{v}_0(\omega)\mu(\omega)\sinh(x\mu(\omega)), \quad 0 < x < x_s.$$ (7.34)

It remains only to invert these transforms. As high frequency noise in the measurement of v_0 may undermine this transform we introduce a cut-off frequency, Ω, in our representation

$$v(x_s,t) = \int_{-\Omega}^{\Omega} \hat{v}_0(\omega)\cosh(x_s\mu(\omega))\exp(2\pi i t\omega)\,d\omega,$$

$$v_x(x_s^-,t) = \int_{-\Omega}^{\Omega} \hat{v}_0(\omega)\mu(\omega)\sinh(x_s\mu(\omega))\exp(2\pi i t\omega)\,d\omega.$$ (7.35)

The choice of Ω is dictated by examination of the frequency content of the measured end potentials. In a similar fashion the transformed (distal) cable equation reads

$$\lambda^2 \hat{v}_{xx}(x,\omega) = (2\pi i \tau\omega + 1)\hat{v}(x,\omega) \quad x_s < x < \ell, \quad \hat{v}(\ell,\omega) = \hat{v}_1(\omega), \quad \hat{v}_x(\ell,\omega) = 0,$$

and so, arguing as above,

$$\hat{v}(x,\omega) = \hat{v}_1(\omega)\cosh((\ell - x)\mu(\omega)),$$

from which we deduce that

$$v(x_s, t) = \int_{-\Omega}^{\Omega} \hat{v}_1(\omega)\cosh((\ell - x_s)\mu(\omega))\exp(2\pi it\omega)\,d\omega,$$

(7.36)

$$v_x(x_s^+, t) = \int_{-\Omega}^{\Omega} \hat{v}_1(\omega)\mu(\omega)\sinh((\ell - x_s)\mu(\omega))\exp(2\pi it\omega)\,d\omega.$$

We compute the quantities in Eqs. (7.35) and (7.36) in the manner discussed in our band-pass example. Namely, $\mathbf{FMF}^{-1}$, where the mask matrix implements low-pass filtered discrete versions of $\cosh(x_s\mu(\omega))$, $\mu(\omega)\sinh(x_s\mu(\omega))$, and $\mu(\omega)\sinh((\ell - x_s)\mu(\omega))$. We have coded this in `trapcabsyninv.m` and illustrated its use in Figure 7.5.

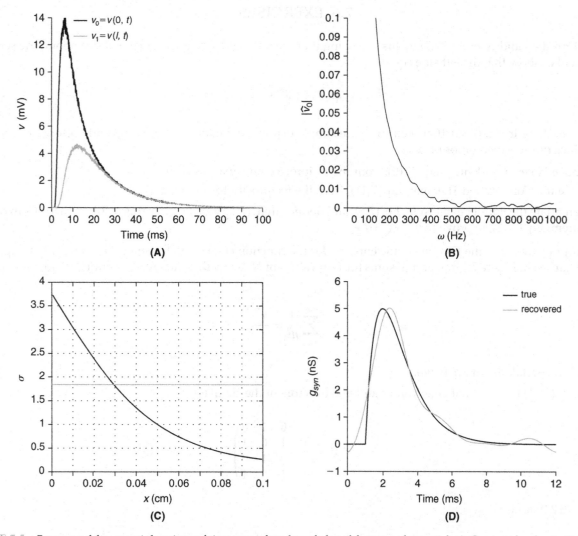

FIGURE 7.5   Recovery of the synaptic location and time course from knowledge of the two end potentials. **A.** Computed end potentials, sullied by multiplicative Gaussian noise, for the cable described by Eq. (6.17) with an α-synapse at $x_s = 0.03$ cm with $\overline{g}_{syn} = 5$ nA and $\tau_\alpha = 1$ ms. **B.** The magnitude of the Fourier transform of the end potential. This suggests a cut-off frequency near 350 Hz. **C.** The σ-function (black) and the computed strength ratio (red) cross at the synapse location as predicted by Eq. (6.81). **D.** The true g_{syn} and that recovered through Eqs. (7.31), (7.35), and (7.36) using a cut-off frequency of $\Omega = 350$ Hz. (`trapcabsyninv.m`)

7.5 SUMMARY AND SOURCES

We have defined Fourier series and transforms, considered numerous analytical as well as computational examples, derived their most basic properties and offered a taste of their applicability to neuroscience data and models. We will see many more examples in the chapters to come. In particular, we will see in Chapter 16 how Fourier methods can be extended to study random functions and in Chapters 20 and 21 how Fourier transforms are applied to characterize the receptive fields of sensory neurons. The role of the cochlea in discerning the frequency components of sound is expounded in the text of von Bekesy (1960). He was awarded the 1961 Nobel Prize in Physiology or Medicine for his contributions to these discoveries. Our application of Fourier analysis to the estimation of the time course of distal synaptic conductance is drawn from Cox (2004). Regarding the analytical scope of these tools, we note that convergence of the Fourier series, Eq. (7.3), is not well defined for functions with unbounded oscillations and that convergence of the Fourier transform, Eq. (7.26), is not well defined for functions that do not decay sufficiently fast at ∞. These matters are resolved in Pinsky (2002). For a detailed treatment of Fourier transforms and series, see also Rudin (1991) and Zygmund (1959). See Briggs and Henson (1987) for further development of the discrete Fourier transform. See Strauss (2007) for an introduction to distributions and their derivatives, as briefly touched upon in Exercises 20 and 21 below. Further references include Rudin (1991) or the original work of Schwartz (1966).

7.6 EXERCISES

1. Confirm the validity of Eq. (7.7) by first showing that the left hand side is proportional to a geometric series. In particular, show that the left side equals

$$e^{-2\pi i N x}(1+e^{2\pi i x}+e^{2\pi i 2x}+\cdots+e^{2\pi i 2N x}).$$

Now recall, as in Eq. (7.16), that such sums are simply expressed. Finally, multiply top and bottom by $e^{-2\pi i x/2}$ to produce the specified ratios of sines.

2. [†]Deduce Parseval's identity, Eq. (7.10), from the reciprocity formula, Eq. (7.9).

3. Deduce the Convolution Theorem, Eq. (7.11), from the reciprocity formula, Eq. (7.9).

4. Differentiate the Fourier expansion, Eq. (7.3), and deduce that, $\widehat{(f')}_n = 2\pi i n \hat{f}_n$. Use this result with the Convolution Theorem, Eq. (7.11), to prove that $f' \star g = (f \star g)'$.

5. [†]Compute, by hand, the Fourier coefficients, $\hat{f}_m$, for the function $f(x) = x$ on the interval $[-1/2, 1/2]$. Graphically compare, as in Figure 7.1, the partial sums for two values of N. Show that Parseval's identity, in this case, reveals that

$$\sum_{n=1}^{\infty} \frac{1}{n^2} = \frac{\pi^2}{6}. \tag{7.37}$$

This is a special case of Eq. (6.66).

6. Use Eq. (7.24) to show that eigenvalues and eigenvectors of the circulant matrix

$$\mathbf{B} = \begin{pmatrix} 1 & 0 & 1 & 0 \\ 0 & 1 & 0 & 1 \\ 1 & 0 & 1 & 0 \\ 0 & 1 & 0 & 1 \end{pmatrix}$$

are $(2\ 0\ 2\ 0)$ and

$$\begin{pmatrix} 1 \\ 1 \\ 1 \\ 1 \end{pmatrix} \quad \begin{pmatrix} 1 \\ i \\ -1 \\ -i \end{pmatrix} \quad \begin{pmatrix} 1 \\ -1 \\ 1 \\ -1 \end{pmatrix} \quad \begin{pmatrix} 1 \\ -i \\ -1 \\ i \end{pmatrix}. \tag{7.38}$$

Argue that as **B** and its eigenvalues are real then the real and imaginary parts (when nontrivial) of the vectors in Eq. (7.38) are also eigenvectors. Show that this permits you to garner a set of four real eigenvectors (two corresponding to $\lambda=2$ and two to $\lambda=0$) that is complete in the sense that each is orthogonal to the other three.

7. †Establish the validity of the two statements in Eq. (7.23).

8. Establish the validity of the transform derivative formula, Eq. (7.28), by arguing along the lines used in Eqs. (3.15) and (3.16).

9. †Establish the validity of the Convolution Theorem, Eq. (7.29), by arguing along the lines used in Eq. (3.22).

10. Argue, based on the Convolution Theorem, Eq. (7.29), that the convolution operation is commutative and associative:

$$u \star v = v \star u \quad \text{and} \quad u \star (v \star w) = (u \star v) \star w.$$

11. Show that the Fourier transform of $\cos(2\pi at)$ is $\frac{1}{2}(\delta(a-\omega)+\delta(a+\omega))$. Hint: Use Eq. (7.1) to represent the cosine as a sum of complex exponentials and then argue as in Eq. (7.27). What is the corresponding expression for $\sin(2\pi at)$?

12. †Show that the Fourier, like the Laplace, transform follows the simple scaling laws:

(i) If $g(t)=f(t-a)$ then $\hat{g}(\omega)=\hat{f}(\omega)e^{-2\pi ia\omega}$.

(ii) If $g(t)=f(t/a)$ then $\hat{g}(\omega)=a\hat{f}(a\omega)$.

13. Show that if $u(t)$ is real then its Fourier transform satisfies $\hat{u}(\omega)=\hat{u}(-\omega)^*$, where * denotes complex conjugation. Hint: Use the fact that $(\int f(x)\,dx)^* = \int f(x)^*\,dx$.

14. †Show that if u is even, i.e., $u(t)=u(-t)$, then so too is its Fourier transform, i.e., $\hat{u}(\omega)=\hat{u}(-\omega)$.

15. †Show that the Fourier transform of the Gaussian,

$$u(t)=e^{-t^2/2}$$

is the Gaussian

$$\hat{u}(\omega)=\sqrt{2\pi}e^{-(2\pi\omega)^2/2}$$

by completing

(i) Show that u obeys the differential equation $u'(t)=-tu(t)$.

(ii) Differentiate the Fourier transform, with respect to its only variable, ω, and find

$$\hat{u}'(\omega)=-2\pi i\int_{-\infty}^{\infty}e^{-2\pi i\omega t}tu(t)\,dt,$$

(iii) Now replace $-tu$ with u' per (i), integrate by parts, and arrive at the differential equation $\hat{u}'(\omega)=-4\pi^2\omega\hat{u}(\omega)$.

(iv) Conclude that $\hat{u}(\omega)=\hat{u}(0)e^{-(2\pi\omega)^2/2}$ and prove the gorgeous identity

$$\int_{-\infty}^{\infty}e^{-t^2/2}\,dt=\sqrt{2\pi}, \tag{7.39}$$

to complete the exercise. Hint: By squaring each side of Eq. (7.39) arrive at the equivalent identity

$$\int_{-\infty}^{\infty}e^{-(x^2+y^2)/2}\,dx\,dy=2\pi.$$

Compute the left hand side by transforming to polar coordinates.

16. †Assume that $V_{Cl}=0$ in Eq. (3.2). How must the function $w(t)$ be defined so that $V(T)$ can be written as the convolution of $I_{stim}(t)$ with $w(t)$, that is,

$$V(T) = \int_{-\infty}^{\infty} w(T-t)I_{stim}(t)\,\mathrm{d}t$$

(Hint: Use $I_{stim}(t)=0$ for $t<0$)? Compute the Fourier transform of $w(t)$. If $m(\omega)$ and $\phi(\omega)$ are the modulus and phase of $\hat{w}(\omega)$, i.e., $\hat{w}(\omega)=m(\omega)e^{i\phi(\omega)}$ show that $m(\omega)$ is equal to Eq. (3.7) and that $\phi(\omega)=-\tan^{-1}(2\pi\tau\omega)$.

17. †Now show that

$$V_f(T) = \int_{-\infty}^{\infty} w(T-t)f(t)\,\mathrm{d}t$$

defines a linear and time invariant mapping from f to V_f, that is

$$V_{\alpha f+\beta g}(T) = \alpha V_f(T) + \beta V_g(T)$$

and if $g(t)=f(t+t_0)$, then $V_g(T)=V_f(T+t_0)$.

18. †Next, compute numerically the Fourier transform of $w(t)$ using fft in MATLAB and reproduce the graphs of Figure 3.1. Use the following parameters: $A=4\pi\,10^{-6}$ cm^2, $C_m=1$ μF/cm^2, and $g_{Cl}=0.3$ mS/cm^2. To compute the discrete Fourier transform, use a sampling step of 1/8 ms, and 8192 time samples.

19. †Prove the identity

$$\sum_{k=0}^{N-1} e^{2\pi ik(m-l)/N} = N\delta_{ml}, \tag{7.40}$$

where δ_{ml} is the Kronecker delta. Use it to show directly that

$$g_l = \frac{1}{N}\sum_{k=0}^{N-1} \hat{g}_k e^{2\pi ilk/N}, \quad l=0,\dots,N-1 \tag{7.41}$$

is the inverse transform of

$$\hat{g}_k = \sum_{l=0}^{N-1} g_l e^{-2\pi ikl/N}, \quad k=0,\dots,N-1. \tag{7.42}$$

20. Although the Dirac impulse cannot be defined as a continuous function, it can be defined as a linear *mapping* from a set of functions to the real (or complex) numbers. Such a mapping is usually called a *functional* or *distribution*. Let $\mathcal{D}$ be the set of differentiable functions that vanish outside of a closed, bounded interval.

Definition. For a function $f(t)\in\mathcal{D}$ define $\delta(f)=f(0)$.
Show that this functional is linear, i.e., $\delta(\alpha f+\beta g)=\alpha\delta(f)+\beta\delta(g)$, for functions $f,g\in\mathcal{D}$ and $\alpha,\beta\in\mathbb{R}$.

We can now formally write the Dirac distribution in integral form,

$$\delta(f) = \int_{-\infty}^{\infty} \delta(t)f(t)\,\mathrm{d}t$$

and the corresponding integrand behaves in many ways as a regular function. For example, show that if we define the distribution $\delta_\tau(f) = f(\tau)$ we can identify it with $\delta(t - \tau)$. (Hint: Change of variables).

For a differentiable function $g(t)$ define

$$D_g(f) = \int_{-\infty}^{\infty} g(t)f(t)\,dt, \quad f \in \mathcal{D}.$$

Show that D_g is a distribution.

21. For a distribution d define its derivative through

$$d'(f) = d(-f'), \quad f \in \mathcal{D}.$$

Show that d' is a distribution as well and that this definition generalizes the derivative of a differentiable function in the sense that

$$D_g' = D_{g'}.$$

(Hint: Integration by parts). Define the Heaviside distribution through

$$\mathbb{1}(f) = \int_{-\infty}^{\infty} \mathbb{1}(x)f(x)\,dx = \int_{0}^{\infty} f(x)\,dx,$$

where $\mathbb{1}(x)$ is the Heaviside function, Eq. (1.6). Show that the derivative of the Heaviside distribution is the Dirac distribution, i.e., $\mathbb{1}' = \delta$.

The Passive Dendritic Tree

OUTLINE

8.1	The Discrete Passive Tree	103	8.5	The Equivalent Cylinder*	111
8.2	Eigenvector Expansion	105	8.6	Branched Eigenfunctions*	113
8.3	Numerical Methods	107	8.7	Summary and Sources	115
8.4	The Passive Dendrite Equation	110	8.8	Exercises	115

As we observed at the outset of Chapter 6, the straight cable is an idealization. In reality, neurons exhibit an incredible variety of branching patterns. We offer six representatives in Figure 8.1 and note that though they vary greatly in both size and number of dendritic branches, each cell is a tree (no closed loops) with a well-defined cell body, or soma. In this chapter we append a soma and a pair of branches to the simple passive cable of Chapter 6. We demonstrate that each of the mathematical and computational tools developed for the cable have natural extensions to the tree. We proceed to investigate synaptic integration and attenuation, with particular attention to the role played by tree eigenfunctions. We also specify and analyze the conditions under which the response of the tree may be well approximated by that of a simple straight cable.

8.1 THE DISCRETE PASSIVE TREE

We work in the concrete context of Figure 8.2 on the way to a more general understanding. We have indexed the compartments, following an observation of Hines, in a manner that leads to minimal fill-in in the LU factorization, Exercise 5.2, of the resulting linear system associated with the backward Euler and trapezoid schemes. The physical lengths and radii of the three fibers are

$$\ell_1, \ell_2, \ell_3 \quad \text{and} \quad a_1, a_2, a_3$$

respectively, while the length of each compartment, except the soma, is $\mathrm{d}x$. The soma is presumed to have surface area A_s and is not typically further compartmentalized.

If we inject I_{stim} at the soma then Kirchhoff's Current Law, at the node with potential $v_{3,4}$, requires

$$I_{stim} = C_m A_s v'_{3,4} + g_{Cl} A_s v_{3,4} + a_3^2 \pi (v_{3,4} - v_{3,3})/(\mathrm{d}x R_a) \tag{8.1}$$

where, as in §6.1, $v_{i,j} = V_{i,j} - V_{Cl}$, while at the branch point $(v_{3,1})$ we find

$$\frac{\pi a_3^2 (v_{3,2} - v_{3,1})}{R_a \mathrm{d}x} = \frac{\pi a_2^2 (v_{3,1} - v_{2,4})}{R_a \mathrm{d}x} + \frac{\pi a_1^2 (v_{3,1} - v_{1,4})}{R_a \mathrm{d}x} + 2\pi a_3 \mathrm{d}x (C_m v'_{3,1} + g_{Cl} v_{3,1}).$$

Mathematics for Neuroscientists. DOI: 10.1016/B978-0-12-374882-9.00008-3

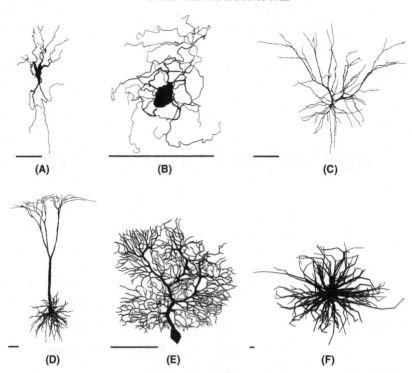

(A)   **(B)**   **(C)**

(D)   **(E)**   **(F)**

FIGURE 8.1   Dendritic diversity. **A**. A neuron of the vagal motor pathway, part of the autonomic nervous system. **B**. A neuron of the olivary body in the brainstem. **C**. A pyramidal cell of the cortex, from layer 2/3. **D**. A pyramidal cell of the cortex, from layer 5. **E**. A Purkinje cell from the cerebellum. **F**. An α-motorneuron from the spinal cord. Each scale bar is $100\,\mu$m long. Adapted from Segev (1998).

Current balance at the remaining nodes proceeds exactly as before, recall Eq. (6.5). In particular, with $\lambda_j^2 \equiv a_j/(2R_a g_{Cl})$, the squared space constant of branch j, we find

$$\tau v'_{1,1} + v_{1,1} - \lambda_1^2(v_{1,2} - v_{1,1})/\mathrm{d}x^2 = 0$$

$$\tau v'_{1,2} + v_{1,2} - \lambda_1^2(v_{1,3} - 2v_{1,2} + v_{1,1})/\mathrm{d}x^2 = 0$$

$$\tau v'_{1,3} + v_{1,3} - \lambda_1^2(v_{1,4} - 2v_{1,3} + v_{1,2})/\mathrm{d}x^2 = 0$$

$$\tau v'_{1,4} + v_{1,4} - \lambda_1^2(v_{3,1} - 2v_{1,4} + v_{1,3})/\mathrm{d}x^2 = 0$$

$$\tau v'_{2,1} + v_{2,1} - \lambda_2^2(v_{2,2} - v_{2,1})/\mathrm{d}x^2 = 0$$

$$\tau v'_{2,2} + v_{2,2} - \lambda_2^2(v_{2,3} - 2v_{2,2} + v_{2,1})/\mathrm{d}x^2 = 0$$

$$\tau v'_{2,3} + v_{2,3} - \lambda_2^2(v_{2,4} - 2v_{2,3} + v_{2,2})/\mathrm{d}x^2 = 0 \qquad (8.2)$$

$$\tau v'_{2,4} + v_{2,4} - \lambda_2^2(v_{3,1} - 2v_{2,4} - v_{2,3})/\mathrm{d}x^2 = 0$$

$$\tau v'_{3,1} + v_{3,1} + \frac{a_2 \lambda_2^2(v_{3,1} - v_{2,4}) - a_3 \lambda_3^2(v_{3,2} - v_{3,1}) + a_1 \lambda_1^2(v_{3,1} - v_{1,4})}{a_3 \mathrm{d}x^2} = 0$$

$$\tau v'_{3,2} + v_{3,2} - \lambda_2^2(v_{3,3} - 2v_{3,2} + v_{3,1})/\mathrm{d}x^2 = 0$$

$$\tau v'_{3,3} + v_{3,3} - \lambda_3^2(v_{3,4} - 2v_{3,3} + v_{3,2})/\mathrm{d}x^2 = 0$$

$$\tau v'_{3,4} + v_{3,4} - (A_3/A_s)\lambda_3^2(v_{3,3} - v_{3,4})/\mathrm{d}x^2 - I_{stim}/(g_{Cl}A_s) = 0$$

where $A_3 = 2\pi a_3 \mathrm{d}x$. We write this collection of equations as the linear system

$$\mathbf{v}'(t) = \mathbf{B}\mathbf{v}(t) + \mathbf{f}(t), \quad \mathbf{B} = (\mathbf{H} - \mathbf{I})/\tau, \quad \mathbf{f}(t) = I_{stim}(t)\mathbf{e}_{12}/(C_m A_s) \qquad (8.3)$$

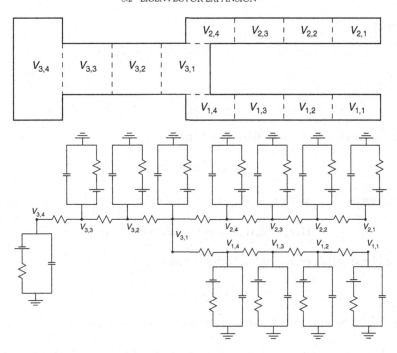

FIGURE 8.2   The compartmentalization of a branched cell with soma, and its associated circuit diagram.

and $\mathbf{H}$ is the Hines matrix

$$\mathbf{H} = \frac{1}{dx^2} \begin{pmatrix} -\lambda_1^2 & \lambda_1^2 & 0 & 0 & 0 & 0 & 0 & 0 & 0 & 0 & 0 & 0 \\ \lambda_1^2 & -2\lambda_1^2 & \lambda_1^2 & 0 & 0 & 0 & 0 & 0 & 0 & 0 & 0 & 0 \\ 0 & \lambda_1^2 & -2\lambda_1^2 & \lambda_1^2 & 0 & 0 & 0 & 0 & 0 & 0 & 0 & 0 \\ 0 & 0 & \lambda_1^2 & -2\lambda_1^2 & 0 & 0 & 0 & 0 & \lambda_1^2 & 0 & 0 & 0 \\ 0 & 0 & 0 & 0 & -\lambda_2^2 & \lambda_2^2 & 0 & 0 & 0 & 0 & 0 & 0 \\ 0 & 0 & 0 & 0 & \lambda_2^2 & -2\lambda_2^2 & \lambda_2^2 & 0 & 0 & 0 & 0 & 0 \\ 0 & 0 & 0 & 0 & 0 & \lambda_2^2 & -2\lambda_2^2 & \lambda_2^2 & 0 & 0 & 0 & 0 \\ 0 & 0 & 0 & 0 & 0 & 0 & \lambda_2^2 & -2\lambda_2^2 & \lambda_2^2 & 0 & 0 & 0 \\ 0 & 0 & 0 & r_1\lambda_1^2 & 0 & 0 & 0 & r_2\lambda_2^2 & -c & \lambda_3^2 & 0 & 0 \\ 0 & 0 & 0 & 0 & 0 & 0 & 0 & 0 & \lambda_3^2 & -2\lambda_3^2 & \lambda_3^2 & 0 \\ 0 & 0 & 0 & 0 & 0 & 0 & 0 & 0 & 0 & \lambda_3^2 & -2\lambda_3^2 & \lambda_3^2 \\ 0 & 0 & 0 & 0 & 0 & 0 & 0 & 0 & 0 & 0 & \rho\lambda_3^2 & -\rho\lambda_3^2 \end{pmatrix}$$

where

$$r_1 = a_1/a_3, \quad r_2 = a_2/a_3, \quad c = r_1\lambda_1^2 + r_2\lambda_2^2 + \lambda_3^2, \quad \text{and} \quad \rho = A_3/A_s.$$

The genius of $\mathbf{H}$ is at least double – it factors easily and is similar to a symmetric matrix. Regarding the former, we note that, as in the tridiagonal $\mathbf{S}$ of Chapter 6, Gaussian Elimination applied to this matrix requires only one elimination per column.

8.2 EIGENVECTOR EXPANSION

We now describe the solution of Eq. (8.3) in terms of a series expansion in the eigenvectors of $\mathbf{B}$. Our expansion in the single fiber case made great use of the symmetry of $\mathbf{S}$ and the resulting orthonormality of its eigenvectors. We recognize that although the soma and the branch point have rendered $\mathbf{H}$ asymmetric it is nonetheless **similar** to a symmetric matrix. Let us unpack that last remark in the slightly more general context in which fiber j has N_j

compartments. We note that

$$dx = \ell_j / N_j \quad \text{and} \quad N \equiv N_1 + N_2 + N_3 + 1,$$

define the diagonal matrix

$$\texttt{D=diag([a1 ones(N1,1) a2ones(N2,1) a3ones(N3,1) a3/}\rho\texttt{])}$$

and note that $\mathbf{DH} = (\mathbf{DH})^T = \mathbf{H}^T\mathbf{D}$. This implies (Exercise 1) that

$$\mathbf{A} \equiv \mathbf{D}^{1/2}\mathbf{H}\mathbf{D}^{-1/2} \tag{8.4}$$

is symmetric. It follows, (Exercise 2), that if $\{\mu_n, \mathbf{q}_n\}_{n=1}^N$ is the sequence of eigenpairs of $\mathbf{A}$, i.e., $\mathbf{A}\mathbf{q}_n = \mu_n\mathbf{q}_n$ then

$$\mathbf{H}\mathbf{w}_n = \mu_n\mathbf{w}_n \quad \text{where} \quad \mathbf{w}_n = \mathbf{D}^{-1/2}\mathbf{q}_n \tag{8.5}$$

and so the eigenvectors of $\mathbf{H}$ are orthonormal in the weighted sense,

$$\mathbf{w}_n^T\mathbf{D}\mathbf{w}_m = \delta_{mn}. \tag{8.6}$$

We illustrate, in Figure 8.3, the first nine nonconstant eigenvectors for the symmetric fork with

$$a_1 = a_2 = a_3 = 1\,\mu\text{m}, \quad \ell_1 = \ell_2 = \ell_3 = 250\,\mu\text{m}, \quad \text{and} \quad A_s = 400\pi\,\mu\text{m}^2. \tag{8.7}$$

and passive cable parameters

$$C_m = 1\,\mu\text{F/cm}^2, \quad g_{Cl} = 1/15\,\text{mS/cm}^2, \quad \text{and} \quad R_a = 0.3\,\text{k}\Omega\,\text{cm}. \tag{8.8}$$

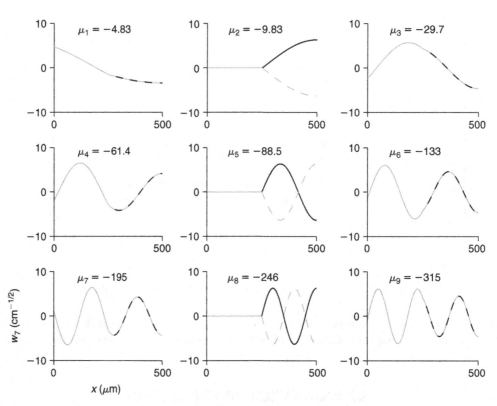

FIGURE 8.3 The first nine (nonconstant) eigenvectors, $\mathbf{w}_n$, and associated eigenvalues, μ_n, arranged in decreasing order of the Hines matrix $\mathbf{H}$ for the cell described by Eqs. (8.7) and (8.8) and $dx = 1\,\mu\text{m}$. Here the mother, branch 3, is depicted in red over the initial $250\,\mu\text{m}$ segment and the daughters, branch 1 in black and branch 2 in dashed red, are plotted over the second $250\,\mu\text{m}$. These eigenvectors appear in two varieties. Either the two daughters are equal and opposite and the mother silent, or the daughters coincide and the mother plays along (in which case her slope at the soma is nonzero). (bevec.m)

Regarding the representation of $\mathbf{f}$ in terms of $\mathbf{w}$, we write

$$\mathbf{f}(t) = \sum_{n=0}^{N-1} c_n(t)\mathbf{w}_n = \mathbf{D}^{-1/2} \sum_{n=0}^{N-1} c_n(t)\mathbf{q}_n$$

and so find that $\mathbf{c} = \mathbf{W}^T \mathbf{Df}$. Hence, with $z_n = (\mu_n - 1)/\tau$, and $\mathbf{f}(t) = I_{stim}(t)\mathbf{e}_N/(C_m A_s)$, it follows from Eq. (5.21) that

$$\boxed{\mathbf{v}(t) = \frac{1}{2\pi \, dx C_m} \sum_{n=0}^{N-1} \mathbf{w}_n w_{n,N} \int_0^t I_{stim}(s) \exp((t-s)z_n) ds} \tag{8.9}$$

is the solution of the discrete passive dendrite equation, Eq. (8.3), with current injection at the soma. If we instead inject $I_m(t)$ at compartment c_m, where $m = 1, \ldots, M$, then the above takes the form

$$\mathbf{v}(t) = \frac{1}{2\pi \, dx C_m} \sum_{n=0}^{N-1} \mathbf{w}_n \sum_{m=1}^{M} w_{n,c_m} \int_0^t I_m(s) \exp((t-s)z_n) ds.$$

With this we investigate the interaction of pairs of simple inputs. In particular if we place the pair of equal impulses

$$I_1(t) = I_2(t) = \gamma \delta(t - t_1)$$

at compartments c_1 and c_2 then

$$\mathbf{v}(t) = \frac{\gamma \mathbb{1}_{(t_1, \infty)}(t)}{2\pi \, dx C_m} \sum_{n=0}^{N-1} \mathbf{w}_n (w_{n,c_1} + w_{n,c_2}) \exp((t-t_1)z_n). \tag{8.10}$$

We quantify their interaction by considering the strength of the soma response

$$S(c_1, c_2) \equiv \int_0^\infty v_N(t) \, dt = \frac{-\gamma}{2\pi \, dx C_m} \sum_{n=0}^{N-1} \frac{w_{n,N}}{z_n} (w_{n,c_1} + w_{n,c_2}). \tag{8.11}$$

We see that the strength at the soma, associated with simultaneous impulsive current injections, is a weighted average of the individual eigeninteractions, $w_{n,N}(w_{n,c_1} + w_{n,c_2})$, of the input elements, c_1 and c_2, and the output element, N. We can "see" these terms, for small n, in the eigenvectors plotted in Figure 8.3. Note that the Nth component, corresponding to the soma, appears at the far left in each plot. As $w_{2,N} = w_{5,N} = w_{8,N} = 0$ and the other $w_{n,N}$ are small compared to $w_{1,N}$ we may be able to capture the salient interactions by retaining only the $\mathbf{w}_0$ and $\mathbf{w}_1$ terms in Eq. (8.11). This surmise is further supported by the fact that the interactions are scaled by $z_n = (\mu_n - 1)/\tau$ where the μ_n are eigenvalues, see Figure 8.3, that increase rapidly in magnitude. It follows that $w_{1,N}/z_1$ is more than 20 times its next term, $w_{3,N}/z_3$. We exploit these observations in Figure 8.4 where we contrast the full strength, Eq. (8.11), with the leading order strength associated with retaining the $n=0$ and $n=1$ terms.

8.3 NUMERICAL METHODS

We may solve Eq. (8.3) via the trapezoid rule, precisely as in Eq. (6.24). As an application we investigate the integration of 10 current pulses at distinct times and places. More precisely, we suppose that our right hand side takes the form

$$\mathbf{f}(t) = \frac{I_0}{2\pi a_1 \, dx C_m} \sum_{k=1}^{10} \mathbf{e}_{c_k} \mathbb{1}_{(t_k, t_k+1)}(t) \tag{8.12}$$

where c_k denotes the compartment number of the kth stimulus, $\mathbf{e}_{c_k}$ is defined as in Eq. (6.10), and compute, see Figure 8.5, the response at the cell body.

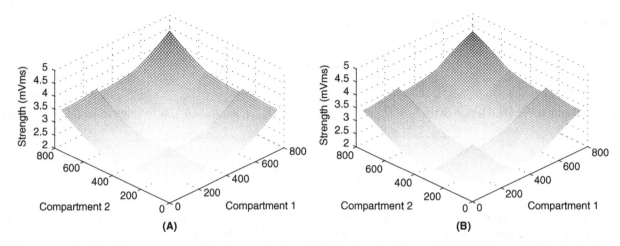

FIGURE 8.4 The strength as a function of input location for the cell described by Eqs. (8.7) and (8.8). Compartments 1 to 250 correspond to daughter 1, 251 to 500 to daughter 2, and 501 to $750+1$ to the mother and soma. We see that the strongest interactions occur for proximal (close to soma) inputs. For a fixed choice of c_1 the strength increases as c_2 approaches the soma. **A.** The full strength, Eq. (8.11). **B.** The strength computed by retaining only the $n=0$ and $n=1$ terms. We see that the leading order strength indeed captures all of the important detail of the full strength, and hence the first nonconstant eigenvector, $\mathbf{w}_1$, is seen as the arbiter of synaptic integration. (bevec.m)

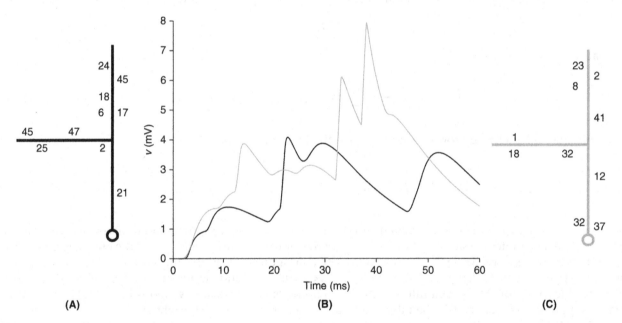

FIGURE 8.5 The somatic response, in **B**, of the cell described by Eqs. (8.7) and (8.8) to current injection of the form Eq. (8.12) of amplitude $I_0=100$ pA at the sites and times indicated in **A** and **C**. We observe smooth integration of distal early inputs punctuated by sharp increases immediately following proximal input. (trapfork.m)

If rather than multisite current injection we suppose polysynaptic input then we must solve

$$\mathbf{v}'(t) + \sum_{k=1}^{K} c_{syn,k}(t)(\mathbf{v}(t) - v_{syn})\mathbf{e}_{c_k} = \mathbf{B}\mathbf{v}(t) \qquad (8.13)$$

where, with a_{b_k} denoting the radius of the branch that receives the kth input,

$$c_{syn,k}(t) = \frac{g_{syn,k}(t)}{2\pi a_{b_k} dx C_m}.$$

We solve this via the trapezoid rule precisely as we did in §6.5. In particular, we implement Eq. (6.55) where, now, $\mathbf{B} = (\mathbf{H} - \mathbf{I})/\tau$, and $g_{syn,k}(t)$ is an α-function

$$g_{syn,k}(t,t_k) = \overline{g}_{syn}((t-t_k)/\tau_\alpha)\exp(1-(t-t_k)/\tau_\alpha)\mathbb{1}_{(t_k,\infty)}(t)$$

that commences from t_k. We illustrate our findings in Figure 8.6.

We observe, in Figure 8.6, that the early stimulus into branch 1 indeed depolarizes branch 2 and that the combined response attenuates as it approaches the soma. We investigate, in Figure 8.7, the difference between peak synaptic and peak somatic potentials as the synapse moves away from the soma.

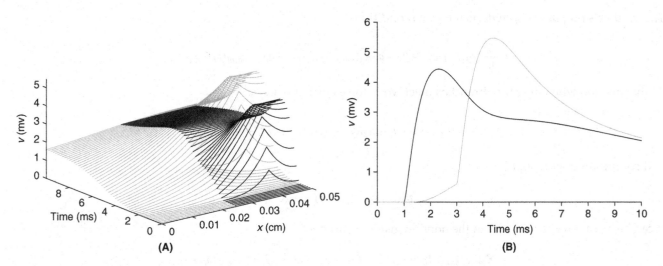

(A) **(B)**

FIGURE 8.6   The response of the cell described by Eqs. (8.7) and (8.8) to α-synaptic input onto the two daughter branches, with $\overline{g}_{syn} = 1$ nS, $\tau_\alpha = 1$ ms, $t_1 = 1$, and $t_2 = 3$ ms and reversal potential $v_{syn,k} = 70$ mV. Both inputs are located 100 μm from the branch ends. **A.** Full space-time response. The response of the mother (branch 3) is plotted in red over the first 250 μm. The response of the two daughters is plotted over the second 250 μm with the response of branch 1 in black and that of branch 2 in red. **B.** The response in time at the two sites of stimulation, with black and red denoting branches 1 and 2 respectively, as in **A.** (trapforksyn.m)

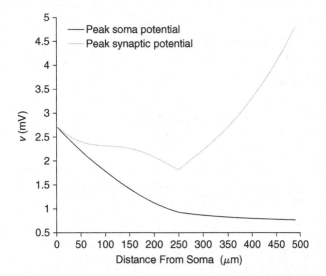

FIGURE 8.7   Peak somatic and synaptic potentials for the cell described by Eqs. (8.7) and (8.8), as a function of the distance from the soma to the site of a single α-synapse, with $\overline{g}_{syn} = 0.5$ nS and $\tau_\alpha = t_1 = 1$ ms. The steep decrease in peak soma potential as the synapse travels away from the soma diminishes as the synapse enters a daughter branch and the peak synaptic potential grows as the synapse approaches the sealed end. We have seen such "end effects" before in Figure 6.3A. (trapforksyngain.m)

8.4 THE PASSIVE DENDRITE EQUATION

As we pass to the limit of infinitely many infinitely short compartments we arrive (precisely as in §6.4) at three cable equations

$$\tau\frac{\partial v_j}{\partial t}(x,t)+v_j(x,t)=\lambda_j^2\frac{\partial^2 v_j}{\partial x^2}(x,t), \quad 0<x<\ell_j, \quad j=1,2,3,$$

for the three space-time potential functions, v_1, v_2, and v_3. The two daughters are sealed at their distal ends, i.e.,

$$\frac{\partial v_1}{\partial x}(0,t)=\frac{\partial v_2}{\partial x}(0,t)=0.$$

The mother's proximal end reflects the soma condition

$$\tau\frac{\partial v_3}{\partial t}(\ell_3,t)+v_3(\ell_3,t)+a_3\lambda_3^2(2\pi/A_s)\frac{\partial v_3}{\partial x}(\ell_3,t)=I_{stim}(t)/(g_{Cl}A_s).$$

At the junction where the three branches meet we enforce current balance

$$a_1\lambda_1^2\frac{\partial v_1}{\partial x}(\ell_1,t)+a_2\lambda_2^2\frac{\partial v_2}{\partial x}(\ell_2,t)=a_3\lambda_3^2\frac{\partial v_3}{\partial x}(0,t),$$

and continuity of potential

$$v_1(\ell_1,t)=v_2(\ell_2,t)=v_3(0,t).$$

It can be advantageous to work in the nondimensional variables

$$X\equiv x/\lambda_j, \quad L_j\equiv\ell_j/\lambda_j, \quad T\equiv t/\tau, \quad \text{and} \quad h\equiv a_3\lambda_3(2\pi/A_s). \tag{8.14}$$

For then the associated response and stimulus,

$$u_j(X,T)\equiv v_j(x,t), \qquad J(T)\equiv I_{stim}(t)$$

obey

$$\frac{\partial u_j}{\partial T}(X,T)+u_j(X,T)=\frac{\partial^2 u_j}{\partial X^2}(X,T), \quad 0<X<L_j \tag{8.15}$$

subject to the two sealed end conditions

$$\frac{\partial u_1}{\partial X}(0,T)=\frac{\partial u_2}{\partial X}(0,T)=0, \tag{8.16}$$

the soma condition

$$\frac{\partial u_3}{\partial T}(L_3,T)+u_3(L_3,T)+h\frac{\partial u_3}{\partial X}(L_3,T)=J(T)/(g_{Cl}A_s), \tag{8.17}$$

and the junction conditions

$$a_1^{3/2}\frac{\partial u_1}{\partial X}(L_1,T)+a_2^{3/2}\frac{\partial u_2}{\partial X}(L_2,T)=a_3^{3/2}\frac{\partial u_3}{\partial X}(0,T)$$

$$u_1(L_1,T)=u_2(L_2,T)=u_3(0,T). \tag{8.18}$$

Before proceeding to solve this general problem we pause to consider an important special case.

8.5 THE EQUIVALENT CYLINDER*

We observe that the fork can be collapsed to a single cable, or cylinder, under a pair of simple geometric assumptions. We assume, for ease of presentation, that the only stimulus is current into the soma.

(**EC1**) If the two daughters have equal electrotonic lengths, i.e., $L_1 = L_2$, we may define

$$U(X,T) = \begin{cases} \dfrac{a_1^{3/2} u_1(X,T) + a_2^{3/2} u_2(X,T)}{a_1^{3/2} + a_2^{3/2}}, & 0 < X < L_1 \\[2mm] u_3(X - L_1, T), & L_1 < X < L_1 + L_3 \end{cases} \tag{8.19}$$

and note that it obeys, with $L \equiv L_1 + L_3$,

$$\frac{\partial U}{\partial T}(X,T) + U(X,T) = \frac{\partial^2 U}{\partial X^2}(X,T), \quad 0 < X < L_1, \, L_1 < X < L$$

$$U(L_1^-, T) = U(L_1^+, T)$$

$$(a_1^{3/2} + a_2^{3/2}) \frac{\partial U}{\partial X}(L_1^-, T) = a_3^{3/2} \frac{\partial U}{\partial X}(L_1^+, T)$$

$$\frac{\partial U}{\partial X}(0,T) = 0, \quad \frac{\partial U}{\partial T}(L,T) + U(L,T) + h \frac{\partial U}{\partial X}(L,T) = J(T)/(g_{Cl} A_s).$$

The third condition predicts a break in the slope of U if $a_1^{3/2} + a_2^{3/2} \neq a_3^{3/2}$.

(**EC2**) If the cell obeys the "3/2 law," i.e., $a_1^{3/2} + a_2^{3/2} = a_3^{3/2}$ then U is simply the solution to

$$\frac{\partial U}{\partial T}(X,T) + U(X,T) = \frac{\partial^2 U}{\partial X^2}(X,T), \quad 0 < X < L, \, 0 < T$$

$$\frac{\partial U}{\partial X}(0,T) = 0, \quad 0 < T$$

$$\frac{\partial U}{\partial T}(L,T) + U(L,T) + h \frac{\partial U}{\partial X}(L,T) = J(T)/(g_{Cl} A_s), \quad 0 < T \tag{8.20}$$

$$U(X,0) = 0, \quad 0 < X < L.$$

This system, Eq. (8.20), is known as the **equivalent cylinder problem**. We solve it, as in §6.4, by proceeding from the hope that $U(X,T) = q(X)p(T)$. This hope necessitates

$$p'(T)/p(T) + 1 = q''(X)/q(X), \quad 0 < X < L$$

$$q'(0) = 0, \quad p'(T)/p(T) + 1 + hq'(L)/q(L) = J(T)/(g_{Cl} A_s p(T)q(0)).$$

If, as in §6.4, we label by ϑ the common value of $q''(X)/q(X)$ and $p'(T)/p(T) + 1$ then we see that it too must appear in the boundary condition for q. That is, we are compelled to consider

$$q''(X) = \vartheta q(X), \quad q'(0) = 0, \quad \text{and} \quad hq'(L) + \vartheta q(L) = 0. \tag{8.21}$$

This produces only a minor inconvenience, for the eigenfunction must still be of the form

$$q_n(X) = b_n \cos(\sqrt{-\vartheta_n} X) \tag{8.22}$$

and ϑ_n is chosen to guarantee $hq_n'(L) = -\vartheta_n q_n(L)$. More precisely, ϑ_n is the negative of the square of each root of

$$F(z) \equiv z + h \tan(zL). \tag{8.23}$$

We shall demonstrate (in Exercise 5) that these roots are simple and deduce (in Exercise 6) that

$$(\vartheta_m - \vartheta_n)\left(q_m(L)q_n(L)/h + \int_0^L q_m(X)q_n(X)\,dX\right) = 0, \tag{8.24}$$

and hence that the eigenfunctions are orthogonal with respect to the inner product

$$\langle f,g\rangle \equiv f(L)g(L)/h + \int_0^L f(X)g(X)\,dX. \tag{8.25}$$

We next normalize these eigenfunctions by choosing the b_n in Eq. (8.22) such that $\langle q_n,q_n\rangle = 1$, i.e., such that

$$b_n^2\left(\cos^2(\sqrt{-\vartheta_n}L)/h + \int_0^L \cos^2(\sqrt{-\vartheta_n}X)\,dX\right) = 1. \tag{8.26}$$

As with the straight cable, the naive guess that $U(X,T) = q(X)p(T)$ has led us to the better guess

$$U(X,T) = \sum_{m=0}^{\infty} p_m(T)q_m(X). \tag{8.27}$$

On taking the inner product, Eq. (8.25), of each side with q_n we deduce from $\langle q_m,q_n\rangle = \delta_{mn}$ that

$$\langle U,q_n\rangle = U(L,T)q_n(L)/h + \int_0^L U(X,T)q_n(X)\,dX = p_n(T)\langle q_n,q_n\rangle = p_n(T). \tag{8.28}$$

We now differentiate this with respect to time, T, and use Eq. (8.20) to replace time derivatives of U with space derivatives of U, and arrive at

$$p_n'(T) = \frac{\partial U}{\partial T}(L,T)q_n(L)/h + \int_0^L \frac{\partial U}{\partial T}(X,T)q_n(X)\,dX$$

$$= \left\{J(T)/(g_{Cl}A_s) - U(L,T) - h\frac{\partial U}{\partial X}(L,T)\right\}q_n(L)/h + \int_0^L \left\{\frac{\partial^2 U}{\partial X^2}(X,T) - U(X,T)\right\}q_n(X)\,dX$$

$$= \left\{J(T)/(g_{Cl}A_s) - h\frac{\partial U}{\partial X}(L,T)\right\}q_n(L)/h - p_n(T) + \int_0^L \frac{\partial^2 U}{\partial X^2}(X,T)q_n(X)\,dX.$$

To this we apply integration by parts, in Exercise 7, to shift derivatives from U onto q_n and so find

$$\int_0^L \frac{\partial^2 U}{\partial X^2}(X,T)q_n(X)\,dX = \frac{\partial U}{\partial X}(L,T)q_n(L) + \vartheta_n p_n(T). \tag{8.29}$$

It then follows that p_n obeys the familiar, Eq. (2.12), ordinary differential equation

$$p_n'(T) + (1 - \vartheta_n)p_n(T) = J(T)q_n(L)/(g_{Cl}A_s h). \tag{8.30}$$

Its solution, per Eq. (3.2), is the simple convolution,

$$p_n(T) = \frac{q_n(L)}{g_{Cl}A_s h}\int_0^T J(s)\exp((T-s)(\vartheta_n - 1))\,ds.$$

On inserting this into Eq. (8.27) we find that

$$U(X,T) = \sum_{n=0}^{\infty} \frac{q_n(L)q_n(X)}{g_{Cl}A_s h} \int_0^T J(s) \exp((T-s)(\vartheta_n - 1)) \, ds$$

(8.31)

solves the equivalent cylinder with soma problem, Eq. (8.20).

8.6 BRANCHED EIGENFUNCTIONS*

We return to the full nondimensional system of §8.4 and pose and solve the eigenproblem for

$$\mathbf{q}(X) = (q_1(X) \; q_2(X) \; q_3(X))^T.$$

Each component obeys the elemental branch condition

$$q_j''(X) = \vartheta q_j(X), \quad 0 < X < L_j$$

(8.32)

subject to the joint and seal conditions

$$q_1'(0) = q_2'(0) = h q_3'(L_3) + \vartheta q_3(L_3) = 0$$

$$q_1(L_1) = q_2(L_2) = q_3(0)$$

(8.33)

$$a_1^{3/2} q_1'(L_1) + a_2^{3/2} q_2'(L_2) = a_3^{3/2} q_3'(0).$$

Just as eigenvectors of the Hines matrix were orthogonal in the weighted sense, Eq. (8.6), we find (Exercise 10) that $\mathbf{q}_m$ is orthogonal to $\mathbf{q}_n$ in the weighted inner product

$$\langle (f_1 \, f_2 \, f_3), (g_1 \, g_2 \, g_3) \rangle \equiv a_3^{3/2} f_3(L_3) g_3(L_3)/h + \sum_{j=1}^{3} a_j^{3/2} \int_0^{L_j} f_j(X) g_j(X) \, dX.$$

(8.34)

Arguing in precisely the same fashion as the previous section, we find that the full solution of the passive dendrite, subject to somatic current injection, may be expressed as

$$u(X,T) = \sum_{n=0}^{\infty} \frac{\mathbf{q}_n(X) q_{n,3}(L_3)}{g_{Cl}A_s h} \int_0^T J(s) \exp((T-s)(\vartheta_n - 1)) \, ds.$$

(8.35)

This is the natural three-dimensional analog of the response, Eq. (8.31), of the equivalent cylinder. To help fix ideas we now compute these branched eigenfunctions for dendrites whose branches have equal electrotonic lengths, i.e., $L_1 = L_2 = L_3 = L$.

Without soma. We begin, for simplicity, by removing the soma. As $A_s \to 0$ we find $h \to \infty$ and so $q_3'(L) = 0$. In this case,

$$q_1 = b_1 \cos(\sqrt{-\vartheta} X), \quad q_2 = b_2 \cos(\sqrt{-\vartheta} X), \quad \text{and} \quad q_3 = b_3 \cos(\sqrt{-\vartheta}(L - X))$$

and so continuity at the joint requires

$$b_1 \cos(\sqrt{-\vartheta} L) = b_2 \cos(\sqrt{-\vartheta} L) = b_3 \cos(\sqrt{-\vartheta} L)$$

(8.36)

while Kirchhoff's Current Law at the joint requires

$$-a_1^{3/2} \sqrt{-\vartheta} b_1 \sin(\sqrt{-\vartheta} L) - a_2^{3/2} \sqrt{-\vartheta} b_2 \sin(\sqrt{-\vartheta} L) = a_3^{3/2} \sqrt{-\vartheta} b_3 \sin(\sqrt{-\vartheta} L).$$

(8.37)

There now appears a natural splitting. In particular, if $\cos(\sqrt{-\vartheta}L) = 0$ then Eq. (8.36) holds and the b_j are constrained by Eq. (8.37). This is one linear equation in three unknowns and so defines a plane. The upshot is that each eigenvalue has two linearly independent eigenfunctions. To be precise

$$\vartheta_n = -\frac{n^2\pi^2}{4L^2}, \quad \mathbf{q}_n(X) = b_n^1 \mathbf{q}_n^1(X) + b_n^2 \mathbf{q}_n^2(X) \quad n = 1,3,5,\ldots \tag{8.38}$$

where

$$\mathbf{q}_n^1(X) = \begin{pmatrix} \cos(\sqrt{-\vartheta_n}X) \\ 0 \\ -(a_1/a_3)^{3/2}\cos(\sqrt{-\vartheta_n}(L-X)) \end{pmatrix}$$

and

$$\mathbf{q}_n^2(X) = \begin{pmatrix} 0 \\ \cos(\sqrt{-\vartheta_n}X) \\ -(a_2/a_3)^{3/2}\cos(\sqrt{-\vartheta_n}(L-X)) \end{pmatrix}. \tag{8.39}$$

We note that the continuity equation is satisfied by the vanishing of each term in the second condition of Eq. (8.33). The analogous satisfaction of current balance at the joint, Eq. (8.37), requires $\sin(\sqrt{-\vartheta}L) = 0$ in which case continuity requires $b_1 = b_2 = b_3$ and we find

$$\vartheta_n = -\frac{n^2\pi^2}{4L^2} \quad n = 2,4,6,\ldots$$

$$\mathbf{q}_n(X) = b\begin{pmatrix} \cos(\sqrt{-\vartheta_n}X) \\ \cos(\sqrt{-\vartheta_n}X) \\ \cos(\sqrt{-\vartheta_n}(L-X)) \end{pmatrix}$$

where b is the arbitrary normalization constant. In summary, we note that the eigenvalues are $-n^2\pi^2/(2L)^2$ for $n = 0,1,2,\ldots$ and that these are simple for even n and double for odd n.

With soma. If we now attach the soma we find that the eigenfunction of branch 3 must be of the form

$$q_3(X) = b_3\{\cos(\sqrt{-\vartheta}(L-X)) + (\sqrt{-\vartheta}/h)\sin(\sqrt{-\vartheta}(L-X))\}.$$

It follows that continuity at the joint requires

$$b_1\cos(\sqrt{-\vartheta}L) = b_2\cos(\sqrt{-\vartheta}L) = b_3\{\cos(\sqrt{-\vartheta}L) + (\sqrt{-\vartheta}/h)\sin(\sqrt{-\vartheta}L)\} \tag{8.40}$$

while Kirchhoff's Current Law there requires

$$-a_1^{3/2}b_1\sin(\sqrt{-\vartheta}L) - a_2^{3/2}b_2\sin(\sqrt{-\vartheta}L) = a_3^{3/2}b_3\{\sin(\sqrt{-\vartheta}L) - (\sqrt{-\vartheta}/h)\cos(\sqrt{-\vartheta}L)\}. \tag{8.41}$$

As above, there is a natural splitting. If $\cos(\sqrt{-\vartheta}L) = 0$ then Eq. (8.40) implies that $b_3 = 0$ and Eq. (8.41) then requires that $a_1^{3/2}b_1 + a_2^{3/2}b_2 = 0$ and so, with b an arbitrary normalization constant,

$$\vartheta_n = -\frac{n^2\pi^2}{4L^2} \quad n = 1,3,5,\ldots$$

$$\mathbf{q}_n(X) = b\cos(\sqrt{-\vartheta_n}X)\begin{pmatrix} 1 \\ -(a_1/a_2)^{3/2} \\ 0 \end{pmatrix}.$$

We recognize these eigenfunctions in panels μ_2, μ_5, and μ_8 in Figure 8.3. The zero in $\mathbf{q}_n$ (third component) has interesting consequences for branch to branch communication. In particular, any stimulus of the form

$$J(X,T) = \sum_{m=1}^{\infty} J_m(T) \mathbf{q}_{2m-1}(X), \tag{8.42}$$

with $J_m(T)$ arbitrary, will be invisible to the mother and therefore the soma. See Exercise 9.

Next, if $\cos(\sqrt{-\vartheta}L) \neq 0$ then Eq. (8.40) implies that

$$b_1 = b_2 = b_3(1 + (\sqrt{-\vartheta}/h)\tan(\sqrt{-\vartheta}L))$$

and Eq. (8.41) that

$$-a_1^{3/2}b_1\tan(\sqrt{-\vartheta}L) - a_2^{3/2}b_2\tan(\sqrt{-\vartheta}L) = a_3^{3/2}b_3(\tan(\sqrt{-\vartheta}L) - \sqrt{-\vartheta}/h).$$

Combining these two we find that ϑ is the negative of the square of each root of

$$F(z) \equiv (1 + (z/h)\tan(zL))\tan(zL)(a_1^{3/2} + a_2^{3/2}) + a_3^{3/2}(\tan(zL) - z/h),$$

the branched analog of Eq. (8.23). The associated eigenfunction is

$$\mathbf{q}_n(X) = b \begin{pmatrix} \cos(\sqrt{-\vartheta_n}X) \\ \cos(\sqrt{-\vartheta_n}X) \\ \frac{\cos(\sqrt{-\vartheta_n}(L-X))}{1 + (\sqrt{-\vartheta_n}/h)\tan(\sqrt{-\vartheta_n}L)} \end{pmatrix}$$

where b is the normalization constant. We recognize these eigenfunctions in panels μ_1, μ_3, μ_4, μ_6, μ_7, and μ_9 in Figure 8.3.

8.7 SUMMARY AND SOURCES

We have added a soma and a pair of branches to our passive cable and demonstrated that each of the analytical and computational approaches developed for the cable apply, with little change, to the passive dendrite with soma. The only real change is the replacement of the second difference matrix with the Hines matrix and the fact that the eigenvectors of the latter are considerably more complicated than those of the straight cable. We have restricted attention to the three branched fork solely for reasons of exposition. For each of the fundamental constructs makes perfect sense in larger trees. In particular, Hines (1984), solves the compartmental ordering problem for general trees. Rall, see Segev et al. (1994), solves the equivalent cylinder problem for reducible trees and von Below (1988) establishes the inner product in which the branched eigenfunctions of general trees are orthogonal. Exercise 11 is drawn from Nicaise (1987).

8.8 EXERCISES

1. Regarding the lead up to Eq. (8.4), show that **DH** is indeed symmetric and deduce the symmetry of **A** from this. Do this by hand (without numbers) by drawing and exploiting the block structure of **H**.

2. †Show that Eq. (8.5) and Eq. (8.6) indeed follow from Eq. (8.4).

3. †Integrate the response of the soma component to dual simultaneous current impulses and explain how Eq. (8.11) arises from Eq. (8.10).

4. †Although dendritic cable diameters and branching do not permit one to space-clamp an extended cell, it is not uncommon for experimentalists to employ voltage clamps at one or more sites. The most common site is the soma. With regard to our concrete compartmental system, Eq. (8.2), note that if we clamp the soma potential, $v_{3,4}$, to the value v_c, then the penultimate equation in Eq. (8.2) takes the form

$$\tau v'_{3,3} + v_{3,3} - \lambda_3^2(-2v_{3,3} + v_{3,2}) = \lambda_3^2 v_c/\mathrm{d}x^2, \tag{8.43}$$

and that the final equation in Eq. (8.2) is no longer a constraint on the system (for $v_{3,4}$ is already constrained) but is rather an expression for the current, I_c, that is necessary to hold $v_{3,4}$ at v_c. In particular

$$I_c = g_{Cl} A_s v_c - g_{Cl} A_3 \lambda_3^2 (v_{3,3} - v_c)/dx^2. \tag{8.44}$$

The upshot of these two equations is that we now remove the last row and column of the Hines matrix, $\mathbf{H}$, and replace the stimulus vector, $\mathbf{f}$ in Eq. (8.3) with

$$\mathbf{f}(t) = (\lambda_3/dx)^2 v_c \mathbf{e}_{11}/\tau.$$

Please modify `trapforksyn.m` to permit a somatic voltage clamp and produce results like Figure 8.8.
Hint: Note that the rest potential is nonzero and decreases away from the clamp. To find it, return to Eq. (8.3) and solve $\mathbf{B} v_r + \mathbf{f} = 0$. This nonzero rest also has implications for the initialization of our trapezoid rule. Return to Eq. (6.23) to get it right.

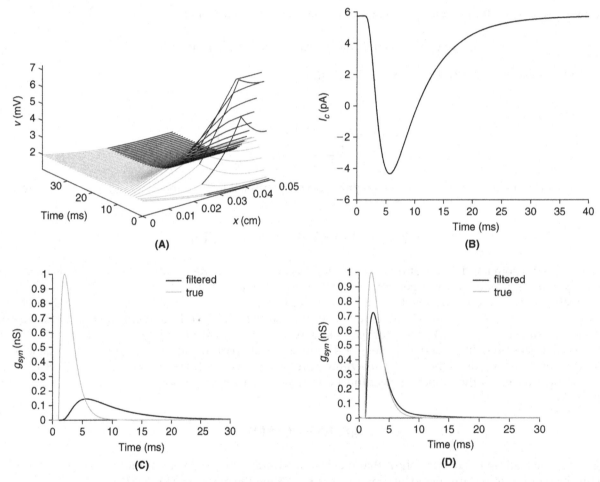

(A)   **(B)**   **(C)**   **(D)**

FIGURE 8.8   **A**. Space-time illustration of the potential in the fork with the soma potential clamped at $v_c = 2$ mV, and a distal (400 μm) α-synapse with $\bar{g}_{syn} = 1$ nS, $\tau_\alpha = t_1 = 1$ ms and $v_{syn} = 70$ mV. Color scheme as in Figure 8.6A. **B**. The associated clamp current at the soma, as computed by Eq. (8.44). This is a beautiful signature of the distal excitatory input. On dividing it by the clamp potential we arrive, as in Chapter 4, at an estimate of the time varying conductance. In particular, in **C** and **D** we plot (in black) the "received" conductance $g(t) = (I_c(t) - I_c(0))/(v_c - v_{syn})$. **C** corresponds to the synapse of **A** while **D** is the same conductance but placed proximal (50 μm). For comparison purposes we have included the true synaptic conductance, in red. The figures provide yet another window on the attenuation, or dendritic filtering, of synaptic inputs. (`trapforksynclamp.m`)

5. The eigenvalues, ϑ_n, of the equivalent cylinder with soma are determined by z_n, the roots of $z/h + \tan(zL)$, via $\vartheta_n = -z_n^2$. For representative L and h carefully graph the functions $f(z) = \tan(zL)$ and $g(z) = -z/h$ and argue that these two graphs intersect at infinitely many points, $0 = z_0 < z_1 < z_2 < \cdots$. What number is z_n close to for large n?

6. Establish the orthogonality, Eq. (8.24), of the eigenfunctions of the equivalent cylinder with soma by demonstrating that

$$\vartheta_n \int_0^L q_n(X)q_m(X)\mathrm{d}X = \int_0^L q_n''(X)q_m(X)\mathrm{d}X$$

$$= q_m(L)q_n(L)(\vartheta_m - \vartheta_n)/h + \vartheta_m \int_0^L q_n(X)q_m(X)\mathrm{d}X.$$

7. [†]Establish the validity of Eq. (8.29).

8. Consider a cell that satisfies the equivalent cylinder conditions. Rather than injecting current at the soma, we now inject equal current into the two daughters. In particular, we suppose

$$\frac{\partial u_j}{\partial T}(X,T) + u_j(X,T) - \frac{\partial^2 u_j}{\partial X^2}(X,T) = I_{stim}(X,T), \quad j=1,2$$

for some function I_{stim}. Derive a system of equations for the U of Eq. (8.19).

9. Modify `trapfork.m` to accept distributed current input. Assume equal electrotonic branch lengths and apply a stimulus of the form Eq. (8.42) and show, as in Figure 8.9, that the mother is indeed kept in the dark.

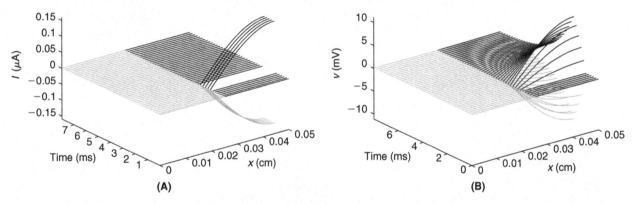

FIGURE 8.9 An example of a stimulus (A) that does not reach the soma, see response in B. Color scheme as in Figure 8.8A. (`trapforkd.m`)

10. [†]Establish the orthogonality of the branched eigenfunctions, $\mathbf{q}_n$ obeying Eqs. (8.32) and (8.33), with regard to the inner product defined in Eq. (8.34).

11. It can be shown under fairly general hypotheses that the eigenvalues of a branched tree fall in two camps, $\vartheta = -n^2\pi^2$ and $\cos(\sqrt{-\vartheta}) = z_j$ where z_j is an eigenvalue, less than 1 in magnitude, of the **adjacency matrix** associated with the tree. For our simple fork, the adjacency matrix is

$$\mathbf{A} = \frac{1}{\sqrt{a_1^{3/2} + a_2^{3/2} + a_3^{3/2}}} \begin{pmatrix} 0 & 0 & 0 & a_1^{3/4} \\ 0 & 0 & 0 & a_2^{3/4} \\ 0 & 0 & 0 & a_3^{3/4} \\ a_1^{3/4} & a_2^{3/4} & a_3^{3/4} & 0 \end{pmatrix}.$$

Confirm, using, e.g., the symbolic toolbox in MATLAB, that $0, 0, 1, -1$ are the eigenvalues of $\mathbf{A}$. Reconcile this result with our findings in Eqs. (8.38)–(8.39).

The Active Dendritic Tree

OUTLINE

9.1   The Active Uniform Cable   120

9.2   On the Interaction of Active Uniform Cables*   122

9.3   The Active Nonuniform Cable   125

9.4   The Quasi-Active Cable*   130

9.5   The Active Dendritic Tree   134

9.6   Summary and Sources   136

9.7   Exercises   136

We are now prepared to assemble models that are capable of reproducing the great variety of responses, seen in the laboratory, to synaptic input distributed in space and time. This requires only that we add ion channels to our passive dendrite. A combination of the numerical methods of Chapters 4 and 8 will permit us to generate the action potential launched by suprathreshold current injection and to study its propagation from the spike initiation zone down the cell's axon and back up into the soma and the dendritic tree, in agreement with the recordings in Figure 9.1.

We then build a model for determining the extracellular current induced by such traveling action potentials and study its effect on neighboring cables like axons or dendrites. We next move on to synaptic initiation of somatic spikes and investigate the role of a specialized glutamate receptor, called the NMDA receptor, in acknowledging action

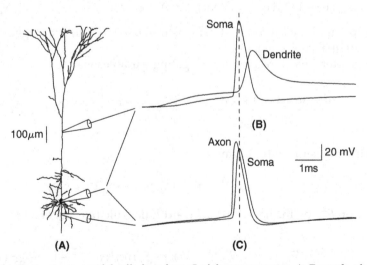

FIGURE 9.1   Action potential initiation in pyramidal cells from layer 5 of the rat neocortex. **A.** Example of a reconstructed cell and approximate location of two electrodes in two separate recordings. Electrodes were placed either in dendrite and soma (**B**) or in axon and soma (**C**). **B.** Simultaneous recordings of action potential initiation by synaptic stimulation indicates that the action potential propagates from the soma, with attenuation, back into the dendrites $\approx 270\,\mu$m in ≈ 1 ms. **C.** Simultaneous recordings from soma and axon shows that the action potential originates in the axon and propagates back to the soma $\approx 17\,\mu$m in ≈ 0.1 ms, before reaching the dendrites (see **B**).

Mathematics for Neuroscientists. DOI: 10.1016/B978-0-12-374882-9.00009-5

potential back propagation into the dendrites. We next develop and study the quasi-active cable and demonstrate its ability to capture the cell's subthreshold response and resonant frequency. We then investigate synaptic attenuation and integration on our active fork prior to introducing and demonstrating MATLAB tools for the simulation of arbitrarily branched cells. Finally, we move on to the fully branched case, where we study synaptic integration.

9.1 THE ACTIVE UNIFORM CABLE

If we add the sodium and potassium currents of Chapter 4 to the passive cable of Chapter 6 we arrive at the active cable system

$$
\begin{aligned}
C_m \frac{\partial V}{\partial t} &= G_a \frac{\partial^2 V}{\partial x^2} - \bar{g}_{Na} m^3 h (V - V_{Na}) - \bar{g}_K n^4 (V - V_K) - g_{Cl}(V - V_{Cl}) + I_{stim}/(2\pi a) \\
m_t &= \alpha_m(V)(1-m) - \beta_m(V)m \\
h_t &= \alpha_h(V)(1-h) - \beta_h(V)h \\
n_t &= \alpha_n(V)(1-n) - \beta_n(V)n
\end{aligned}
\tag{9.1}
$$

where $G_a = a/(2R_a)$ is the axial conductance. We assume that the cable is sealed

$$
\frac{\partial V}{\partial x}(0,t) = \frac{\partial V}{\partial x}(\ell,t) = 0,
$$

and that it begins at rest

$$
V(x,0) = V_r, \ m(x,0) = m_\infty(V_r), \ h(x,0) = h_\infty(V_r), \ n(x,0) = n_\infty(V_r).
$$

If the ionic conductances are uniformly distributed, i.e., their conductance densities do not vary with position, then the rest potential is in fact the same V_r as that in Eq. (4.16).

As Eq. (9.1) does not yield to elementary mathematical analysis we pursue its approximate solution. In particular, we choose a space step, dx, and so study a cable with $N_x = \ell/dx$ compartments, and then choose a time step, dt, and final time T and so march through $N_t = T/dt$ units of time. We evaluate our stimulus and approximate the response on the associated space-time grid

$$
\begin{aligned}
\mathsf{v}_i^j &\approx V((i-1/2)dx, (j-1)dt) \\
\mathsf{m}_i^j &\approx m((i-1/2)dx, (j-3/2)dt) \\
\mathsf{I}_i^j &= I_{stim}((i-1/2)dx, (j-3/2)dt)/(2\pi a), \quad i=1,\ldots,N_x, \quad j=1,\ldots,N_t
\end{aligned}
\tag{9.2}
$$

where $(i-1/2)dx$ is the midpoint of the ith compartment, as in Eq. (6.53), and the staggering of voltage and gating time grids conforms to our original choice, Eq. (4.17).

Arguing precisely as in Chapter 4 we may advance the gating variables via

$$
\mathsf{m}_i^j = \frac{(1/dt - (\alpha_m(\mathsf{v}_i^{j-1}) + \beta_m(\mathsf{v}_i^{j-1}))/2)\mathsf{m}_i^{j-1} + \alpha_m(\mathsf{v}_i^{j-1})}{1/dt + (\alpha_m(\mathsf{v}_i^{j-1}) + \beta_m(\mathsf{v}_i^{j-1}))/2} \quad i=1,\ldots,N_x.
\tag{9.3}
$$

We now collect the compartmental terms into columns

$$
\mathsf{v}^j = (\mathsf{v}_1^j \ \mathsf{v}_2^j \ \cdots \ \mathsf{v}_{N_x}^j)^T, \quad \mathsf{m}^j = (\mathsf{m}_1^j \ \mathsf{m}_2^j \ \cdots \ \mathsf{m}_{N_x}^j)^T, \quad \text{etc.,}
$$

and advance the voltage vector v^{j-1} by the half-step backward Euler rule (per Eq. (4.20))

$$
C_m \frac{\mathsf{v}^{j-1/2} - \mathsf{v}^{j-1}}{dt/2} = G_a \mathsf{S} \mathsf{v}^{j-1/2} - \bar{g}_{Na}(\mathsf{m}^j)^3 \mathsf{h}^j (\mathsf{v}^{j-1/2} - V_{Na}) - \bar{g}_K(\mathsf{n}^j)^4 (\mathsf{v}^{j-1/2} - V_K) - g_{Cl}(\mathsf{v}^{j-1/2} - V_{Cl}) + \mathsf{I}^j
$$

where S is our standard second difference matrix, Eq. (6.9). We write this as a linear system for $\mathsf{v}^{j-1/2}$,

$$
(\text{diag}(\mathsf{d}^j + 2C_m/dt) + G_a\mathsf{S})\mathsf{v}^{j-1/2} = (2C_m/dt)\mathsf{v}^{j-1} + \mathsf{f}^j
\tag{9.4}
$$

where the elements of d and f are

$$d_i^j = \overline{g}_{Na}(m_i^j)^3 h_i^j + \overline{g}_K(n_i^j)^4 + g_{Cl} \quad \text{and} \quad f_i^j = \overline{g}_{Na}(m_i^j)^3 h_i^j V_{Na} + \overline{g}_K(n_i^j)^4 V_K + g_{Cl} V_{Cl} + I_i^j$$

respectively. We conclude, as in Eq. (4.21), with the final additional half-step update

$$v^j = 2v^{j-1/2} - v^{j-1}. \tag{9.5}$$

We have coded this and illustrated its use in Figure 9.2 on the cable with size and passive parameters as in Eq. (6.17), active parameters and functionals as detailed in §§4.1 and 4.2, and a 1 ms stimulus

$$I_{stim}(x,t) = I_0 \mathbb{1}_{(1,2)}(t)\delta(x - x_s) \tag{9.6}$$

of amplitude I_0 delivered at $x = x_s$. We see that a 1 ms current pulse at midcable ignites an action potential when I_0 exceeds the threshold, I_θ, of approximately 150 pA and we note that the V_{max}/I_0 curve differs very little from the isopotential case, Figure 4.7B. In the case of a cable, however, stimulus location can also play a major role. For current delivered near a sealed end sees a greater resistance and hence yields a greater depolarization. We make this precise in Figure 9.3.

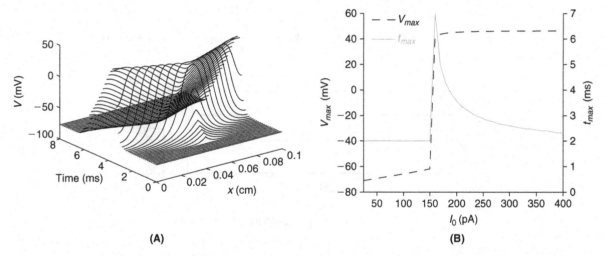

| (A) | (B) |

FIGURE 9.2 Response of the active cable described by Eqs. (6.17), (4.8), (4.9), (4.13), and (4.14) to a current pulse described by Eq. (9.6) with $x_s = 0.05$ cm. **A.** Full space-time response to suprathreshold input, $I_0 = 400$ pA. This stimulus has initiated an action potential that propagates at constant velocity in each direction. (stEcab.m) **B.** A plot of the maximum depolarization at x_s, and the time at which it occurred, as a function of stimulus amplitude, I_0. (stEcabthresh.m)

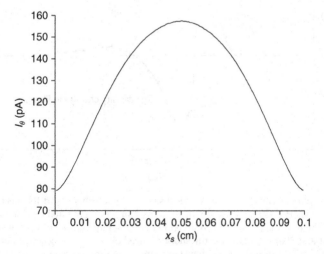

FIGURE 9.3 A plot of stimulus threshold, I_θ, as a function of stimulus location, x_s, for the cable described by Eqs. (6.17), (4.8), (4.9), (4.13), and (4.14) and a current pulse of the form Eq. (9.6). (stEcabthreshloc.m)

The speed of the action potential wave illustrated in Figure 9.2A depends on both the geometry of the cable and the mix of currents crossing its lateral surface. We will investigate these dependencies in the exercises.

9.2 ON THE INTERACTION OF ACTIVE UNIFORM CABLES*

There is ample evidence, see Figure 9.4, to support the investigation of the nonsynaptic influence that an action potential traveling down a cable may have on its neighbors. These interactions are often deemed "ephaptic" and arise, e.g., from extracellular currents and excess extracellular potassium associated with traveling action potentials.

In Exercise 4.5 we demonstrated that increased extracellular potassium depolarizes nearby cells. We here build and analyze a model, see Figure 9.5, of two parallel cables of radii a_1 and a_{-1}, separated by a distance $2a_0$, in which extracellular current may flow. If dx is the length of a compartment then current balance at the nodes marked $\phi_{2,1}$ and $\phi_{2,-1}$ yields

$$2\pi a_1 dx\{C_m(\phi_{2,1} - \phi_{2,0})' + I_{ion}(\phi_{2,1} - \phi_{2,0})\} = \frac{\pi a_1^2}{R_a dx}(\phi_{1,1} - 2\phi_{2,1} + \phi_{3,1})$$

$$2\pi a_{-1} dx\{C_m(\phi_{2,-1} - \phi_{2,0})' + I_{ion}(\phi_{2,-1} - \phi_{2,0})\} = \frac{\pi a_{-1}^2}{R_a dx}(\phi_{1,-1} - 2\phi_{2,-1} + \phi_{3,-1}).$$

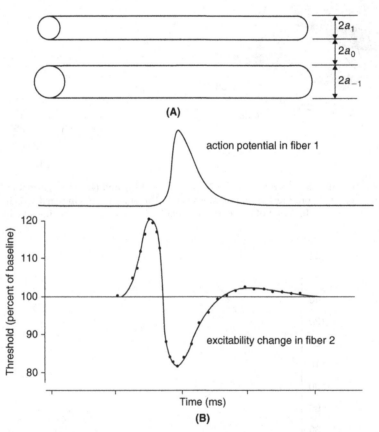

(A)

(B)

FIGURE 9.4 **A.** A schematic of two parallel cables. **B.** The electrical stimulation of fiber 1 and its effect on the threshold of fiber 2. Action potentials in fibers 1 and 2 are elicited by short electric pulses. An illustration of an action potential recorded from fiber 1 is on top. The threshold change is expressed as a percentage of the baseline value (100) observed in fiber 2 without stimulation of fiber 1 and is measured as a function of the stimulation interval between fiber 1 and fiber 2. Initially the threshold is raised by the traveling action potential in fiber 1, but then the second fiber becomes more excitable followed by a period of slightly reduced excitability. In vitro preparation of a limb nerve of the crab. Adapted from Katz and Schmitt (1940).

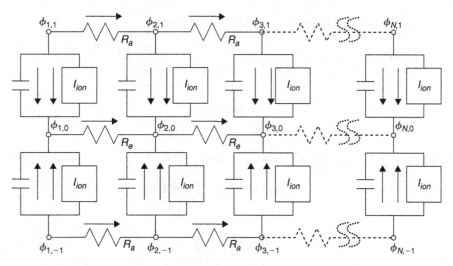

FIGURE 9.5 A circuit diagram, corresponding to Figure 9.4A, of two cables and the extracellular fluid that separates them. Here R_e is the effective axial resistance of the extracellular fluid, $\phi_{j,\pm1}$ denote the intracellular potentials of the respective cables, $\phi_{0,\pm1}$ denote the associated extracellular potentials, and the membrane currents, at each compartment, have been lumped into the I_{ion} boxes.

Next, as the fibers are separated by a distance of $2a_0$, current balance at the node marked $\phi_{2,0}$ yields

$$2\pi a_1 dx\{C_m(\phi_{2,1}-\phi_{2,0})'+I_{ion}(\phi_{2,1}-\phi_{2,0})\}+2\pi a_{-1}dx\{C_m(\phi_{2,0}-\phi_{2,-1})'+I_{ion}(\phi_{2,0}-\phi_{2,-1})\}$$
$$=-\frac{\pi a_0^2}{R_e dx}(\phi_{1,0}-2\phi_{2,0}+\phi_{3,0}).$$

If we now define the transmembrane potentials

$$V_n \equiv \phi_{n,1}-\phi_{n,0} \quad \text{and} \quad W_n \equiv \phi_{n,-1}-\phi_{n,0}$$

the above become

$$C_m V_2' + I_{ion}(V_2) = \frac{a_1}{2R_a}\frac{V_1-2V_2+V_3}{dx^2}+\frac{a_1}{2R_a}\frac{\phi_{1,0}-2\phi_{2,0}+\phi_{3,0}}{dx^2} \tag{9.7}$$

$$C_m W_2' + I_{ion}(W_2) = \frac{a_{-1}}{2R_a}\frac{W_1-2W_2+W_3}{dx^2}+\frac{a_{-1}}{2R_a}\frac{\phi_{1,0}-2\phi_{2,0}+\phi_{3,0}}{dx^2} \tag{9.8}$$

and

$$a_1\{C_m V_2'+I_{ion}(V_2)\}+a_{-1}\{C_m W_2'+I_{ion}(W_2)\}=-\frac{a_0^2}{2R_e}\frac{\phi_{1,0}-2\phi_{2,0}+\phi_{3,0}}{dx^2}.$$

On substituting this equation into Eqs. (9.7) and (9.8) we find

$$\frac{a_0^2 R_a+a_1^2 R_e}{a_0^2 R_a}\{C_m V_2'+I_{ion}(V_2)\}+\frac{a_1 a_{-1}R_e}{a_0^2 R_a}\{C_m W_2'+I_{ion}(W_2)\}=\frac{a_1}{2R_a}\frac{V_1-2V_2+V_3}{dx^2} \tag{9.9}$$

$$\frac{a_0^2 R_a+a_{-1}^2 R_e}{a_0^2 R_a}\{C_m W_2'+I_{ion}(W_2)\}+\frac{a_{-1}a_1 R_e}{a_0^2 R_a}\{C_m V_2'+I_{ion}(V_2)\}=\frac{a_{-1}}{2R_a}\frac{W_1-2W_2+W_3}{dx^2}. \tag{9.10}$$

Now $(a_0^2 R_a+a_{-1}^2 R_e)/(a_1 a_{-1}R_e)$ times Eq. (9.9) minus Eq. (9.10) brings

$$C_m V_2'+I_{ion}(V_2)=c_1\frac{a_1}{2R_a}\frac{V_1-2V_2+V_3}{dx^2}-c_2\frac{a_{-1}}{2R_a}\frac{W_1-2W_2+W_3}{dx^2}, \tag{9.11}$$

where the coupling parameters are

$$c_1=\frac{a_0^2 R_a+a_{-1}^2 R_e}{a_0^2 R_a+(a_1^2+a_{-1}^2)R_e} \quad \text{and} \quad c_2=\frac{a_1 a_{-1}R_e}{a_0^2 R_a+(a_1^2+a_{-1}^2)R_e}. \tag{9.12}$$

Similarly, $(a_0^2 R_a + a_1^2 R_e)/(a_1 a_{-1} R_e)$ times Eq. (9.10) minus Eq. (9.9) brings

$$C_m W_2' + I_{ion}(W_2) = c_{-1}\frac{a_{-1}}{2R_a}\frac{W_1 - 2W_2 + W_3}{dx^2} - c_2\frac{a_1}{2R_a}\frac{V_1 - 2V_2 + V_3}{dx^2}, \tag{9.13}$$

where

$$c_{-1} = \frac{a_0^2 R_a + a_1^2 R_e}{a_0^2 R_a + (a_1^2 + a_{-1}^2)R_e}.$$

Current balance at the remaining nodes proceeds exactly as above. As such we may express the full coupled system as

$$C_m \mathbf{u}'(t) + g_{Cl}(\mathbf{u}(t) - V_{Cl}) + \bar{g}_K \mathbf{n}^4(\mathbf{u} - V_K) + \bar{g}_{Na}\mathbf{m}^3\mathbf{h}(\mathbf{u} - V_{Na}) = \mathbf{B}\mathbf{u}(t) + \mathbf{f}(t), \tag{9.14}$$

where

$$\mathbf{u}(t) = \begin{pmatrix} \mathbf{v}(t) \\ \mathbf{w}(t) \end{pmatrix}$$

with $\mathbf{v}(t) = (V_1(t), \ldots, V_n(t))^T$ and $\mathbf{w}(t) = (W_1(t), \ldots, W_n(t))^T$. The matrix $\mathbf{B}$ is defined by

$$\mathbf{B} = \begin{pmatrix} c_1 G_1 \mathbf{S} & -c_2 G_{-1} \mathbf{S} \\ -c_2 G_1 \mathbf{S} & c_{-1} G_{-1} \mathbf{S} \end{pmatrix},$$

with $G_{\pm 1} = a_{\pm 1}/(2R_a)$ and $\mathbf{S}$ is our familiar second difference matrix. The gating variables continue to obey equations of the form

$$\mathbf{m}'(t) = \frac{m_\infty(\mathbf{u}(t)) - \mathbf{m}(t)}{\tau_m(\mathbf{u}(t))}$$

where

$$m_\infty(\mathbf{u}(t)) = (m_\infty(u_1(t)), \ldots, m_\infty(u_n(t)))^T \quad \text{and} \quad \tau_m(\mathbf{u}(t)) = (\tau_m(u_1(t)), \ldots, \tau_m(u_n(t)))^T.$$

We recognize that the off-diagonal elements of $\mathbf{B}$ capture the interaction of the two cables. In particular, each cable "stimulates" the other through a current that is proportional to the spatial second difference of its membrane potential. In addition, as $c_{\pm 1} < 1$, we note that the effective individual axial conductances, $c_{\pm 1}G_{\pm 1}$, are each smaller than their original values.

We may proceed, as in the case of a single cable, to apply the staggered Euler scheme to Eq. (9.14). We have implemented this in stE2cab.m and demonstrate its findings in Figure 9.6. In reality both cables would be receiving independent input and rather than the first cable fully exciting the second, it is more likely that activity in the first serves to lower the second's threshold for excitation. This is the scenario illustrated in Figure 9.4 and we will investigate it further in the exercises.

It may perhaps be easier to visualize the interaction terms by passing to the limit, $dx \to 0$, in Eq. (9.14) and so arriving at the coupled active cable equations

$$C_m \frac{\partial V}{\partial t} + g_{Cl}(V - V_{Cl}) + \bar{g}_K n_1^4(V - V_K) + \bar{g}_{Na}m_1^3 h_1(V - V_{Na}) = c_1 G_1 \frac{\partial^2 V}{\partial x^2} - c_2 G_{-1}\frac{\partial^2 W}{\partial x^2} + I_{stim}/(2\pi a_1)$$

$$C_m \frac{\partial W}{\partial t} + g_{Cl}(W - V_{Cl}) + \bar{g}_K n_2^4(W - V_K) + \bar{g}_{Na}m_2^3 h_2(W - V_{Na}) = c_{-1}G_{-1}\frac{\partial^2 W}{\partial x^2} - c_2 G_1 \frac{\partial^2 V}{\partial x^2}$$

where

$$\partial_t m_1 = \frac{m_\infty(V) - m_1}{\tau_m(V)} \quad \text{and} \quad \partial_t m_2 = \frac{m_\infty(W) - m_2}{\tau_m(W)},$$

and similarly for the remaining gating equations. The two potential equations now make it clear that it is the axial current in a cable that stimulates its neighboring cables. In particular, with regard to Figure 9.6E, we see that as the top cable fires, its membrane potential, V, at fixed time t, progresses from a single concave bump to two concave bumps traveling away from the site of initiation. Where V is concave we know that $\partial^2 V/\partial x^2 \leq 0$ and so the stimulus to the lower cable is positive. Hence, as the V wave travels in the upper cable it reinforces, and is likewise reinforced by, the W wave in the lower cable.

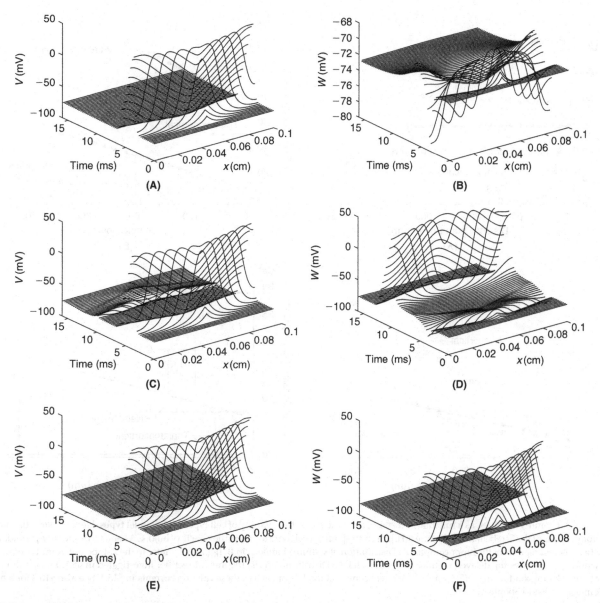

FIGURE 9.6 The full space-time potentials of the two cables (top at left and bottom at right) separated by $2a_0$. Each cable is identical to that examined above in Figure 9.2 and the resistivity of the extracellular medium is $R_e = 0.1$ kΩcm. We stimulate the top cable with a suprathreshold pulse as in Eq. (9.6) with $I_0 = 400$ pA. This causes an action potential traveling wave in the cable. A. With $a_0 = 1.5\,\mu$m the wave in the top cable delivers a complex, but ultimately subthreshold stimulus to the lower cable, as illustrated in B. The influence of this upon the top cable appears negligible. C. With $a_0 = 1\,\mu$m the wave in the top cable produces a small disturbance in the bottom cable that eventually brings its two ends to threshold. These two end waves travel inward and annihilate each other at the midpoint, see D. This latter wave causes a notable, but subthreshold, disturbance in the top cable. E. With $a = 0.5\,\mu$m the wave in the top cable quickly ignites a wave in the bottom cable, see F. The bottom wave likely lies in the refractory wake of the top wave and therefore provides negligible feedback. (stE2cab.m)

9.3 THE ACTIVE NONUNIFORM CABLE

Neurons are not simply nonuniform in their geometry and branching patterns, they are also highly nonuniform with regard to their distribution of channels. One simple nonuniformity stems from the observation that many cells partition their "input end" from their "output end" for the obvious reasons that action potentials have a metabolic cost and several inputs ought to arrive in a small window if the subsequent output spike is to mean anything. This partition is often achieved by distributing channels in such a way as to create a weakly excitable dendrite and a strongly excitable cell body and axon initial segment. For example, see Figure 9.7, Purkinje and CA3 cells achieve this by decreasing $\bar{g}_{Na}$ with distance from the soma, while CA1 and mitral cells achieve this by increasing $\bar{g}_K$ with distance from the soma.

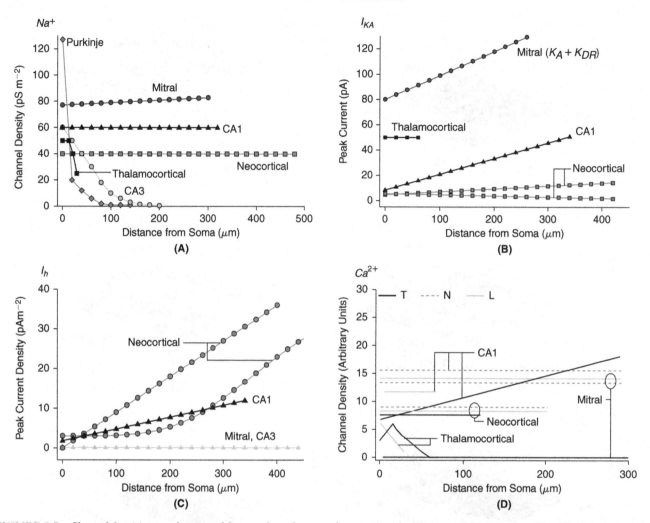

FIGURE 9.7   Channel densities, as a function of distance from the soma, for a variety of cell types and channel types. Here Purkinje denotes the large inhibitory cells of the cerebellum (see Figure 8.1E), the mitral cell is a cell type found in the olfactory bulb, CA1 and CA3 refer to pyramidal cells found in two distinct regions of the hippocampus. **A**. Distribution of sodium channels. In **B**, I_{KA} and K_A refer to the A-type potassium conductance of §4.4, while K_{DR} signifies the delayed rectifier current of §4.3. **C**. Distribution of I_h, the inward rectifier investigated in §5.5. **D**. Distribution of three types of calcium conductances (T, N, and L). We will construct models of each of these calcium currents in §13.1. See also §10.3 for a model of I_T. From Migliore and Shepherd (2002).

Before opening the door to wildly branched cells with exotic channel distributions we focus on the straight cable and mimic a weakly excitable dendrite and a highly excitable cell body by assuming that both sodium and potassium peak conductances are constant, except for an excitable "hot spot":

$$\bar{g}_K(x) = 40 - 20\mathbb{1}_{siz}(x) \quad \text{and} \quad \bar{g}_{Na}(x) = 44 + 560\mathbb{1}_{siz}(x) \quad \text{where} \quad siz = (0.005, 0.01) \tag{9.15}$$

denotes the spike initiation zone and the cable has length $\ell = 0.1$ cm. We first compute the associated nonuniform rest potential by solving $G_a V_r''(x) = I^{ss}(x)$ where

$$I^{ss}(x, V_r) \equiv \bar{g}_{Na}(x)m_\infty^3(V_r)h_\infty(V_r)(V_r - V_{Na}) + \bar{g}_K(x)n_\infty^4(V_r)(V_r - V_K) + g_{Cl}(V_r - V_{Cl}), \tag{9.16}$$

subject to $V_r'(0) = V_r'(\ell) = 0$. We solve this, as before, via Newton's method with `fsolve` in MATLAB, although here, with perhaps thousands of compartments, this is a much more difficult task. The Jacobian, $\nabla I^{ss} \in \mathbb{R}^{N_x \times N_x}$,

$$(\nabla I^{ss})_{ij} = \frac{\partial I_i^{ss}(V)}{\partial V_j} \tag{9.17}$$

that springs from the quasi-active counterpart (see §9.4) greatly eases the burden. In particular, writing the discretized rest equation as $G_a\mathbf{S}\mathbf{V} - \mathbf{I}^{ss}(\mathbf{V}) = 0$ we note that Newton's method converges to the (discrete) rest potential via the update rule

$$\mathbf{V}^{k+1} = \mathbf{V}^k - (G_a\mathbf{S} - \nabla\mathbf{I}^{ss}(\mathbf{V}^k))\backslash(G_a\mathbf{S}\mathbf{V}^k - \mathbf{I}^{ss}(\mathbf{V}^k)).$$

We have coded this in `stEcabnon.m` and illustrate its use in Figure 9.8.

We see in both panels of Figure 9.8 a direct reflection of the cable's nonuniform channel distribution. To better appreciate the impact of Figure 9.8B we show in Figure 9.9 the full spatio-temporal response to a stimulus that is subthreshold when delivered distally but suprathreshold when delivered proximally.

Although the stimulus in Figure 9.9B was delivered to a weak segment of the cable we see that the entire cable is excitable enough to support a traveling action potential. In addition, as in Figure 9.1, we note that the action potential in the distal region is smaller than that at the siz.

We now focus on the synaptic machinery that detects the presence of such a back-propagating action potential in the postsynaptic cell shortly following presynaptic activity. In particular, we place a spine (recall §6.5) at x_s and endow its head with two types, AMPA and NMDA, of glutamate receptors. The abbreviation NMDA stands for N-methyl-D-aspartic acid, which is a selective activator (or agonist) of the NMDA receptor (NMDAR), just as AMPA is for the AMPA receptor. We built a model for AMPA receptors in §2.5. The methodology for NMDARs is similar to a point, for the associated conductance has a strong voltage dependence. If W denotes the spine head transmembrane

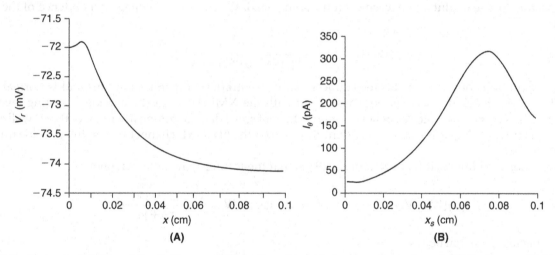

FIGURE 9.8 Rest potential (**A**) and threshold current (**B**) for the cable with the nonuniform channel distribution specified in Eq. (9.15). (`stEcabnon.m` and `stEcabthreshloc.m`)

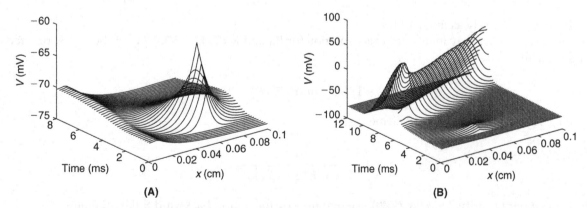

FIGURE 9.9 Response to injection of 200 pA for 1 ms at $x = 0.06$, (**A**), and $x = 0.04$ cm, (**B**). This is not merely a three-dimensional view of Figure 9.8B, for here we see that the proximal stimulus did not elicit an action potential at the stimulation site (where the cable is only weakly excitable), but rather was sufficiently strong that it eventually reached the highly excitable zone. (`stEcabnon.m`)

potential our cable equation takes the form

$$C_m \frac{\partial V}{\partial t} = G_a \frac{\partial^2 V}{\partial x^2} - \bar{g}_{Na} m^3 h (V - V_{Na}) - \bar{g}_K n^4 (V - V_K) - g_{Cl}(V - V_{Cl}) + \gamma_2 (W(t) - V(x,t)) \delta(x - x_s)$$

while the spine potential, W, obeys

$$C_m W'(t) + g_{Cl}(W(t) - V_{Cl}) + (g_A(t) + g_N(t) M(W(t)))(W(t) - V_{syn}) = \gamma_1 (V(x_s, t) - W(t)). \tag{9.18}$$

The coupling parameters, as in §6.5, are

$$\gamma_1 = 1/(R_{sn} A_{sh}) \quad \text{and} \quad \gamma_2 = 1/(R_{sn} 2\pi a)$$

while the AMPA and NMDA conductances obey

$$g_A(t) = \bar{g}_A R_A(t) \quad \text{and} \quad g_N(t) = \bar{g}_N R_N(t) \tag{9.19}$$

where R_A and R_N are the respective fractions of activated AMPA and NMDA receptors. We suppose, as in Eq. (2.20), that they obey the first order equations

$$R_A'(t) = k_A^+ T(t)(1 - R_A(t)) - k_A^- R_A(t) \quad \text{and} \quad R_N'(t) = k_N^+ T(t)(1 - R_N(t)) - k_N^- R_N(t)$$

where $T(t)$ is the dosage of glutamate received at the spine head. We encode the voltage dependence of the NMDA receptor in

$$M(W) = \frac{1}{1 + [Mg^{2+}]_e \exp(-0.062W)/3.57}, \tag{9.20}$$

where $[Mg^{2+}]_e$ (in units of mM) denotes the extracellular concentration of magnesium ions and is normally equal to 2 mM. These ions block the channel pore associated with the NMDAR from the outside at resting levels of W (Figure 9.10A). This magnesium block is relieved upon sufficient spine depolarization in a manner that is well captured by Eq. (9.20) (Figure 9.10B). As a result, the current flow across the NMDAR channel is a highly nonlinear function of W (Figure 9.10C).

Regarding initial conditions, it follows from Eq. (9.18) that the resting spine potential obeys

$$g_{Cl}(W_r - V_{Cl}) = \gamma_1 (V_r(x_s) - W_r), \quad \text{e.g.,} \quad W_r = \frac{g_{Cl} V_{Cl} + \gamma_1 V_r(x_s)}{g_{Cl} + \gamma_1}$$

and so the cable rest potential obeys

$$G_a V_r'' = \bar{g}_{Na} m_\infty^3(V_r) h_\infty(V_r)(V_r - V_{Na}) + \bar{g}_K n_\infty^4(V_r)(V_r - V_K) + g_{Cl}(V_r - V_{Cl}) - \frac{\gamma_2 g_{Cl}}{g_{Cl} + \gamma_1}(V_{Cl} - V_r) \delta(x - x_s).$$

We solve this for V_r precisely as in Eq. (9.17).

If T is simply a pulse we may invoke the exact solution for R_A and R_N in Eq. (3.36). Let us, however, proceed more generally and define

$$T^j = T((j-1)dt), \quad \text{and} \quad R_A^j \approx R_A((j-1)dt),$$

and update R_A via the backward Euler scheme

$$R_A^j = \frac{R_A^{j-1} + dt k_A^+ T^j}{1 + (k_A^+ T^j + k_A^-)dt}.$$

Given the explicit nonlinearity, M in Eq. (9.20), we update W by the hybrid backward Euler scheme

$$C_m(W^j - W^{j-1})/dt + g_{Cl}(W^j - V_{Cl}) + (g_A^j + g_N^j M(W^{j-1}))(W^j - V_{syn}) = \gamma_1 (V_k^{j-1} - W^j)$$

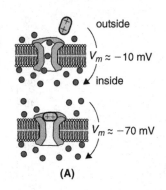

(A)

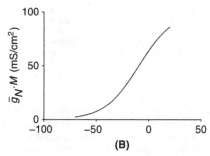

(B)

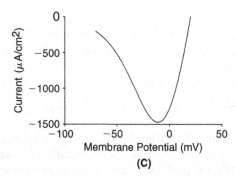

(C)

FIGURE 9.10 **A.** Schematic illustration of the block of the NMDA receptor channel by magnesium. At potentials near rest, magnesium enters the pore and blocks the channel (bottom). At depolarized potentials the magnesium is ejected and the channel is free to pass Na$^+$, K$^+$, and, most importantly, Ca^{2+}. **B.** Dependence of $\bar{g}_N M$ on W. **C.** Dependence of $\bar{g}_N M(W)(W - V_{syn})$ on W.

or

$$W^j = \frac{(C_m/dt)W^{j-1} + g_{Cl}V_{Cl} + (g_A^j + g_N^j M(W^{j-1}))V_{syn} + \gamma_1 V_k^{j-1}}{(C_m/dt) + g_{Cl} + g_A^j + g_N^j M(W^{j-1}) + \gamma_1}.$$

We apply the same scheme to the gating variables, e.g.,

$$m_i^j = \frac{m_i^{j-1} + dt\,\alpha_m(V_i^{j-1})}{1 + dt(\alpha_m(V_i^{j-1}) + \beta_m(V_i^{j-1}))},$$

and finally update the cable potential via an honest backward Euler scheme

$$C_m(V^j - V^{j-1})/dt = (G_a \mathbf{S} - \mathrm{diag}\,(d^j))V^j + f^j$$

where the elements of d^j and f^j are

$$d_i^j = \bar{g}_{Na}(m_i^j)^3 h^j + \bar{g}_K(n_i^j)^4 + g_{Cl} + \gamma_2\delta_{ik} \quad \text{and}$$

$$f_i^j = \bar{g}_{Na}(m_i^j)^3 h^j V_{Na} + \bar{g}_K(n_i^j)^4 V_K + g_{Cl}V_{Cl} + \gamma_2 W^j \delta_{ik}$$

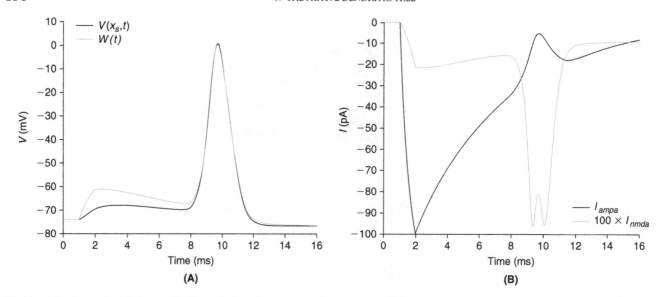

FIGURE 9.11   Potentials (**A**), and currents (**B**), at the spine, on the nonuniform active cable. Following the BPAP, we see the strong late depolarization of the spine head free the magnesium block at the NMDAR and so permit a sizable, inward, NMDA current. This current is the signature of near coincident pre- and postsynaptic activity, and as such forms a natural substrate for the Hebbian learning algorithm of §12.6. To lend it even greater specificity, this current is rich in calcium ions. We will take a careful look at the complex role of Ca^{2+} in spine heads in Chapter 13. (stEcabspine.m)

and k is the number of the compartment at which the spine is attached. We now consider a concrete example. We place a spine at $x_s = 0.04$ cm, with the geometric parameters as in Eq. (6.57), and receptor and conductance parameters

$$k_A^+ = 1.1 \;(\text{mMms})^{-1}, \quad k_A^- = 0.19 \;\text{ms}^{-1}, \quad \text{and} \quad \overline{g}_A = 200 \;\text{mS/cm}^2,$$

$$k_N^+ = 0.072 \;(\text{mMms})^{-1}, \quad k_N^- = 0.0066 \;\text{ms}^{-1}, \quad \text{and} \quad \overline{g}_N = 100 \;\text{mS/cm}^2,$$

and synaptic reversal potential $V_{syn} = 20$ mV. On stimulating the spine with a 1 ms pulse of 1 mM glutamate we find, as in Figure 9.9B, slow progression of subthreshold depolarization toward the hot zone followed by a rapid back-propagating action potential (BPAP). We plot the salient features in Figure 9.11.

9.4 THE QUASI-ACTIVE CABLE*

If the injected current is small, say εI_{stim}, we may develop V and its gating variables in power series, as in Eq. (5.1), in ε. For example, $V(x,t) = V_r(x) + \varepsilon \tilde{V}(x,t) + O(\varepsilon^2)$, where $V_r(x)$ is the rest potential. As in Eq. (5.2), the linear terms in this expansion obey what we call the quasi-active system

$$\frac{\partial \tilde{m}}{\partial t} = (\overline{m}'_\infty \tilde{V} - \tilde{m})/\overline{\tau}_m$$

$$\frac{\partial \tilde{h}}{\partial t} = (\overline{h}'_\infty \tilde{V} - \tilde{h})/\overline{\tau}_h$$

$$\frac{\partial \tilde{n}}{\partial t} = (\overline{n}'_\infty \tilde{V} - \tilde{n})/\overline{\tau}_n \tag{9.21}$$

$$C_m \frac{\partial \tilde{V}}{\partial t} = \lambda^2 \frac{\partial^2 \tilde{V}}{\partial x^2} - \overline{g}_{Na}\{\overline{m}^3 \overline{h} \tilde{V} + (3\tilde{m}\overline{m}^2 \overline{h} + \overline{m}^3 \tilde{h})v_{Na}\} - \overline{g}_K\{\overline{n}^4 \tilde{V} + 4\tilde{n}\overline{n}^3 v_K\}$$
$$- g_{Cl}\tilde{V} + I_{stim}(x,t)/(2\pi a),$$

where $\overline{m}(x) \equiv m_\infty(V_r(x))$, $\overline{\tau}_m \equiv \tau_m(V_r(x))$, and $\overline{m}'_\infty \equiv m'_\infty(V_r(x))$. We gather the unknowns in $\mathbf{y} \equiv (\tilde{m} \; \tilde{h} \; \tilde{n} \; \tilde{V})^T$ and represent Eq. (9.21) as

$$\frac{\partial \mathbf{y}}{\partial t} = \mathbf{B}\mathbf{y} + \mathbf{f} \tag{9.22}$$

where $\mathbf{f} = I_{stim}(x,t)/(2\pi a C_m)(0\ 0\ 0\ 1)^T$ and $\mathbf{B}$ is the matrix differential operator

$$\mathbf{B} = \begin{pmatrix} -1/\overline{\tau}_m & 0 & 0 & \overline{m}'_\infty/\overline{\tau}_m \\ 0 & -1/\overline{\tau}_h & 0 & \overline{h}'_\infty/\overline{\tau}_h \\ 0 & 0 & -1/\overline{\tau}_n & \overline{n}'_\infty/\overline{\tau}_n \\ -3\overline{m}^2\overline{h}v_{Na}/\tau_{Na} & -\overline{m}^3 v_{Na}/\tau_{Na} & -4\overline{n}^3 v_K/\tau_K & (\lambda^2/\tau)\partial_{xx} - \gamma \end{pmatrix} \tag{9.23}$$

where $\gamma = \overline{m}^3\overline{h}/\tau_{Na} + \overline{n}^4/\tau_K + 1/\tau_{Cl}$. We have discretized (precisely as in the past three sections) and coded this system in stEQcab.m. We contrast the quasi-active and active responses of the uniform cable to random current stimuli in stEcabQandA.m and illustrate our findings in Figure 9.12.

Figure 9.12 indicates that the quasi-active model is an accurate predictor of the cumulative response to subthreshold spatio-temporal input. We next investigate its ability to predict the cell's resonant frequency.

Resonance. We expect the resonant frequencies of the active cable to be reflected in the imaginary parts of the eigenvalues of $\mathbf{B}$. As in §5.3 we write

$$\mathbf{B}\mathbf{w}(x) = \zeta\mathbf{w}(x) \quad \text{with} \quad \mathbf{w} \equiv (\mu(x)\ \eta(x)\ \nu(x)\ q(x))^T$$

and deduce that

$$\overline{m}'_\infty q - \mu = \zeta\overline{\tau}_m\mu \quad \text{so} \quad \mu = \frac{\overline{m}'_\infty}{1 + \zeta\overline{\tau}_m}q.$$

The other gating variables follow suit, namely

$$\eta = \frac{\overline{h}'_\infty}{1 + \zeta\overline{\tau}_h}q \quad \text{and} \quad \nu = \frac{\overline{n}'_\infty}{1 + \zeta\overline{\tau}_n}q$$

and so the equation for the quasi-potential, q, reads

$$(\lambda^2/\tau)q'' - \left(\gamma + \frac{3\overline{m}^2\overline{h}v_{Na}\overline{m}'_\infty}{\tau_{Na}(1 + \zeta\overline{\tau}_m)} + \frac{\overline{m}^3 v_{Na}\overline{h}'_\infty}{\tau_{Na}(1 + \zeta\overline{\tau}_h)} + \frac{4\overline{n}^3 v_K\overline{n}'_\infty}{\tau_K(1 + \zeta\overline{\tau}_n)}\right)q = \zeta q. \tag{9.24}$$

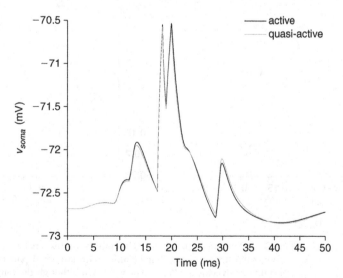

FIGURE 9.12   The voltage response at $x = 0$, for both the active and quasi-active uniform cable, to 10 current stimuli, each 1 ms in duration and 20 pA in amplitude, with random start times and locations. Compare with Figure 5.1. (stEcabQandA.m)

If the cable is uniform then the large bracketed term is independent of x and we may choose q to be the nth eigenfunction, Eq. (6.39), of the passive uniform cable. As $q_n'' = \vartheta_n q_n$ Eq. (9.24) becomes

$$(\lambda^2/\tau)\vartheta_n q_n - \left(\gamma + \frac{3\overline{m}^2 \overline{h} v_{Na} \overline{m}_\infty'}{\tau_{Na}(1+\zeta\overline{\tau}_m)} + \frac{\overline{m}^3 v_{Na} \overline{h}_\infty'}{\tau_{Na}(1+\zeta\overline{\tau}_h)} + \frac{4\overline{n}^3 v_K \overline{n}_\infty'}{\tau_K(1+\zeta\overline{\tau}_n)}\right)q_n = \zeta q_n.$$

On canceling the common q_n we find that the eigenvalue, ζ, must be a root of the quartic

$$\begin{aligned}
P_n(\zeta) = & (\zeta + \gamma - (\lambda^2/\tau)\vartheta_n)(1+\zeta\overline{\tau}_m)(1+\zeta\overline{\tau}_h)(1+\zeta\overline{\tau}_n) + 3\overline{m}^2\overline{h}v_{Na}\overline{m}_\infty'(1+\zeta\overline{\tau}_h)(1+\zeta\overline{\tau}_n)/\tau_{Na} \\
& + \overline{m}^3 v_{Na}\overline{h}_\infty'(1+\zeta\overline{\tau}_m)(1+\zeta\overline{\tau}_n)/\tau_{Na} + 4\overline{n}^3 v_K \overline{n}_\infty'(1+\zeta\overline{\tau}_m)(1+\zeta\overline{\tau}_h)/\tau_K.
\end{aligned} \tag{9.25}$$

We label these roots

$$\zeta_{n,j}, \quad n = 0,1,2,\dots, \quad j = 1,2,3,4$$

and illustrate them in Figure 9.13 for uniform cables of differing lengths. As $\vartheta_0 = 0$ it follows that the roots of P_0 are precisely those of the space-clamped isopotential cable (recall Eq. (5.24)). As in §5.3, the associated eigenfunctions of **B** for the uniform cable are

$$\mathbf{w}_{n,j}(x) = \left(\frac{\overline{m}_\infty'}{1+\zeta_{n,j}\overline{\tau}_m}q_n(x) \quad \frac{\overline{h}_\infty'}{1+\zeta_{n,j}\overline{\tau}_h}q_n(x) \quad \frac{\overline{n}_\infty'}{1+\zeta_{n,j}\overline{\tau}_n}q_n(x) \quad q_n(x)\right)^T \tag{9.26}$$

and so if

$$I_{stim}(x,t) = \sum_{n=0}^{\infty} I_{stim,n}(t)q_n(x), \quad \text{i.e.,} \quad I_{stim,n}(t) = \int_0^{\ell} I_{stim}(x,t)q_n(x)\,dx,$$

then the full stimulus vector enjoys the expansion

$$\mathbf{f} = \sum_{n=0}^{\infty}\sum_{j=1}^{4} c_{n,j}(t)\mathbf{w}_{n,j}(x)$$

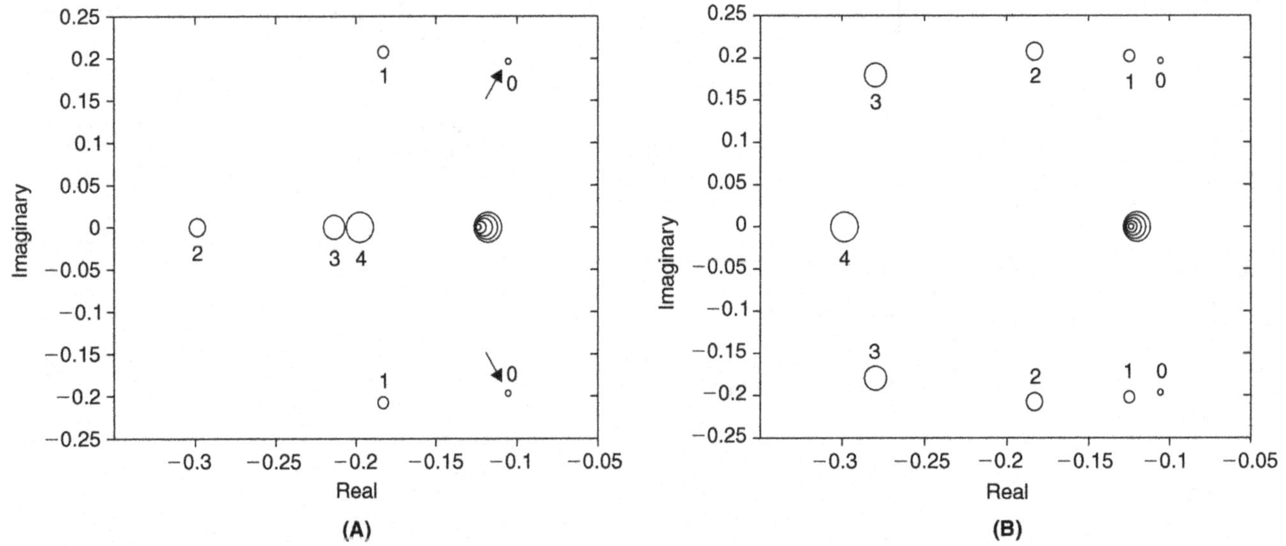

FIGURE 9.13 The roots of the quartic P_n, Eq. (9.25), for $n = 0,1,2,3,4$. The radius of the enclosing circle is proportional to $n+1$. A. $\ell = 1$ mm. B. $\ell = 2$ mm. Regarding resonance, our interest is in nonreal eigenvalues with large real part (arrows on plot). We observe that these occur for $n = 0$ and so correspond to the constant eigenvector, q_0. We also observe that although the longer cable possesses more nonreal eigenvalues, the nonreal eigenvalue with the largest real part is the same in the two cases. Note that the cable length, ℓ, enters P_n via $\vartheta_n = -(n\pi/\ell)^2$ and so is not seen by P_0. (quasicabspec.m)

where, recalling Eq. (5.26),

$$c_{n,j}(t) = \frac{I_{stim,n}(t)}{2\pi a C_m} \frac{(1 + \zeta_{n,j}\bar{\tau}_m)(1 + \zeta_{n,j}\bar{\tau}_h)(1 + \zeta_{n,j}\bar{\tau}_n)}{\bar{\tau}_m\bar{\tau}_h\bar{\tau}_n \prod_{k\neq j}(\zeta_{n,j} - \zeta_{n,k})}. \tag{9.27}$$

It follows that

$$\tilde{V}(x,t) = \sum_{n=0}^{\infty} q_n(x) \sum_{j=0}^{3} \int_0^t c_{n,j}(s)\exp((s-t)\zeta_{n,j})\,\mathrm{d}s \tag{9.28}$$

is the response, with respect to rest, of the quasi-active uniform cable.

We next investigate, in Figure 9.14, the impact of nonuniform channel distribution on the eigenvalues and eigenvectors of the quasi-active system. In this case, although the eigenvectors retain the functional form in Eq. (9.26), the nonuniformity of the coefficients in Eq. (9.24) prohibit its exact solution. We therefore turn to numerical means. We have coded the discretized nonuniform eigenvalue problem in Qcabnon.m.

We now investigate the correspondence between the spectra of the uniform and nonuniform quasi-active cables and the associated resonance, or input resistance, curves of the corresponding active cables. In particular, we drive the uniform and nonuniform active cables with the distributed current

$$I_{stim}(x,t) = I_0 \sin(2\pi\omega t)\Re(q_0(x)) \tag{9.29}$$

where $\Re(q_0)$ is the real part of the eigenvector of **B** associated with the nonreal eigenvalue of greatest real part for the uniform, and nonuniform quasi-active cables, respectively. These two spatial distributions of current will maximize the respective resonances. We drive the cable until time T, where T is large enough to get past the initial transient, then compute

$$V_{max,\infty} \equiv \max_{\substack{0\leq x\leq \ell \\ t>T/2}} V(x,t) \tag{9.30}$$

and examine, in Figure 9.15, the dependence of the associated input resistance on input frequency.

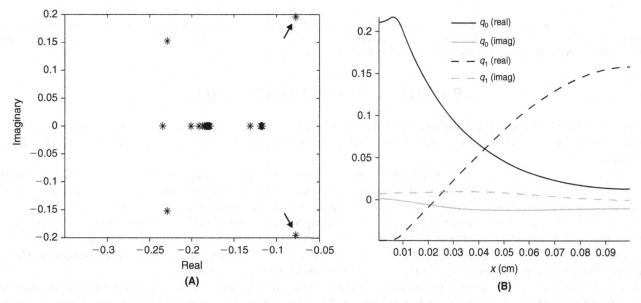

(A)

(B)

FIGURE 9.14   Eigenvalues (**A**), and eigenvectors (**B**), of the quasi-active operator **B** when the active conductances are distributed per Eq. (9.15). Regarding panel **A**: since the nonreal eigenvalue with the greatest real part has moved right in comparison to Figure 9.13 (see arrows on plot), we expect the associated input resistance to have a sharper peak. The eigenvectors in **B**, labeled q_0 and q_1, correspond to the two pair of nonreal eigenvalues in **A**, with q_0 associated with the nonreal eigenvalue of greatest real part. Compare Figure 6.2. (Qcabnon.m)

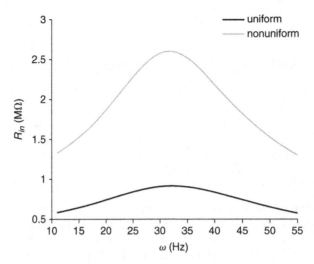

FIGURE 9.15   Input resistance, $R_{in}(\omega) = V_{max,\infty}/I_0$, of the active cable where $I_0 = 10$ pA and ω are prescribed in Eq. (9.29) and $V_{max,\infty}$ in Eq. (9.30). As predicted by the two quasi-active spectra, the nonuniformity has yielded a sharper resonant peak. (stEcabResdrive.m)

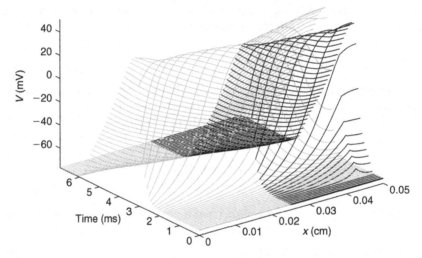

FIGURE 9.16   Action potential propagation in the active uniform fork. A 1 ms suprathreshold current pulse was delivered near the distal end of the black daughter at 0.5 ms. We see her depolarize and initiate a wave that travels in both directions. As it reaches the branch point the wave splits and travels down the mother and up the other daughter (both in red). (stEfork.m)

9.5 THE ACTIVE DENDRITIC TREE

We return to the forked cell with geometric and passive parameters as in Eq. (8.7) and Eq. (8.8). To this we add the standard Hodgkin–Huxley channels and investigate action potential wave propagation (see Figure 9.16), threshold, attenuation, and synaptic integration.

The minimum current required to elicit such a wave is revealed in Figure 9.17A. We next repeat the experiment of Figure 8.7. That is, we compute the maximal somatic and synaptic potentials arising from a single α-synaptic input, as the synapse is placed at successively more distal locations. We illustrate our findings in Figure 9.17B.

We next investigate the active tree's integration of two synaptic inputs. For simplicity we will illustrate our findings for the uniform active tree. In each case, each synapse will be described by an α-function with $\bar{g}_{syn} = 0.5$ nS and $\tau_\alpha = 1$ ms, though typically inhibitory GABA synapses have longer time constants (≈ 5 ms) than excitatory AMPA synapses. For excitatory synapses we use $V_{syn} = 0$ and for inhibitory $V_{syn} = -70$ mV.

In our first simulation we contrast the response at the soma to simultaneous excitatory input into the two daughters with the sum of the responses to individual input. The placement of the synapses is illustrated in the inset to Figure 9.18A. The corresponding curves demonstrate the cell's strong nonlinear amplification of the two inputs.

In our second simulation we contrast distal and proximal inhibition of a fixed excitatory input. The placement is illustrated in the inset to Figure 9.18B. The red diamond marks the excitatory synapse while the inhibitory synapse

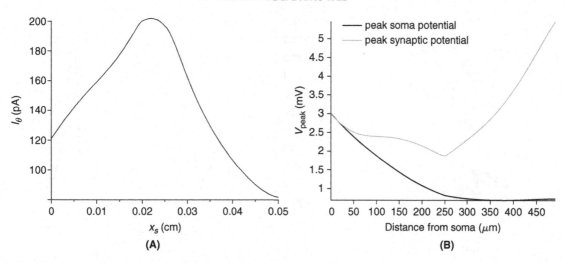

FIGURE 9.17   The active uniform fork. **A.** Threshold at which a 1 ms current pulse will generate an action potential, as a function of stimulation site. **B.** Peak somatic and synaptic potentials. (`stEforksyngain.m` and `stEforkthreshloc.m`)

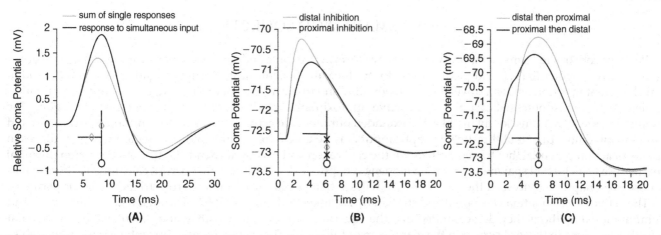

FIGURE 9.18   The response at the cell body of the active uniform fork to a pair of synaptic inputs. **A.** Comparison of response to simultaneous dual excitation (red) to the sum of the responses to individual excitations (black). In these two cases we report the relative soma potential, $V(\ell_3, t) - V_r(\ell_3)$. **B.** Comparison of response to distal (red) and proximal (black) inhibition of a fixed excitatory input. **C.** Comparison of distal before proximal excitatory input to proximal before distal excitatory input. (`stEforksyndrive.m`)

is placed at either, but not both, the proximal or distal black x. The corresponding curves demonstrate that proximal inhibition offers significantly more attenuation.

In our two previous examples our two synapses were presumed to fire simultaneously. For our third simulation we contrast the timing of distal and proximal excitatory input. The placement of the synapses is illustrated in the inset to Figure 9.18C. The two inputs were separated in time by 2 ms. The corresponding curves demonstrate that distal before proximal offers a greater boost than proximal before distal.

Using the active fork we have been able to illustrate the basic notions of action potential propagation and synaptic integration. Most cells, recall Figure 8.1, however, possess tens and often hundreds of tapered branches. The modeling of such structures proceeds as above, i.e., we compartmentalize, balance currents, and construct the associated Hines matrix. The compartmentalization is, however, preceded by a manual or automatic "tracing" of the cell's morphology. There are now two standard formats, `asc` and `swc`, for files that represent these tracings, see Cannon et al. (1998). We have included converters for both types, `ascconverter.m` and `swcconverter.m`, as well as routines that make the common morphology data structure and Hines matrix, `makemd.m` and `makeH.m`, and finally a routine for viewing the tree, `treeplot.m`. With these we may extend `stEforksyn.m` to `stEtreesyn.m` and so permit the MATLAB simulation of practically all traced cells. For example, we examine in Figure 9.19 a pyramidal cell from the CA1 region of the rodent hippocampus.

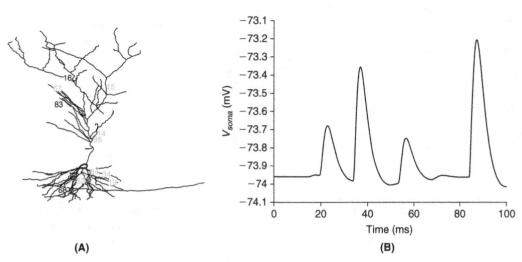

(A)   **(B)**

FIGURE 9.19   The response at the cell body to 12 synaptic inputs. The cell model is weakly excitable, $\bar{g}_K = 40$, $\bar{g}_{Na} = 40$ mS/cm^2, with a highly excitable cell body $\bar{g}_K = 20$ and $\bar{g}_{Na} = 600$ mS/cm^2. **A.** Alpha synapses, $\bar{g}_{syn} = 0.75$ nS and $\tau_\alpha = 1$ ms, are placed at the locations shown. Red for excitatory, $V_{syn} = 0$, and black for inhibitory, $V_{syn} = -70$ mV. The number indicates the activation time (in ms). **B.** The resulting response at the cell body. (stEtreesyn.m)

9.6 SUMMARY AND SOURCES

We have constructed a mathematical model of a uniform active cable and combined our computational approaches to the active isopotential cell and passive cable to produce an efficient means for investigating (a) the threshold at which current injection ignites a traveling action potential and (b) the impact of this traveling wave upon neighboring cables. As in the isopotential case the quasi-active approximation performs well in the subthreshold regime. We examine this system more closely in §14.4. We extended our model to active, branched, nonuniform, spiny cables and demonstrated how distal subthreshold synaptic input may be transferred by the cable to a region where it suffices to ignite an action potential that travels both down the cell's axon and up into its dendritic tree. As the action potential reaches the spine(s) that spawned its ignition it opens synaptic NMDA channels that permit calcium into those spines whose presynaptic activity lead the cell to fire. We will see that spinal calcium may in turn trigger synaptic plasticity.

The active cable equation was posed and studied by Hodgkin and Huxley (1952). Through a mix of analytical and computational methods they demonstrated that the equation was consistent with action potentials that traveled at speeds very close to those observed in the giant axon of the squid. The section on ephaptic interaction of two cables was suggested by Scott (2002). For further background see Jefferys (1995). The kinetic schemes and parameters of the AMPA and NMDA receptors in §9.3 are drawn from Destexhe et al. (1998). Although we have adopted MATLAB as a platform for modeling, simulation, and analysis, there are excellent software tools that are tailored for both modeling and simulation of single neurons as well as circuits. The two most commonly used are GENESIS, see Bower and Beeman (1998), and NEURON, see Carnevale and Hines (2006). We examine the impact of myelin on axonal wave propagation in Exercises 3–5. FitzHugh (1962) is one of the first models of the myelinated axon. For a recent historical review of myelin, see Hartline and Colman (2007). Exercise 6 considers large scale synaptic input into a finely branched cell in a manner motivated by Destexhe et al. (2001).

9.7 EXERCISES

1. Investigate the impact of cable radius and $\bar{g}_{Na}$ on the velocity of the action potential that propagates down the active uniform cable. In particular, modify stEcab.m to produce Figure 9.20.

2. †Investigate the extent to which an excited cable lowers the threshold of its neighbors. In particular, modify stE2cab.m to produce Figure 9.21.

3. We have seen that wave speed along cables can be increased by increasing either the cable radius or the density of sodium channels. As each of these comes with high metabolic costs a third way, based on insulation, has evolved. Many long axons in the nervous system of vertebrates (and invertebrates as well) are wrapped with layers of fat, known as myelin.

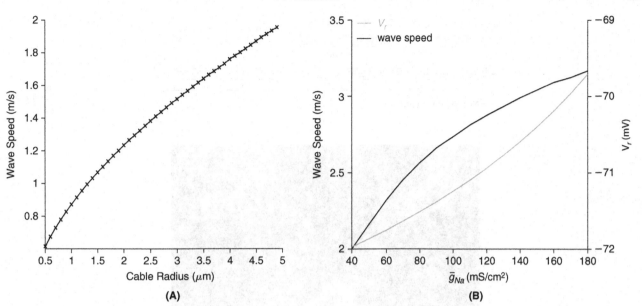

FIGURE 9.20 **A.** Travelling action potential wave speed of the active uniform cable of Figure 9.2 as a function of cable radius. **B.** Rest potential and action potential wave speed of the active uniform cable of Figure 9.2 as a function of maximal sodium conductance, $\bar{g}_{Na}$. (`stEcabsdriver.m` and `stEcabgNadriver.m`)

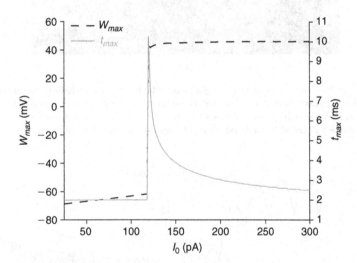

FIGURE 9.21 The maximum midcable depolarization, and the time at which it occurs, in an active uniform cable of radius $1\,\mu$m, e.g., $2\,\mu$m away from a second cable of radius $1\,\mu$m. This second cable receives a midcable, $1\,$ms, $400\,$pA current stimulus, while the first cable receives a midcable, $1\,$ms current injection of amplitude I_0. On comparing with Figure 9.2B we find that the active neighbor lowers the threshold from 150 to 120 pA. (`stE2cabthresh.m`)

These layers are outgrowths of neighboring glial cells. As myelin is only a passive conductor, in order for the wrapped axon to support a traveling action potential the myelin is periodically perforated, exposing the underlying cable at what are known as nodes of Ranvier, see Figure 9.22A. The distribution of Na$^+$ and K$^+$ channels at nodes of Ranvier is highly specific, as illustrated in Figure 9.22B. We will build and investigate, in a series of exercises, a simple model of a myelinated cable. In particular, we will assume that the roughly 100 layers of myelin serve to decrease both the membrane capacitance and conductance by a factor of 100 and that the cable expresses active conductances only at the nodes of Ranvier. Modify `stEcab.m` to accept two new parameters, `id`, the internodal distance, and `nnor`, the number of nodes of Ranvier and so reproduce Figure 9.23.

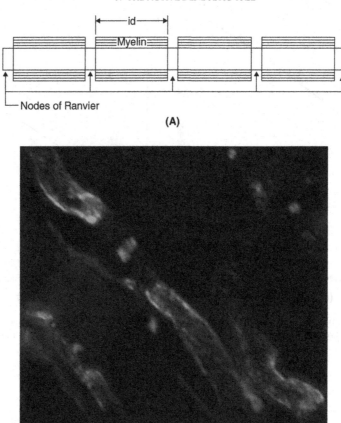

(A)

(B)

FIGURE 9.22   **A.** Schematic cross section of a segment of myelinated cable. **B.** Double-labeled micrograph of myelinated axons in the optic nerve illustrating the distribution of channels at nodes of Ranvier. The staining is for Na^+ channels in red, and Kv1.2 K^+ channels in gray. The Na^+ channels are localized at the nodes which typically measure $1\,\mu m$ in length along the nerve fiber. The K^+ channels are localized in the paranodal region. Micrograph courtesy of Dr. M.N. Rasband, Dept. of Neuroscience, Baylor College of Medicine, Houston, TX.

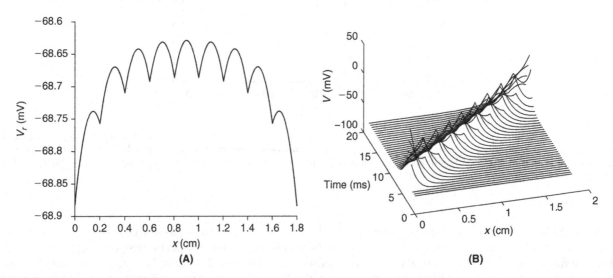

(A)   **(B)**

FIGURE 9.23   The rest potential, **(A)**, and traveling action potential, **(B)**, in a myelinated cable of radius $1\,\mu m$ with 10 nodes, an internodal distance $id = 2$ mm, a node length of $2\,\mu m$, and a step size $dx = 1\,\mu m$. Two of the ten nodes appear at the cable's two ends. The cable was driven with a 1 ms, 50 pA current pulse at the first node. The membrane capacitance was $1\,\mu F/cm^2$ in each nodal compartment and 0.01 in each internodal compartment. The membrane conductance was 0.3 mS/cm^2 in each nodal compartment and 0.003 in each internodal compartment. The sodium conductance density was 120 mS/cm^2 in each nodal compartment and 0 in each internodal compartment. The potassium conductance density was 36 mS/cm^2 in each nodal compartment and 0 in each internodal compartment. (myelins.m)

4. †We note in Figure 9.23B that the potential dips between nodes. Please modify your code from the previous exercise in order to ascertain, as in Figure 9.24, the dependence of action potential wave speed on internodal distance and cable radius.

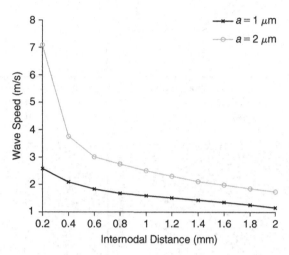

FIGURE 9.24   Action potential wave speed of the myelinated cable. The wave slows as the internodal distance grows. (myelinsdriver.m)

5. Diseases such as multiple sclerosis are characterized by the systematic, and typically irreversible, loss of myelin. To understand how this can lead to loss of function please modify your code from Exercise 3 to reflect the loss of the sixth segment of myelin and so reproduce the findings of Figure 9.25.

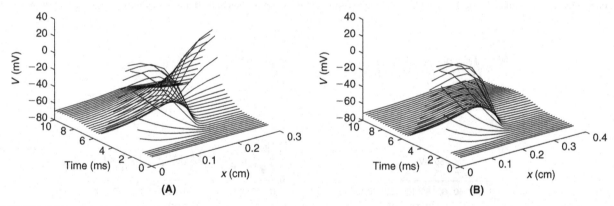

FIGURE 9.25   Conduction block in a partial demyelinated cable. This is the cable used in Figure 9.23 except that $C_m = 1\,\mu F/cm^2$ and $g_{Cl} = 0.3$ mS/cm² in the sixth internodal segment. **A**. With an internodal distance $id = 300\,\mu m$ we see conduction slow in the demyelinated segment and then recover. **B**. With an internodal distance of $id = 400\,\mu m$ the wave stagnates in the demyelinated segment. (demyelin.m)

6. We now consider the impact of large scale synaptic input onto a realistic cell. The cell's asc file is called sep12a.asc and has been plotted using treeplot.m in Figure 9.26A. Please modify stEtreesyn.m to reproduce the remaining panels in Figure 9.26 and Figure 9.27.

With a compartment size of $2\,\mu m$ the cell is subdivided in 945 compartments. We assume the branches to be weakly excitable, $\bar{g}_K = \bar{g}_{Na} = 40$ mS/cm², and the cell body to be strongly excitable, $\bar{g}_K = 20$ and $\bar{g}_{Na} = 600$ mS/cm². The leakage conductance is everywhere $1/15$ mS/cm². We place an α-synapse at every compartment. Eighty percent are presumed excitatory, $V_e = 0$ mV and $\tau_e = 0.5$ ms, and the remainder are inhibitory, $V_i = -80$ mV and $\tau_i = 1$ ms. Their locations and start times are randomly chosen from the uniform distribution. The maximal excitatory conductance, $\bar{g}_e$, is normally distributed with mean 1 nS and variance 0.01 nS, while the maximal inhibitory conductance, $\bar{g}_i$, is normally distributed with mean 2 nS and variance 0.01 nS. We illustrate the cell and the mean conductance waveforms and their activation in space and time in Figure 9.26.

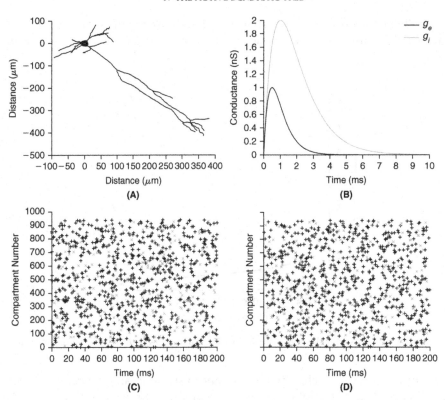

FIGURE 9.26 **A.** Pyramidal cell from the rat entorhinal cortex. **B.** Unitary excitatory and inhibitory conductance time courses. **C** and **D**. Two instances of random synaptic input into the cell of **A**. Each black + corresponds to an excitatory input, g_e as in **B**, at the associated compartment at the designated time. Each red x corresponds to an inhibitory input, g_i as in **B**, at the associated compartment at the designated time. (drfsenoper.m)

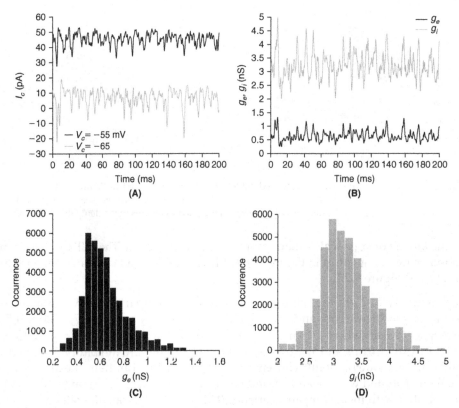

FIGURE 9.27 **A.** The current required to clamp the soma at $V = V_c$ throughout synaptic bombardment. When clamped at -65 mV we used the synaptic schedule of Figure 9.26C while when clamping at -55 mV we used the synaptic schedule of Figure 9.26D. **B.** Effective excitatory and inhibitory conductances derived from **A** and Eq. (9.31). **C** and **D**. Histograms of the solution to Eq. (9.31) associated with the data in **A**. (drfsenoper.m)

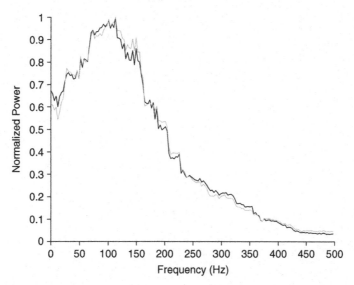

FIGURE 9.28 Power spectra of the excitatory and inhibitory conductances plotted in black and red, respectively. The peak value has been normalized to one. (`drfsenoper.m`)

In order to discern the "effective" synaptic impact we clamp the soma, as in Exercise 8.4, at $V_{c,1}$ and record the ensuing clamp current, $I_{c,1}(t)$, and then repeat this at a second clamp potential, $V_{c,2}$, and record the ensuing clamp current, $I_{c,2}(t)$. These currents are plotted in Figure 9.27A. With this data we may reverse engineer the effective conductances by solving

$$g_e(t)(V_{c,1} - V_e) + g_i(t)(V_{c,1} - V_i) = I_{c,1}(t)$$
$$g_e(t)(V_{c,2} - V_e) + g_i(t)(V_{c,2} - V_i) = I_{c,2}(t)$$

(9.31)

for g_e and g_i. The results are presented in Figure 9.27B, C, and D. As a preview of §17.4 we also record the associated power spectra in Figure 9.28.

10

Reduced Single Neuron Models

OUTLINE

10.1 The Leaky Integrate-and-Fire Neuron   143   10.4 Summary and Sources   152

10.2 Bursting Neurons   146   10.5 Exercises   153

10.3 Simplified Models of Bursting Neurons   147

A principle that has proven fruitful in modeling neural systems is to consider the simplest model capable of predicting the experimental phenomenon under consideration. This approach allows one to capture the essential points of a particular phenomenon without obscuring the picture with unnecessary details. This is precisely the approach taken by Hodgkin and Huxley to model action potential propagation along the squid giant axon in terms of sodium and potassium conductances. We have also seen how a simplification of the Hodgkin–Huxley model to a two-variable reduced FitzHugh model allows one to characterize the firing properties of the Hodgkin–Huxley system in terms of phase plane analysis (Exercise 4.6). A set of simplified models are often used as a first pass to study issues related to synaptic integration or the impact of subthreshold membrane conductances on the processing of sensory inputs by neurons. In this chapter, we first present the most elementary model usually employed to simulate neurons, called the leaky integrate-and-fire model. Next, we introduce a class of neurons that have the ability to fire short bursts of spikes and briefly discuss their role in information processing in the nervous system. Finally, we analyze two simplified models of bursting neurons that highlight different mechanisms of burst generation within a single neuron.

10.1 THE LEAKY INTEGRATE-AND-FIRE NEURON

The most widespread simplified model for the activity of single neurons in response to various inputs is the *leaky integrate-and-fire neuron* (LIF neuron). In this model, the conductances responsible for spike generation (g_{Na} and g_K in the Hodgkin–Huxley model) are ignored and the spiking mechanism is replaced by a potential threshold, v_{thres}. This means that the membrane potential follows the differential equation,

$$C\frac{dv}{dt} = -\frac{v}{R} + I, \quad t > 0, \tag{10.1}$$

where $I = I(t)$ is some stimulation current and we adopt the initial condition $v(0) = 0$. When $v(t_1) = v_{thres}$ reaches threshold, a spike is emitted at t_1 and the potential is reset to zero. Note that at steady state and without input current the membrane potential is equal to zero which corresponds to the resting membrane potential value of the model.

Subthreshold behavior. Below threshold, the membrane potential satisfies a linear differential equation that is none other than the passive patch equation of Chapters 2 and 3 (e.g., Eqs. (2.12) and (3.1)). Thus, the approximation made in the leaky integrate-and-fire model amounts to neglecting all active membrane conductances as well as the electrotonic structure of a neuron's dendritic tree. Furthermore, the subthreshold membrane potential of the LIF neuron is a low-pass filtered version of its input, as in the example of §3.1.

f-I curve for constant current injection. We now compute the steady-state firing rate in response to a constant current pulse starting at $t = 0$. Eq. (10.1) implies an exponential relaxation to the steady-state value $v_\infty = IR$,

$$v(t) = IR(1 - \exp(-t/\tau))$$

with $\tau = RC$, the membrane time constant in Eq. (2.14). Thus, the injected current I has to be larger than the threshold current $I_{thres} = v_{thres}/R$ if the cell is to fire. For current above this value, the threshold potential is reached at that time, t_{thres}, for which $v_{thres} = IR(1 - \exp(-t_{thres}/\tau))$. That is, at

$$t_{thres} = -\tau \log(1 - v_{thres}/(IR)).$$

To mimic the refractory period observed in real neurons and in the Hodgkin–Huxley model, recalling Exercise 4.2, we enforce a period t_{ref} after the spike during which the membrane potential remains fixed at its reset value. If the model is endowed with such an absolute refractory period, t_{ref}, the firing rate is obtained from

$$f = \frac{1}{t_{ref} + t_{thres}} = \frac{1}{t_{ref} - \tau \log(1 - v_{thres}/(IR))}. \tag{10.2}$$

We infer from this formula that the firing rate saturates at a frequency $f_\infty = 1/t_{ref}$ in the limit of large injected currents (Figure 10.1).

Perfect integrator limit. In the limit of very high membrane resistance, we obtain a perfect integrator, or integrate-and-fire (IF) neuron, governed by the differential equation

$$C\frac{dv}{dt} = I(t).$$

In this case, past inputs are not forgotten over time and sum up perfectly. Under constant current injection the membrane potential grows at a rate I/C and thus reaches threshold when $v_{thres} = It_{thres}/C$ or equivalently the firing rate (without refractory period) is given by $f = I/Cv_{thres}$. When is the perfect integrator a reasonable approximation to the leaky integrate-and-fire neuron? This is only the case when the average time interval between inputs is small compared to the leaky integrate-and-fire membrane time constant τ, so that the output firing rate of the model is large compared to $1/\tau$. In this case, the capacitance does not have time to discharge significantly so that inputs do not get forgotten.

Synaptic inputs. Synaptic inputs to a LIF neuron can be simulated as simple instantaneous current inputs,

$$I_{syn}(t) = \sum_{n=1}^{n_{ex}} q_{ex}\delta(t - t_{ex,n}) + \sum_{n=1}^{n_{in}} q_{in}\delta(t - t_{in,n}). \tag{10.3}$$

This corresponds to n_{ex} excitatory inputs at times $t_{ex,n}$ and n_{in} inhibitory inputs at times $t_{in,n}$. Here q_{ex} and q_{in} represent the charge transferred instantaneously to the membrane capacitance by an excitatory or inhibitory input, respectively.

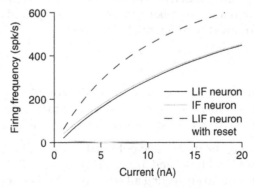

FIGURE 10.1   Firing frequency of a LIF neuron (black solid line; $R = 20\,\text{M}\Omega$, $\tau = 30\,\text{ms}$, $t_{ref} = 1\,\text{ms}$, $v_{thres} = 16\,\text{mV}$), the corresponding IF neuron (red line) and an LIF with $v_{reset} = 8\,\text{mV}$. (fi_curves.m)

On recalling Eq. (3.4) we note that each excitatory input spike increments the potential by q_{ex}/C. In order to compute the corresponding response we choose a time step, dt, and apply the backward Euler scheme to Eq. (10.1), with increments when an input spike has arrived in the last dt interval, and checks on refractoriness and threshold. More precisely, with $v_j \approx v((j-1)dt)$, we march according to

$$\text{If not refractory then } v_j = v_{j-1}/(1 + dt/\tau).$$
$$\text{If fresh input has arrived then } v_j = v_j + (q/C)/(1 + dt/\tau).$$
$$\text{If } v_j \geq v_{thres} \text{ then } v_j = v_{reset}. \tag{10.4}$$

The reader will have an opportunity to code this in Exercises 1 and 2 and so reproduce panels A and B in Figure 10.2. As synaptic input is more accurately modeled as a conductance change, we also consider stimuli of the form

$$I_{syn}(t) = \sum_{n=1}^{n_{ex}} g_{ex}(t, t_{ex,n})(v - v_{ex}) + \sum_{n=1}^{n_{in}} g_{in}(t, t_{in,n})(v - v_{in}), \tag{10.5}$$

where, e.g., each g is an α-function as in Eq. (2.17). Integration of this stimulus, in Exercises 3 and 4, will produce panels C and D in Figure 10.2.

Membrane potential reset after an action potential. The usual choice for the reset membrane potential v_{reset} after an action potential is the resting membrane potential, v_{rest}, which is equal to zero in Eq. (10.1). However, nothing forbids us from choosing a different reset value. If $v_{reset} \neq v_{rest}$, then the f-I curve of Eq. (10.2) depends on $\theta = v_{thres} - v_{reset}$ and its slope for high step currents is $\approx 1/C\theta$ (assuming $t_{ref} = 0$ and using $\log(1+x) \approx x$ for x small). Thus, the value of the reset potential allows one to control the slope of the f-I curve independently of v_{thres}. A second consequence of a high reset value is that the membrane potential hovers close to threshold and is thus much more sensitive to transient coincident inputs. This typically increases the variability of the spike train under random inputs.

Relative refractory period and threshold fatigue. Real neurons typically exhibit an absolute refractory period during which they will not fire and a relative refractory period during which the threshold for firing is elevated (Exercise 4.2 and Figure 15.3). A relative refractory period is sometimes implemented by incrementing the threshold after each

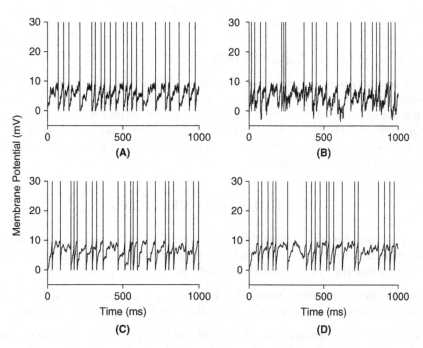

FIGURE 10.2 LIF membrane potential in response to random excitatory current-type synaptic inputs (**A**), a mixture of excitatory and inhibitory current-type synaptic inputs (**B**), excitatory conductance-type synaptic inputs (**C**) and a mixture of excitatory and inhibitory conductance-type inputs (**D**). See Exercises 1–4 for model parameters. Size of spikes is arbitrarily set 30 mV above rest. (lif_rand_inp.m)

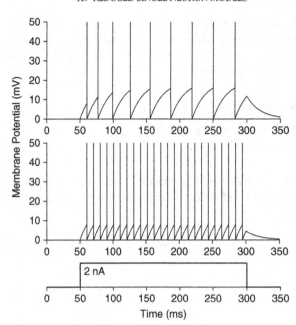

FIGURE 10.3   Response of a LIF with threshold fatigue (top) and without (middle) to a 2 nA current pulse (bottom; see Exercise 5 for model parameters). Spike height has been arbitrarily set to 50 mV above rest. (thresh_fatigue.m)

action potential and letting it decay towards its steady-state value. More precisely,

If spiked

$$v_{thres} = v_{thres} + \delta v_{thres}$$

else   (10.6)

$$\frac{\mathrm{d}v_{thres}}{\mathrm{d}t} = -\frac{v_{thres} - v_{thres0}}{\tau_{v_{thres}}}$$

end.

We will put this scheme to use in Exercise 5 and achieve Figure 10.3.

Additional subthreshold conductances. Another common practice is to add additional subthreshold conductances to the LIF neuron to study their effect on the firing characteristics of the model. For example, instead of modeling a relative refractory period as explained above, one can introduce a conductance that hyperpolarizes the cell following an action potential (abbreviated AHP for after-hyperpolarization) with a dependence on a slow varying variable like the calcium concentration. We will encounter such a conductance in our model of CA3 hippocampal pyramidal neurons in the next section, as well as in Figure 13.8.

10.2 BURSTING NEURONS

An important property of many neurons is their ability to generate short bursts of spikes. This points to the existence of ionic conductances that are able to activate and deactivate periodically on a time scale much slower than the action potential duration and thus drive the firing of small "packets" or bursts of spikes.

Intrinsic properties lead to different bursting behaviors. The ionic conductances responsible for bursting have been investigated in different cell types. It is now clear that several distinct mechanisms are at play.

1. Bursting can be caused by the activation of low-threshold conductances that are usually inactivated or closed at rest, such as the calcium permeable *T conductance* (I_T). Hyperpolarization of the membrane potential removes the inactivation or opens the channels and allows a depolarizing current to turn on, leading to "rebound excitation." A prominent example of this bursting mechanism are relay neurons in the thalamus discussed in the next section. In

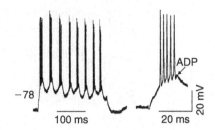

FIGURE 10.4   Intracellular recording from a chattering neuron in the visual cortex of the cat. In response to a depolarizing current pulse (0.9 nA) the cell generates a repetitive burst discharge of action potentials. The panel on the right is at an expanded time scale and shows an after-depolarization following the burst. Adapted from Gray and McCormick (1996).

addition, other low-threshold conductances such as, e.g., the I_h current of §5.5 can play a similar role (see Figures 5.6 and 10.9 below).

2. A second widespread mechanism of bursting involves spatial interactions between the soma and dendritic compartments of a neuron. An example is given by CA3 pyramidal cells of the hippocampus that possess calcium channels localized in the dendritic compartments, but not the soma. A two-compartment model of this bursting mechanism is analyzed in the next section. Upon current injection in the soma, the depolarization of the dendritic compartment is delayed in time with respect to the soma, causing significant current flow to and from the soma. Delayed activation of dendritic calcium conductances eventually sustains the depolarization of the soma causing the cell to burst (see Figures 10.10–10.12 below). A similar mechanism of bursting has been described in cortical neurons called *chattering cells* (Figure 10.4). In these neurons the burst frequency can be unusually high (up to 40 Hz) and relies on an interaction between soma and dendrites based on fast sodium conductances, instead of calcium conductances.

3. Dendritic morphology can play an important role in determining firing characteristics given a fixed set and distribution of conductances in various functional compartments of a neuron. An example that has been investigated in some detail includes various types of excitatory neurons of the cerebral cortex (pyramidal cells of different sizes, smooth, and stellate cells). It has been shown by simulations that larger neurons with decoupled somatic and dendritic compartments are more prone to bursting than more compact neurons (Figure 10.5).

4. Although intrinsic properties can cause cells to burst, such effects are typically observed within networks of cells and the properties of bursts are thus in part determined by interactions among different neurons of a network (Figure 10.6).

Functional role of bursts. Bursts are thought to fulfill various functional roles in the nervous system. These include:

1. *Rhythm generation.* Many tasks such as, e.g., locomotion, swimming, or digestion of food involve the rhythmic activation of muscles. Such rhythms are typically generated by networks of neurons activated in definite sequences. Thus, both the intrinsic properties of nerve cells and their pattern of synaptic connections influence the generation of rhythms.

2. *Safety against unreliable synapses.* Bursts have long been thought to be effective at safely signalling important events. One reason is that synaptic transmission is stochastic and therefore often unreliable. Thus, stimulating repetitively a synaptic target offers a way to overcome this problem and assure that a message is delivered reliably. Therefore bursts of spikes could represent a "safety factor" in synaptic transmission. In cortex, e.g., layer 5 pyramidal cells are those most prone to burst and typically send long range connections toward other cortical or subcortical areas.

3. *Detection of sensory events.* Bursts could be used in sensory systems to signal important events; e.g., the occurrence of a salient object in the visual field (Figure 10.7).

10.3 SIMPLIFIED MODELS OF BURSTING NEURONS

We analyze two models in detail. The first one is a single-compartment model of bursting in thalamic relay neurons that receive inputs from the sensory periphery and send their axons to cortical neurons. The second model is a two-compartment model of pyramidal neurons of the hippocampus, a structure at the edge of the cerebral cortex that is thought to be involved in learning and memory as well as navigation.

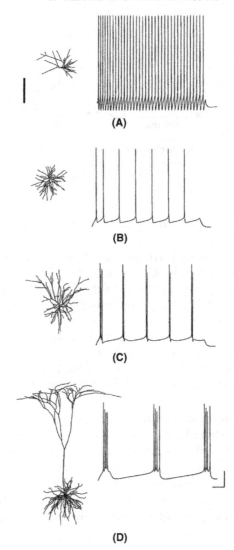

(A)

(B)

(C)

(D)

FIGURE 10.5   Model neurons with identical ion channel distributions generate distinct firing patterns according to their morphology. **A.** Layer 3 spiny stellate cell of the rat somatosensory cortex. **B–D.** Layer 4 spiny stellate cell, layer 3 pyramidal cell, and layer 5 pyramidal cell of the cat visual cortex, respectively. Scale bars: 250 μm, 100 ms, 25 mV. Adapted from Mainen and Sejnowski (1996).

Model of thalamic relay neuron bursting. Thalamic relay neurons have been extensively investigated as a model of bursting. We consider a single-compartment model comprising several active conductances generating distinct currents: the fast sodium, I_{Na}, and delayed rectifier currents, I_K, that are responsible for action potentials, as well as a persistent sodium current, I_{NaP}, a low-threshold calcium current, I_T, and a hyperpolarization activated mixed sodium/potassium current, I_h, like that encountered in §5.5. The differential equation governing the model is thus,

$$C_m \frac{dV}{dt} = -I_T - I_h - I_{Na} - I_K - I_{NaP} - I_L + I_{inj},   \tag{10.7}$$

where I_L is a leak (passive) current and I_{inj} represents the current injected through an electrode in the model.

The steady-state activation, s_∞, and inactivation, h_∞, variables for the low-threshold calcium current, I_T, are plotted in Figure 10.8 (Exercise 6). I_T is excitatory with a reversal potential $V_{Ca} = 120$ mV. Furthermore, I_T is essentially inactivated around the resting membrane potential of the model (≈ -65 mV), and thus does not influence the neuron's response to depolarizing inputs.

The steady-state activation, q_∞, and time constant, τ_q, functionals associated with I_h are plotted in Figure 5.6A. We recall, §5.5, that I_h is excitatory as well, since its reversal potential is above rest ($V_h = -40$ mV). However, it is only partially activated at rest. It also has the unusual property of further closing at depolarizing potentials and therefore plays a minor role in shaping the spike pattern of the neuron when it is depolarized from rest. Consequently, a constant, positive current pulse will mainly activate I_{Na} and I_K (and I_{NaP} to a lesser extent), causing regular spiking

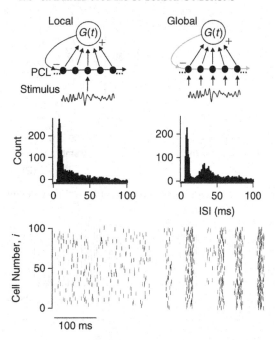

FIGURE 10.6   In the weakly electric fish *Apteronotus*, pyramidal neurons in the pyramidal cell layer (PCL) of a hindbrain structure called the electrosensory lateral line lobe encode information on random amplitude modulations of an external electric field (Stimulus). If a single cell is stimulated locally, it fires action potentials that are irregular, leading to an interspike interval distribution with a single peak (middle left). In contrast, simultaneous activation of many pyramidal cells through an extended (Global) stimulus, leads to two peaks in the interspike interval distribution resulting from bursting patterns of action potentials (middle right). This is caused by activation of strong inhibitory feedback (top left, red). Feedback activation by global stimuli also causes the pyramidal cells to synchronize or oscillate (bottom panels). These simulations summarize experimental results on the role of feedback described in Doiron et al. (2003).

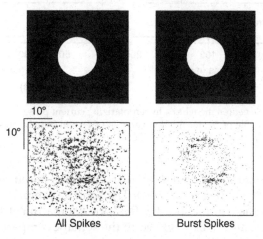

FIGURE 10.7   Burst spikes of visual cortical neurons recorded in monkeys reflect more clearly than all spikes what the animal was seeing. Bursts are defined as events consisting of two spikes less than 10 ms apart. The object was a static white disk on a black background (top). The screen of the video monitor covered 60 by 45 degrees of visual angle. The monkey was rewarded for following a fixation point, so that the receptive field of the cell could be positioned over the stimulus. Spikes were mapped in the lower panels according to the position of the recorded neuron's receptive field in space at their moment of occurrence. Adapted from Livingstone et al. (1996).

(Figure 10.9B; Exercise 7). In contrast a negative current pulse will activate I_h and relieve I_T from inactivation, causing a rebound depolarization leading to a burst of spikes well after termination of the current pulse (Figure 10.9A).

Note that since bursting can be described by a single-compartment model it does not involve the more complex somatodendritic interactions necessary to describe bursting in other cell types. In addition bursting in the model occurs on two different time scales: 7–14 Hz and 0.5–4 Hz, respectively, as observed in real neurons. These time scales correlate well with the kinetics of the T-type calcium current and the h-type mixed sodium/potassium current, respectively. Thus, the model suggests that activation of these currents is sufficient to explain the intrinsic bursting properties of thalamic relay neurons.

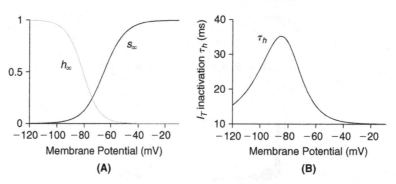

FIGURE 10.8   **A.** Steady-state activation, s_∞, and inactivation, h_∞, of I_T. **B.** Time constant of inactivation of I_T. (wang_ss.m)

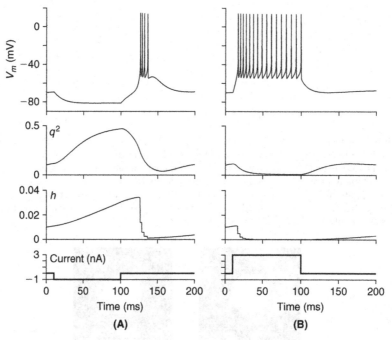

FIGURE 10.9   **A.** Response of the thalamic neuron model to a hyperpolarizing current pulse ($-1\ \mu A/cm^2$, 90 ms long). From top to bottom: membrane potential, squared activation variable of I_h, inactivation variable of I_T and current pulse as a function of time. **B.** Response to a depolarizing current pulse ($+3\ \mu A/cm^2$). (wang_mod.m)

Model of CA3 hippocampal pyramidal neuron bursting. This model is based on two compartments representing the soma and dendritic tree, respectively (Figure 10.10A). The somatic compartment corresponds to a fraction p of the total membrane surface area of the neuron and the dendritic compartment to $(1-p)$. To fit experimental data, the model requires $1/2$ of the surface area to be assigned to the somatic compartment. The somatic compartment is endowed with fast sodium and delayed rectifier conductances that can generate action potentials while the dendritic compartment has a voltage-activated calcium conductance that can generate calcium spikes on a much slower time scale (Figure 10.10B). The differential equations for the somatic, V_s, and dendritic, V_d, potentials are as follows:

$$C_m V_s' = -g_L(V_s - V_L) - I_{Na}(V_s) - I_K(V_s) + \frac{g_c(V_d - V_s) + I_s}{p}$$

$$C_m V_d' = -g_L(V_d - V_L) - I_{Ca}(V_d) - I_{K,AHP}(V_d) - I_{K,C}(V_d) - \frac{I_{syn} - g_c(V_s - V_d) - I_d}{1-p}. \tag{10.8}$$

All currents and conductances are expressed as densities, in units of $\mu A/cm^2$ and mS/cm^2, respectively. Thus, the coupling current between the two compartments that is proportional to $V_d - V_s$ and the injected somatic, I_s, and dendritic, I_d, currents, as well as the synaptic current, I_{syn}, are scaled by the fractional area of their respective compartments (p and $1-p$ for soma and dendrite, respectively). The parameters of the model are given in Exercise 8.

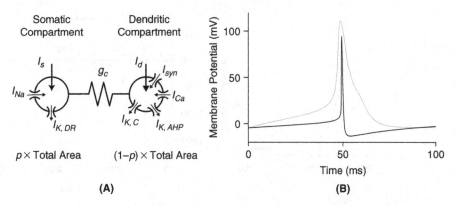

FIGURE 10.10   **A.** Schematic of the model, leak currents have been omitted for clarity. I_d and I_s represent currents injected through an electrode. **B.** Sodium (black) and calcium (red) spikes elicited in the isolated somatic and dendritic compartments ($g_c = 0$). The calcium spike was obtained by injecting a current of $0.68\ \mu\mathrm{A/cm^2}$, while the somatic spike results spontaneously. (pr_sodca_spike.m)

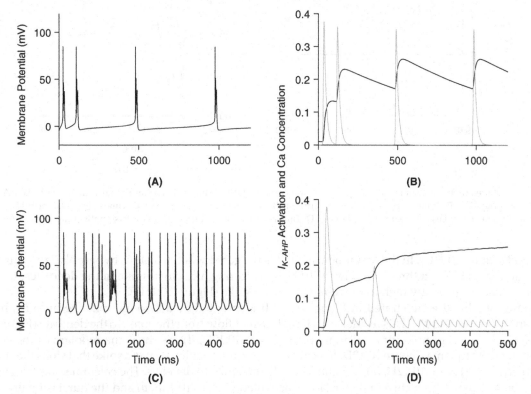

FIGURE 10.11   **A.** Somatic membrane potential in response to a somatic current injection ($0.75\ \mu\mathrm{A/cm^2}$). **B.** Time course of the q variable governing activation of $I_{K,AHP}$ (in black) and calcium concentration (in red, arbitrary units, scaled down by a factor one thousand). **C, D.** Same as A, B but for a current injection of $2.5\ \mu\mathrm{A/cm^2}$. (pr_modes.m)

In the dendritic compartment, both potassium currents, $I_{K,C}$ and $I_{K,AHP}$, depend on the intracellular calcium concentration of the dendritic compartment, $c = [\mathrm{Ca^{2+}}]_d$. We suppose, for simplicity, that it is dimensionless. Its rate of change increases with $-I_{Ca}$ and decreases, e.g., through pumping mechanisms (see §13.2), that depend on c itself. To be precise, we suppose

$$c' = -0.13 I_{Ca} - 0.075c. \tag{10.9}$$

The leading minus sign reflects the convention that inward currents are negative. In the absence of calcium current, c decreases exponentially towards zero with a time constant of $1/0.075 = 13$ ms.

The model possesses several distinct firing modes. For low somatic current injections, the model generates low frequency bursts (Figure 10.11A), whereas for higher currents the model generates regular spiking after an initial

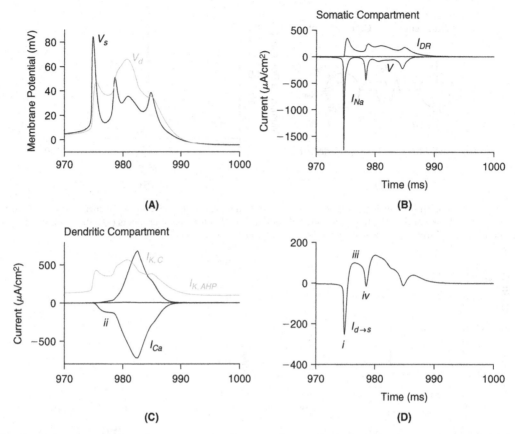

FIGURE 10.12   Detailed time course of membrane potential and currents during a burst. Same simulation as in Figure 10.11A. **A**. Somatic and dendritic membrane potentials. **B**. Time course of the somatic currents (leak current too small to see). **C**. Time course of dendritic currents. $I_{K,AHP}$ has been scaled up by a factor 50. Leak current too small to see. **D**. Time course of current from dendritic to somatic compartment. (`pr_complex.m`)

transient period (Figure 10.11C). In the first mode, a burst is triggered when the slow, hyperpolarizing current activation variable decreases below a threshold (Figure 10.11B), triggering a calcium spike in the dendrites. In the second mode, $I_{K,AHP}$ remains sufficiently high to prevent a dendritic spike (Figure 10.11D).

The dynamics of a burst is illustrated in Figure 10.12. It is initiated by a somatic spike because I_{Na} has a lower threshold than I_{Ca} (Figure 10.10B). This results in an initial current flow from the soma to the dendrite (Figure 10.12D, i) that activates I_{Ca}, below threshold for a calcium spike (Figure 10.12C, ii). As the soma repolarizes the current flow reverses from dendrite to soma (Figure 10.12D, iii), causing a second, smaller, somatic spike that stops the current drain from dendrite to soma (Figure 10.12D, iv) and allows a calcium spike to develop. The calcium spike triggers damped spikes in the soma as the sodium current is partially inactivated (Figure 10.12B, v) and the burst is finally terminated by the calcium-dependent current $I_{K,C}$. After the burst, when the more powerful active conductances are turned off, the much smaller current $I_{K,AHP}$ controls again the dynamics of the interburst interval. Thus, in hippocampal CA3 pyramidal cells, bursting results from a complex interaction between active conductances in somatic and dendritic compartments.

10.4 SUMMARY AND SOURCES

In this chapter, we have introduced several reduced single cell models. The leaky integrate-and-fire model goes back to Lapicque (1907). See Gerstner and Kistler (1992) for a thorough treatment. The leaky integrate-and-fire model is a basic workhorse used in countless theoretical studies of single neurons. The two bursting models of §10.3 capture the essence of bursting based on two distinct biophysical mechanisms. The model of thalamic relay neurons is taken from Wang (1994) and that of CA3 pyramidal cells from Pinsky and Rinzel (1994). Both models are based on several decades of experimental and theoretical work. For extensive modeling of the hippocampus network, see Traub and Miles (1991). For a review of cellular and network mechanisms underlying thalamic activity see McCormick and Bal (1997). Bursting in thalamic relay neurons was originally studied by Jahnsen and Llinàs (1984). Weakly electric fish is one of the systems where the mechanisms, the information content, and the behavioral implications of bursting have been best studied. See Turner et al. (1994) and Fernandez et al. (2005) for the biophysics of bursts in pyramidal cells and Laing et al. (2003) for a dynamical system perspective. For the implications of bursting on information coding and behavior, see Doiron et al. (2003), Oswald et al. (2004), Chacron and Bastian (2008), and Marsat et al. (2009). Krahe and Gabbiani (2004) reviews bursting across several sensory systems. We will return to simplified neuron models in §14.4 where we introduce a principled way of reducing the complexity of a high-dimensional compartmental model. The impact of random synaptic input on the membrane potential and firing rate of leaky integrate-and-fire neurons was briefly touched upon in Figure 10.2. We will study again the impact of random synaptic inputs on neuronal firing properties in Chapter 15 and with the help of reduced models in §17.4, once we have more powerful modeling tools at hand.

10.5 EXERCISES

1. Simulate an LIF neuron receiving random excitatory current-type synaptic inputs with parameters $\tau = 20$ ms, $R = 10$ MΩ, $v_{thres} = 10$ mV, $t_{ref} = 0$, and $v_{reset} = 0$. Simulate the model over 1 s, with a time step of 0.05 ms and assume that it receives $n_{ex} = 500$ excitatory inputs whose activation times are uniformly distributed over that interval, each with an associated charge $q_{ex} = 2$ pCb. Use the marching scheme of Eq. (10.4) to reproduce Figure 10.2A.

2. Modify the model of the previous exercise to include current-type inhibition. Use the same model parameters, but assume that $q_{in} = 4$ pCb and that the number of excitatory and inhibitory inputs over the 1 s interval is $n_{ex} = 660$ and $n_{in} = 100$, respectively (Figure 10.2B).

3. Replace the current-type synapse of Exercise 1 by an α-synapse. Assume $\tau_\alpha = 1$ ms and a reversal potential $v_{ex} = 70$ mV above rest. Use a peak conductance $g_{max} = Kq_{ex}$, where K is such that the total charge transferred by the synapse equals q_{ex} when the potential is clamped at its resting value. Use $n_{ex} = 600$ (Figure 10.2C).

4. Add inhibitory α-synapses. Use the same factor K as in the previous exercise and $q_{in} = 4$ pCb as in Exercise 2. Assume $v_{in} = 0$ mV, $n_{ex} = 690$, and $n_{in} = 100$ (Figure 10.2D).

5. Simulate the response of a LIF neuron with threshold fatigue to a 250 ms long, 2 nA current pulse. Assume $C = 2$ nF, $\tau = 20$ ms, $v_{thres0} = 8$ mV, $\delta v_{thres} = 4$ mV, $\tau_{v_{thres}} = 80$ ms (Figure 10.3, top). Hint: Use a simple forward Euler integration scheme with $dt = 0.1$ ms.

6. Plot the steady-state activation and inactivation variables for I_T, given by $s_\infty(V) = 1/(1 + \exp(-(V + 65)/7.8))$ and $h_\infty(V) = 1/(1 + \exp((V - \theta_h)/k_h))$, with $\theta_h = -81$ mV and $k_h = 6.25$ mV^{-1}. Plot the effective inactivation time constant, τ_h/ϕ_h, with $\tau_h(V) = h_\infty(V) \exp((V + 162.3)/17.8) + 20.0$, and $\phi_h = 2$.

7. Implement the model of Eq. (10.7) using a hybrid Euler scheme. Compute the response to 90 ms long -1 μA/cm^2 and $+3$ μA/cm^2 current pulses, respectively (Figure 10.9). In Eq. (10.7), $C_m = 1$ μF/cm^2 and all variables are normalized per unit area (e.g., in the case of I_{inj}, μA/cm^2).

   The T-type calcium current is described by $I_T = \bar{g}_T s_\infty^3(V)h(V - V_{Ca})$, where the activation s is assumed to be instantaneously at equilibrium. The inactivation h and the other activation and inactivation variables described below are governed by the differential equation

$$dX/dt = \phi_X(X_\infty - X)/\tau_X(V) \qquad (10.10)$$

with $X = h, q, n$. ϕ_X is a temperature scaling factor that determines the effective time constant, τ_X/ϕ_X, of X. Assume $\bar{g}_T = 0.3$ mS/cm^2, $V_{Ca} = 120$ mV and see Exercise 6 for other values.

   The h-current is described by $I_h = \bar{g}_h q^2(V - V_h)$ with $\bar{g}_h = 0.04$ mS/cm^2 and $V_h = -40$ mV. The steady-state activation and time constant functionals are specified in Eq. (5.33). We assume $\phi_h = 1$.

   The potassium current is given by $I_K = \bar{g}_K n^4(V - V_K)$, with

$$\alpha_n(V) = \frac{0.01(V + 45.7 - \sigma_K)}{1 - \exp(-0.1(V + 45.7 - \sigma_K))} \quad \text{and} \quad \beta_n(V) = 0.125 \exp(-(V + 55.7 - \sigma_K)/80)$$

with $\phi_n = 200/7$, $\bar{g}_K = 30$ mS/cm^2, $V_K = -80$ mV, and $\sigma_K = 10$ mV.

   The sodium current is given by $I_{Na} = \bar{g}_{Na} m_\infty^3(V)(0.85 - n)(V - V_{Na})$. The activation is assumed to be instantaneous and is replaced by its steady-state value. The inactivation h has been replaced by $(0.85 - n)$ as per Exercise 4.6. The constituents of m_∞ are

$$\alpha_m(V) = \frac{0.1(V + 29.7 - \sigma_{Na})}{1 - \exp(-0.1(V + 29.7 - \sigma_{Na}))}$$

(10.11)

$$\beta_m(V) = 4\exp(-(V + 54.7 - \sigma_{Na})/18)$$

with $\bar{g}_{Na} = 42$ mS/cm^2, $V_{Na} = 55$ mV, and $\sigma_{Na} = 3$ mV.

The persistent sodium current is given by $I_{NaP} = \bar{g}_{NaP} m_\infty^3(V) V - V_{Na})$ with $\bar{g}_{NaP} = 9$ mS/cm^2 and $\sigma_{Na} = -5$ mV in Eq. (10.11).

The leak current is given by $I_L = g_L(V - V_L)$ with $g_L = 0.1$ mS/cm^2.

8. Implement the CA3 model of Eq. (10.8) using the MATLAB function ODE23 based on a Runge–Kutta integration scheme. The various currents of the model are defined as follows:

$$I_{Na}(V_s) = \bar{g}_{Na} m_\infty^2(V_s) h(V_s - V_{Na}), \quad I_K(V_s) = \bar{g}_K n(V_s - V_K), \quad I_{Ca}(V_d) = \bar{g}_{Ca} s^2(V_d - V_{Ca}),$$

and two calcium-dependent potassium currents

$$I_{K,C}(V_d) = \bar{g}_{K,C} \chi(c) r(V_d - V_K) \quad \text{and} \quad I_{K,AHP}(V_d) = \bar{g}_{K,AHP} q(V_d - V_K).$$

The activation and inactivation variables obey

$$w'(V) = (w_\infty(V) - w)/\tau_w(V), \quad w_\infty(V) = \alpha_w(V)/(\alpha_w(V) + \beta_w(V)), \quad \tau_w(V) = 1/(\alpha_w(V) + \beta_w(V)),$$

with $w = h, n, s, r$, and q, respectively. The functions α_w and β_w are

$$\alpha_m = \frac{0.32(13.1 - V_s)}{\exp((13.1 - V_s)/4) - 1} \quad \text{and} \quad \beta_m = \frac{0.28(V_s - 40.1)}{\exp((V_s - 40.1)/5) - 1}$$

$$\alpha_n = \frac{0.016(35.1 - V_s)}{\exp((35.1 - V_s)/5) - 1} \quad \text{and} \quad \beta_n = 0.25\exp(0.5 - 0.025V_s)$$

$$\alpha_h = 0.128\exp((17 - V_s)/18) \quad \text{and} \quad \beta_h = \frac{4}{1 + \exp((40 - V_s)/4)}$$

$$\alpha_s = \frac{1.6}{1 + \exp(-0.072(V_d - 65))} \quad \text{and} \quad \beta_s = \frac{0.02(V_d - 51.1)}{\exp((V_d - 51.1)/5) - 1}$$

and

$$\alpha_c = \begin{cases} \exp((V_d - 10)/11 - (V_d - 6.5)/27)/18.975 & \text{when} \quad V_d \le 50 \\ 2\exp((6.5 - V_d)/27) & \text{otherwise} \end{cases}$$

$$\beta_c = \begin{cases} 2\exp((6.5 - V_d)/27) - \alpha_c & \text{when} \quad V_d \le 50 \\ 0 & \text{otherwise} \end{cases}$$

with $\alpha_q = \min(0.00002c, 0.01)$, and $\beta_q = 0.001$ and maximal conductances (in mS/cm^2)

$$g_L = 0.1, \bar{g}_{Na} = 30, \bar{g}_K = 15, \bar{g}_{Ca} = 10, \bar{g}_{K,AHP} = 0.8, \bar{g}_{K,C} = 15,$$

and reversal potentials (in mV),

$$V_{Na} = 120, V_{Ca} = 140, V_K = -15, \quad \text{and} \quad V_L = 0.$$

The coupling parameters are $p = 0.5$, and $g_c = 2.1$ mS/cm^2. The capacitance is $C_m = 3$ μF/cm^2 and $\chi(c) = \min(c/250, 1)$. The stable rest state of the model is at the state-variable values of $(V_s, V_d, h, n, s, r, q, c) = (-4.6, -4.5, 0.999, 0.001, 0.009, 0.007, 0.01, 0.2)$, with the membrane potentials V_s and V_d relative to -60 mV.

Use the model to reproduce Figures 10.10B, 10.11, and 10.12 using the parameters given in the figure legends.

Probability and Random Variables

11.1 Events and Random Variables	155	11.8 Transformation of Random Variables* 163
11.2 Binomial Random Variables	157	11.9 Random Vectors* 164
11.3 Poisson Random Variables	159	11.10 Exponential and Gamma Distributed Random
11.4 Gaussian Random Variables	159	Variables 167
11.5 Cumulative Distribution Functions	160	11.11 The Homogeneous Poisson Process 168
11.6 Conditional Probabilities*	161	11.12 Summary and Sources 170
11.7 Sum of Independent Random Variables*	162	11.13 Exercises 170

OUTLINE

A fundamental property of nervous systems is that their components do not often operate reliably. Thus, the release of neurotransmitter at synapses is usually stochastic, and so is the generation of action potentials in neurons operating within their natural, *in vivo*, environment. At the level of whole animals, behavior under identical conditions also exhibits random components. To describe this "randomness" and study it, we need the tools of probability theory. This chapter introduces random variables and their basic properties as well as the homogeneous Poisson process, that is the most basic tool to describe random events occurring over extended time periods.

11.1 EVENTS AND RANDOM VARIABLES

Probabilities are essential to describe experiments whose outcome is uncertain. The first required ingredient is the *sample space of events*, Ω, or possible outcomes of an experiment. For concreteness we consider the case of a single synaptic vesicle, filled with neurotransmitter molecules and docked at a presynaptic terminal, that can either be released or not in the synaptic cleft upon arrival of an action potential (Figure 11.2). In this simple example, Ω consists of two elementary events,

$$\Omega = \{\text{released, not-released}\}.$$

Each event is assigned a probability, P, of occurrence. The assignment has to satisfy several constraints to be meaningful:

1. $P(\Omega) = 1$. The space Ω represents all possible outcomes: in the previous example, either the vesicle is released following an action potential or not. Thus, the probability of the vesicle being either released or not must be equal to one.

Mathematics for Neuroscientists. DOI: 10.1016/B978-0-12-374882-9.00011-3

2. If an event consists of two (or more) mutually exclusive or disjoint events, then their probabilities add. In the previous example, a vesicle is either released or not following an action potential, thus

$$P(\{\text{released, not-released}\}) = P(\{\text{released}\}) + P(\{\text{not-released}\}).$$

According to property 1 the left hand side of this equation is equal to 1. In the following we will abbreviate the "released" event by r, the "not-released" event by $\bar{r}$ and their probabilities by $P(\{r\}) = p$, $P(\{\bar{r}\}) = q$ with $q = 1 - p$.

A *random variable* is a function that maps events in Ω onto real numbers. In the above example, we can define a random variable X as the number of released vesicles, or equivalently

$$X(\{r\}) \equiv 1, \quad X(\{\bar{r}\}) \equiv 0.$$

In this simple case, the probability that X equals 1 or 0 is immediately determined from the above definition to be

$$P(X = 1) = p, \quad P(X = 0) = q.$$

We can now define the *mean*, m_X, or *expected* number, $E[X]$, of released vesicles by

$$m_X = E[X] \equiv 0 \cdot q + 1 \cdot p = p. \tag{11.1}$$

The *variance*, σ_X^2, is defined as the expected value of the squared difference between X and its mean:

$$\sigma_X^2 = E[(X - m_X)^2] \equiv (0 - p)^2 \cdot q + (1 - p)^2 \cdot p = p \cdot q. \tag{11.2}$$

In other words, the variance is a measure of the fluctuation of a random variable around its mean, because it measures the average squared deviation from the random variable's mean.

More generally, let $\Omega = \{e_1, \ldots, e_n\}$ be a probability space consisting of n distinct events, each of probability p_{e_i} and such that $\sum_{i=1}^{n} p_{e_i} = 1$. Let X be a random variable mapping Ω into a set of real numbers $a_1, \ldots, a_k$. We denote by $\{X = a_1\}$ the subset of events e_i such that $X(e_i) = a_1$. Then $p_j = P(X = a_j)$ can be obtained by summing the probabilities p_{e_i} of each individual event $e_i \in \{X = a_j\}$ and

$$m_X = E[X] = \sum_{i=1}^{k} a_i p_i, \qquad \sigma_X^2 = \sum_{i=1}^{k} (a_i - m_X)^2 p_i$$

(see Figure 11.1).

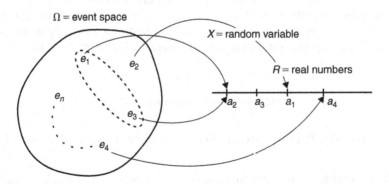

FIGURE 11.1 Schematic illustration of the relation between an event space, Ω, a random variable, X, and its target values (real numbers a_1, a_2, etc). In this example $\{X = a_2\} = \{e_1, e_3\}$ (dashed ellipse).

11.2 BINOMIAL RANDOM VARIABLES

A synapse often contains more than one release site (Figure 11.2). In the general case of n release sites, the sample space of events, Ω, consists of all n-tuplets such as $(r_1, \bar{r}_2, \ldots, r_n)$, where r_i or $\bar{r}_i$ specifies whether the i-th vesicle has been released or not following an action potential. Thus, the sample space, Ω, contains 2^n elements, since each component of a n-tuplet in Ω can take either one of the two values r or $\bar{r}$. If we assume that the release of the i-th vesicle is *independent* of the release of the other vesicles in the releasable pool and that each vesicle has the same probability of release p, the probability of an event $(r_1, \bar{r}_2, \ldots, r_n)$ is given by

$$P(\{(r_1, \bar{r}_2, \ldots, r_k)\}) = p^l q^m, \tag{11.3}$$

where l is equal to the number of released vesicles (the number of r's in the n-tuplet $(r_1, \bar{r}_2, \ldots, r_n)$) and m is the number of vesicles not released (the number of $\bar{r}$'s), with $l + m = n$. In general, two events A and B in Ω are *independent* if their probabilities satisfy the equation

$$P(A \cap B) = P(A)P(B). \tag{11.4}$$

This equation states that the probability of events A and B occurring in conjunction ($A \cap B$) is given by multiplying the probabilities of A and B occurring separately. To illustrate this point and how Eq. (11.3) arises, consider the case of a synapse containing two release sites, i.e., $k = 2$. The events $A = \{(r_1, r_2); (r_1, \bar{r}_2)\}$ and $B = \{(r_1, r_2); (\bar{r}_1, r_2)\}$ correspond respectively to the first or second vesicle being released, regardless of what happens to the remaining one. By assumption, both $P(A)$ and $P(B)$ equal p, since this is the probability of release of a single vesicle. The event $A \cap B = \{(r_1, r_2)\}$ corresponds to the simultaneous release of both vesicles and according to (11.4) has probability $p \cdot p$. Eq. (11.3) can be derived by similar arguments.

The concept of independence generalizes naturally to random variables. Let X and Y be two random variables taking values $a_1, \ldots, a_n$, and $b_1, \ldots, b_m$, respectively. X and Y are said to be independent if

$$P(X = a_k, Y = b_l) = P(X = a_k)P(Y = b_l)$$

for all a_k's and b_l's. For example, let X_1, X_2, and X_3 denote three random variables that take the values 1 or 0 depending on whether vesicle 1, 2, or 3 is released or not for three independent release sites. By definition, X_1 is independent of $X_2 + X_3$ but not of $X_1 + X_3$. An equivalent definition of independence states that

$$P(X \leq a, Y \leq b) = P(X \leq a)P(Y \leq b)$$

for a and b arbitrary. In this equation, $X \leq a, Y \leq b$ is a short hand for the event $\{X \leq a\} \cap \{Y \leq b\}$. This latter definition generalizes to continuous random variables such as those that we will encounter in §11.4.

The random variable representing the total number of vesicles or quanta released, S_n, is given by

$$S_n = X_1 + \cdots + X_n,$$

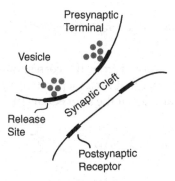

MATHEMATICS FOR NEUROSCIENTISTS

FIGURE 11.2   Schematic illustration of a synapse between two cells. In this example, the synapse has two release sites, each able to release one vesicle into the synaptic cleft when an action potential invades the presynaptic terminal.

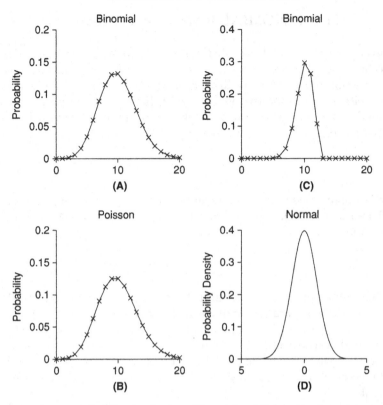

FIGURE 11.3 Illustration of two discrete probability distributions (binomial and Poisson) and a continuous probability density function (normal, or Gaussian with zero mean, unit standard deviation). **A.** Binomial distribution with parameters $n = 100$, $p = 0.1$. **B.** Poisson distribution with parameter $\lambda = 100 \cdot 0.1$. **C.** Binomial with parameters $n = 12$, $p = 0.83$. **D.** Normal distribution ($\mu = 0$, $\sigma = 1$). (`prob_pdfs.m`)

where X_i is defined as above to be 1 if vesicle i is released and 0 otherwise. Thus, the number of quanta that can be released ranges from $S_n = 0$ (for the event $(\bar{r}_1, \ldots, \bar{r}_n) \in \Omega$) to $S_n = n$ (for the event $(r_1, \ldots, r_n) \in \Omega$). When the number of released vesicles lies between 0 and n, say 3, there are several possible elementary events in Ω that lead to $S_n = 3$, e.g., the release of vesicles 1, 2, and 3 or 2, 3, and 4 and so on. The probability of k vesicles being released, i.e., $P(S_n = k) = p_k$ for $0 \leq k \leq n$ is given by the *binomial theorem*:

$$p_k = \frac{n!}{k!(n-k)!} p^k q^{n-k}, \quad k = 0, \ldots, n \tag{11.5}$$

(Exercise 1). The corresponding probability distribution is called *the binomial distribution* of size n and parameter p (Figure 11.3A and C).

Two important properties of the binomial random variable S_n are its mean and variance, corresponding in the case of a synapse with n release sites to the mean and variance of the number of released quanta,

$$m_{S_n} = E[S_n] = \sum_{k=0}^{n} k p_k \quad \text{and} \quad \sigma_{S_n}^2 = E[(S_n - m_{S_n})^2] = \sum_{k=0}^{n} (k - m_{S_n})^2 p_k,$$

respectively. These two quantities can be computed from the corresponding values for X in the single release site example (see Eqs. (11.1) and (11.2)), and the fact that for independent random variables $X_1, \ldots, X_n$ the mean of the sum equals the sum of the means and the variance of the sum equals the sum of the variances (Exercise 2),

$$m_{S_n} = \sum_{k=1}^{n} m_{X_k}, \quad \sigma_{S_n}^2 = \sum_{k=1}^{n} \sigma_{X_k}^2. \tag{11.6}$$

Thus, $m_{S_n} = np$, as expected: on average the number of vesicles released should be n times the release probability of a single site, p. The variance is given by: $\sigma_{S_n}^2 = npq$.

11.3 POISSON RANDOM VARIABLES

In the limit where the number of release sites n is large and the release probability per release site, p, is small, the binomial distribution can be approximated by the *Poisson distribution* (Exercise 3). This limit is of interest because certain synapses like the neuromuscular junction discussed in the next chapter possess a large number of release sites and some experiments characterizing it were performed under conditions where the release probability p was very low. Let us denote by S the random variable representing the number of released quanta. In the case of a Poisson distribution, S depends only on one parameter, λ, and is given by

$$P(S=k) = e^{-\lambda} \frac{\lambda^k}{k!}, \quad k \in \mathbb{N} \tag{11.7}$$

(Figure 11.3B). Note that in this equation, the number of released quanta is unrestricted (k can be arbitrarily large), in contrast to the binomial random variable. Thus, the Poisson random variable can only approximate the binomial random variable in the limit of large n. The probability of a high number of quanta being released decays, however, very fast because of the factorial term, $k!$, in the denominator of Eq. (11.7). The mean and variance of this distribution can be computed directly (Exercise 4),

$$m_S = E[S] = \sum_{k=0}^{\infty} k e^{-\lambda} \frac{\lambda^k}{k!} = \lambda,$$

$$\sigma_S^2 = E[(S-\lambda)^2] = E[S^2] - E[S]^2 = (\lambda^2 + \lambda) - \lambda^2 = \lambda.$$

Thus, λ is the mean of S or the mean number of released quanta and corresponds to np in the binomial model. The parameter λ is often called the *quantal content*. The variance in the number of released quanta is equal to the mean. In contrast, in the binomial model mean and variance are different.

A quantity that will be important in comparing the Poisson model to experimental data is the *coefficient of variation*, defined as the ratio of the standard deviation, σ_S (the square root of the variance) and the mean m_S,

$$C_{V_{Poisson}} \equiv \frac{\sigma_S}{m_S} = \frac{1}{\sqrt{\lambda}}. \tag{11.8}$$

The coefficient of variation is thus a measure of variability of a probability distribution, normalized by its mean.

11.4 GAUSSIAN RANDOM VARIABLES

The random variables encountered up to now only took discrete values, such as $0, 1, 2, \ldots$. In many cases, random variables take a continuum of values. Consider, e.g., the postsynaptic depolarization elicited in a neuron or at the neuromuscular junction by the release of a single vesicle of neurotransmitter. The measure used in such a case is often the peak depolarization recorded by the intracellular electrode, and is variable from one trial to the next. The recorded values typically follow a distribution similar to that of Figure 11.3D (see the inset of Figure 12.4A). This variability could be due to many factors. For example, variations in the number of neurotransmitter molecules contained in individual synaptic vesicles and reaching the postsynaptic receptors or variability in the properties of postsynaptic channels. Modeling this variability requires the use of a *probability density function* because the membrane potential is a continuous variable. By definition, the probability density function, $p(v)$, allows us to write the probability of the membrane potential, V, taking a value between v_0 and v_1 as,

$$P(v_0 < V \le v_1) = \int_{v_0}^{v_1} p(v) \, dv. \tag{11.9}$$

The probability density of the random variable V is thus the probability per unit membrane potential. A satisfactory description is usually obtained by assuming that the membrane potential in response to the release of single vesicle follows the distribution of a *Gaussian random variable*. The Gaussian density is given by,

$$p(v) = \frac{1}{\sigma\sqrt{2\pi}} \exp(-(v-\mu)^2/(2\sigma^2)), \tag{11.10}$$

(see Figure 11.3D). The Gaussian density depends on two parameters, μ and σ^2. We will prove shortly that they represent the mean and variance of the distribution of membrane potential values, respectively. Thus the Gaussian density is uniquely characterized by its mean and variance. The Gaussian density is also often called the normal density and a random variable X that follows such a density is also called a *normal* random variable, abbreviated by $X \sim \mathcal{N}(\mu, \sigma^2)$. When $X \sim \mathcal{N}(0,1)$ we say that X is a *standard* Gaussian (normal) random variable.

To show that μ and σ^2 represent the mean and variance of the Gaussian distribution, we first need to define the mean and variance of a continuous random variable. The definition is analogous to the one used for discrete random variables, but now the sum over probabilities is replaced by the integral over the probability density, since the range of values is continuous:

$$m_X = E[X] \equiv \int\limits_{-\infty}^{\infty} x p(x) \, dx,$$

$$\sigma_X^2 = E[(X - m_X)^2] \equiv \int\limits_{-\infty}^{\infty} (x - m_X)^2 p(x) \, dx,$$

$$= E[X^2] - m_X^2.$$

Proof that μ and σ^2 are the mean and variance of X. First, one shows by direct calculation that the mean and variance of a standard normal variable ($X \sim \mathcal{N}(0,1)$) are equal to 0 and 1, respectively,

$$m_X = 0, \quad \sigma_X^2 = 1, \qquad [X \sim \mathcal{N}(0,1)]$$

(Exercise 6(i)).

Second, one shows that a Gaussian random variable with parameters μ and σ can be obtained from a standard Gaussian random variable by translation and scaling and vice-versa. In other words, if X is standard normal, $X \sim \mathcal{N}(0,1)$, then $Y = \sigma X + \mu \sim \mathcal{N}(\mu, \sigma^2)$. Conversely, if $Y \sim \mathcal{N}(\mu, \sigma^2)$, then $X = (Y - \mu)/\sigma \sim \mathcal{N}(0,1)$ (Exercise 6(ii)).

Third, one shows that when any random variable (i.e., not necessarily Gaussian) is scaled and translated by constant factors, $Y = aX + b$, then the mean scales and translates accordingly: $m_Y = a m_X + b$, and the variance is given by $\sigma_Y^2 = a^2 \sigma_X^2$ (Exercise 6(iii)).

Summing up these three facts, we obtain

$$m_X = \mu, \quad \sigma_X^2 = \sigma^2, \quad \text{or} \quad X \sim \mathcal{N}(\mu, \sigma^2).$$

11.5 CUMULATIVE DISTRIBUTION FUNCTIONS

The *cumulative distribution function* of a random variable X is defined by

$$F(x) \equiv P(X \leq x).$$

The cumulative distribution function is *monotone increasing*, meaning that $x_1 \leq x_2$ implies $F(x_1) \leq F(x_2)$. This follows simply from the fact that $\{X \leq x_2\} = \{X \leq x_1\} \cup \{x_1 < X \leq x_2\}$ and the additivity of probabilities for disjoint events. Furthermore, if X takes values between $-\infty$ and ∞, like the Gaussian random variable, then $F(-\infty) = 0$ and $F(\infty) = 1$. If the random variable X is continuous and possesses a density, $p(x)$, like the Gaussian random variable does, it follows immediately from the definition of F, and since $F(-\infty) = 0$, that

$$F(x) = \int\limits_{-\infty}^{x} p(y) \, dy.$$

Conversely, according to the fundamental theorem of calculus, Eq. (1.7), $p(x) = F'(x)$. Thus, the probability density is the derivative of the cumulative distribution function. This in turn implies that the probability density is always nonnegative, $p(x) \geq 0$, because F is monotone increasing. The cumulative distribution function of the standard normal distribution is, up to constant factors, the *error function*,

$$\text{erf}(x) \equiv \frac{2}{\sqrt{\pi}} \int_0^x \exp(-y^2) \, dy,$$

(Exercise 7). The error function is not an elementary function, meaning that it cannot be built explicitly in terms of simple functions like the exponential, the logarithm or n*th* roots by means of the four elementary operations (addition, subtraction, multiplication, and division).

11.6 CONDITIONAL PROBABILITIES*

If B is an event in a probability space Ω such that $P(B) \neq 0$ we define the *conditional probability* of event A given B as

$$P(A|B) \equiv \frac{P(A \cap B)}{P(B)}.$$

Note first that $P(\cdot|B)$ is a *bona fide* probability measure on the event space Ω since it satisfies properties 1 and 2 enumerated in §11.1. For example,

$$P(\Omega|B) = \frac{P(\Omega \cap B)}{P(B)} = \frac{P(B)}{P(B)} = 1.$$

Property 2 is also easily verified. The conditional probability $P(A|B)$ of an event A is a measure of its dependence on B. If A and B are independent, $P(A \cap B) = P(A)P(B)$, Eq. (11.4), then

$$P(A|B) = \frac{P(A \cap B)}{P(B)} = P(A).$$

Consider, e.g., two adjacent release sites with the following release probabilities upon arrival of an action potential:

$P(\cdot\,;\cdot)$	r_2	$\bar{r}_2$
r_1	$pq + \varepsilon$	$p(1-q) - \varepsilon$
$\bar{r}_1$	$(1-p)q - \varepsilon$	$(1-p)(1-q) + \varepsilon$

with $p = 1/3$, $q = 1/4$, and $\varepsilon = 1/6$. What is the probability of release of vesicle 1 given that vesicle 2 has been released? By summing the columns and rows of the table we see that $P(\{r_1\}) = p$, $P(\{\bar{r}_1\}) = 1 - p$, $P(\{r_2\}) = q$, and $P(\{\bar{r}_2\}) = 1 - q$. The conditional probability for release of vesicle 1 given the release of vesicle 2 is

$$P(\{r_1\}|\{r_2\}) = \frac{P(\{r_1, r_2\})}{P(\{r_2\})} = \frac{pq + \varepsilon}{q} = p + \frac{\varepsilon}{q}.$$

We substitute the values $p = 1/3$, $q = 1/4$, and $\varepsilon = 1/6$ into this equation and conclude that $P(\{r_1\}|\{r_2\}) = 1$. Therefore the release of vesicle 1 is not independent of the release of vesicle 2.

An important property of conditional probabilities is known as *Bayes formula* stating that

$$P(A|B) = P(B|A) \cdot \frac{P(A)}{P(B)}. \tag{11.11}$$

Bayes formula can be immediately derived from the definition of $P(A|B)$ and is often used to infer posterior probabilities of events. The *posterior probability* of an event is its conditional probability, given the knowledge of events affecting its occurrence. For example, assume that we know the probability of an action potential (event B) in a postsynaptic neuron given the release of a vesicle (A) from a presynaptic neuron, i.e., $P(B|A)$. If we know the unconditional probability of release, $P(A)$, as well as that of action potential generation, $P(B)$, we can compute the probability that release actually occurred given an action potential in the postsynaptic neuron using Eq. (11.11).

In the case of continuous random variables X and Y possessing a joint probability density $p(x,y)$, we may define the conditional probability density of y given x as $p(y|x) \equiv p(x,y)/p(x)$, provided $p(x) \neq 0$. The probability density, $p(x)$, is obtained from $p(x,y)$ by integrating out the y dependence, $p(x) = \int p(x,y)\,dy$ and is often called the *marginal density* of X. We will see in §11.9 that in the case of two random variables that are jointly Gaussian, the conditional density of one given the other is again Gaussian.

11.7 SUM OF INDEPENDENT RANDOM VARIABLES*

We now turn to the question of determining the distribution function of the sum $Z = X + Y$ of two independent random variables X and Y. If X and Y take only nonnegative values $(0, 1, \dots)$ like the binomial or Poisson distribution then

$$P(Z = k) = \sum_{n=0}^{k} P(X = n, Y = k - n),$$

since the events $X = n, Y = k - n$, $n = 0, \dots, k$ are mutually exclusive. Because X and Y are independent, $P(X = n, Y = k - n) = P(X = n)P(Y = k - n)$ and setting $P(X = k) = p_{Xk}$, $P(Y = k) = p_{Yk}$, and $P(Z = k) = p_{Zk}$ we obtain the *convolution formula*

$$p_{Zk} = \sum_{n=0}^{k} p_{Xn} p_{Yk-n}. \tag{11.12}$$

For two independent Poisson random variables X and Y with parameters λ and μ, respectively, this formula allows us to conclude that Z is Poisson as well, with parameter $\lambda + \mu$ (Exercise 5). If X and Y are two independent continuous random variables with probability densities $p_X(x)$, $p_Y(y)$, we obtain the probability density $p_Z(z)$ of $Z = X + Y$ from the continuous version of the convolution formula,

$$p_Z(z) = \int_{-\infty}^{\infty} p_X(x) p_Y(z - x)\,dx = \int_{-\infty}^{\infty} p_X(z - y) p_Y(y)\,dy.$$

The continuous convolution formula may be derived by computing the cumulative distribution $F_Z(z) = P(Z \leq z)$ of Z using the joint density $p(x,y)$ of X and Y:

$$F_Z(z) = \int_{-\infty}^{z} p_Z(t)\,dt = \int_{-\infty}^{+\infty} \int_{-\infty}^{z-x} p(x,y)\,dy\,dx,$$

where $p(x,y)$ is the joint probability density of X and Y. The last equality follows from the fact that for each value of x, $Z = X + Y$ will be smaller than z if and only if $y \leq z - x$. The fundamental theorem of calculus, Eq. (1.7), tells us that

$$\frac{d}{dz} \int_{-\infty}^{z-x} p(x,y)\,dy = p(x, z - x).$$

Therefore,

$$p_Z(z) = \int_{-\infty}^{\infty} p(x, z - x)\,dx, \tag{11.13}$$

and since X and Y are independent, $p(x, z - x) = p_X(x) p_Y(z - x)$.

If X and Y are Gaussian random variables with zero means and standard deviations σ_1, σ_2, then

$$p(x, z-x) = p_X(x) p_Y(z-x) = \frac{1}{2\pi\sigma_1\sigma_2} \exp\left(-\frac{x^2}{2\sigma_1^2} - \frac{(z-x)^2}{2\sigma_2^2}\right), \tag{11.14}$$

and the convolution formula allows us to compute the probability density of the sum exactly. In this case, Z is a Gaussian random variable as well, with mean (resp. variance) equal to the sum of the means (resp. variances) of X and Y (Exercise 8).

11.8 TRANSFORMATION OF RANDOM VARIABLES*

Let X be a continuous random variable with probability density $p_X(x)$ taking values over the interval $I = (a,b)$ (with possibly infinite boundary values a and b). If $g(x)$ is a smooth function we can define a new random variable $Y = g(X)$. Y is the transform of X through the function g. One question arises: what is the probability distribution of Y given that of X? Let us assume first that $g(I) = (c,d)$ and that $dg/dx \neq 0$ over I (e.g., $g(x) = \alpha x$). According to the inverse function theorem, g is invertible over (a,b) and $dg^{-1}(g(x))/dy = 1/g'(x)$ over (c,d). We are looking for an explicit formula for the probability density,

$$P(Y \leq y_0) = \int_c^{y_0} p_Y(y)\, dy, \tag{11.15}$$

in terms of the probability density of X. The probability that $Y \leq y_0$ is given by the probability (over the random variable X) that the characteristic function (recall Eq. (1.6)), $\mathbb{1}_{(c,y_0)}(g(x))$, is equal to 1. That is

$$P(Y \leq y_0) = \int_a^b \mathbb{1}_{(c,y_0)}(g(x)) p_X(x)\, dx.$$

We now perform the change of variable $x \to y = g(x)$ so that $dx \to |dx/dy|dy = dy/|g'(x)|$ and hence

$$P(Y \leq y_0) = \int_c^d \mathbb{1}_{(c,y_0)}(y) \frac{p_X(g^{-1}(y))}{|g'(g^{-1}(y))|}\, dy$$

$$= \int_c^{y_0} \frac{p_X(g^{-1}(y))}{|g'(g^{-1}(y))|}\, dy.$$

Comparing with Eq. (11.15) we obtain

$$p_Y(y) = \frac{p_X(g^{-1}(y))}{|g'(g^{-1}(y))|}. \tag{11.16}$$

This equation can be generalized to the case where g is locally invertible over an open set I. For example, if X is a random variable taking values in the interval $(-b,b)$ (with $b > 0$) and $g(x) = \alpha x^2$ then $dg/dx \neq 0$ over $(-b,0) \cup (0,b)$ where g can be inverted (Figure 11.4). Let $f_\pm(y) = \pm\sqrt{y/\alpha}$ denote these local inverses. For $y_0 > 0$,

$$P(Y \leq y_0) = \int_{-b}^0 \mathbb{1}_{(c,y_0)}(g(x)) p_X(x)\, dx + \int_0^b \mathbb{1}_{(c,y_0)}(g(x)) p_X(x)\, dx,$$

and by the arguments presented above,

$$p_Y(y) = p_X(f_-(y)) \left|\frac{df_-}{dy}\right| + p_X(f_+(y)) \left|\frac{df_+}{dy}\right|.$$

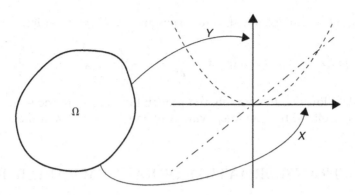

FIGURE 11.4 Schematic illustration of a transformation of random variables. In the first example, $Y = g(X)$ is a linear function of X ($Y = \alpha X$, dash dotted line). In the second example, Y is a quadratic function of X ($Y = \alpha X^2$, dashed line).

11.9 RANDOM VECTORS*

In §11.2, we considered a synapse consisting of n release sites that could either release or not release a synaptic vesicle upon arrival of an action potential. The associated random variables X_i took the value of 0 or 1 depending on whether vesicle i was released or not. In this case, the random vector $\mathbf{v}_X = (X_1, \dots, X_n)^T$ describes all possible release outcomes triggered by the action potential. More generally, if $X_1, \dots, X_n$ is a collection of jointly defined random variables, then $\mathbf{v}_X = (X_1, \dots, X_n)^T$ is called a *random vector*. The function $F_{\mathbf{v}_X}(x_1, \dots, x_n) = P(X_1 \leq x_1, \dots, X_n \leq x_n)$ is called the distribution function of $\mathbf{v}_X$ and is a direct generalization of the distribution function of random variables defined in §11.4. In the case of continuous random variables and when there exists a function $p_{\mathbf{v}_X}(x_1, \dots, x_n)$ such that

$$F_{\mathbf{v}_X}(x_1, \dots, x_n) = \int\limits_{-\infty}^{x_1} \cdots \int\limits_{-\infty}^{x_n} p_{\mathbf{v}_X}(y_1, \dots, y_n) \, dy_1 \cdots dy_n,$$

we call $p_{\mathbf{v}_X}$ the *probability density* of $\mathbf{v}_X$.

Transformation of random vectors. If $\mathbf{z} = \mathbf{g}(\mathbf{x}) = (g_1(\mathbf{x}), \dots, g_n(\mathbf{x}))^T$ is a transformation of the vector $\mathbf{x} = (x_1, \dots, x_n)^T$ onto $\mathbf{z} = (z_1, \dots, z_n)^T$ over the open set $U \subseteq \mathbb{R}^n$, then just as in the one-dimensional case, using the transformation of variables formula for multidimensional integrals,

$$p_{\mathbf{v}_Z}(\mathbf{z}) = p_{\mathbf{v}_X}(\mathbf{g}^{-1}(\mathbf{z}))|\det \nabla \mathbf{g}^{-1}(\mathbf{z})|, \tag{11.17}$$

where det is the determinant defined in Eq. (5.45) and $\nabla \mathbf{g}^{-1}$ is the so-called Jacobian matrix with entries

$$(\nabla \mathbf{g}^{-1}(\mathbf{z}))_{ij} \equiv \frac{\partial g_i^{-1}(\mathbf{z})}{\partial z_j}.$$

Two-dimensional Gaussian random vectors. For concreteness, we will consider the example of a two-dimensional *Gaussian* random vector $(X_1, X_2)^T$ with probability density

$$p(x_1, x_2) = \frac{1}{2\pi(\det \mathbf{C})^{1/2}} \exp(-(\mathbf{x} - \mathbf{m})^T \mathbf{C}^{-1}(\mathbf{x} - \mathbf{m})/2), \tag{11.18}$$

where

$$\mathbf{x} = \begin{pmatrix} x_1 \\ x_2 \end{pmatrix}, \quad \mathbf{m} = \begin{pmatrix} m_1 \\ m_2 \end{pmatrix}, \quad \text{and} \quad \mathbf{C} = \begin{pmatrix} \sigma_1^2 & \sigma_{12} \\ \sigma_{12} & \sigma_2^2 \end{pmatrix}.$$

Note that the matrix $\mathbf{C}$ in Eq. (11.18) is assumed to be symmetric, $\mathbf{C} = \mathbf{C}^T$, and invertible, $\det \mathbf{C} \neq 0$ (Exercise 5.8). We will also see shortly that $\mathbf{C}$ is required to be nonnegative, meaning that its two eigenvalues $\lambda_1, \lambda_2 \geq 0$. The probability density (11.18) is plotted in Figure 11.5C and D for $m_1 = -1$, $m_2 = -2$, $\sigma_1 = 2$, $\sigma_2 = 3$, and $\sigma_{12} = 1$. From the figure, it is clear that the expected value of the random vector $\mathbf{v}_X = (X_1, X_2)^T$ is $E[\mathbf{v}_X] = \mathbf{m}$.

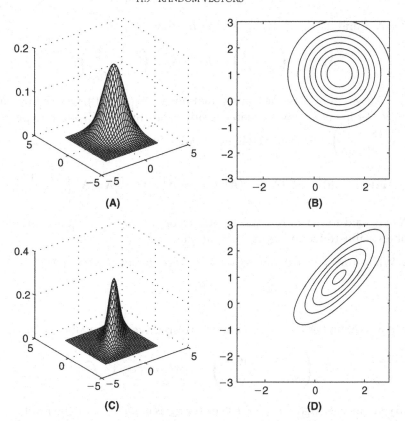

FIGURE 11.5 Probability densities of two-dimensional Gaussian random vectors. The two-dimensional density is a product of two 1-dimensional densities in **A**, but not in **C** ($\rho = 0.8$). The two-dimensional contour lines of constant density are plotted in **B** and **D**, respectively. (gauss_fig.m)

To understand the significance of **C**, consider first the case where $\sigma_{12} = 0$. The corresponding density is plotted in Figure 11.5A and B. As is clear from the figure, $p(x_1, x_2)$ is the product of two 1-dimensional Gaussian densities with means m_1, m_2 and variances σ_1^2, σ_2^2, respectively: $p(x_1, x_2) = p_{X_1}(x_1) p_{X_2}(x_2)$. In this case, the random variables X_1 and X_2 are independent since $P_{\mathbf{v}_X} = P_{X_1} \cdot P_{X_2}$, where P_{X_1} and P_{X_2} are the one-dimensional probabilities associated with the densities p_{X_1} and p_{X_2}, see Eq. (11.9). Furthermore,

$$\mathbf{C} = \begin{pmatrix} \sigma_1^2 & 0 \\ 0 & \sigma_2^2 \end{pmatrix} = \begin{pmatrix} E[(X_1 - m_1)^2] & 0 \\ 0 & E[(X_2 - m_2)^2] \end{pmatrix} = E[(\mathbf{v}_X - \mathbf{m})(\mathbf{v}_X - \mathbf{m})^T]. \tag{11.19}$$

The matrix $E[(\mathbf{v}_X - \mathbf{m})(\mathbf{v}_X - \mathbf{m})^T]$ is called the *covariance* of $\mathbf{v}_X$. Its off-diagonal element $E[(X_1 - m_1)(X_2 - m_2)] = 0$ for two independent Gaussian random variables. Conversely, Eq. (11.19) implies that if the off-diagonal element of the covariance matrix is equal to zero for a two-dimensional Gaussian random vector, then its components X_1 and X_2 are independent. Note that according to Eq. (11.19) $\lambda_1 = \sigma_1^2 \geq 0$ and $\lambda_2 = \sigma_2^2 \geq 0$. The case $\lambda_i = \sigma_i^2 = 0, i = 1, 2$, corresponds to *degenerate* random variables X_i, that are essentially identical to their means, m_i. If either one of $X_i, i = 1, 2$ is degenerate, then the random vector (X_1, X_2) does not possess a probability density according to Eq. (11.18), since the associated matrix **C** is not invertible.

The relation $E[(\mathbf{v}_X - \mathbf{m})(\mathbf{v}_X - \mathbf{m})^T] = \mathbf{C}$ remains valid for a two-dimensional Gaussian random vector, even if $\sigma_{12} \neq 0$. To see this, consider first a linear, invertible transformation $\mathbf{z} = \mathbf{A}\mathbf{x} + \mathbf{b}$. The probability density of $\mathbf{v}_Z$ is obtained by applying the transformation rules for densities under the integral sign (Eq. (11.17) and §11.8),

$$p_{\mathbf{v}_Z}(\mathbf{z}) = \frac{1}{|\det \mathbf{A}|} p_{\mathbf{v}_X}(\mathbf{A}^{-1}(\mathbf{z} - \mathbf{b})). \tag{11.20}$$

Thus, $\mathbf{v}_Z$ is again a two-dimensional Gaussian random vector, since its probability density is of the same functional form as in Eq. (11.18), with **C** replaced by $\mathbf{A}\mathbf{C}\mathbf{A}^T$. Since **C** is symmetric, we now choose **A** to be a rotation (an orthogonal transformation with $\mathbf{A}^T = \mathbf{A}^{-1}$ and det $\mathbf{A} = 1$, Exercise 14) such that

$$\mathbf{A}\mathbf{C}\mathbf{A}^T = \begin{pmatrix} \lambda_1 & 0 \\ 0 & \lambda_2 \end{pmatrix}, \quad \mathbf{A}\mathbf{C}^{-1}\mathbf{A}^T = \begin{pmatrix} \lambda_1^{-1} & 0 \\ 0 & \lambda_2^{-1} \end{pmatrix},$$

and $\mathbf{b} = -\mathbf{A}\mathbf{m}$ so that $\mathbf{v}_Z = \mathbf{A}(\mathbf{v}_X - \mathbf{m})$. Using the transformation law, Eq. (11.20), we see immediately that the density of $\mathbf{v}_Z$ is the product of two 1-dimensional Gaussian densities and thus Z_1, Z_2 are independent Gaussian random variables with covariance $\begin{pmatrix} \lambda_1 & 0 \\ 0 & \lambda_2 \end{pmatrix}$. Just as in §11.4, $\mathbf{m}_{\mathbf{v}_Z} = \mathbf{A}\mathbf{m} + \mathbf{b}$ and

$$E[(\mathbf{v}_X - \mathbf{m})(\mathbf{v}_X - \mathbf{m})^T] = E[(\mathbf{A}^T\mathbf{v}_Z)(\mathbf{A}^T\mathbf{v}_Z)^T] = \mathbf{A}^T E[\mathbf{v}_Z\mathbf{v}_Z^T]\mathbf{A} = \mathbf{A}^T \begin{pmatrix} \lambda_1 & 0 \\ 0 & \lambda_2 \end{pmatrix}\mathbf{A} = \mathbf{C}.$$

When $\sigma_{12} \neq 0$ X_1 and X_2 are said to *covary* or equivalently to be *correlated*. The joint density of correlated pairs of Gaussian random variables is illustrated in Figure 11.5C and D.

Correlation coefficient. When $\sigma_1\sigma_2 \neq 0$ we define the *correlation coefficient* of X_1 and X_2 as

$$\rho \equiv \frac{\sigma_{12}}{\sigma_1\sigma_2}.$$

An important property of ρ is that it lies between -1 and 1 irrespective of the values of σ_1, σ_2. To see this, note that

$$\mathbf{C} = \begin{pmatrix} \sigma_1^2 & \sigma_1\sigma_2\rho \\ \sigma_1\sigma_2\rho & \sigma_2^2 \end{pmatrix}, \quad \det\mathbf{C} = \sigma_1^2\sigma_2^2(1-\rho^2). \tag{11.21}$$

Thus, det $\mathbf{C} > 0$ ($\sigma_1 \neq 0$, $\sigma_2 \neq 0$) implies that $-1 < \rho < 1$. If σ_1 (or σ_2) is equal to zero, the random vector $\mathbf{v}_X$ is *degenerate*, as explained above. In this case X_1 (or X_2) is essentially equal to its mean value and the vector $\mathbf{v}_X = (X_1, X_2)^T$ does not have a proper density since $\mathbf{C}$ is not invertible (see Eq. (11.18)). If $\sigma_1, \sigma_2 \neq 0$, and $\rho = \pm 1$ then det $\mathbf{C} = 0$ and $\mathbf{v}_X$ is degenerate as well. In this case, a rotation matrix $\mathbf{A}$ that diagonalizes $\mathbf{C}$ will yield an eigenvalue λ_1 (or λ_2) equal to zero. The corresponding random variable Z_1 (or Z_2) is then essentially equal to its mean or equivalently X_1 and X_2 are proportional to each other. For example, if $\rho = 1$ and $\sigma_1 \neq 0$ it is easy to see that $E[(\frac{\sigma_2}{\sigma_1}(X_1 - m_1) - (X_2 - m_2))^2] = 0$, meaning that $X_1 - m_1$ is proportional to $X_2 - m_2$. The above arguments can be summarized as follows: let ρ be the correlation coefficient between two jointly Gaussian random variables X_1 and X_2. Then $-1 \leq \rho \leq 1$. If $\rho = 1$ then $X_1 - m_1$ is proportional to $X_2 - m_2$ and if $\rho = -1$ then $X_1 - m_1$ is proportional to $m_2 - X_2$. Thus, the correlation coefficient is a measure of *linearity* between the two Gaussian random variables.

Conditionally Gaussian random variable. If det $\mathbf{C} \neq 0$ we may compute $\mathbf{C}^{-1}$ in term of its components, Eq. (11.21), and arrive at the following alternate expression for the probability density of $\mathbf{v}_X$, Eq. (11.18),

$$p(x_1, x_2) = \frac{1}{2\pi\sigma_1\sigma_2\sqrt{1-\rho^2}}e^{\frac{-1}{2(1-\rho^2)}\left(\frac{(x_1-m_1)^2}{\sigma_1^2} + \frac{(x_2-m_2)^2}{\sigma_2^2} - \frac{2\rho(x_1-m_1)(x_2-m_2)}{\sigma_1\sigma_2}\right)}. \tag{11.22}$$

This expression allows us to compute the conditional probability density $p(x_2|x_1)$ and to conclude that X_2 is Gaussian conditional on the value of X_1, following the distribution $\mathcal{N}(m_2 + \frac{\rho\sigma_2}{\sigma_1}(x_1 - m_1), \sigma_2(1 - \rho^2))$ (Exercise 11).

Sum of two jointly Gaussian correlated random variables. An important generalization of the result described in §11.7 is that the linear combination $\alpha_1 X_1 + \alpha_2 X_2$ of two jointly Gaussian random variables is again Gaussian. This can be seen by first noting that if X_1, X_2 are jointly Gaussian (means m_i, variances σ_i^2, $i = 1, 2$, and covariance σ_{12}) then $\alpha_1 X_1$ and $\alpha_2 X_2$ are jointly Gaussian as well, with means $\alpha_i m_i$, variances $\alpha_i^2\sigma_i^2$, $i = 1, 2$, and covariance $\alpha_1\alpha_2\sigma_{12}$, respectively (Exercise 10). Thus, it is sufficient to prove that for X_1, X_2 jointly Gaussian, $X_1 + X_2$ is Gaussian with mean $m_1 + m_2$ and variance $\sigma_1^2 + 2\rho\sigma_1\sigma_2 + \sigma_2^2$ (Exercise 12).

n-dimensional Gaussian random vectors. The probability density of an n-dimensional Gaussian random vector $\mathbf{v}_X = (X_1, \ldots, X_n)^T$ is defined similarly as in Eq. (11.18) above. The matrix $\mathbf{C}$ is now $n \times n$ dimensional and represents the covariance of $\mathbf{v}_X$ as in the two-dimensional case. The significance of its elements is identical to the two-dimensional case, C_{ii} is the variance of X_i and C_{ij} ($i \neq j$) is the covariance of X_i and X_j. The results described above for two-dimensional Gaussian random vectors carry over at once to multidimensional Gaussian random vectors. Thus, if any two components of a multidimensional Gaussian random vector are uncorrelated, $E[(X_i - m_i)(X_j - m_j)] = 0$, then they are also independent random variables. This is not true in general for random vectors that are not Gaussian. Similarly, any linear combination of their components, $a_1 X_1 + \cdots + a_n X_n$, is a Gaussian random variable.

Non-Gaussian random vectors. For an arbitrary random vector, the covariance matrix is still defined by $\mathbf{C} \equiv E[(\mathbf{v}_X - \mathbf{m})(\mathbf{v}_X - \mathbf{m})^T]$ and is symmetric by definition, although no explicit formula for the probability density of the random vector exists in general. The eigenvalues of $\mathbf{C}$ are positive or zero, $\lambda_i \geq 0$, $i = 1, \ldots, n$, just as in the Gaussian case (Exercise 15). The off-diagonal elements of the covariance matrix remain a measure of the statistical relation between their corresponding random variables. In general, X_1 and X_2 are said to be *uncorrelated* when $\sigma_{12} = 0$, although this does not imply their independence as in the Gaussian case. The *coefficient of correlation* of X_1 and X_2 is defined as usual, $\rho \equiv \sigma_{12}/\sigma_1\sigma_2$. By definition, ρ is the covariance of the centered and normalized random vector associated with $\mathbf{v}_X$: define $\mathbf{v}_Z = (Z_1, Z_2)^T$, with $Z_1 = (X_1 - m_1)/\sigma_1$, $Z_2 = (X_2 - m_2)/\sigma_2$ then the covariance of Z is given by

$$\mathbf{C}_Z = \begin{pmatrix} 1 & \rho \\ \rho & 1 \end{pmatrix}. \tag{11.23}$$

As in the Gaussian case, the coefficient of correlation ρ is confined to values between -1 and 1: $-1 \leq \rho \leq 1$. It can also be shown that when $\rho = 1$ the two random variables X_1 and X_2 are linearly related, $X_2 = aX_1 + b$ with $a \geq 0$. Conversely, $\rho = -1$ implies $X_2 = aX_1 + b$ with $a \leq 0$ (Exercise 16). Thus, in general the correlation coefficient is a measure of *linearity* between two random variables.

11.10 EXPONENTIAL AND GAMMA DISTRIBUTED RANDOM VARIABLES

We now introduce a family of positive random variables used to describe the time intervals separating two random events such as the time interval between successive releases at a synaptic site, for example. The first of these random variables has an *exponential distribution*, given by

$$p_1(t) = \varrho \exp(-\varrho t) \mathbb{1}(t). \tag{11.24}$$

Note that the density is equal to zero for negative values of t. This is expected for the probability distribution of a time interval, since time intervals cannot be negative. The parameter ϱ of the exponential distribution determines its mean value:

$$m_t = \int_0^\infty t p_1(t) \, dt = 1/\varrho. \tag{11.25}$$

Thus, if $1/\varrho$ is the mean value separating two events, ϱ is the rate at which the events occur. The cumulative distribution function corresponding to the exponential density is given by

$$F(t) = (1 - \exp(-\varrho t)) \mathbb{1}(t).$$

A family of probability densities that generalizes the exponential density is given by:

$$p_n(t) = \frac{\varrho(\varrho t)^{n-1}}{(n-1)!} \exp(-\varrho t) \mathbb{1}(t), \quad n = 2, 3, \ldots.$$

Each such density is called a *gamma density* with parameters ϱ and n (Figure 11.6). The gamma density is similar to an exponential distribution (which corresponds to the special case $n = 1$) in that it decays exponentially fast for large t. For small values of t it differs from the exponential density by increasing from a value of 0 for $t = 0$ because of the power term, t^{n-1}. The mean of the gamma distribution is given by:

$$m_t = n/\varrho.$$

An important distinction between gamma distributions with different n values is their relative variability: the larger n, the smaller the variability. This can be seen by computing the variance of the distribution,

$$\sigma_t^2 = n/\varrho^2,$$

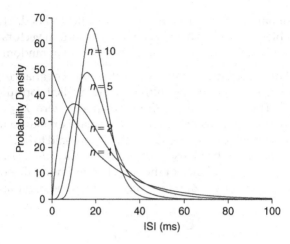

FIGURE 11.6   Plot of gamma distributions of order $n = 1, 2, 5$, and 10 with identical mean equal to 20 ms. (`gamma_distr.m`)

and the coefficient of variation,

$$CV_{gamma} = \frac{\sigma_t}{m_t} = \frac{1}{\sqrt{n}}.$$

Thus, we see that for an exponential distribution, the coefficient of variation is equal to 1, whereas for a gamma distribution with $n = 4$ and the same mean value, the coefficient of variation is only equal to 1/2. In §15.4 and Exercise 15.7 we will show that the sum of n independent and identically distributed exponential random variables is a gamma random variable of order n.

11.11 THE HOMOGENEOUS POISSON PROCESS

The *homogenous Poisson process* is a model describing the occurrence of random events in time. As we will see in the next chapters, it is often used to describe spontaneous synaptic release or the spontaneous activity of neurons. The model is based on the following two assumptions:

1. Each event is isolated, i.e., no two (or more) events can occur at the same moment in time.
2. Events are generated randomly and independently of each other with a mean rate ϱ that is uniform in time. Specifically, for each interval $(a, b]$ the mean number of events is given by $\varrho(b - a)$ and follows a Poisson distribution,

$$P(N(a, b) = k) = e^{-\varrho(b-a)} \frac{(\varrho(b-a))^k}{k!}.$$

Independence is guaranteed if the number of events generated in any two disjoint intervals $(a, b]$ and $(c, d]$ (i.e., $(a, b] \cap (c, d] = \emptyset$) are independent random variables. Thus,

$$P(N(a, b), N(c, d)) = P(N(a, b))P(N(c, d)).$$

Ten samples from such a Poisson process are illustrated in Figure 11.7.

From assumptions 1 and 2 we first derive a formula for the probability density of the interevent distribution of the homogeneous Poisson process. Let us assume that we observe an event at time a. The probability that the interval Δt_0 to the next event is greater than $(b - a)$ is simply the probability that no new event occurs in the interval $(a, b]$, i.e., $P(\Delta t_0 > (b - a)) = P(N(a, b) = 0)$. Since $P(\Delta t_0 \leq (b - a)) = 1 - P(\Delta t_0 > (b - a))$, we have

$$P(\Delta t_0 \leq (b - a)) = 1 - e^{-\varrho(b-a)}.$$

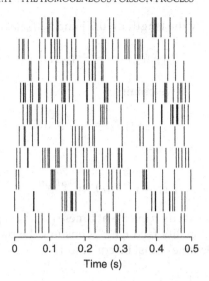

FIGURE 11.7   Plot of ten spike trains belonging to a Poisson process with a mean rate of 50 Hz. (plot_pp.m)

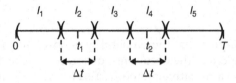

FIGURE 11.8   Schematic illustration of the intervals $I_1, \ldots, I_5$ used in the proof of Eq. (11.26). The intervals I_2 and I_4 are centered around t_1 and t_2, respectively, and of length $\Delta t \to 0$.

But the probability density is the derivative of this probability distribution,

$$P(\Delta t_0 \le (b-a)) = \int_0^{b-a} p(\Delta t_0) \, d\Delta t_0.$$

For simplicity set $\Delta t = b - a$ in the previous two equations and take the derivative:

$$p(\Delta t) = \varrho e^{-\varrho \Delta t} \quad \text{for} \quad \Delta t > 0.$$

In other words, the interevent distribution of a homogeneous Poisson process is exponential, just as in §11.10.

Let us now compute the probability density of registering exactly n events at times $t_1, \ldots, t_n$ (with $t_1 < t_2 < \cdots < t_n$), during the observation interval $(0, T]$. We call this probability density $p_{(0,T]}(t_1, \ldots, t_n)$. For this purpose we consider a sufficiently small interval Δt around each t_i and compute the probability of observing one event in each of these intervals and no event outside these intervals. We then take the limit for $\Delta t \to 0$. For simplicity, we derive only the formula for $p_{(0,T]}(t_1, t_2)$, the general formula can be derived in exactly the same manner. We set $h = (\Delta t)/2$ and consider the five intervals $I_1 = (0, t_1 - h]$, $I_2 = (t_1 - h, t_1 + h]$, $I_3 = (t_1 + h, t_2 - h]$, $I_4 = (t_2 - h, t_2 + h]$, and $I_5 = (t_2 + h, T]$ (Figure 11.8). Because these intervals are disjoint, the event probabilities are independent and

$$P_{(0,T]}(t_1, t_2) = P(N(I_1) = 0)P(N(I_2) = 1)P(N(I_3) = 0)P(N(I_4) = 1)P(N(I_5) = 0).$$

We can now set the probabilities for each interval according to the Poisson distribution. For notational simplicity let us write $|I|$ for the length of interval I. For example: $|I_3| = (t_1 + h) - (t_2 - h) = t_1 - t_2 - \Delta t$. We obtain

$$P_{(0,T]}(t_1, t_2) = e^{-\varrho|I_1|} e^{-\varrho|I_2|} (\varrho|I_2|) e^{-\varrho|I_3|} e^{-\varrho|I_4|} (\varrho|I_4|) e^{-\varrho|I_5|}.$$

Rearranging,

$$P_{(0,T]}(t_1, t_2) = e^{-\varrho(|I_1| + |I_2| + |I_3| + |I_4| + |I_5|)} (\varrho|I_2|)(\varrho|I_4|).$$

But the sum of all interval lengths is simply the length of $(0, T]$ and I_2, I_4 have length Δt. Therefore,

$$P_{(0,T]}(t_1, t_2) = e^{-\varrho T} (\varrho \Delta t)^2.$$

Dividing by Δt^2 (and taking the limit $\Delta t \to 0$) we obtain,

$$p_{(0,T]}(t_1, t_2) = e^{-\varrho T} \varrho^2.$$

This formula immediately generalizes to

$$p_{(0,T]}(t_1, \ldots, t_n) = e^{-\varrho T} \varrho^n. \tag{11.26}$$

Thus the probability density of observing exactly n events at times $t_1, \ldots, t_n$ is proportional to the product of the event rate, ϱ, at those time points. The proportionality factor, $e^{-\varrho T}$, ensures the proper normalization since the sum of all possible spike observations at all possible times must be equal to 1,

$$\sum_{n=0}^{\infty} \int_0^T \int_{t_1}^T \int_{t_{n-1}}^T p_{(0,T]}(s_1, \ldots, s_n) \, ds_1 \cdots ds_n = 1 \tag{11.27}$$

(Exercise 13). When $n = 1$, Eq. (11.26) implies that the probability of observing a spike in any small interval of length Δt is proportional to $\varrho \Delta t$ and independent of the occurrence of spikes outside Δt. This fact may be used to simulate a homogeneous Poisson process, but an alternative method is discussed in Exercise 21.

11.12 SUMMARY AND SOURCES

This chapter provided a general overview of the tools of probability theory. We will use these tools extensively in the subsequent chapters and extend their scope in Chapter 16. Several additional constraints, besides those given in §11.1, are required to obtain a mathematically complete theory of probability. There are many books available on probability theory that will fill in the gaps in our presentation. For the mathematically inclined, we recommend Brémaud (1994) or Chung (2000). Feller (1968) is a classic with many historical references. See Papoulis and Pillai (2002) or Bendat and Piersol (2000) for an engineering perspective. Regarding conditional probability densities, we will see in §22.2 that the conditional distribution of a subset $X_1, \ldots, X_m$ of jointly Gaussian random variables $X_1, \ldots, X_n$ ($m < n$) is again Gaussian, a result that generalizes that of Exercise 11.

11.13 EXERCISES

1. Show that $P(S_n = k) = p_k$, as given in Eq. (11.5).
2. Let X and Y be two random variables taking values $x_1, \ldots, x_n$ and $y_1, \ldots, y_m$, with probabilities $P(x_i, y_j)$. Show that

$$E[X + Y] = E[X] + E[Y].$$

Assume furthermore that X and Y are independent. Show that

$$E[(X + Y - m_X - m_Y)^2] = E[(X - m_X)^2] + E[(Y - m_Y)^2],$$

where $E[X] = m_X$ and $E[Y] = m_Y$.

3. Compute the probability distribution of a Poisson random variable from that of a binomial random variable under the assumption that $\lambda = n \cdot p$ with $n \to \infty$, $p \to 0$ for λ fixed. Hint: Compute first $\log p_0$ under the assumption $p \to 0$ by using the power series

$$\log(1 - x) = -x - x^2/2 + O(x^3)$$

and compute p_k / p_{k+1} under the same assumption to recursively derive $p_1, p_2, \ldots$.

4. Compute the mean and variance of the Poisson distribution.

5. Show that the sum of two independent Poisson random variables of parameters λ and μ is again Poisson with parameter $\lambda + \mu$. Hint: Use the discrete convolution formula, Eq. (11.12), after deriving the identity

$$(\lambda + \mu)^k = \sum_{n=1}^{k} \frac{k!}{n!(k-n)!} \lambda^n \mu^{k-n}. \tag{11.28}$$

6. (i) Compute the mean and variance of the standard normal distribution.

   (ii) Show that if $Y = aX + b$ and $X \sim \mathcal{N}(0,1)$ then $Y \sim \mathcal{N}(b, a^2)$ and vice-versa. Hint: Use the results of §11.8.

   (iii) Show that for arbitrary random variables X and $Y = aX + b$, we have $m_Y = am_X + b$ and $\sigma_Y^2 = a^2 \sigma_X^2$. Hint: The expectation is a linear function.

7. †Show that the cumulative distribution function of the standard normal distribution is given by: $\Phi(x) = (1/2)(1 + \mathrm{erf}(x/\sqrt{2}))$.

8. Show using the convolution formula that the probability density of the sum of two independent Gaussian random variables with means m_1, m_2 and variances σ_1^2, σ_2^2 is Gaussian with mean $m_1 + m_2$ and variance $\sigma_1^2 + \sigma_2^2$. Hint: First use Exercises 7.12 and 7.15 to show that if $X \sim \mathcal{N}(\mu, \sigma)$ then

$$\hat{p}(\omega) = E[e^{-2\pi i \omega X}] = \int_{-\infty}^{\infty} e^{-2\pi i \omega x} p(x) \, dx$$

$$= e^{-2\pi i \omega \mu} e^{-4\pi^2 \sigma^2 \omega^2 / 2}.$$

Next note that the convolution formula implies that $\hat{p}_Z(\omega) = \hat{p}_X(\omega) \cdot \hat{p}_Y(\omega)$.

9. †If $X \sim \mathcal{N}(0,1)$ is standard normal then $Y = X^2$ is called a *chi-squared* random variable. Compute $p_Y(y)$ and show that $E[Y] = 1$ and $\sigma_Y^2 = 2$. Hint: Use the results of §11.8 and the easily derived properties of the Gamma function

$$\Gamma(t) = \int_0^{\infty} x^{t-1} e^{-x} \, dx,$$

$\Gamma(3/2) = \sqrt{\pi}/2$, $\Gamma(t+1) = t\Gamma(t)$ for $t > 0$.

10. †Show that if $\mathbf{v}_X = (X_1, X_2)^T$ is a Gaussian random vector with mean $\mathbf{m} = (m_1, m_2)^T$ and covariance matrix

$$\mathbf{C} = \begin{pmatrix} \sigma_1^2 & \sigma_{12} \\ \sigma_{12} & \sigma_2 \end{pmatrix}$$

then $\mathbf{v}_Z = (\alpha_1 X_1, \alpha_2 X_2)^T$ is Gaussian with mean $(\alpha_1 m_1, \alpha_2 m_2)^T$ and covariance matrix

$$\begin{pmatrix} \alpha_1^2 \sigma_1^2 & \alpha_1 \alpha_2 \sigma_{12} \\ \alpha_1 \alpha_2 \sigma_{12} & \alpha_2^2 \sigma_2 \end{pmatrix}.$$

11. Derive Eq. (11.22) from Eqs. (11.18) and (11.21). Show next that

$$p(x_2 | x_1) = \frac{1}{\sqrt{2\pi} \sigma_2 \sqrt{1 - \rho^2}} \exp\left(-\frac{1}{2\sigma_2^2 (1-\rho^2)} \left((x_2 - m_2) - \frac{\rho \sigma_2}{\sigma_1}(x_1 - m_1) \right)^2 \right).$$

12. Show by integrating directly the convolution formula, Eq. (11.13), that the sum of two correlated Gaussian random variables is again Gaussian, with mean $m_1 + m_2$ and variance $\sigma_1^2 + 2\rho\sigma_1\sigma_2 + \sigma_2^2$. Hint: First convince yourself that it is sufficient to prove the assertion in the case $m_1 = m_2 = 0$. Next, start with the simple case $\sigma_1 = \sigma_2$ and $\rho = 0$. Carry out the integration of the density, Eq. (11.14), by "completing the square" for the integration variable x. Finally, treat the general case in the same manner.

13. Prove Eq. (11.27).

14. Show that if $\mathbf{A} \in \mathbb{R}^{2 \times 2}$ and $\mathbf{A}\mathbf{A}^T = \mathbf{I}$ and $\det \mathbf{A} = 1$ then

$$\mathbf{A} = \mathbf{R}(\theta) \quad \text{with} \quad \mathbf{R}(\theta) = \begin{pmatrix} \cos\theta & \sin\theta \\ -\sin\theta & \cos\theta \end{pmatrix} \quad \text{with} \quad \theta \in [0; 2\pi).$$

Hint: Recall Exercise 5.6.

15. Show that the covariance matrix of a random vector is positive definite. Hint: Proceed as in Exercises 6.1–6.3.

16. Show that in general, the correlation coefficient between two random variables satisfies $-1 \leq \rho \leq 1$ and that values of ± 1 correspond to $X_2 = aX_1 + b$ with $a \gtrless 0$, respectively.

17. †Plot a bar histogram of the binomial probability distribution for $n = 200$ release sites and single release site probabilities $p = 0.01, 0.05$, and 0.1. What are the parameters of the associated Poisson limit distribution? Add to each of these three graphs a bar histogram of the corresponding Poisson distribution. Compute in each case the maximal relative absolute error between both distributions for probability values of the binomial distribution exceeding 0.05 (i.e., if p_k is the probability of k vesicles being released under the binomial distribution and q_k the corresponding value for the Poisson distribution, compute $\max_{\{k \mid p_k \geq 0.05\}} |p_k - q_k|/p_k$). Explain the results. Repeat in the case of $n = 4$ and $p = 0.1, 0.5$, and 0.75. Compare the results in both cases. Hint: Take advantage of the following MATLAB functions: `poisspdf`, `binopdf`, `bar`.

18. †If X is a random variable with density $p_X(x)$, show that the random variable

$$Z(X) = \int_{-\infty}^{X} p_X(y)\, dy$$

is uniformly distributed between 0 and 1. Use this formula to generate random samples of an exponentially distributed random variable from those of a uniformly distributed one. Generate 1000 random samples of the exponential distribution with mean interval 10 ms and compute from these samples an estimate of the probability density between 0 and 50 ms by sampling in 10 bins centered at $0, 5, \ldots, 45$ ms. Compare your estimate with the true density, Eq. (11.24), by plotting them simultaneously, as in Figure 11.9. Finally, compare your inversion formula with the MATLAB code for generating exponentially distributed random variates by typing `type exprnd` at the MATLAB prompt. Can you explain the difference with your formula? Hint: Use the results of §§11.8 and 11.5 to compute the density of Z. Invert the transformation between X and Z and use `rand` to generate uniformly distributed (pseudo-)random numbers.

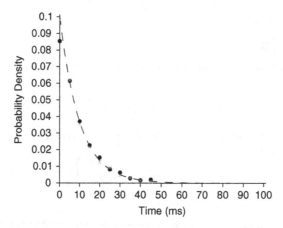

FIGURE 11.9 Plot of the theoretical exponential distribution, the numerical estimate based on MATLAB's `exprnd` function (red crosses) and the estimate obtained as in Exercise 18 (black dots). (`exp_rand.m`)

19. †(i) Show that if $\mathbf{v}_X \sim \mathcal{N}(\mathbf{0}, \mathbf{I})$ then $\mathbf{v}_Z = \mathbf{L}\mathbf{v}_X + \mathbf{m} \sim \mathcal{N}(\mathbf{m}, \mathbf{D})$ where $\mathbf{D} = \mathbf{L}\mathbf{L}^T$ is the Cholesky factorization of $\mathbf{D}$ (recall Exercise 6.7). Hint: Use the transformation formula, Eq. (11.20).

    (ii) Compute by hand the Cholesky factorization of the covariance matrix

$$\mathbf{D} = \begin{pmatrix} 4 & 2 \\ 2 & 25 \end{pmatrix}.$$

    and compare your result with that of the MATLAB function `chol`.

    (iii) Use this result and the MATLAB function `randn` to generate and plot $n_s = 1000$ random samples of $\mathbf{v}_Z$ with mean $\mathbf{m} = (1\ 2)^T$ and covariance $\mathbf{D}$. Plot on the same graph the ellipse of constant probability $\mathbf{x}^T \mathbf{D}^{-1} \mathbf{x} = 1$, as in Figure 11.10A below.

(iv) Compute from the n_s samples $\mathbf{a}_1, \ldots, \mathbf{a}_{n_s}$ an estimate of $\mathbf{m}$ and $\mathbf{D}$ according to the formulas

$$\breve{\mathbf{m}} = \frac{1}{n_s} \sum_{i=1}^{n_s} \mathbf{a}_i, \qquad \breve{\mathbf{D}} = \frac{1}{n_s} \sum_{i=1}^{n_s} (\mathbf{a}_i - \breve{\mathbf{m}})(\mathbf{a}_i - \breve{\mathbf{m}})^T.$$

(v) Plot the mean squared error $(1/2) \sum_{i=1}^{2} (m_i - \breve{m}_i)^2$ and $(1/4) \sum_{i,j=1}^{2} (D_{ij} - \breve{D}_{ij})^2$ as a function of the number of samples $n_s = 10^2, \ldots, 10^5$ to arrive at plots like those in Figure 11.10B and C.

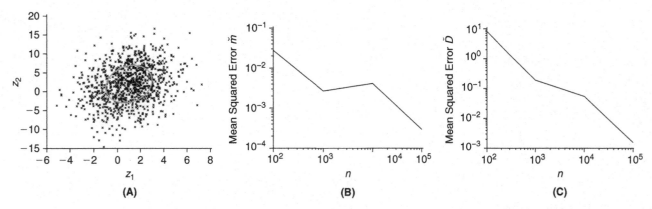

(A)　　　　　　　　**(B)**　　　　　　　　**(C)**

FIGURE 11.10　**A.** Samples of $\mathbf{v}_Z$ and contour of constant probability density (as specified in Exercise 19). **B, C.** Mean square error in the estimate of $\breve{\mathbf{m}}$ and $\breve{\mathbf{D}}$ as a function of the number of samples. (`chol_gauss.m`)

20. Let X_1 and X_2 be nonnegative, independent random variables with densities $p_1(x)$ and $p_2(x)$, respectively. If $Y = X_1 + X_2$ has density $q(x)$, show that the Laplace transform of q obeys

$$\mathcal{L}(q)(s) = \mathcal{L}(p_1)(s)\mathcal{L}(p_2)(s).$$

Hint: Use the fact that $\mathcal{L}(q)(s) = E[e^{-sY}]$. Generalize this result to the sum of an arbitrary number of such random variables, $Y = X_1 + \cdots + X_n$.

21. Plot 10 sample Poisson spike trains with a mean rate of 50 Hz and of duration 0.5 s, as in Figure 11.7. Hint: Generate a sufficient number of exponentially distributed interspike intervals and use the MATLAB function `cumsum`.

22. Show that the sum of two homogeneous Poisson processes of rates ϱ_1 and ϱ_2 is a homogeneous Poisson process of rate $\varrho_3 = \varrho_1 + \varrho_2$. Hint: Use the result of Exercise 5 to verify directly properties 1 and 2 of §11.11.

12

Synaptic Transmission and Quantal Release

OUTLINE

12.1 Basic Synaptic Structure and Physiology 175

12.2 Discovery of Quantal Release 177

12.3 Compound Poisson Model of Synaptic Release 178

12.4 Comparison with Experimental Data 180

12.5 Quantal Analysis at Central Synapses 181

12.6 Facilitation, Potentiation, and Depression of Synaptic Transmission 183

12.7 Models of Short-Term Synaptic Plasticity 186

12.8 Summary and Sources 189

12.9 Exercises 190

Up to now, we have essentially described synaptic transmission as a deterministic process, by which a presynaptic neuron usually excites its postsynaptic target through activation of an α-conductance. There is, however, much more to synaptic transmission than α-conductances. As briefly alluded to in the previous chapter, neurotransmitter molecules are packed in vesicles and their release is stochastic (Figure 11.2). After an overview in §12.1, we present in §§12.2–12.5 the classical work that characterized this fundamental aspect of synaptic transmission. We cover first the neuromuscular junction and then synapses in the central nervous system. In addition to being stochastic, synaptic transmission is dynamic: §§12.6 and 12.7 describe how the strength of synapses varies over time.

12.1 BASIC SYNAPTIC STRUCTURE AND PHYSIOLOGY

Neurons are isolated from each other and from the extracellular environment by a high resistance, high capacitance lipid bilayer membrane. Synapses are the specialized structures that allow one neuron to influence the electrical and biochemical activity of another neuron. We have encountered a few examples in the previous chapters, but synapses come in a large variety of configurations: the two main classes are electrical and chemical. In electrical synapses (also called *gap junctions*), a channel allows intracellular ions to flow directly from one neuron to the next following electrochemical gradients. Current flow can either be bidirectional, or unidirectional when electrical gap junctions are "rectifying." Chemical synapses, in contrast, are essentially unidirectional allowing chemical neurotransmitter substances released by the presynaptic neuron to influence its postsynaptic target.

Chemical synapses are often, but not exclusively, found between the axonal terminal endings of the presynaptic neuron and dendrites of postsynaptic neurons (Figure 2.1). At the electron microscopic level, they consist of a presynaptic ending that contains synaptic vesicles (about 50 nm in size), a synaptic cleft separating the presynaptic and postsynaptic endings and the postsynaptic membrane that contains specialized receptor proteins. The width of the synaptic cleft is 20–30 nm at synapses between neurons in the central nervous system and about 50 nm at the neuromuscular junction. Chemical synaptic transmission occurs when one or more synaptic vesicles in the presynaptic ending fuse with the cellular membrane and release their chemical content in the synaptic cleft, a process called *exocytosis*. This process is calcium dependent: lowering the extracellular calcium concentration (this is usually done by replacing Ca^{2+} with Mg^{2+} ions to keep the total concentration of divalent cations constant) reduces the release of

Mathematics for Neuroscientists. DOI: 10.1016/B978-0-12-374882-9.00012-5

neurotransmitter. Following exocytosis, the neurotransmitter molecules diffuse in the cleft toward the postsynaptic membrane where they bind at the receptor sites.

The effect of neurotransmitters on their target neurons upon binding to receptors can be mediated by several distinct mechanisms. In the simplest case, the receptor site is directly attached to an ion-selective channel (or *ionotropic receptor*) and binding causes the channel to open, thus allowing ions to flow in or out of the cell. In other cases, the receptors will activate second messenger pathways that mediate their action indirectly by phosphorylating other membrane channels, for example. Some such pathways are sketched in Figure 12.1. An important aspect of chemical transmission is that the same transmitter molecule can activate distinct pathways depending on the type of receptors inserted in the postsynaptic membrane. Thus, glutamate, the most common excitatory neurotransmitter of the vertebrate central nervous system, activates various types of receptors directly coupled to ion permeable channels (iGluRs) such as AMPA (§2.5), NMDA (§9.3), and kainate/quisqualate receptors. In addition, *metabotropic* or G-protein coupled receptors (mGluRs) couple to various intracellular second messenger pathways.

The effect of neurotransmitters on postsynaptic terminals is terminated either by degradation of the neurotransmitter substance in the synaptic cleft or by reuptake mechanisms in both neurons and glial cells. Acetylcholine, the neurotransmitter released at the neuromuscular junction of vertebrates and a major excitatory neurotransmitter in the central nervous system of invertebrates, is degraded by acetylcholinesterase into two components, one of which

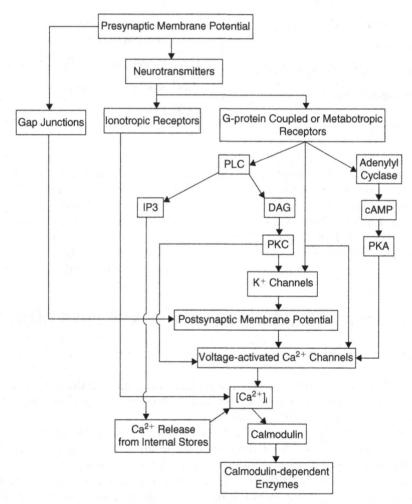

FIGURE 12.1　Overview of synaptic transmission mechanisms. Gap junctions (left) directly couple the presynaptic and postsynaptic membrane potentials. Ionotropic receptors open ion-selective channels that can modify the postsynaptic membrane potential as well as pass calcium ions, which play an important role in intracellular second messenger pathways. G-protein coupled receptors, also called metabotropic receptors, can directly affect the properties of ion channels such as K^+ or Ca^{2+} channels. They can also cause calcium to be released from internal stores through activation of phospholipase C (PLC) and generation of inositol 1,4,5-triphosphate (IP3). In addition, diacylglycerol (DAG) can activate protein kinase C (PKC) which in turns affects the function of K^+ and Ca^{2+} channels. Finally, protein kinase A (PKA) can affect the function of Ca^{2+} channels following activation by adenylyl cyclase and cyclic AMP (cAMP). Intracellular calcium can in turn activate calmodulin and a range of calmodulin-dependent enzymes. Adapted from Nicholls (1994).

is taken up again by the presynaptic nerve terminal and used to synthesize new neurotransmitter molecules. GABA, a major inhibitory neurotransmitter both in vertebrate and invertebrate central nervous systems, is taken up directly from the synaptic cleft by an efficient sodium-dependent transporter.

Release of neurotransmitters can also have a direct effect on the presynaptic terminal itself when receptors for the released neurotransmitter are present on the presynaptic membrane as well. This turns out to be rather common both at excitatory and inhibitory central synapses in vertebrates and invertebrates. Presynaptic receptors are thought to provide feedback mechanisms to the presynaptic terminal.

It should be clear from this brief summary that the mechanisms of synaptic transmission in the central nervous system can be complex. Further illustrations of the technical complexity hampering the study of synaptic transmission at central synapses will be presented in the following sections.

12.2 DISCOVERY OF QUANTAL RELEASE

The first detailed studies of synaptic transmission were performed in the 1950s by Katz and colleagues on a preparation somewhat simpler and more accessible than synapses between neurons. They studied the neuromuscular junction in frogs, typically using leg muscles such as the sartorius and gastrocnemius. The neuromuscular junction is responsible for triggering muscle fiber contractions upon arrival of action potentials at the axonal endings of presynaptic motor neurons. The neuromuscular junction is a synapse between a neuron and a muscle fiber; therefore not all the experimental results gathered from such a preparation extend without changes to synapses between neurons. By recording with intracellular electrodes the membrane potential of single muscle fibers (Figure 12.2), Katz and colleagues were able to make the following observations.

1. The membrane potential of muscle fibers fluctuates in time: small depolarizations were observable in the absence of nervous activity and were particularly evident close to the junction of the nerve fiber with the muscle fiber. Because of its plate-shaped structure in mammals and lizards, this junction is also called an *end-plate*. They therefore called these membrane potential fluctuations *miniature end-plate potentials* (m.e.p.p.s) and concluded that neurotransmitter "leaks" or is released spontaneously from the nerve terminal. The release process appeared to be completely random with a probability of release constant in time. Subsequent releases occurred independently of each other without any clear refractory period (i.e., no dead time between individual release events).

2. Synaptic release was known to be dependent on the availability of extracellular calcium. By decreasing the extra-cellular calcium concentration, they were able to reduce the amount of spontaneous release. However, the size of individual miniature end-plate potentials did not change and was observed to occur in discrete steps. Evoked potentials obtained by stimulating the nerve under these conditions were multiples of the miniature end-plate potentials.

Figure 12.3 shows a schematic drawing of a vertebrate neuromuscular junction. Synaptic vesicles cluster around dense cytoplasmic formations and face on the other side the postsynaptic end-plates on the muscle fibers. Katz and colleagues formulated the hypothesis that acetylcholine is contained in the vesicles and that during a spontaneous event, triggered by calcium entry in the presynaptic terminal, the content of one or more of these vesicles was released

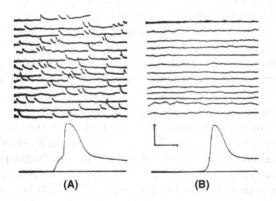

(A)   (B)

FIGURE 12.2 **A.** Spontaneous activity recorded from a muscle fiber at the end-plate of the frog neuromuscular junction (top). The response to a nerve impulse is shown at the bottom. **B.** Same as in A, but recorded 2 mm away from the end-plate. Scale bars: 50 mV and 2 ms (bottom), 3.6 mV and 47 ms (top). Adapted from Fatt and Katz (1952).

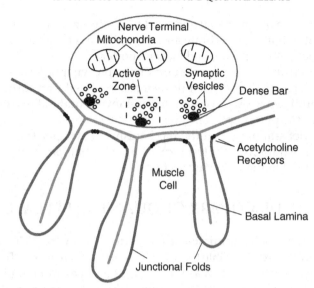

FIGURE 12.3   Schematic drawing of the neuromuscular junction. The presynaptic terminal contains synaptic vesicles filled with acetylcholine. The dense bars represent active zones where synaptic vesicles are released in the synaptic cleft. Acetylcholine receptors are located opposite to the active zones in the muscle cell membrane. Acetylcholine esterase is contained in the postsynaptic folds of the synaptic cleft. The basal lamina is part of the extracellular matrix material coating the muscle fiber.

in the cleft. Variability in miniature end-plate potentials would then correspond to variability in the number of vesicles released and would therefore naturally occur in steps. This is the *quantum hypothesis of synaptic release*.

Some additional information on the experimental results of Fatt and Katz and a quick calculation can immediately give us a better idea of what is going on at the end-plate following nerve activation. The usual miniature end-plate potentials measured by Fatt and Katz typically ranged from 0.4–1.0 mV in size. A typical end-plate potential elicited by stimulation of the nerve reached at least 50 mV, with typical values closer to 70–80 mV. Thus, during normal function, according to the quantum hypothesis, the nerve ending must release >100 vesicles to generate the normal end-plate potential. This suggests that there are at least 100 release zones, and probably more, if the release probability is smaller than 1, as suggested by the random events observed spontaneously.

12.3 COMPOUND POISSON MODEL OF SYNAPTIC RELEASE

The observations described in the previous section provide the experimental basis for a model describing the statistical properties of synaptic release at the neuromuscular junction. As explained in §11.2, each synapse is assumed to have *n release sites* (also called *active zones*) and during a spontaneous or evoked event, each site is assumed to release a single synaptic vesicle independently of other sites, with probability p. Since the synapse has n release sites, the total number of quanta released, S_n, is a binomial random variable.

In the limit where the number of release sites is large and the release probability per release site is small, the binomial distribution is well approximated by the *Poisson distribution* (§11.3). This limit is of interest because synapses at the neuromuscular junction possess a large number of release sites (probably more than 200) and some studies, including the ones summarized above, were performed under conditions where the release probability was very low. The Poisson distribution is given in Eq. (11.7) and depends only on one parameter, λ, the *quantal content*. If S denotes the number of released quanta, its mean is equal to its variance: $m_S = \lambda$ and $\sigma_S^2 = \lambda$.

In conditions where only single quanta are released from the end-plate, the size of miniature end-plate potentials, typically measured as the peak depolarization recorded by the intracellular electrode, is variable from one trial to the next. Thus, there is not only variability in the number of quanta released by the presynaptic terminal, but also in the postsynaptic response to a single quantum. This variability could be due to many factors. For example, it could be due to variations in the number of neurotransmitter molecules contained in individual synaptic vesicles and reaching the postsynaptic receptors or to variability in the properties of postsynaptic receptors or channels. The unitary miniature end-plate potentials typically follow the distribution of a Gaussian random variable, given in Eqs. (11.9) and (11.10) (Figure 12.4A inset). Recall that the Gaussian density depends on two parameters, its mean μ and variance σ^2.

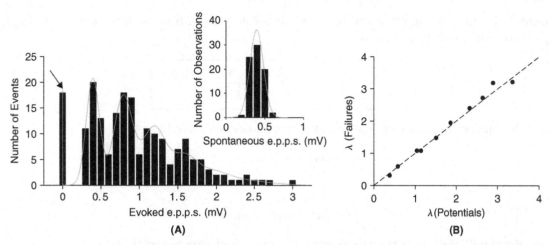

FIGURE 12.4 **A.** Histograms of e.p.p.s and spontaneous potential amplitude distribution (inset) in a fiber in which neuromuscular transmission was blocked by increasing the magnesium concentration to 12.5 mM. Red lines indicate the model fit described in §12.4. Arrow indicates expected number of failures in response to nerve stimuli. **B.** Comparison of the two methods of obtaining the quantal content λ according to Eqs. (12.5) (abscissa) and (12.7) (ordinate). Adapted from Boyd and Martin (1956). (boyd_martin2.m)

We can now combine the Poisson model of vesicle release with the Gaussian description of unitary miniature end-plate potential events to obtain the probability distribution of the postsynaptic potential during evoked release. We discuss only the Poisson presynaptic model, but the binomial model could be handled in the same way. The postsynaptic membrane potential is assumed to be the sum of the response evoked by each released quantum,

$$V = \begin{cases} 0, & \text{if } S=0, \\ V_1 + V_2 + \cdots + V_S, & \text{if } S > 0. \end{cases} \tag{12.1}$$

Both the number of quanta released, S, and the membrane potential depolarization in response to each quantum, V_i, are random variables. We can write the probability density for the membrane potential, $p(v)$, as a function of the probability of k quanta being released, $P(S=k)$, and the probability density of the membrane potential given that k quanta were released, $p(v|S=k)$. The probability densities $p(v|S=k)$ are conditional probability densities (§11.6). The formula is:

$$p(v) = p(v|S=0)P(S=0) + p(v|S=1)P(S=1) + p(v|S=2)P(S=2) + \cdots$$

In this equation the individual terms add because the events $S=0, S=1$, and so on, are mutually exclusive (i.e., either 1 quanta is released or 2, and so on; see §11.1). The values $P(S=k)$ are obtained from the Poisson distribution (Eq. (11.7)) and it remains only to compute the $p(v|S=k)$ for $k \in \mathbb{N}$. If no quanta are released ($S=0$) the membrane potential is equal to 0 with probability 1 (Eq. (12.1)); as we will see, this is a very convenient fact that can be used to test explicitly the validity of the Poisson model. We represent this by a Dirac "density" $\delta(v)$ that is zero for every value of v except for $v=0$ where it is infinite but integrates to 1:

$$\int_{-\infty}^{\infty} \delta(v)\,dv = 1$$

(Eq. (3.6), Exercise 7.20). The probability density $p(v|S=1)$ is the Gaussian density (Eq. (11.10)). When two quanta are released $p(v|S=2)$ is the sum of two independent Gaussian variables ($V=V_1+V_2$), each with mean μ and variance σ^2. We already know (Eq. (11.6)) that this variable has mean 2μ and variance $2\sigma^2$. As explained in §11.9, an important property of Gaussian random variables is that their sum V is also Gaussian and thus its density is given by

$$p(v|S=2) = \frac{1}{\sqrt{2}\sigma\sqrt{2\pi}} e^{-\frac{(v-2\mu)^2}{2\cdot 2\sigma^2}}.$$

The same result holds for $S=3$, in other words, $p(v|S=3)$ is Gaussian with mean 3μ and variance $3\sigma^2$, and so on. Combining these results together we obtain:

$$p(v) = e^{-\lambda}\delta(v) + e^{-\lambda}\sum_{k=1}^{\infty}\frac{\lambda^k}{k!}\frac{1}{\sqrt{2\pi k\sigma^2}}e^{-\frac{(v-k\mu)^2}{2k\sigma^2}}. \tag{12.2}$$

The mean and the variance of the membrane potential distribution are given by:

$$m_V = m_S\mu = \lambda\mu, \tag{12.3}$$

and

$$\sigma_V^2 = \sigma_S^2\mu^2 + m_S\sigma^2 = \lambda(\mu^2 + \sigma^2). \tag{12.4}$$

These two equations will prove important to compare the model with experimental data.

12.4 COMPARISON WITH EXPERIMENTAL DATA

Eq. (12.2) represents the prediction for the distribution of end-plate potentials in response to nerve stimulation at the neuromuscular junction under the following assumptions:

1. Release is quantal and follows a Poisson distribution.
2. The postsynaptic effects of quanta are independent and sum linearly.

To compare the prediction of Eq. (12.2) with experimental data we need to compute the parameters λ that represents the mean number of quanta released per nerve stimulation as well as the mean, μ, and the variance, σ^2, of a single unitary miniature end-plate potential. This program was first carried out at the neuromuscular junction in conditions where the probability of release was diminished. Under these conditions, spontaneous release consists essentially of single quanta with typical mean depolarizations μ of 0.4–1.0 mV and standard deviations σ equal to about $0.2 \cdot \mu$ (i.e., the coefficient of variation of the m.e.p.p.s is approximately of 0.2; Figure 12.4A, inset). To compute the quantal content λ during evoked synaptic release one can now take advantage of Eq. (12.3) above. This equation tells us that the mean membrane potential depolarization during nerve stimulation should be proportional to the quantal content and the proportionality constant is none other than μ, the mean spontaneous depolarization for a single spontaneous quantal event. Thus,

$$\lambda = \frac{\text{mean amplitude of the e.p.p. response}}{\text{mean amplitude of spontaneous potentials}}. \tag{12.5}$$

From these three measurements (two from spontaneously occurring miniature end-plate potentials and one from evoked release) we can now fit the probability density distribution of evoked end-plate potentials (Figure 12.4). The validity of the Poisson assumption can be verified by two additional tests sometimes called the *method of failures* and *CV method*.

The method of failures. Once the quantal content λ has been obtained from experimental data, the Poisson distribution is in principle completely determined, since it depends only on the value of λ (see Eq. (11.7)). Thus, it is possible to test the validity of the Poisson assumption by comparing the probability of k packets being released with the prediction of Eq. (11.7). In practice, the quantity most easily compared with the theoretical prediction is the probability of failures, $P(S=0)$, since a failure to respond to nerve stimulation is easy to observe and record (no deflection of the postsynaptic end-plate potential after electrical stimulation of the nerve). More precisely, it follows from Eqs. (11.7) and (12.5) that

$$\log(\text{fraction of failures}) = -\frac{\text{mean amplitude of the e.p.p. response}}{\text{mean amplitude of spontaneous potentials}}. \tag{12.6}$$

To compare this prediction with experimental data, a series of experiments is done with different nerve fibers to obtain a range of failure values. The negative logarithm of the fraction of failures is plotted against the experimentally determined quantal content (according to Eq. (12.5)). If the prediction of Eq. (12.6) is right, the points should fall on a straight line of slope 1 through the origin (Figure 12.4B).

The CV method. The starting point for the second method consists in computing the coefficient of variation of the evoked end-plate potentials, $C_{V_{epps}}$. From Eqs. (12.3) and (12.4) it follows that,

$$C_{V_{epps}} = \frac{1}{\sqrt{\lambda}} \sqrt{1 + \sigma^2/\mu^2}. \tag{12.7}$$

Recalling the value of the CV of the Poisson distribution (Eq. (11.8)), we see that, up to a constant $K = \sqrt{1 + \sigma^2/\mu^2}$, it coincides with the CV of the e.p.p.s:

$$C_{V_{epps}} = C_{V_{Poisson}} K.$$

Taking the logarithm on both sides of Eq. (12.7), we see that:

$$\log C_{V_{epps}} = -\frac{1}{2} \log \lambda + \log(K). \tag{12.8}$$

Therefore, if one performs a series of experiments, computes for each experiment the coefficient of variation of the evoked e.p.p.s, and plots them as a function of the quantal content, λ (computed from Eq. (12.5)) on a logarithmic scale, they should fall on a straight line of slope $-1/2$. Fatt and Katz proceeded slightly differently: instead of computing the coefficient of variation of the e.p.p.s directly, they first assigned each e.p.p. to its class (i.e., decide from the value of the e.p.p. whether a single quantum was released or two quanta and so on) and they computed the coefficient of variation from the resulting distribution. This corresponds to (artificially) setting the variability of e.p.p.s to zero (i.e., set σ equal to 0 in Eq. (12.7)), which is equivalent to setting the constant $\log(K)$ to zero in Eq. (12.8). Their results support the Poisson hypothesis, at least in the case of fibers that have a quantal content smaller than ≈ 10. For larger quantal contents, the predictions of the compound Poisson model start to fail. One possible reason is that the assumption of linear summation of m.e.p.p.s (see Eq. (12.1)) is incorrect for larger depolarizations. In other words, the second assumption formulated at the beginning of this paragraph is violated.

12.5 QUANTAL ANALYSIS AT CENTRAL SYNAPSES

Following the success of quantal analysis at the neuromuscular junction, quantal analysis has also been performed at many central synapses in the nervous system. The first objective has been to assess whether the quantal theory also holds there. The second objective has been to estimate the quantal parameters governing release at single central synapses, that is, the number of release sites, the probability of release (quantal content), and the size of the postsynaptic response elicited by a single release (quantal size).

Technically, the application of quantal analysis to central synapses is much more difficult than at the neuromuscular junction. One reason is that neurons typically receive thousands of input synapses at various positions in their dendritic tree. Isolating a single synapse and its miniature excitatory or inhibitory postsynaptic potentials (mepsps and mipsps, respectively) is thus difficult. In many cases the size of mepsps or mipsps falls within the range of background noise in the recordings. When mepsps or mipsps cannot be isolated from background noise, three critical parameters of the Poisson (and binomial) model cannot be estimated (the quantal size, its variance, and the rate of failures) complicating significantly the analysis. The situation has been improved by the invention of the *patch-clamp technique* (Figures 13.21 and 17.1B) that allows for considerably lower access resistances to the intracellular potential as compared to sharp electrodes and thus results in much higher signal-to-noise ratios in the recordings. In some cases, this technique could also be used to voltage-clamp the neuron and the postsynaptic terminal, thus giving direct access to miniature excitatory or inhibitory postsynaptic currents. This is a significant advantage over recording mepsps/mipsps because postsynaptic currents allow one to circumvent one of the assumptions of the release model, namely that postsynaptic potentials add linearly. This assumption cannot be true for large depolarizations, whereas currents always add linearly.

Quantal analysis has in general been most powerful at central synapses when combined with complementary anatomical or pharmacological techniques. We illustrate this with the example of the release statistics at input synapses to the Mauthner cell, a neuron in fish involved in generating fast tail-flips underlying turning and escape responses. One of the first outcomes of quantal analysis on Mauthner cell synapses that has often been verified at other central synapses is that the Poisson limit is not an appropriate description of quantal release. Hence the more general binomial model with its two parameters N and p has to be used. Structural studies of the same synapses used for quantal

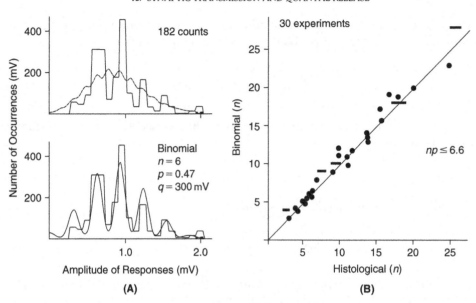

FIGURE 12.5   **A.** Fits with binomial and Poisson distributions of inhibitory postsynaptic potentials elicited by stimulation of interneurons onto the Mauthner cell of goldfish. Adapted from Korn et al. (1982). **B.** Summary plot of the number of release sites determined from the binomial model as a function of histologically determined release sites in the same neurons. Adapted from Korn (1984).

analysis were also made using electron microscopy. This allowed the investigators to count the number of release sites N_{anat} and to compare it with the value of N obtained by fitting the binomial model to spontaneous and evoked synaptic potentials. In most cases, the two turned out to be close, $N \approx N_{anat}$, thus leading to the *one release-site one quantum* hypothesis, stipulating that each active zone in a synaptic contact releases exactly one quantum (or one vesicle) per action potential (Figure 12.5). Here it is important to note that the use of electron microscopy is crucial: *synaptic boutons*, the apposition of presynaptic and postsynaptic elements between two neurons can be determined by light-microscopic methods, but the identification of synaptic vesicles and the zones where they are released requires electron microscopy (Figure 12.6). Although in many cases each bouton contains a single release site, it is possible for a synaptic bouton to contain more than one release site.

The reason for the failure of the Poisson approximation at many central synapses is that both the assumption of a large number of release sites and a low probability of release are violated.

1. The number of release sites, N, per synaptic contact between two neurons can be very low. In some cases, it is thought that only one synaptic release site exists between two cells. This is the case between CA3 pyramidal cells in the hippocampus and their target inhibitory interneurons, for example. At the other extreme, synapses like the calyx of Held (in the cochlear nucleus of the auditory system) or the climbing fiber synapse made by inferior olive axons on Purkinje cells of the cerebellum are estimated to contain ≈ 500 release sites, a situation similar to the neuromuscular junction.

2. The probability of release, p, is often variable across synapses and is in many cases quite high. The range of synaptic release probabilities estimated for central synapses ranges from $p = 0.05$ to p close to 1, depending on the junction studied. Even in single neurons release probabilities of individual synapses can be highly variable.

Another important aspect of quantal analysis at central synapses is that there is evidence for violation of some of the central assumptions underlying the model:

1. The release probability at different release sites of a single synaptic contact is not always uniform. When this is the case the assumption of a single p value for all release sites is violated. Under these conditions both the Poisson and binomial models are no longer valid approximations to the synaptic release process.

2. Release of vesicles is assumed to be independent at different release sites. There is evidence that this is probably not true at several central synapses.

3. There is evidence that a single release site can in some instances release more than one vesicle per action potential.

4. In some cases, the variability of postsynaptic responses is much lower than what would be expected from addition of independent mepsps. This has been suggested to be due to saturation of postsynaptic receptor sites by the

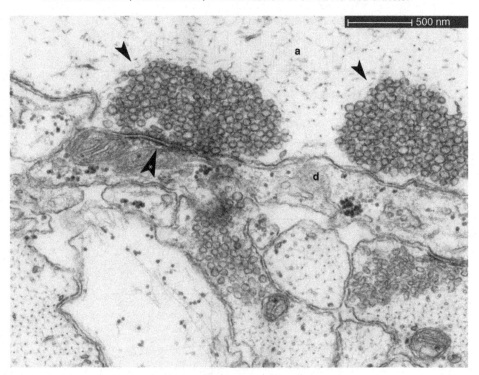

FIGURE 12.6 Electron micrograph of a giant reticulospinal synapse in the lamprey. The axon is on top (**a**) and the dendrite below it (**d**). Two large clusters of synaptic vesicles are visible in the presynaptic axon (arrow heads) and an active zone is indicated by the asterisked arrow head. The scale bar on top is about twice the size of the smallest resolvable extent by light microscopy (200–300 nm). Courtesy of A.E. Foldes and Dr. J. Morgan, Molecular Cell and Developmental Biology Department, University of Texas at Austin.

neurotransmitter released from the vesicles. When this is the case, the quantization of the postsynaptic response is likely to be determined in part by the number of postsynaptic receptors rather than the number of released vesicles.

Because of this, the use of quantal models has to be considered with care, since the interpretation of results depends critically on these assumptions.

12.6 FACILITATION, POTENTIATION, AND DEPRESSION OF SYNAPTIC TRANSMISSION

Synaptic transmission is not static in time: in cases where sequences of action potentials arrive at the presynaptic terminal, the strength of the responses measured postsynaptically varies. The time course of these variations depends on the specific synapse studied. Three main types of synaptic changes have been described (Figure 12.7):

1. *Facilitation* is used to describe the progressive increase in response during a short train of action potentials, typically lasting a few seconds. Facilitation is observed at central synapses but also at the neuromuscular junction. As explained in more detail below, facilitation is thought to be due to an accumulation of calcium in the presynaptic terminal that increases the probability of transmitter release. Recovery from facilitation is rapid, arising in few hundreds of milliseconds following the termination of stimulation.

2. *Potentiation* describes an increase in response following repetitive stimulation of a synapse. Potentiation is more slow to develop than facilitation and typically outlasts the stimulus. A protocol that is able to elicit potentiation of synaptic transmission is to deliver a short train of high frequency action potentials to the presynaptic terminal, which is often called a *tetanus*. The potentiation observed following such a pulse is therefore called *posttetanic potentiation* (PTP). This type of synaptic transmission change is observed at central synapses and also at the neuromuscular junction. Under certain conditions potentiation at central synapses can last for a very long amount of time, typically over the entire course of an experiment (i.e., hours). This phenomenon is thought to represent a permanent change in synaptic strength and is termed *long-term potentiation* (LTP). The mechanisms underlying LTP are thought to be different from those underlying PTP.

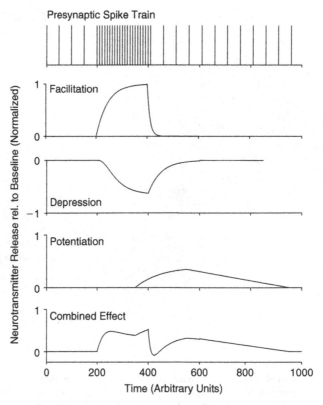

FIGURE 12.7   Schematic illustration of the hypothetical time course of facilitation, potentiation, and depression of neurotransmitter release at a synapse. These effects can occur simultaneously, leading to a complex time-dependent modulation of synaptic release.

3. *Depression* is the opposite of potentiation and describes a progressive decrease in response over the course of stimulation. Long-term synaptic depression (LTD) has been described at central synapses and can also last over long periods of time.

Quantal analysis has been used to investigate these changes in synaptic transmission and in particular to clarify whether they are due to presynaptic changes such as an increase or decrease in release probability or to postsynaptic changes such as in increase or decrease in postsynaptic response strength. The methods used are very similar to the ones described above and will be summarized here using the binomial model of synaptic transmission, since this model is usually more appropriate to describe synaptic transmission at central synapses.

Recall from §11.2 that for the binomial model, the mean number of vesicles released is $m_{S_n} = np$, and the variance in the number of released vesicles is given by $\sigma^2_{S_n} = np(1-p)$. Assuming, as in the Poisson model, a mean quantal postsynaptic response μ with variance σ^2, the mean evoked response is the product of the number of packets released and the mean quantal response,

$$m_V = m_{S_n}\mu = np\mu. \tag{12.9}$$

The variance of the postsynaptic response is attributable to both the variance in the number of released packets and the variance of unitary potentials,

$$\sigma^2_V = \sigma^2_{S_n}\mu^2 + m_{S_n}\sigma^2. \tag{12.10}$$

Direct determination of release parameters.   One can use Eqs. (12.9) and (12.10) to study changes in synaptic transmission by determining the parameters n, p, and μ before and after a protocol that elicits a change in synaptic transmission. If, e.g., a protocol is used that induces LTP at a given synapse, one can investigate whether strengthening of the synapse corresponds to changes in the number of release sites n, or the probability of release, p, or the response to a single quantum, μ. The analysis proceeds as follows: μ, σ^2, m_V, and σ^2_V are determined directly by experiments before and after applying the protocol. The mean number of released vesicles can then be obtained from Eq. (12.9). From here we determine the variability in the release process, $\sigma^2_{S_n}$, using Eq. (12.10). The release probability is then obtained from $\sigma^2_{S_n} = npq = np(1-p)$. Finally the number of release sites is computed from $m_{S_n} = np$.

Method of failures. A second method that can be used to demonstrate changes in release probability is to monitor the fraction of failures before and after the protocol used to elicit changes in synaptic transmission. In the binomial model, the probability of a failure to respond is given by

$$p_0 = (1-p)^n.$$

Thus, if the probability of release changes, the failure rate should change accordingly. This method is only applicable if transmission failures can be reliably established, i.e., unitary responses are well above the recording noise.

Variants of the CV method. If we neglect the variability in postsynaptic responses (i.e., assume $\sigma = 0$) we see from Eq. (12.10) that

$$\frac{1}{\sigma_{S_n}^2} = \frac{\mu^2}{\sigma_V^2}.$$

Multiplying both sides of this equation by $(np)^2$ and using Eq. (12.9) we see that

$$\frac{m_V^2}{\sigma_V^2} = \frac{np}{1-p}.$$

The left hand side of this equation is equal to $1/C_{V_{ev.resp.}}^2$, i.e., the squared reciprocal of the coefficient of variation of the evoked synaptic responses. This quantity can be measured directly by recording the activity of a postsynaptic neuron. The right hand side shows that this quantity depends only on presynaptic parameters, under the assumption that the binomial model of release is correct. Thus a change in $1/C_{V_{ev.resp.}}^2$ after a protocol used to induce changes in synaptic transmission is interpreted as evidence for a presynaptic change in synaptic efficacy. Assuming n fixed, this corresponds to a change in release probability (Figure 12.8).

We can use Eq. (12.9) to rewrite Eq. (12.10) for the variability of the postsynaptic response in terms of the mean postsynaptic response,

$$\sigma_V^2 = \mu\left(1 + C_{V_{minis}}^2\right) m_V - \frac{m_V^2}{n}, \tag{12.11}$$

where $C_{V_{minis}}$ is the coefficient of variation of the quantal response, equal to σ/μ. Because the coefficient of variation $C_{V_{minis}}$ is typically of the order of $0.2-0.4$, its square represents a small (5–15%) correction to the quantal size μ. This equation states that variance in evoked responses is a parabola whose slope for low responses (m_V) is proportional to the quantal size μ. Thus one can monitor changes in quantal size by monitoring changes in the slope of the relation between σ_V^2 and m_V before and after a protocol inducing changes in synaptic transmission. Typically, several pairs of (m_V, σ_V^2) values are sampled by varying the Ca^{2+}/Mg^{2+} concentration resulting in increased release and thus increased m_V. Figure 12.9 illustrates the process in a voltage-clamp experiment which allows one to extract the peak synaptic conductance from the measured peak current and to bypass the nonlinear effects mentioned at the beginning of this section.

Comparison with experimental data. The methods described above have been applied on experimental data in a number of different preparations. It has been found that many changes in synaptic strength are consistent with changes in presynaptic release. In particular facilitation, depression, and potentiation are often thought to be due to presynaptic changes in the release probability or in the number of released vesicles. The models described in the next section illustrate this point. Short-term depression has also been attributed in part to postsynaptic effects such as desensitization of postsynaptic receptors under repeated stimulation. LTP appears to rely on several distinct presynaptic and postsynaptic mechanisms. Postsynaptically, the activation of the NMDA receptor often plays an important role in triggering LTP. Since NMDA receptor activation requires coincident presynaptic and postsynaptic activity (§9.3), the resulting synaptic plasticity is termed to be *Hebbian*, after D.O. Hebb who postulated that coincident presynaptic and postsynaptic activity should lead to synaptic strengthening. Following NMDA receptor activation, the best described postsynaptic mechanism involves the insertion of new receptors in the postsynaptic membrane, thus converting synapses that are "silent," because no AMPA receptors are present, into active ones. In addition, biochemical pathways can enhance the efficacy of AMPA receptors already present in the postsynaptic membrane by phosphorylating them. We will present a model of the biochemical pathway involved in this process in §13.4.

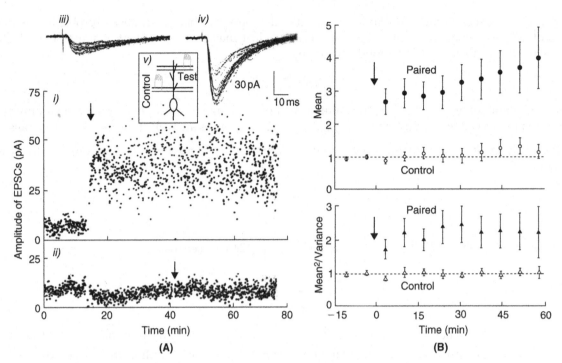

FIGURE 12.8 **A**. Induction of LTP by paired stimulation (40 times, twice a second) and postsynaptic depolarization (from −70 mV to 0 mV) of a CA1 pyramidal cell in the hippocampus. Excitatory postsynaptic currents (EPSCs) measured by stimulating the "test" pathway at low frequency are illustrated in *i)*. The arrow indicates the time at which this pathway is tetanically stimulated while the postsynaptic cell is simultaneously depolarized. EPSCs measured as the "control" pathway is stimulated at low frequency are illustrated in *ii)*. The arrow indicates the time of tetanic stimulation without simultaneous postsynaptic depolarization. Representative EPSCs in the test pathway before, *iii)*, and after, *iv)*, tetanic stimulation are illustrated on top. The boxed inset, *v)*, is a schematic illustration of the recorded cell and the two stimulated axonal pathways (stimulation electrodes illustrated in red). **B**. The paired "test" pathway shows increased synaptic currents (top, mean) and increased squared mean-to-variance ratio, consistent with a presynaptic change in transmitter release parameters. Adapted from Malinow and Tsien (1990).

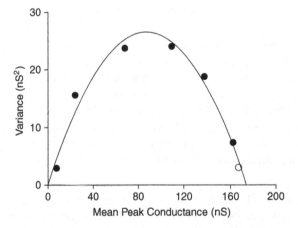

FIGURE 12.9   Change in variance as a function of mean conductance at the climbing fiber synapse onto a cerebellar Purkinje cell. Mean conductance and variance were measured at the peak of the EPSC obtained by stimulating repeatedly the climbing fiber at 0.2 Hz (black circles) and 0.033 Hz (white circle). Different mean conductances were obtained by changing the calcium to magnesium ratio ($[Ca^{2+}]/[Mg^{2+}]$) from 0.1 to 8 ($[Ca^{2+}]$ from 4 mM to 0.05 mM). Solid line is fit with the binomial model (Eq. (12.11) with $C_{V_{minis}} = 0$, $\mu = 0.61$ nS, and $n = 285$). Adapted from Silver et al. (1998).

12.7 MODELS OF SHORT-TERM SYNAPTIC PLASTICITY

As discussed above, synapses between neurons exhibit short-term plasticity. In addition, when a neuron makes synapses on several different cells, each synapse can be expected to have its own characteristic time-varying properties, as illustrated in Figure 12.10. Some synapses may be facilitating while others, synapsing onto adjacent neurons will be depressing. The biophysical basis underlying this diversity is thought to originate in the existence of two distinct

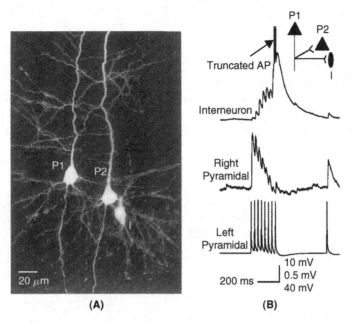

(A) **(B)**

FIGURE 12.10   **A.** Biocytin stain of three neurons recorded simultaneously in the rat somatosensory cortex. Pyramidal neuron P1 projects to pyramidal neuron P2 and bipolar interneuron I. **B.** Simultaneous response of both target neurons to a train of action potentials elicited in pyramidal neuron P1. The pyramidal neuron to interneuron synapse facilitates, eventually leading to an action potential (AP), while the pyramidal to pyramidal neuron synapse depresses rapidly. Note the different vertical scales for the three plots. Adapted from Markram et al. (1998).

pools of synaptic vesicles in the presynaptic terminal, the readily releasable pool, or RRP, and the slowly releasable pool, or SRP. The relative size and dynamics of their release probabilities, as well as the rate of replenishment and vesicle conversion between the pools is thought to underlie this diversity. The involvement of the RRP and SRP in vesicle release will be investigated in §13.5.

Here, we confine our attention to a simple model of short-term depression that successfully describes this phenomenon at many synapses. Subsequently, the model will be extended to include short-term facilitation. We will for simplicity neglect the variability in synaptic release that has been the focus of the previous sections and track only the average number of vesicles released as a function of time. Let $n(t)$ denote the average number of vesicles available for release at time t and u_0 the fraction that is effectively released on average as an action potential invades the presynaptic terminal. Thus, immediately after the action potential $n(t)$ is updated to $n(t^+) = n(t) - u_0 n(t)$ (i.e., the average number of available vesicles minus the average number of released ones). In addition, we assume that the pool of available vesicles slowly recovers towards its equilibrium value, n_{max} between action potentials with a time constant τ_{rec}. Equivalently, $n'(t) = (n_{max} - n)/\tau_{rec}$. To simplify the notation, we define the fraction of available vesicles or resources as $r(t) \equiv n(t)/n_{max}$, and note that it satisfies the differential equation

$$\frac{dr}{dt} = \frac{1 - r(t)}{\tau_{rec}}. \tag{12.12}$$

Immediately after an action potential at time t, $r(t)$ is reset to the value $r(t^+) = r(t) - u_0 r(t)$. We also assume that the release of neurotransmitter, $u_0 r(t)$, results in an instantaneous current or charge input $q(t) = q_{max} u_0 r(t)$ on the postsynaptic cell. Thus the synaptic depression model has three parameters: the time constant of vesicle recovery, τ_{rec}, the synaptic use of resources per action potential, u_0, and the maximal postsynaptic charge, q_{max}. The postsynaptic cell is modeled as a leaky integrate-and-fire neuron with membrane time constant τ and input resistance R_{in}. Thus,

$$\tau v' = -v + R_{in} I_{syn}(t), \quad I_{syn}(t) = \sum_{i=1}^{N} q(t_i)\delta(t - t_i). \tag{12.13}$$

Equivalently, v satisfies the differential equation $\tau v' = -v$ and immediately after an action potential at time t_i, the membrane potential v is instantaneously reset to the value $v(t_i^+) = v(t_i) + (R_{in}/\tau)q(t_i)$.

Figure 12.11A illustrates the response of the model to a constant train of action potentials. The available resources start at their maximal value of one and gradually decrease towards a steady-state value within a few hundred

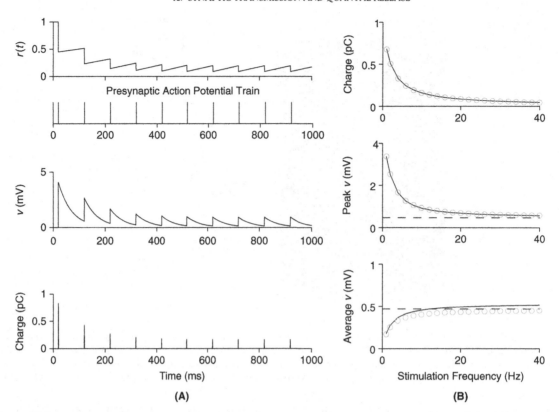

FIGURE 12.11   Synaptic depression model. **A.** The top panel illustrates the time course of $r(t)$ during a train of action potentials delivered at 10 Hz. The third and fourth panel from top illustrate the postsynaptic membrane potential and the synaptic charge, respectively. **B.** From top to bottom, the three panels depict the steady-state charge, the steady-state peak membrane depolarization, and the steady-state average membrane depolarization as a function of the presynaptic action potential frequency. The solid black curves are obtained by numerical simulation (Exercise 2) and the red dots correspond to analytical predictions. The dashed solid lines are limit values for the average and peak membrane potential obtained from the analytical predictions (Exercise 3). (mt_mod6.m)

milliseconds following the train onset. Consequently, both the charge delivered to the postsynaptic membrane and the peak depolarization converge to a steady-state value as well. Figure 12.11B plots as a function of the presynaptic action potential frequency, the steady-state values of the charge delivered by the synapse, the peak membrane potential following each release event, and the time-averaged membrane potential. Since the model consists of a pair of linear differential equations with varying jump conditions, the steady-state values of these variables can be computed analytically and are plotted in Figure 12.11B as well (Exercise 3). For large values of the stimulation frequency, the steady-state charge delivered by the synapse decays as $1/f$ (top panel of Figure 12.11B; Exercise 3). Consequently, both the peak and average postsynaptic membrane depolarization converge towards a constant value independent of f. This means that a depressing synapse operating in this regime does not convey changes in the presynaptic action potential frequency to the postsynaptic cell in its steady state. However, such a synapse will initially generate a few transient EPSPs as the presynaptic frequency is switched, as illustrated in the third panel of Figure 12.11A and can therefore best signal changes in the presynaptic firing rate by transient changes in the postsynaptic depolarization.

The synaptic depression model described in the previous paragraph can easily be modified to generate facilitation in the release of neurotransmitter. Although this is most likely not the only reason, facilitation is often thought to be caused by residual calcium in the presynaptic terminal. During a single action potential, calcium enters the presynaptic terminal and causes vesicle release. It is then cleared by various mechanisms such as pumps and buffers that will be studied in §13.2. If, however, a small fraction of the calcium remains in the terminal (residual calcium), it will add to the calcium entering upon the next action potential, causing an increase in release. This mechanism fits well with the observation that the amount of vesicle release depends nonlinearly on the external calcium concentration, and thus presumably also on the internal calcium concentration. To illustrate this point, let's assume that the calcium concentration is normalized in such a way that at rest it is equal to zero and rises to one immediately after an action potential. If synaptic release depends, e.g., on the fourth power of the calcium concentration, then a residual calcium concentration of 5% will have a negligible effect on spontaneous vesicle release after the action potential

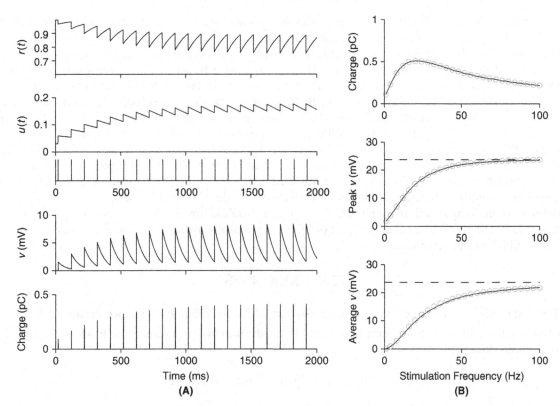

FIGURE 12.12 Synaptic facilitation model. **A.** The top two panels illustrate the time course of $r(t)$ and $u(t)$ in response to the spike train depicted in the third panel (stimulation frequency: 10 Hz). The last two panels illustrate the membrane potential and the synaptic charge, respectively. **B.** From top to bottom, the three panels depict the steady-state charge, the steady-state peak membrane depolarization, and the steady-state average membrane depolarization as a function of the presynaptic action potential frequency. The solid black curves are obtained by numerical simulation (Exercise 4) and the red dots correspond to analytical predictions. The dashed solid lines are limit values for the average and peak membrane potential obtained from the analytical predictions (Exercise 5). (mt_mod12.m)

$(0.05^4 = 6.25 \cdot 10^{-6})$, but will have a large effect on evoked release upon the next action potential $((1+0.05)^4 = 1.22)$. To model facilitation we assume that the synaptic use term, which was constant and equal to u_0, is now dynamic as well,

$$\frac{du}{dt} = \frac{u_0 - u}{\tau_{facil}}. \tag{12.14}$$

Immediately after an action potential, u is increased from its current value, $u(t)$, to $u(t^+) = u(t) + u_0(1 - u(t))$ and decays back towards its baseline value u_0 with a time constant τ_{facil} between action potentials (Eq. (12.14)). Note that the update rule guarantees that $u(t) < 1$. Figure 12.12A illustrates a simulation of this model. As the synaptic resources, $r(t)$, decrease, the use term, $u(t)$, increases and both reach a steady state after approximately 1500 ms. Both the membrane potential and charge transferred by the synapse increase over the course of the pulse. Figure 12.12B shows that the dependence of the charge, peak depolarization, and average depolarization at steady state is qualitatively different from that of the depression model of Figure 12.11. There is now an optimal nonzero frequency for the synaptic charge transferred by the synapse at steady state. In addition, both the peak and average steady state membrane potential are linearly dependent on the stimulation frequency before saturating at frequencies above 30 Hz. Thus, in this example, a facilitating synapse is able to encode linearly at steady state the presynaptic action potential frequency in the average peak membrane depolarization of the postsynaptic cell.

12.8 SUMMARY AND SOURCES

This chapter described basic models for various aspects of synaptic transmission and quantal release. We will consider more detailed models, including coupling to calcium signalling pathways, in the next chapter (§§13.4 and 13.5). Katz shared the 1970 Nobel Prize in Medicine for his work on quantal synaptic release. Figure 12.7 is inspired by the book of Levitan and Kaczmarek (2001) which provides many additional biological details on synaptic transmission. A recent confirmation of the one release-site one quantum hypothesis is given by Silver et al. (2003). This article also contains references on multivesicular release, postsynaptic receptor saturation, and the CA3 to interneuron synapse properties discussed in §12.5. See Rosenmund et al. (1993) and Murthy et al. (1997) for studies of nonuniform release probability at central synapses. See Toth et al. (2000) for a study on the differences between synapses made onto distinct postsynaptic target neurons. Postsynaptic receptor saturation is reported, e.g., in Edwards et al. (1990). Synaptic transmission at the calyx of Held is described in Scheuss et al. (2002) and at the climbing fiber synapse in Silver et al. (1998). Our treatment of synaptic facilitation and depression at neocortical synapses is based on Tsodyks and Markram (1997) and Markram et al. (1998). These two articles provide references to earlier work reporting similar phenomena at a variety of synapses, including the neuromuscular junction. See §5.8 in Abbott and Dayan (2001) for an introduction to short-term synaptic plasticity from a different perspective. The mechanisms and implications of long-term potentiation for memory formation have been extensively studied. We recommend the following three recent review articles for their complementary perspectives: Blundon and Zakharenko (2008), Malinow and Malenka (2002), and Feldman (2009). The consequences of synaptic plasticity on neuronal processing within networks of neurons will be addressed in §14.3 and in Chapter 27.

12.9 EXERCISES

1. Fit the Poisson model to the experimental data of Boyd and Martin (1956) to reproduce Figure 12.4.

   (i) Fit the spontaneous data histogram to a normal distribution and reproduce the inset of Figure 12.4A. The spontaneous data histogram is

   $$\{(0.2\ 1)\,(0.3\ 25)\,(0.4\ 30)\,(0.5\ 20)\,(0.6\ 2)\},$$

   where each pair consists of a measured depolarization (in mV) and the number of observations.

   (ii) Estimate the quantal size using the standard method (Eq. (12.5)) and the method of failures (Eq. (12.6)). What is the relative error of the method of failures (with respect to the standard method)? Which one of those two methods would you expect to be more accurate? Use the following evoked data histogram:

   $$\{(0\ 18)\,(0.3\ 11)\,(0.4\ 20)\,(0.5\ 13)\,(0.6\ 6)\,(0.7\ 14)\,(0.8\ 18)\,(0.9\ 17)\,(1.0\ 6)$$
   $$(1.1\ 11)\,(1.2\ 10)\,(1.3\ 9)\,(1.4\ 4)\,(1.5\ 7)\,(1.6\ 9)\,(1.7\ 5)\,(1.8\ 5)\,(1.9\ 3)\,(2.0\ 2)$$
   $$(2.1\ 2)\,(2.2\ 1)\,(2.3\ 1)\,(2.4\ 2)\,(2.5\ 1)\,(2.6\ 1)\,(2.7\ 1)\,(2.8\ 0)\,(2.9\ 0)\,(3.0\ 1)\}.$$

   (iii) Fit the evoked activity histogram using the results of (i) and (ii) and reproduce the main plot of Figure 12.4.

2. Implement the synaptic depression model of Eqs. (12.12) and (12.13) using a backward Euler numerical integration scheme and reproduce the solid black curves in Figure 12.11A and B. The model parameters are $\tau_{rec} = 800$ ms, $u_0 = 0.55$, $q_{max} = 1.5$ pCb, $\tau = 50$ ms, and $R_{in} = 250$ MΩ. The initial conditions are $r(0) = 1$ and $v(0) = 0$. Time of first presynaptic action potential: 20 ms. Hint: Use Eq. (10.4) as the basic recipe for setting up your model.

3. Show that in response to a presynaptic spike train of frequency f, the steady-state resources r_{ss} are given by

$$r_{ss} = \frac{1 - e^{-\frac{\Delta t}{\tau_{rec}}}}{1 - (1 - u_0)e^{-\frac{\Delta t}{\tau_{rec}}}},$$

where $\Delta t = 1/f$ is the time interval between two presynaptic action potentials. Use this result to derive similar expressions for the steady-state charge delivered by the synapse, q_{ss}, the steady-state peak depolarization, $v_{peak,ss}$, and the corresponding time-averaged depolarization, $v_{av,ss}$. Use these analytical formulas to show that when $\Delta t \ll \tau_{rec}$ and τ,

$$q_{ss} \approx \frac{q_{max}\,\Delta t}{\tau_{rec}} \quad v_{peak,ss} \approx \frac{q_{max}R_{in}}{\tau_{rec}}, \quad v_{av,ss} \approx \frac{q_{max}R_{in}}{\tau_{rec}}.$$

Use these results to reproduce the red dots as well as the dashed lines on Figure 12.11B. Hint: Use the solution to the differential equation (12.12) to write down a formula for the resources r_{n+1} at the time, t_{n+1}, of the $n+1$st action potential as a function of the resources, r_n, at the time, t_n, of the nth action potential. Note that at steady state, $r_{ss} = r_{n+1} = r_n$. Proceed similarly for $v_{peak,ss}$. To compute $v_{av,ss}$ compute the mean of the steady-state potential over the time interval Δt between two presynaptic action potentials.

4. Modify the synaptic depression model (Exercise 2) to implement synaptic facilitation as in Eq. (12.14). Use the model to reproduce the solid black traces in Figure 12.12. Use the following parameters: $\tau_{rec} = 130$ ms, $u_0 = 0.03$, $q_{max} = 3.08$ pCb, $\tau = 60$ ms, and $R_{in} = 1$ GΩ. The initial conditions are $r(0) = 1$, $u(0) = u_0$, and $v(0) = 0$. Time of the first presynaptic action potential: 20 ms. Hint: As in Exercise 2, use Eq. (10.4) as the basic recipe for setting up your model.

5. Show that under the synaptic facilitation model

$$u_{ss} = \frac{u_0}{1 - (1 - u_0)e^{-\frac{\Delta t}{\tau_{facil}}}}, \quad r_{ss} = \frac{1 - e^{-\frac{\Delta t}{\tau_{rec}}}}{1 - (1 - u_{ss})e^{-\frac{\Delta t}{\tau_{rec}}}}.$$

Use these results to reproduce the red circles and dashed lines on Figure 12.12B.

13

Neuronal Calcium Signaling*

OUTLINE

13.1 Voltage-Gated Calcium Channels   195

13.2 Diffusion, Buffering, and Extraction of
      Cytosolic Calcium   198

13.3 Calcium Release from the ER   201

13.4 Calcium in Spines   209

13.5 Presynaptic Calcium and Transmitter Release 213

13.6 Summary and Sources   217

13.7 Exercises   217

We learned in the previous chapter that neurotransmitter released into the synaptic cleft is the initial, often noisy, messenger of presynaptic information to the postsynaptic cell. Although this message is transcribed into a transient conductance change its effect remains transient unless supported by the postsynaptic cell's network of second messengers. Ca^{2+}, the most important of the second messengers, triggers change that activates a host of biochemical pathways (recall Figure 12.1) that have been found necessary for many (but not all) forms of presynaptic and postsynaptic plasticity. In this chapter we will work from the outside in. In the first section we develop and illustrate the principal types of currents that carry calcium across the plasma membrane. In the subsequent section we discuss the buffering, diffusion, exchange, and extraction of cytosolic calcium and its modulatory effect on the cell's firing rate. We then consider the remarkable ability of cytosolic calcium to trigger its own release from the cell's endoplasmic reticulum (ER), see Figures 13.1 and 13.2. We then build and integrate models of ryanodine, IP_3, and metabotropic glutamate receptors and demonstrate that the ER functions as a "neuron within a neuron" in the sense that it supports the active propagation of intracellular calcium waves.

In the final two sections of this chapter we focus on the crucial role played by calcium at both the postsynaptic and presynaptic terminals. On the postsynaptic side we demonstrate how buffered calcium in the spine head may trigger the autophosphorylation of an important Ca^{2+}/calmodulin-dependent kinase of type II, CaMKII, and so extend the duration of a calcium signal long after it has returned to its resting level. On the presynaptic side we investigate a model of calcium's role in orchestrating the release of two distinct pools of synaptic vesicles.

Our goal throughout this chapter is to first develop and then integrate *representative* models of the key components in the cell's calcium handling machinery. We emphasize representative because we do not pause to consider the large variation within individual components.

Mathematics for Neuroscientists. DOI: 10.1016/B978-0-12-374882-9.00013-7
Copyright © 2010 Elsevier Inc. All rights reserved.

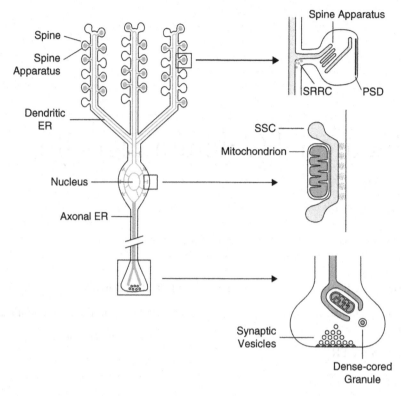

FIGURE 13.1 The ER, red, forms a continuous network within a neuron that reaches up into the dendritic tree, down through its axonal tree and even into spines and presynaptic terminals. The insets on the right illustrate various specializations of the ER. Top: the ER forms the spine apparatus in $\approx 50\%$ of spines (PSD, postsynaptic density; SRRC, synapse-associated polyribosome complex, involved in local protein synthesis). Middle: the ER comes in close contact with the plasma membrane to form subsurface cisterns (SSC). Bottom: in the axon, the ER extends up to the presynaptic terminal where it is often associated with a mitochondrion. Adapted from Berridge (1998).

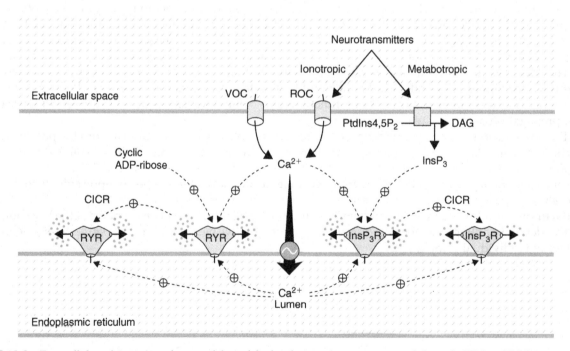

FIGURE 13.2 Extracellular calcium enters the cytosol through both voltage and receptor operated channels, VOC and ROC respectively. Once there it is pumped into the ER and released from the ER via ryanodine and IP$_3$ receptors, RYR and InsP$_3$R respectively. As the rate of release depends strongly on the presence of cytosolic calcium (in conjunction with two other second messengers, cyclic ADP-ribose and InsP$_3$) this process is termed "calcium induced calcium release," or CICR. Adapted from Berridge (1998).

13.1 VOLTAGE-GATED CALCIUM CHANNELS

As in Chapter 4 we will model calcium currents as the product of a driving force and a gating mechanism. While the gating functionals will echo those developed earlier for sodium and potassium currents, the driving force will here take on a different form. This difference arises from the dramatic disparity between the nominal extracellular and intracellular concentrations of Ca^{2+},

$$c_o \equiv [Ca^{2+}]_{ext} = 1 \text{ mM} \quad \text{and} \quad c_i \equiv [Ca^{2+}]_{int} = 0.05 \ \mu M. \tag{13.1}$$

At these levels one may not expect to discern any outward current at physiological membrane potentials. In other words, there is no practically discernable reversal potential for the calcium current. As such we must modify the simple Ohmic assumption that $I_{Ca} = g_{Ca}(V - V_{Ca})$. To accomplish this we return to the Nernst–Planck equation,

$$J(r) = -\mu k T \frac{dc}{dr}(r) - \mu z e c(r) \frac{d\phi}{dr}(r) \tag{13.2}$$

for the flux, J, arising from the concentration gradient, dc/dr, and potential gradient, $d\phi/dr$, of Ca^{2+}. Here, as in §2.2, e is the elementary charge, $z = 2$ is the valence, μ is mobility, k is Boltzman's constant, and T is temperature. Where in §2.2 we were interested solely in computing the potential gradient associated with rest, i.e., at $J = 0$, we here prescribe the potential gradient

$$\phi'(r) = -V/\delta, \quad 0 < r < \delta, \tag{13.3}$$

where δ is the thickness of the membrane, and compute the associated J. This approach will yield an $I - V$ relationship that we may use to supplant Ohm's, as J is proportional to current density ($I_{Ca} = z e N_A J$, where N_A is Avogadro's number). On substituting Eq. (13.3) and

$$D = \mu k T \quad \text{and} \quad V_T = kT/e,$$

into Eq. (13.2) it follows that we must solve

$$c'(r) - \frac{zV}{V_T \delta} c = -J/D$$

and so $(c \exp(-zVr/(V_T\delta)))' = -(J/D) \exp(-zVr/(V_T\delta))$ or on integrating from $r = 0$ to $r = \delta$, and using $c(0) = c_i$ and $c(\delta) = c_o$, we find

$$\exp(-zV/V_T)c_o - c_i = -\frac{JV_T}{DzV\delta}(1 - \exp(-zV/V_T)).$$

After slight rearrangement we arrive at

$$J = \frac{D}{\delta} \frac{zV}{V_T} \frac{c_i - \exp(-zV/V_T)c_o}{1 - \exp(-zV/V_T)}.$$

We next factor out c_o, multiply top and bottom by $\exp(zV/V_T)$ and lump the leading constant into the conductance term and so arrive at the Goldman–Hodgkin–Katz equation,

$$I_{Ca} = g_{Ca}\Phi(c_i/c_o, V), \quad \Phi(u, V) \equiv V \frac{1 - u \exp(zV/V_T)}{1 - \exp(zV/V_T)} \tag{13.4}$$

illustrated in Figure 13.3. This plot shows that at negative membrane potentials the current is nearly a linear function of potential, as expected from Ohm's law. As the membrane potential increases beyond 0 mV, however, the slope of the curve dramatically decreases, a phenomenon called *rectification*. The current predicted by Eq. (13.4) equals zero at the Nernst potential for calcium ($V_{Ca} = 128.1$ mV, according to Eqs. (13.1) and (2.7)) but no discernible outward current is experienced beyond that value.

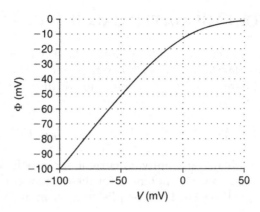

FIGURE 13.3 I-V curve for the non-Ohmic, nonreversing driving force, Eq. (13.4), with $V_T = 25.8$ mV ($T = 27$ °C), $z = 2$, and $u = 5 \times 10^{-5}$ per Eq. (13.1). (ghk.m)

We next turn to the gating properties of calcium currents. Early experiments on a variety of cells led to the identification of several distinct types of calcium currents. We will consider three major ones: $I_{Ca,L}$, where L denotes Long-lasting, $I_{Ca,T}$, where T denotes Transient, and $I_{Ca,N}$, where N denotes Neither L nor T. We distinguish them by their associated conductances

$$g_{Ca,L} = \overline{g}_{Ca,L} m_L^2, \quad g_{Ca,N} = \overline{g}_{Ca,N} m_N^2 h_N, \quad \text{and} \quad g_{Ca,T} = \overline{g}_{Ca,T} m_T^2 h_T$$

where m and h, as in §4.2, signify activation and inactivation respectively. Each of these gating variables obeys the canonical first order rule

$$\tau_{u,X}(V) u'_X = u_{\infty,X}(V) - u_X, \quad u = m \text{ or } h, \quad X = L, N, \text{ or } T,$$

where the associated gating functionals,

$$\tau_{u,X}(V) = \frac{1}{\alpha_{u,X}(V) + \beta_{u,X}(V)} \quad \text{and} \quad u_{\infty,X}(V) = \alpha_{u,X}(V) \tau_{u,X}(V)$$

$$\alpha_{m,X}(V) = \frac{a_X(b_X - V)}{\exp((V - b_X)/10) - 1} \quad \text{and} \quad \beta_{m,X}(V) = c_X \exp(-V/d_X)$$

$$\alpha_{h,X}(V) = e_X \exp(-V/f_X) \quad \text{and} \quad \beta_{h,X}(V) = \frac{1}{1 + \exp((g_X - V)/10)}$$

are parametrized by

$$a_L = 15.69 \text{ (mVms)}^{-1}, \ b_L = 81.5 \text{ mV}, \ c_L = 0.29 \text{ ms}^{-1}, \ d_L = 10.86 \text{ mV},$$

$$a_N = 0.19, \ b_N = 19.88, \ c_N = 0.046, \ d_N = 20.73, \ e_N = 1.6 \times 10^{-4} \text{ ms}^{-1}, \ f_N = 48.46 \text{ mV}, \ g_N = 39 \text{ mV},$$

$$a_T = 0.2, \ b_T = 19.26, \ c_T = 0.009, \ d_T = 22.03, \ e_T = 10^{-6}, \ f_T = 16.26, \ g_T = 29.79,$$

and illustrated in Figure 13.4.

We next add these three channels to our active uniform cable model of §9.1 and assess their associated currents. This application is straightforward, save for the fact that the shift from the linear Ohmic driving force, $V - V_{Ca}$, to the nonlinear driving force, Eq. (13.4), spoils the second-order in time accuracy of our staggered Euler scheme. As a result, we have adopted the hybrid Euler scheme of §4.4. We have coded this in hyEcabCal.m and illustrated its use in Figure 13.5, with conductances

$$\overline{g}_{Ca,T} = 0.25, \quad \overline{g}_{Ca,N} = 2.5, \quad \text{and} \quad \overline{g}_{Ca,L} = 2.5 \text{ mS/cm}^2 \tag{13.5}$$

along the active uniform cable of §9.1.

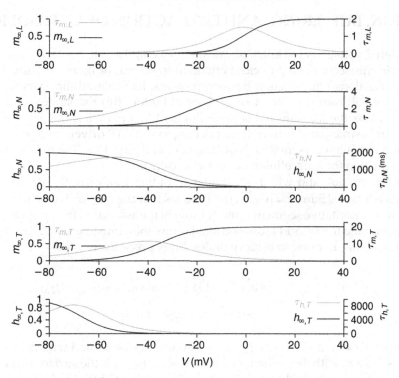

FIGURE 13.4 The gating functionals that govern the L, N, and T type calcium channels. We note that each of the steady-state activation functionals, $m_{\infty,X}$, is close to zero at rest and that they require successively greater depolarization as we move from T to N to L. The associated activation time constant, τ_X, likewise becomes faster as we move from T to N to L. We note that inactivation of the L-type channel is not presumed to be voltage dependent, while the N type deinactivates at a higher potential than the T type. (LNTcurves.m)

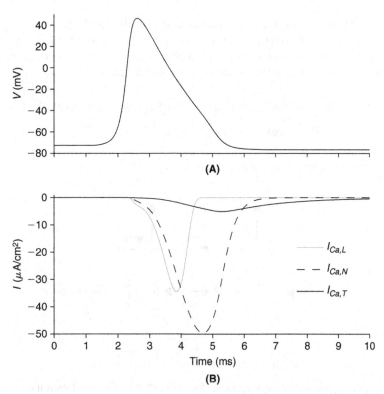

FIGURE 13.5 Midpoint ($x = \ell/2$) response of the active uniform cable of §9.1, now equipped with three calcium channel types, with densities as in Eq. (13.5), to a suprathreshold current pulse delivered at the quarter point ($x = \ell/4$). (hyEcabCa1.m)

13.2 DIFFUSION, BUFFERING, AND EXTRACTION OF CYTOSOLIC CALCIUM

We have so far considered voltage-gated entry of calcium. Once in the cell, however, calcium is subject to a host of regulatory processes. In this section we pay close attention to several of them. (i) Diffusion, via Fick's Law. (ii) Buffering, via first order reactions with calcium binding proteins, like calmodulin, parvalbumin, or calbindin for example. For simplicity, we will consider only a single type of buffer. (iii) Exchange of calcium for sodium, via a membrane protein that exploits the like-directed sodium gradient to replace a single intracellular calcium ion with three sodium ones. And, (iv) extraction of intracellular calcium, via an ATP driven membrane pump. We schematize the principal fluxes in and out of a representative cable segment in Figure 13.6. The balance of these fluxes will lead to a nonlinear diffusion equation for intracellular, or cytosolic, calcium.

We consider calcium flux in, out, and within a cylinder of radius a and length $2dx$. The basic balance law for the concentration of intracellular calcium, $c = [Ca^{2+}]$ (μM), states that the rate of change of the numbers of moles (in nmole/ms) of Ca^{2+} in our representative segment is the net sum of the associated fluxes. As these fluxes enter through volume terms, lateral membrane terms, and cross-sectional terms they must be scaled by their associated volume, $2dx\pi a^2$, or areas, $4\pi a\,dx$, and πa^2, in order to achieve moles. More precisely, we find

$$(\pi a^2)(2dx)\frac{\partial c}{\partial t}(x,t) = (\pi a^2)(F_1 - F_2) + (4\pi a dx)(J_{Ca} - J_{NaCa} - J_{PMCA})$$
$$+ (\pi a^2)(2dx)(k_2 b - k_1 cB) \tag{13.6}$$

where F_1 and F_2 are the two Fickian axial fluxes, J_{Ca} is the surface flux associated with the total calcium current, I_{Ca}, J_{NaCa} is the surface flux associated with the exchanger current, I_{NaCa}, J_{PMCA} is the surface flux associated with the ATP driven plasma membrane Ca^{2+} pump, and k_1 and k_2 are the rates that calcium binds/unbinds the free buffer, B, to form/unform the complex, b. Here the product term, cB, is a consequence of the law of mass action.

If D_c denotes the diffusivity (in cm^2/ms, §2.2) of free calcium, then Fick's law, at each end, reads

$$F_1 = -D_c \frac{\partial c}{\partial x}(x - dx, t) \quad \text{and} \quad F_2 = -D_c \frac{\partial c}{\partial x}(x + dx, t).$$

The exchange flux, J_{NaCa}, is driven by a membrane protein that exploits the fact that Na^+, like Ca^{2+}, is much more abundant outside the cell than inside. In particular, it exchanges one intracellular Ca^{2+} for three extracellular Na^+. The conformational change that flips the exchange gate is voltage dependent. Moreover, as the exchanger itself will be electrogenic (i.e., alter the membrane potential), we express it as a current

$$I_{NaCa}(c_i, V) = \bar{I}_{NaCa}(([Na^+]_i/[Na^+]_o)^3 \exp(V/(2V_T)) - (c_i/c_o)\exp(-V/(2V_T)))$$
$$\bar{I}_{NaCa} = 100\,\mu A/cm^2, \quad [Na^+]_i/[Na^+]_o = 50/440. \tag{13.7}$$

The exchange of three Na^+ for one Ca^{2+} is apparent in Eq. (13.7).

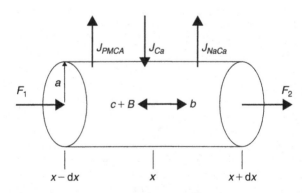

FIGURE 13.6 Calcium fluxes in a representative cable segment. J_{PMCA}: Ca^{2+} flux associated with the plasma membrane calcium pump. J_{NaCa}: Ca^{2+} flux associated with the calcium–sodium exchanger (also located in the plasma membrane). J_{Ca}: Ca^{2+} flux associated with calcium conductances. B, b: free and bound buffer, respectively. F_1 and F_2: diffusion fluxes.

Next, as I_{Ca} and I_{NaCa} are in terms of $\mu A/cm^2$, it follows that

$$J_{Ca} = -\frac{I_{Ca}}{2F} \quad \text{and} \quad J_{NaCa} = -\frac{I_{NaCa}}{2F}.$$

In this equation, Faraday's constant $F = eN_A = 10^5$ C/mole will carry the proper units (nmole/ms/cm^2) and the negative signs reflect our convention that outward currents are positive. Note also that we use I_{Ca} to denote the sum of all voltage-gated calcium currents, e.g., $I_{Ca} = I_{Ca,L} + I_{Ca,T} + I_{Ca,N}$.

Each plasma membrane Ca-ATPase (PMCA) ejects one Ca^{2+} from the cell, against its gradient, at the cost of reducing a molecule of ATP to ADP. This one-to-one stoichiometry yields a behavior that is well represented by the first order Hill function

$$J_{PMCA}(c) = j_{pmca}\frac{c}{1+c}, \quad j_{pmca} = 2 \times 10^{-6}\ \frac{\mu\text{mole}}{\text{cm}^2\text{ms}}.$$

Having established the principal fluxes, we now divide Eq. (13.6) by compartment volume ($2dx\pi a^2$) and arrive at

$$\frac{\partial c}{\partial t}(x,t) = \frac{D_{Ca}}{2dx}\left\{\frac{\partial c}{\partial x}(x+dx,t) - \frac{\partial c}{\partial x}(x-dx,t)\right\} + 2(J_{Ca} - J_{NaCa} - J_{PMCA})/a + k_2 b - k_1 cB.$$

As the compartment size decreases, i.e., $dx \to 0$, we arrive at the nonlinear diffusion equation

$$\frac{\partial c}{\partial t}(x,t) = D_c\frac{\partial^2 c}{\partial x^2}(x,t) + 2(J_{Ca} - J_{NaCa} - J_{PMCA})/a + k_2 b - k_1 cB. \tag{13.8}$$

To "close" this system we must incorporate the evolution of both the buffer, B, and its bound state, b. Arguing as above, we find that mass balance of these two species requires

$$\frac{\partial B}{\partial t}(x,t) = D_B\frac{\partial^2 B}{\partial x^2}(x,t) + k_2 b - k_1 cB,$$

$$\frac{\partial b}{\partial t}(x,t) = D_b\frac{\partial^2 b}{\partial x^2}(x,t) - k_2 b + k_1 cB.$$

As the buffer B, e.g., calmodulin, is typically several orders of magnitude larger than a calcium ion we may presume that its diffusivity is not affected by its binding to Ca^{2+}. Hence, we set $D_B = D_b$ and sum the two equations above to arrive at a simple diffusion equation for the total amount of buffer, $B+b$,

$$\frac{\partial(B+b)}{\partial t} = D_b\frac{\partial^2(B+b)}{\partial x^2}, \quad \frac{\partial(B+b)}{\partial x}(0,t) = \frac{\partial(B+b)}{\partial x}(\ell,t) = 0, \quad (B+b)(x,0) = B_T$$

where B_T is the initial buffer concentration. If B_T is uniform, i.e., independent of x, then in fact $B(x,t) + b(x,t) = B_T$ for all x and t and so we need only keep track of b, for $B = B_T - b$. Our system now takes the form

$$\frac{\partial c}{\partial t}(x,t) = D_c\frac{\partial^2 c}{\partial x^2}(x,t) + k_2 b - k_1 c(B_T - b) + (2/a)(J_{Ca} - J_{NaCa} - J_{PMCA})$$

$$\frac{\partial b}{\partial t}(x,t) = D_b\frac{\partial^2 b}{\partial x^2}(x,t) - k_2 b + k_1 c(B_T - b). \tag{13.9}$$

In order to determine a uniform rest state, $c(x,t) = c_r$ and $b(x,t) = b_r$, this system requires that

$$b_r = B_T\frac{c_r}{c_r + k_2/k_1} \tag{13.10}$$

and

$$J_{Ca}(V_r, c_r) = J_{NaCa}(V_r, c_r) + J_{PMCA}(c_r). \tag{13.11}$$

Although this arguably couples the resting membrane potential, V_r, to the resting level of $[Ca^{2+}]$ we recall from the previous section that each of our calcium currents was negligible near V_r. As such, we compute V_r, as above, assume $J_{Ca}(V_r, c) = 0$ and so determine c_r via the balance of J_{NaCa} and J_{PMCA}. This is sensible, for at small levels of c_i we recognize from Eq. (13.7) that $I_{NaCa} > 0$. That is, the exchanger reverses and brings one Ca^{2+} **into** the cell in return for three Na^+, with a net outward current and a net influx of Ca^{2+}. This influx is balanced by the PMCA efflux, given the parameter set above, when

$$c_r = 0.05 \ \mu M. \tag{13.12}$$

Finally, it is natural to presume that the cable ends are sealed, i.e.,

$$\frac{\partial b}{\partial x}(0, t) = \frac{\partial c}{\partial x}(0, t) = \frac{\partial b}{\partial x}(\ell, t) = \frac{\partial c}{\partial x}(\ell, t) = 0, \tag{13.13}$$

throughout the simulation. We now develop a numerical scheme, to be coupled to our active cable scheme, for approximating the solution to the nonlinear diffusion system, Eq. (13.9), subject to the initial conditions, $c(x, 0) = c_r$ and $b(x, 0) = b_r$, and boundary conditions Eq. (13.13). In particular, we write

$$c_i^j \approx c((i - 1/2)dx, (j - 1)dt) \quad \text{and} \quad b_i^j \approx b((i - 1/2)dx, (j - 1)dt)$$

and use the hybrid trapezoid scheme to represent Eq. (13.9) via

$$(2/dt)\begin{pmatrix} c^j - c^{j-1} \\ b^j - b^{j-1} \end{pmatrix} = \begin{pmatrix} D_c \mathbf{S} - k_1 B_T \mathbf{I} & k_2 \mathbf{I} \\ k_1 B_T \mathbf{I} & D_b \mathbf{S} - k_2 \mathbf{I} \end{pmatrix} \begin{pmatrix} c^j + c^{j-1} \\ b^j + b^{j-1} \end{pmatrix} + 2 \begin{pmatrix} k_1 c^{j-1} b^{j-1} + p(c^{j-1}) \\ -k_1 c^{j-1} b^{j-1} \end{pmatrix}$$

where $\mathbf{S}$ is the standard second difference matrix, Eq. (6.9), and $p = 2(J_{ca} - J_{NaCa} - J_{PMCA})/a$. We rearrange and write this as a system

$$(2 - dt\mathbf{R})\mathbf{u}^j = (2 + dt\mathbf{R})\mathbf{u}^{j-1} + dt\mathbf{f}^{j-1}, \quad \text{for} \quad \mathbf{u}^j \equiv \begin{pmatrix} c^j \\ b^j \end{pmatrix} \tag{13.14}$$

where

$$\mathbf{R} = \begin{pmatrix} D_c \mathbf{S} - k_1 B_T \mathbf{I} & k_2 \mathbf{I} \\ k_1 B_T \mathbf{I} & D_b \mathbf{S} - k_2 \mathbf{I} \end{pmatrix} \quad \text{and} \quad \mathbf{f}^{j-1} = 2 \begin{pmatrix} k_1 c^{j-1} b^{j-1} + p(c^{j-1}) \\ -k_1 c^{j-1} b^{j-1} \end{pmatrix}. \tag{13.15}$$

We have coded this system in `hyEcabCa2drive.m` and illustrated its use in Figure 13.7, given the parameter set

$$\begin{aligned} D_c &= 220 \times 10^{-11} \ cm^2/ms, \quad D_b = 110 \times 10^{-11} \ cm^2/ms, \quad B_T = 500 \ \mu M \\ k_1 &= 1.5 \times 10^{-3} \ 1/ms/\mu M, \quad \text{and} \quad k_2 = 0.3 \times 10^{-3} \ 1/ms. \end{aligned} \tag{13.16}$$

We note that in this case, Eq. (13.10) predicts that Ca^{2+} will be buffered at $b_r = 100 \ \mu M$.

We will consider a number of processes that are triggered by rises in intracellular calcium. Its most immediate consequence is to gate calcium-dependent potassium channels. This produces an outward current that serves to accentuate after hyperpolarization and so decrease the cell's firing rate. Such a current may be modeled by

$$I_{KCa} = \bar{g}_{KCa} m_{KCa}(V - E_K), \quad \bar{g}_{KCa} = 10 \ mS/cm^2,$$

$$\frac{\partial m_{KCa}}{\partial t} = \alpha_{KCa}(V, c)(1 - m_{KCa}) - \beta_{KCa}(V, c)m_{KCa},$$

$$\alpha_{KCa}(V, c) = \frac{0.28c}{c + 0.48\exp(-1.7V/V_T)} \quad \text{and} \quad \beta_{KCa}(V, c) = \frac{0.48}{1 + 7692c\exp(2V/V_T)} \ ms^{-1}.$$

We have plotted the associated activation and time constant functionals in Figure 13.8. We have added this channel to the active uniform cable, see `hyEcabCa3.m`, and illustrated its use in Figure 13.8. Its effect on spike frequency will be investigated in Exercise 1.

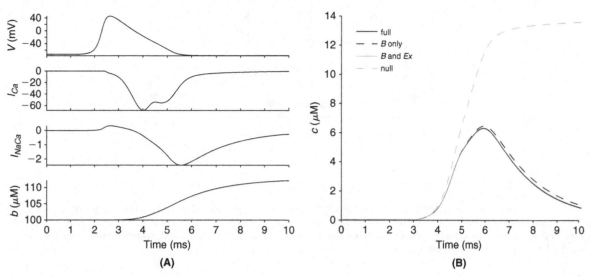

FIGURE 13.7 Calcium influx and regulation at midcable, following a brief suprathreshold injection at the quarter point, to the uniform active cable with calcium channels, exchanger, pump, and buffers. **A**. In viewing top to bottom, the action potential, V, opens calcium channels that bring Ca^{2+} into the cell via the total I_{Ca} ($\mu A/cm^2$). The exchange current, I_{NaCa} ($\mu A/cm^2$), is initially outward but then soon reverses as V decreases and c increases. Finally, the increase in c begets an increase in the amount, b, bound to the intracellular buffer. **B**. Here we tease apart those terms that shape the Ca^{2+} signal. In the absence of buffering, pumping, and exchange, c simply grows and then plateaus (dashed red line). We see that the buffer is a fast effective attenuator and that the pump and exchanger are slower and less dramatic. (hyEcabCa2drive.m)

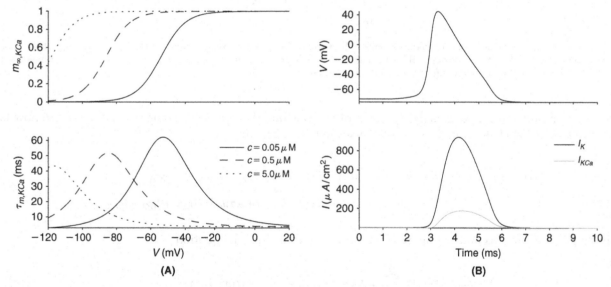

FIGURE 13.8 **A**. Gating functionals for I_{KCa} as functions of membrane potential at three levels of cytosolic Ca^{2+}. (gKCa.m) **B**. The action potential and potassium currents at midcable following a brief suprathreshold current injection at the quarter point. (hyEcabCa3.m)

13.3 CALCIUM RELEASE FROM THE ER

The ER is the organelle in which membrane and secretory proteins are synthesized and folded. As both of these processes are calcium dependent the ER contains a considerable store of calcium. More precisely it is large, roughly 10% of the cell's volume, geometrically contiguous (enveloping the nucleus and reaching into all dendrites and even up into many spines) with a resting level of free calcium concentration near 0.5 mM. This is four orders of magnitude greater than the resting cytosolic level, Eq. (13.12). This source is tapped by two classes of ER membrane bound channels. As the gating of these channels is itself calcium dependent we may view the ER membrane, by analogy with voltage, as an active membrane. Furthermore, as this active membrane is contiguous throughout the cell we may view the ER as a "neuron within a neuron." As the ER also expresses a separate pump mechanism, contains

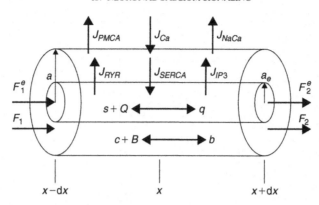

FIGURE 13.9   The principal calcium fluxes in a cable segment of radius a and length $2dx$. The inner cable is a segment of the ER. Its radius is a_e. We use s (for store) to denote the concentration of free ER calcium. We denote the concentrations of free and bound ER Ca^{2+} buffer by Q and q respectively. Calcium diffuses axially along the ER via Fick's law and it may leave the ER via IP_3 and ryanodine receptors and it may enter the ER via sarco-ER Ca^{2+}–ATPase (SERCA) pumps.

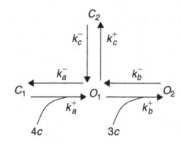

FIGURE 13.10   Kinetic scheme for the ryanodine receptor. The associated channel is closed in states C_1 and C_2 and open in states O_1 and O_2. The transition from C_1 to O_1 requires four cytosolic Ca^{2+} and that from O_1 to O_2 requires an additional three cytosolic Ca^{2+}. When open, the channel permits Ca^{2+} to follow its gradient from ER to cytosol, i.e., from s to c.

distinct calcium buffers, and permits the diffusion of free calcium, the simple flux diagram of Figure 13.6 now takes the form of Figure 13.9. Balancing the cytosolic fluxes in Figure 13.9 requires

$$\pi(a^2 - a_e^2)2dx\frac{\partial c}{\partial t}(x,t) = \pi(a^2 - a_e^2)(F_1 - F_2) + 4\pi a dx(J_{Ca} - J_{NaCa} - J_{PMCA})$$
$$+ \pi(a^2 - a_e^2)2dx(k_2 b - k_1 cB) + 4\pi a_e dx(J_{RYR} + J_{IP3} - J_{SERCA}).$$

On dividing by $(a^2 - a_e^2)2dx$ and letting $dx \to 0$ we arrive at the diffusion equation

$$\frac{\partial c}{\partial t}(x,t) = D_c\frac{\partial^2 c}{\partial x^2} + 2a(J_{Ca} - J_{PMCA} - J_{NaCa})/(a^2 - a_e^2)$$
$$+ k_2 b - k_1 cB + 2a_e(J_{RYR} + J_{IP3} - J_{SERCA})/(a^2 - a_e^2). \tag{13.17}$$

The first three J terms are familiar from the previous section. We develop the new ones one at a time.

The ryanodine flux. The ryanodine receptor is a calcium-gated calcium channel that was first identified with the help of the plant toxin, ryanodine. We will develop and implement a model based on the scheme of Figure 13.10, in which two closed states can transition, in the presence of cytosolic calcium, to two open states.

The driving force for the flux through the associated calcium channel is the ER membrane calcium gradient, $s - c$, and, as we argue in Exercise 4, the gating depicted in Figure 13.10 may be reduced to a single variable. If we denote this variable by w then we arrive at

$$J_{RYR} = v_{ryr}w\frac{1 + (c/K_b)^3}{1 + (K_a/c)^4 + (c/K_b)^3}(s - c) \tag{13.18}$$

where s denotes the ER calcium concentration and w obeys

$$\tau_w(c)w' = w_\infty(c) - w \tag{13.19}$$

with

$$w_\infty(c) = \frac{1 + (K_a/c)^4 + (c/K_b)^3}{1 + (1/K_c) + (K_a/c)^4 + (c/K_b)^3}, \quad \tau_w(c) = 10^4 w_\infty(c). \tag{13.20}$$

The constants are

$$v_{ryr} = 10^{-6}\,\text{cm/ms}, \quad K_a = 0.372\,\mu\text{M}, \quad K_b = 0.636\,\mu\text{M}, \quad \text{and} \quad K_c = 0.057. \tag{13.21}$$

The SERCA flux. The flux, J_{SERCA}, is due to the sarco-ER calcium ATPase that pumps calcium, against its gradient, from the cytosol to the ER, at the price of one molecule of ATP per two calcium ions. This two-for-one stoichiometry is typically represented by a second order Hill function of the form

$$J_{SERCA} = \bar{v}_{serca} \frac{c^2}{K_{serca}^2 + c^2}, \quad K_{serca} = 2\,\mu\text{M}, \quad \bar{v}_{serca} = 2 \times 10^{-4}\,\text{nmole}/(\text{cm}^2\text{ms}). \tag{13.22}$$

We pause to examine the impact of J_{RyR} and J_{SERCA} on c before developing our model for J_{IP3}. As the ryanodine receptor flux depends on store calcium we must first couple our cytosolic system for c and b to the ER system for s and q. This involves no new ideas. In particular we may argue as above and find

$$\frac{\partial s}{\partial t}(x,t) = D_s \frac{\partial^2 s}{\partial x^2} + 2(J_{SERCA} - J_{RYR})/a_e + k_2^e q - k_1^e s(Q_T - q)$$

$$\frac{\partial q}{\partial t}(x,t) = D_q \frac{\partial^2 q}{\partial x^2} - k_2^e q + k_1^e s(Q_T - q) \tag{13.23}$$

where Q_T denotes the total concentration ER calcium buffer. As above, we note that the resting levels of s and q obey

$$q_r = Q_T \frac{s_r}{s_r + k_2^e/k_1^e} \quad \text{and} \quad J_{RYR}(c_r, s_r) = J_{SERCA}(c_r).$$

The latter reads

$$v_{ryr} \frac{1 + (c_r/K_b)^3}{1 + (c_r/K_b)^3 + (1/K_C) + (K_a/c_r)^4}(s_r - c_r) = v_{serca} \frac{c_r^2}{K_{serca}^2 + c_r^2}$$

which, given our parameter set, yields

$$s_r = 500\,\mu\text{M}$$

for the concentration of resting free calcium in the store. We now augment our $\mathbf{u}$ of Eq. (13.14) and $\mathbf{f}$ of Eq. (13.15) to

$$\mathbf{u} = \begin{pmatrix} c \\ b \\ s \\ q \end{pmatrix} \quad \text{and} \quad \mathbf{f} = 2 \begin{pmatrix} k_1 cb + p^i(c,s) \\ -k_1 cb \\ k_1^e sq + p^e(c,s) \\ -k_1^e sq \end{pmatrix}$$

where p^i and p^e encode the nonlinear interactions

$$p^i(c,s) = 2a(J_{Ca}(c) - J_{NaCa}(c) - J_{PMCA}(c))/(a^2 - a_e^2) + 2a_e(J_{RYR}(c,s) - J_{SERCA}(c))/(a^2 - a_e^2)$$
$$p^e(c,s) = 2(J_{SERCA}(c) - J_{RYR}(c,s))/a_e.$$

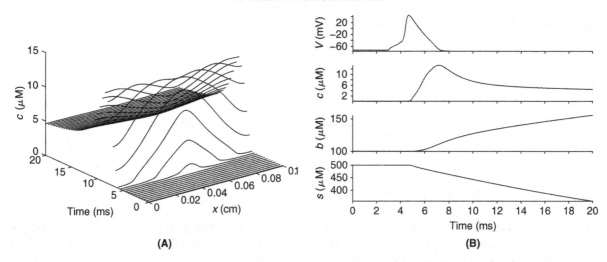

(A)   **(B)**

FIGURE 13.11   Calcium release from the ER associated with an action potential triggered at midcable. **A.** As the action potential travels away from midcable it opens Ca^{2+} channels which in turn induce Ca^{2+} release from the ER through ryanodine receptors. This calcium is simultaneously buffered and pumped out of the cytosol. **B.** We trace the key players in time at midcable. We note the rise in buffered cytosolic calcium, b, and fall of free store calcium, s, as Ca^{2+} enters the cytosol through both plasma membrane calcium channels and ER membrane ryanodine receptors. (hyEcabCa4.m)

Finally, we upgrade our reaction diffusion matrix, **R** of Eq. (13.15), to

$$
\mathbf{R} = \begin{pmatrix} D_c\mathbf{S} - k_1 B_T\mathbf{I} & k_2\mathbf{I} & 0 & 0 \\ k_1 B_T\mathbf{I} & D_b\mathbf{S} - k_2\mathbf{I} & 0 & 0 \\ 0 & 0 & D_s\mathbf{S} - k_1^e Q_T\mathbf{I} & k_2^e\mathbf{I} \\ 0 & 0 & k_1^e Q_T\mathbf{I} & D_q\mathbf{S} - k_2^e\mathbf{I} \end{pmatrix}.
$$

We have coded the (now four dimensional) reaction diffusion system, Eq. (13.14), coupled to the uniform active cable with calcium channels, in hyEcabCa4.m and illustrated its use in Figure 13.11 using the parameters stated above and

$$
a_e = 0.5\ \mu\text{m}, \quad Q_T = B_T, \quad k_j^e = k_j, \quad D_s = D_c, \quad \text{and} \quad D_q = D_b.
$$

To disentangle the contribution of the ER from the electrical events at the cell's plasma membrane one seeks a more controlled stimulus. We here consider the case where the cell has been loaded with calcium bound to a light-sensitive cage. In its bound, or caged, state it does not interact with any of our calcium handling machinery. When light of the proper wavelength is delivered at $x = x_s$ for $t \in (t_1, t_2)$ we arrive at the source term in

$$
\begin{aligned}
\frac{\partial c}{\partial t}(x,t) = D_c \frac{\partial^2 c}{\partial x^2} - 2a(J_{PMCA} + J_{NaCa})/(a^2 - a_e^2) + k_2 b - k_1 cB \\
+ 2a_e(J_{RYR} - J_{SERCA})/(a^2 - a_e^2) + c_0 \mathbb{1}_{(t_1,t_2)}(t)\delta(x - x_s)
\end{aligned}
\tag{13.24}
$$

where the amplitude, c_0, is dependent on the intensity of the light source and the concentration of caged calcium. We solve this system, still coupled to the ER dynamics, Eq. (13.23), and illustrate our findings in Figure 13.12. This propagating calcium wave depends on a subtle balance of calcium induced calcium release from the ER through ryanodine receptors and the delivery, via diffusion and buffering, of fresh cytosolic calcium to neighboring receptors. Its initiation, however, required a spark of calcium. We will now argue that IP_3 receptors are capable of providing such a spark.

The IP_3 flux. Inositol trisphosphate, or IP_3, is a cytosolic second messenger that is produced after the binding of glutamate to a metabotropic glutamate receptor via a pathway whose central constituents interact according to the reaction scheme illustrated in Figure 13.13 and expressed in Eq. (13.25).

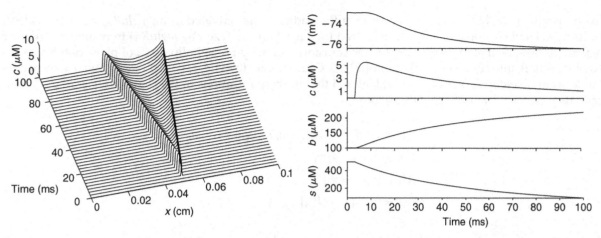

FIGURE 13.12   Release from the ER following a brief calcium stimulus ($t_1 = 3$, $t_2 = 4$ ms, and $c_0 = 1$ μM/ms) at midcable ($x_s = \ell/2$). **A.** We see that Eq. (13.24) coupled to Eq. (13.23) sustains a cytosolic calcium wave. **B.** Although we lack direct electrical stimulus, the calcium machinery effects membrane potential via I_{NaCa} and I_{KCa}. Here we note the inhibitory impact of high cytosolic [Ca^{2+}]. (`hyEcabCa4.m`)

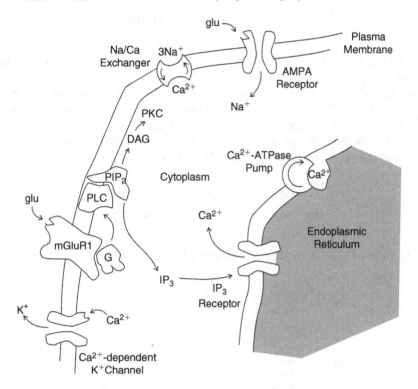

FIGURE 13.13   A schematic, in context, of the synthesis of IP_3 from PIP_2 via PLC following its activation by a G-protein that was itself activated by a metabotropic glutamate receptor following its activation by glutamate. Further context is provided by Figure 12.1. Adapted from Fiala et al. (1996).

$$mgluR_0 + glu \underset{\beta_1}{\overset{\alpha_1}{\rightleftharpoons}} mgluR_A \underset{\beta_2}{\overset{\alpha_2}{\rightleftharpoons}} mgluR_I$$

$$mgluR_A + G_0 \underset{\beta_3}{\overset{\alpha_3}{\rightleftharpoons}} mgluR_A G_0 \overset{\alpha_4}{\rightarrow} mgluR_A + G$$

$$G \overset{\alpha_5}{\rightarrow} G_0$$

$$G + PIP_2 \underset{\beta_6}{\overset{\alpha_6}{\rightleftharpoons}} GPIP_2 \overset{\alpha_7}{\rightarrow} G + IP_3 + DAG$$

$$IP_3 \overset{\alpha_8}{\rightarrow}$$

(13.25)

Here the transmitter, *glu*, binds to the receptor, $mgluR_0$, leading to its activated form, $mgluR_A$, and inactivated form, $mgluR_I$. Its associated G-protein is then transformed (in a reaction catalyzed by $mgluR_A$) from an inactive form, G_0, to an activated form, G, that in turn promotes the transformation, by phospholipase C, of phosphatidylinositol 4,5-bisphosphate (PIP2), into IP_3 and diacylglycerol, *DAG*. G and IP_3 are then degraded at rates α_5 and α_8, respectively. If we assume, as in Exercise 5, that G_0 is abundant and that the concentrations of the complices $mgluR_AG_0$ and $GPIP_2$ are steady then we may translate Eq. (13.25) into

$$m'_A = \gamma_1 [glu](1 - m_A - m_I) - \gamma_2 m_A + \gamma_3 m_I$$
$$m'_I = \gamma_4 m_A - \gamma_3 m_I$$
$$[G]' = \gamma_6 m_A - \gamma_5 [G]$$
$$[IP_3]' = \gamma_8 [G] - \gamma_7 [IP_3]$$

(13.26)

where m_A and m_I denote the respective fractions of active and inactive *mgluR* and the rate constants $\gamma_1, \ldots, \gamma_7$ are derived from the α's and β's of Eq. (13.25). Here $[glu]$ is the transient stimulus and we adopt the rate set

$$\gamma = (0.66\ 20\ 5.3\ 17\ 17\ 7.9\ 5\ 10)$$

(13.27)

where each is in units of $1/s$, except for γ_5 which is in $\mu M/s$. We have discretized this via the Trapezoid rule, see `ip3gen.m`, and illustrated its solution in Figure 13.14.

It remains to develop a model of the IP_3 receptor. The receptor is a trimer and each subunit has three binding sites, one for IP_3 and two for Ca^{2+}. The associated channel opens when IP_3 is bound and Ca^{2+} is bound to one but not both sites. The occupancies of these three sites suggest the eight-state model of Figure 13.15. The network in Figure 13.15 has 24 edges and is therefore parametrized by 24 rates. We reduce this set by supposing first that the rates are independent of whether Ca^{2+} is bound or not to the active site. This yields

$$k_{14} = k_{23},\ k_{41} = k_{32},\ k_{15} = k_{26},\ k_{51} = k_{62}$$
$$k_{58} = k_{67},\ k_{85} = k_{76},\ k_{48} = k_{37},\ k_{84} = k_{73}.$$

(13.28)

We next presume that the rates of Ca^{2+} activation are independent of IP_3 binding and Ca^{2+} inactivation. This yields

$$k_{12} = k_{56} = k_{87} = k_{43} \quad \text{and} \quad k_{21} = k_{65} = k_{78} = k_{34}.$$

(13.29)

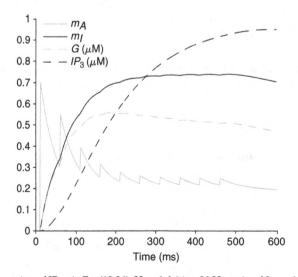

FIGURE 13.14   Generation of IP_3 via Eq. (13.26). Here $[glu]$ is a 20 Hz train of 2 ms, 1 mM doses. (`ip3gen.m`).

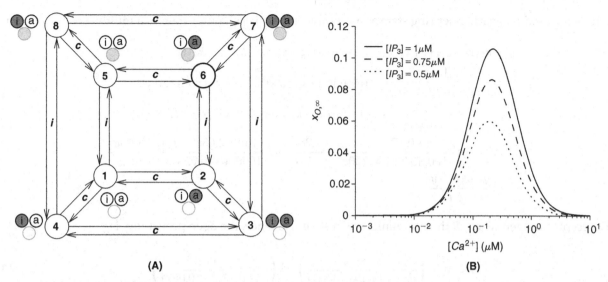

(A) (B)

FIGURE 13.15   **A.** The eight states of the model of the IP$_3$ receptor subunit. Each state is numbered and represented by three circles (black a and i for the active and inactive Ca sites, respectively; red circle for IP$_3$ site). Occupied sites are shaded. The native state is 1. From there it can bind calcium at the activating site and so reach state 2, or the inactivating site and reach state 4, or it may instead bind $i = $[IP$_3$] and achieve state 5. State 6 is the unique state with i bound, c bound to the activating site and not bound to the inactivating site. The subunit transitions from the inner ring to the outer ring when Ca^{2+} binds to the inactivating site. **B.** The probability of achieving state 6 (on all three subunits) as predicted by Eq. (13.34), as a function of [Ca^{2+}] at several fixed levels of IP$_3$. (ip3fundrive.m).

The remaining rates (in ms^{-1}) are fit to data. We obtain, with i denoting the IP$_3$ concentration and c the calcium concentration,

$$k_{15} = k_{48} = 0.4i, \; k_{58} = k_{14} = 2 \times 10^{-4}c, \; k_{12} = 0.02c, \; k_{51} = 0.052,$$
$$k_{85} = 2.1 \times 10^{-4}, \; k_{84} = 0.3772, \; k_{41} = 2.9 \times 10^{-5}, \; k_{21} = 1.64 \cdot 10^{-3}.$$
(13.30)

Some of these rates are much faster than others so we suppose the transitions $1-5-6-2-1$ and $4-8-7-3-4$ to have reached steady state long before the $1-4, 5-8, 6-7$, and $2-3$ transitions. In other words, on the inner ring we find, with differential equations on the left and equilibrium conditions on the right,

$$
\begin{aligned}
x_1' &= k_{41}x_4 - k_{14}x_1, & (k_{15}+k_{12})x_1 &= k_{51}x_5 + k_{21}x_2 \\
x_2' &= k_{32}x_3 - k_{23}x_2, & (k_{21}+k_{26})x_2 &= k_{12}x_1 + k_{62}x_6 \\
x_5' &= k_{85}x_8 - k_{58}x_5, & (k_{51}+k_{56})x_5 &= k_{15}x_1 + k_{65}x_6 \\
x_6' &= k_{76}x_7 - k_{67}x_6, & (k_{62}+k_{65})x_6 &= k_{26}x_2 + k_{56}x_5.
\end{aligned}
$$
(13.31)

Similarly, we find on the outer ring,

$$
\begin{aligned}
x_3' &= k_{23}x_2 - k_{32}x_3, & (k_{34}+k_{37})x_3 &= k_{43}x_4 + k_{73}x_7 \\
x_4' &= k_{14}x_1 - k_{41}x_4, & (k_{43}+k_{48})x_4 &= k_{34}x_3 + k_{84}x_8 \\
x_7' &= k_{67}x_6 - k_{76}x_7, & (k_{73}+k_{78})x_7 &= k_{37}x_3 + k_{87}x_8 \\
x_8' &= k_{58}x_5 - k_{85}x_8, & (k_{84}+k_{87})x_8 &= k_{48}x_4 + k_{78}x_7.
\end{aligned}
$$
(13.32)

We collect their sums in

$$y = x_1 + x_2 + x_5 + x_6 \quad \text{and} \quad 1 - y = x_3 + x_4 + x_7 + x_8.$$

In Exercise 6 we express each inner ring state as a multiple of y and each outer state as a multiple of $1 - y$ and find

$$
\begin{aligned}
y' &= k_{41}x_4 - k_{14}x_1 + k_{32}x_3 - k_{23}x_2 + k_{85}x_8 - k_{58}x_5 + k_{76}x_7 - k_{67}x_6 \\
&= \frac{1-y}{(k_{84}+k_{48})(k_{12}+k_{21})}(k_{41}k_{84}k_{12} + k_{32}k_{21}k_{84} + k_{85}k_{48}k_{12} + k_{76}k_{21}k_{48}) \\
&\quad - \frac{y}{(k_{15}+k_{51})(k_{12}+k_{21})}(k_{14}k_{21}k_{51} + k_{23}k_{51}k_{12} + k_{58}k_{21}k_{15} + k_{67}k_{15}k_{12}) \\
&= (1-y)\frac{2.19c + 0.179 + 16.85ic + 1.38i}{1000(3.77+4i)(20c+1.64)} - y\frac{0.171c + 2.08c^2 + 1.31ic + 16ic^2}{1000(4i+0.52)(20c+1.64)} \\
&\equiv \frac{y_\infty(c,i) - y}{\tau_y(c,i)}.
\end{aligned}
\tag{13.33}
$$

The IP$_3$ receptor is open when *all* three subunits are in state x_6. Hence, the open probability is

$$
x_O = x_6^3 = \left(\frac{k_{15}k_{12}y}{(k_{15}+k_{51})(k_{12}+k_{21})}\right)^3 = \left(\frac{ciy}{(i+0.13)(c+0.082)}\right)^3.
\tag{13.34}
$$

On replacing y with y_∞ we arrive at the steady state functional illustrated in Figure 13.15B. We may now insert the associated flux (with $s \equiv$ calcium concentration in ER)

$$
J_{IP_3} \equiv v_{IP_3}\left(\frac{ciy}{(i+0.13)(c+0.082)}\right)^3 (s-c), \quad v_{IP_3} = 3 \times 10^{-7}\text{cm/ms}
$$

into Eqs. (13.17) and (13.23) and augment this pair of reaction diffusion systems with the associated diffusion equation for IP$_3$,

$$
i_t = D_i i_{xx} + \gamma_8[G](t)\delta(x - x_s) - \gamma_7 i
\tag{13.35}
$$

where $[G](t)$ is the concentration of active G-protein derived from transient stimulation of *mgluRs*, recall Eq. (13.25), at the synapse location, x_s. The associated source and degradation coefficients are expressed in Eq. (13.27). Finally, for purposes of simulation, we have supposed that, D_i, the diffusivity of IP$_3$ coincides with that of Ca^{2+}. We have coupled the resulting five diffusion equations to our active uniform cable in `hyEcabCa5.m` and illustrated its findings, upon focal stimulation of metabotropic glutamate receptors, in Figure 13.16.

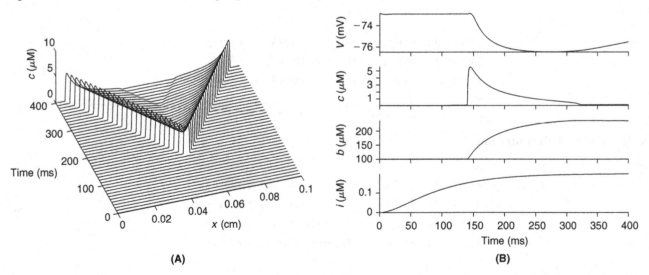

FIGURE 13.16 **A.** An intracellular calcium wave triggered by four 2 ms pulses of glutamate at 50 ms intervals delivered midcable. **B.** We observe that midcable IP$_3$ reaches a critical level at about 140 ms. At this point (compare Figure 13.15B) Ca^{2+} is released by both IP$_3$ and colocalized ryanodine receptors. Via diffusion and mobile buffering this Ca^{2+} is then delivered to neighboring ryanodine receptors and the wave commences. (`hyEcabCa5.m`)

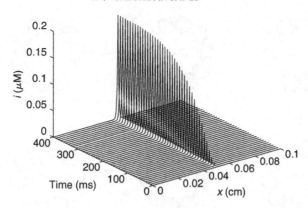

FIGURE 13.17 The space-time evolution of IP$_3$ in the simulation described in Figure 13.16. (hyEcabCa5.m)

We wish to stress that the stimulus, via Eq. (13.35), is delivered only at $x = x_s$ and that we have no influx of calcium from the extracellular environment. Moreover, as IP$_3$ diffuses slowly and is degraded rather than buffered it is not likely to travel far from its source. This observation is supported by Figure 13.17.

We note that intracellular calcium waves have been observed in pyramidal cells in both hippocampal and cortical slices. One proposed function of such waves is the delivery of calcium to the cell body where it may serve to activate transcription factors that regulate the genes that govern the morphological changes associated with long-term synaptic plasticity.

13.4 CALCIUM IN SPINES

We observed in §9.3 that NMDA receptors on the heads of spines, via their dependence on both presynaptic glutamate release and postsynaptic depolarization, serve as exquisite coincidence detectors. The NMDA receptor signals coincidence via the Ca^{2+} component of the resulting NMDA current. The role that this Ca^{2+} signal then plays in modulating the spine's synaptic conductance is one of the central questions in the study of synaptic plasticity. One of the most well-studied forms of plasticity, already introduced in §12.6, is known as long-term potentiation (LTP). It can be induced by several protocols, one being a short (a few seconds) volley of high frequency stimulation, and results in a long (30 or more minutes) sustained enhancement, or potentiation, of the synaptic conductance. The question of how a short burst of activity may have lasting effects receives an answer in the role Ca^{2+} may play in the autophosphorylation of calcium/calmodulin-dependent protein kinase II, or CaMKII. To phosphorylate a protein is to attach a phosphate group to it. An enzyme that catalyzes such an attachment is known as a kinase. This attachment typically requires a conformational change in the recipient which results in a change of function. For example, the activated (autophosphorylated) form of CaMKII may in turn phosphorylate individual AMPA receptors and thereby increase their conductances. We now construct a mathematical model for the autophosphorylation of CaMKII by Ca^{2+}. We will show that this model exhibits a stable steady state in which autophosphorylated CaMKII persists upon transient elevation of the calcium concentration at levels expected from the activation of NMDA receptors. This elevated and persistent level of autophosphorylated CaMKII can in turn maintain AMPA receptors in a high conductance state.

With regard to the block diagram of Figure 12.1, the first step following entry of Ca^{2+} into the spine via NMDA channels, is the binding of four Ca^{2+} to the large mobile buffer calmodulin, CaM, to form the (Ca^{2+})$_4$CaM complex. We will henceforth denote this (Ca^{2+})$_4$CaM complex by C. CaMKII is presumed to possess 10 subunits, with 8–12 being typical. Autophosphorylation involves two adjacent subunits, with one subunit acting as a catalyst and the other as a substrate. A subunit may become catalytic only through either phosphorylation or the binding of C. A subunit may serve as a substrate only after binding C. Moreover, we assume that this process may occur only between neighboring subunits and that it may progress in but one direction. In Figure 13.18 we depict the first two steps of autophosphorylation, propagating clockwise along the CaMKII ring. To move from the inactive kinase, P_0 to the (first) activated level P_1 requires two molecules of C. Each C may bind to CaMKII only after all four Ca^{2+} sites on CaM are filled, and so the rate of binding C to CaMKII is assumed proportional to

$$\frac{([Ca^{2+}]/K_{H1})^4}{1 + ([Ca^{2+}]/K_{H1})^4}.$$

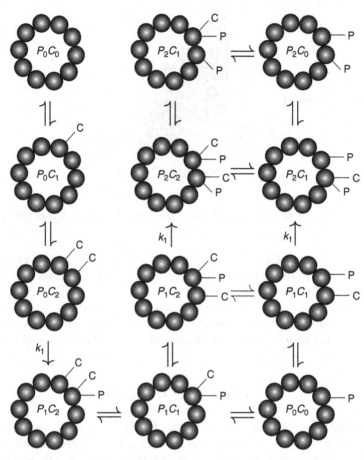

FIGURE 13.18　A schematic of the first two steps in the autophosphorylation of CaMKII. The left column represents the initiation of phosphorylation (from top to bottom). The middle and right columns represent two routes for the propagation of autophosphorylation. Note that the position of the newly added P group is constrained to be clockwise from the first one. Here C denotes the $(Ca^{2+})_4$CaM complex and P denotes orthophosphate.

Here, K_{H1} is the Hill dissociation constant for Ca^{2+} from CaM. As two Cs are required and there are 10 possible adjacent pairs we conclude that

$$P_0 \underset{b_1}{\overset{f_1}{\rightleftharpoons}} P_1 \quad \text{where} \quad f_1 = \frac{10k_1([Ca^{2+}]/K_{H1})^8}{(1+([Ca^{2+}]/K_{H1})^4)^2}.$$

Here k_1 is the rate at which P_0C_2 yields P_1C_2. This is the bottom irreversible reaction in the first column of Figure 13.18.

The binding of one additional C complex to P_1 is enough to trigger a subsequent phosphorylation. The resultant then offers twice the number of targets for dephosphorylation. In symbols,

$$P_1 \underset{b_2}{\overset{f_2}{\rightleftharpoons}} P_2 \quad \text{where} \quad f_2 = \frac{k_1([Ca^{2+}]/K_{H1})^4}{1+([Ca^{2+}]/K_{H1})^4}.$$

Subsequent C driven autophosphorylation also occurs at multiple sites. Namely, P_2 exists in $10(10-1)/2 = 45$ configurations, of which $z_{2,1} = 10$ consist of adjacent phosphorylated sites, as illustrated in the example of Figure 13.18. These configurations offer one new phosphorylation site immediately adjacent in the clockwise direction. The remaining $z_{2,2} = 35$ nonadjacent configurations offer two phosphorylation sites immediately adjacent in the clockwise direction. These configurations arise from the dephosphorylation of CaMKII at random positions through the reaction to be described in Eq. (13.38) below. Hence,

$$P_2 \underset{b_3}{\overset{f_3}{\rightleftharpoons}} P_3 \quad \text{where} \quad f_3 = \frac{z_{2,1}+2z_{2,2}}{z_{2,1}+z_{2,2}}f_2.$$

In general, for $i=2,3,\ldots,9$,

$$P_i \underset{b_{i+1}}{\overset{w_i f_2}{\rightleftharpoons}} P_{i+1} \quad \text{where} \quad w_i = w_{10-i} = \frac{\sum_{j=1}^{i} j z_{i,j}}{\sum_{j=1}^{i} z_{i,j}} \tag{13.36}$$

and $z_{i,j}$ is the number of ways to distribute i items leaving j clockwise neighbors. We offer

$$z = \begin{pmatrix} 10 & \cdot & \cdot & \cdot & \cdot \\ 10 & 35 & \cdot & \cdot & \cdot \\ 10 & 60 & 50 & \cdot & \cdot \\ 10 & 71 & 100 & 29 & \cdot \\ 10 & 80 & 120 & 40 & 2 \end{pmatrix}$$

and so

$$w_1 = w_9 = 1, \ w_2 = 16/9, \ w_3 = 7/3, \ w_4 = 284/105, \ w_5 = 25/9. \tag{13.37}$$

Regarding the reverse reactions characterized by the reverse rates b_i, we suppose that phosphatase, D, strips or dephosphorylates P_i via

$$iP_i + D \underset{d_{-1}}{\overset{d_1}{\rightleftharpoons}} P_i D \overset{d_2}{\rightarrow} P_{i-1} + D \quad i = 1,2,\ldots,10. \tag{13.38}$$

The factor i in front of P_i accounts for the i possible binding sites. If we assume the complex, $P_i D$, achieves rapid equilibrium then

$$P'_{i-1} = d_2[P_i D], \tag{13.39}$$

$$i[P_i][D] = K_M[P_i D], \quad K_M = (d_2 + d_{-1})/d_1, \tag{13.40}$$

where K_M is the Michaelis constant for the phosphatase. Hence, if we define the total active phosphatase concentration

$$[D]_0 = [D] + \sum_{j=1}^{10} [P_j D] \tag{13.41}$$

and use Eq. (13.40) to replace $[D]$, we arrive at the linear system

$$[P_i D] K_M / (i[P_i]) + \sum_{j=1}^{10} [P_j D] = [D]_0, \quad i = 1,2,\ldots,10 \tag{13.42}$$

for $[P_i D]$. This system possesses considerable structure and so permits the simple solution

$$[P_i D] = \frac{i[P_i][D]_0}{K_M + \sum_{j=1}^{10} j[P_j]}. \tag{13.43}$$

Using Eq. (13.39), we may now express the reverse rates

$$b_i = \frac{i d_2[D]_0}{K_M + \sum_{j=1}^{10} j[P_j]}, \tag{13.44}$$

where d_2 is the dephosphorylation rate of Eq. (13.39). We so arrive at the system of ordinary differential equations

$$\begin{aligned} [P_0]' &= b_1[P_1] - f_1[P_0] \\ [P_i]' &= f_i[P_{i-1}] + b_{i+1}[P_{i+1}] - (b_i + f_{i+1})[P_i] \\ [P_{10}]' &= f_{10}[P_9] - b_{10}[P_{10}]. \end{aligned} \tag{13.45}$$

To close this system we must constrain the dynamics of $[D]_0$, the concentration of active phosphatase. We do this via its interaction with I, a $[Ca^{2+}]$-dependent inhibitor of the phosphatase. In particular, we assume a total pool of phosphatase of size $[D]_T$. The phosphatase can bind to the inhibitor through a first order reaction, and $[D]_T - [D]_0$ represents the quantity bound to I. The rates of binding and unbinding are k_3 and k_4, respectively. The inhibitor is produced from its inactive form I_0 by protein kinase A (PKA) at a rate v_{PKA} and inactivated through action of calcineurin at a rate v_{CaN}. Calcineurin itself requires binding of three Ca^{2+} to be active, through binding of three Ca^{2+}/CaM, with Hill coefficient K_{H2}. In symbols,

$$[D]'_0 = -k_3[I][D]_0 + k_4([D]_T - [D]_0)$$

$$[I]' = -k_3[I][D]_0 + k_4([D]_T - [D]_0) + v_{PKA}I_0 - \frac{v_{CaN}[I]([Ca^{2+}]/K_{H2})^3}{1 + ([Ca^{2+}]/K_{H2})^3}. \tag{13.46}$$

Our principle interest is in the number of relevant steady states achievable by Eqs. (13.45) and (13.46). Toward that end, it follows from Eq. (13.46) that the $D - I$ system is steady at

$$[\overline{D}]_0 = \frac{k_4[D]_T}{k_3[\overline{I}] + k_4} \quad \text{and} \quad [\overline{I}] = v_{PKA}I_0 \frac{1 + ([Ca^{2+}]/K_{H2})^3}{v_{CaN}([Ca^{2+}]/K_{H2})^3} \tag{13.47}$$

and that the P system is steady at

$$[\overline{P}_1] = (f_1/b_1)[\overline{P}_0], \quad [\overline{P}_2] = \frac{f_1 f_2}{b_1 b_2}[\overline{P}_0], \quad \text{and} \quad [\overline{P}_j] = \frac{f_1 \cdots f_j}{b_1 \cdots b_j}[\overline{P}_0].$$

On noting that $b_j = jb_1$ and $f_j = w_{j-1}f_2$, we then find

$$[\overline{P}_j] = b_1^{-j} c_j [\overline{P}_0] \quad \text{where} \quad c_j \equiv f_1 f_2^{j-1} w_1 \cdots w_{j-1}/j!. \tag{13.48}$$

Let $[\overline{P}]_T$ be the total amount of CaMKII, i.e.,

$$[\overline{P}]_T = \sum_{j=0}^{10} [\overline{P}_j]. \tag{13.49}$$

If we use this in Eq. (13.48), we may solve for $[\overline{P}_0]$

$$\frac{[\overline{P}]_T}{[\overline{P}_0]} = 1 + \sum_{j=1}^{10} c_j b_1^{-j}, \tag{13.50}$$

and if now we place Eqs. (13.48) and (13.50) in Eq. (13.44) with $i = 1$ we find

$$(k_2[\overline{D}]_0 b_1^{-1} - K_M)\left(1 + \sum_{j=1}^{10} c_j b_1^{-j}\right) = [\overline{P}]_T \sum_{j=1}^{10} j c_j b_1^{-j}$$

which we recognize as an eleventh order polynomial for b_1,

$$(k_2[\overline{D}]_0 - K_M b_1)\left(b_1^{10} + \sum_{j=1}^{10} c_j b_1^{10-j}\right) = [\overline{P}]_T \sum_{j=1}^{10} j c_j b_1^{11-j}, \tag{13.51}$$

where $[\overline{P}]_T$ is the fixed total concentration of CaMKII and $[\overline{D}]_0$, the steady activated level of phosphatase, is set in Eq. (13.47) by $[Ca^{2+}]$. The coefficients, c_j, are likewise set in terms of the forward rates, f_1 and f_2, by $[Ca^{2+}]$. Adopting

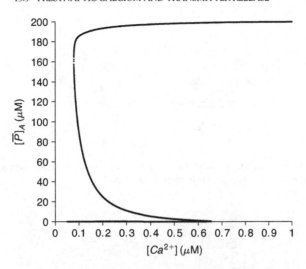

FIGURE 13.19 The bistability curve of Zhabotinsky (2000). For small ($< 0.1~\mu$M) and large ($> 0.7~\mu$M) levels of [Ca^{2+}] there is but one steady state while for $0.1 \le$ [Ca^{2+}] $\le 0.7~\mu$M there are three steady states. The middle state is known to be unstable and so CaMKII is said to be bistable. (camk2ss.m)

the parameters

$$k_1 = 5 \cdot 10^{-1}\,\text{ms}^{-1}, K_{H1} = 4\,\text{mM}, d_2 = 2\,\text{ms}^{-1}, K_M = 0.4\,\text{mM}$$

$$k_3 = 1\,(\text{mMms})^{-1}, k_4 = 1 \cdot 10^{-3}\,\text{ms}^{-1}, K_{H2} = 0.7\,\text{mM}, v_{CaN} = 1\,\text{ms}^{-1}, v_{PKA} = 1\,\text{ms}^{-1} \qquad (13.52)$$

$$[\overline{P}]_T = 20, [\overline{D}]_T = 0.05, \text{and } I_0 = 0.1\,\text{mM}$$

we find that this polynomial has three distinct positive roots for [Ca^{2+}] within a physiologically relevant window. For each such root, the total amount of active CaMKII

$$[\overline{P}]_A \equiv \sum_{j=1}^{10} j[\overline{P}_j] = d_2[\overline{D}]_0 b_1^{-1} - K_M$$

is graphed in Figure 13.19. This curve provides a possible answer to the query that opened this section. More precisely, if a brief high frequency stimulus elevates spinal [Ca^{2+}] above 0.7 μM then CaMKII will reach its high state. Most importantly, as spinal [Ca^{2+}] returns to normal resting levels, the high state of CaMKII persists. The reader will have a chance to test these ideas in Exercise 7.

13.5 PRESYNAPTIC CALCIUM AND TRANSMITTER RELEASE

The previous chapter made numerous references to the fact that transmitter release, through exocytosis, is dependent on the presence of Ca^{2+} in the presynaptic terminal. With regard to the schematic in Figure 13.20, depolarization of the presynaptic terminal opens voltage-gated calcium channels. This calcium binds to a "calcium sensor" on the outer surface of the vesicular membrane. The bound sensor then binds several SNARE (soluble N-ethylmaleimide-sensitive fusion protein receptor) proteins that facilitate the fusion of the vesicular and cellular membranes and the subsequent secretion of neurotransmitter. The goal of this section is to present a mechanistic model of synaptic fusion and experiments suggesting that the protein synaptotagmin-1 is part of the calcium sensor.

We illustrate the experiments that we will model in Figure 13.21, based on recordings from chromaffin cells of the mouse adrenal gland. These are neurosecretory cells that receive synaptic inputs from other neurons, which can cause them to fire an action potential. This, in turn, causes calcium influx and subsequent release of hormones, like epinephrine, stored in secretory vesicles. Rather than using synaptic or electrical stimulation to trigger vesicle release, it is possible to use flash-photolysis to uncage Ca^{2+} that has been previously injected into the cell as a caged compound. The fusion of vesicles can be monitored by measuring changes in membrane capacitance. More precisely, as the vesicular and cellular membranes fuse the resulting surface area of the cell "grows" by one vesicle. As membrane

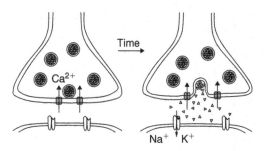

FIGURE 13.20   A depiction of the calcium-dependent exocytotic event. Calcium enters through voltage-gated calcium channels and binds to vesicular proteins that trigger membrane fusion and eventual transmitter secretion.

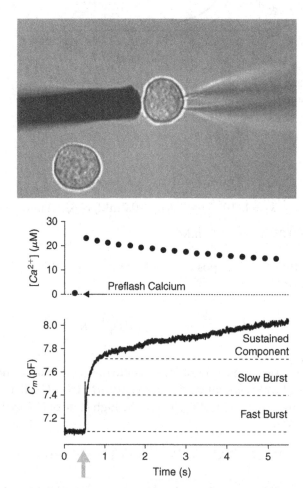

FIGURE 13.21   The top panel shows two isolated chromaffin cells (typical diameter: $\approx 10 - 15\,\mu m$) with the top right one being accessed through a glass electrode visible on its right. This allows delivery of the caged Ca^{2+} compound and measurement of capacitance changes during uncaging. The black electrode on the right is able to measure directly the release of hormones through a technique called amperometry. The middle panel reports the change in calcium concentration immediately before and after the light flash (red arrow at bottom). The bottom panel shows that the change in membrane capacitance has a rapid, a slow, and a sustained component. Adapted from Neher (2006).

capacitance is proportional to surface area, vesicle fusion may be inferred from ΔC_m, the change in membrane capacitance obtained using a recording electrode, by measuring the voltage response to a simple current step. Recall, e.g., that Eqs. (3.10) and (3.12) permit us to write AC_m in terms of strengths and centroids of the stimulus and response. If the recording electrode also contains a calcium indicator, it is possible to simultaneously measure the intracellular calcium concentration, as in Exercise 8. Such measurements show that vesicle release consists of three distinct phases: a fast, a slow, and a sustained phase (Figure 13.21). Since the fast and slow phases appear largely independent of each other, this leads to a two pool model of vesicle release: vesicles either belong to a rapidly releasable pool (RRP) or a slowly releasable pool (SRP) that proceed towards exocytosis largely independently of each other. Such a two pool release model is also thought to capture the properties of synaptic release at presynaptic terminals. The late sustained component corresponds to the release of new vesicles as they are made available by the cell fabrication machinery following depletion of the RRP and SRP pools. We assume that vesicles belonging to the SRP require the binding of three Ca^{2+} ions to be exocytosed while those of the RRP require four.

If we denote the respective steady populations by SRP_0 and RRP_0, and then increment their subscripts when their vesicles bind a calcium ion we obtain the over-all scheme

$$\begin{array}{cc}
\begin{array}{c}k_2(Ca^{2+})\\\rightleftharpoons\\k_{-2}\end{array} SRP_0 \begin{array}{c}k_1\\\rightleftharpoons\\k_{-1}\end{array} RRP_0 & RRP_0+Ca^{2+} \begin{array}{c}4\alpha_r\\\rightleftharpoons\\\beta_r\end{array} RRP_1 \\[2ex]
SRP_0+Ca^{2+} \begin{array}{c}3\alpha_s\\\rightleftharpoons\\\beta_s\end{array} SRP_1 & RRP_1+Ca^{2+} \begin{array}{c}3\alpha_r\\\rightleftharpoons\\2\beta_r b\end{array} RRP_2 \\[2ex]
SRP_1+Ca^{2+} \begin{array}{c}2\alpha_s\\\rightleftharpoons\\2\beta_s\end{array} SRP_2 & RRP_2+Ca^{2+} \begin{array}{c}2\alpha_r\\\rightleftharpoons\\3\beta_r b^2\end{array} RRP_3 \\[2ex]
SRP_2+Ca^{2+} \begin{array}{c}\alpha_s\\\rightleftharpoons\\3\beta_s\end{array} SRP_3 \overset{\gamma_s}{\rightarrow} E_{SRP} & RRP_3+Ca^{2+} \begin{array}{c}\alpha_r\\\rightleftharpoons\\4\beta_r b^3\end{array} RRP_4 \overset{\gamma_r}{\rightarrow} E_{RRP}
\end{array}$$

(13.53)

where E_{SRP} and E_{RRP} denote "exocytosed," from the SRP and RRP respectively. The first two pairs of reactions are associated with pool maintenance, with k_2 credited with "priming" the vesicles, i.e., making them ready for release. The second pair corresponds to the transformation of a vesicle from the SRP to the RRP. The rates are given by

$$k_2 = \frac{r_{max}[Ca^{2+}]}{K_D+[Ca^{2+}]}, \quad r_{max}=55 f\,F/s, \; K_D=2.3, \; k_{-2}=0.005, \; k_1=0.12, \; k_{-1}=0.1$$

where all concentrations are in μM and all rates are in s^{-1}. Note that we measure pool filling rates in femtofarads per second and that the transformation rates k_1 and k_{-1} between the two pools are slow compared to the exocytosis rates given below. As mentioned above, fusing and emptying of the slowly releasable pool is assumed to require the binding of three Ca^{2+} ions, per vesicle, and is parametrized by

$$\alpha_s=0.8 \; (mMs)^{-1}, \quad \beta_s=4 \; s^{-1}, \quad \text{and} \quad \gamma_s=20 \; s^{-1}.$$

(13.54)

The last fusion step and its rate, γ_s, are calcium independent. Fusing and emptying of the readily releasable pool is assumed to require four Ca^{2+} ions, in a cooperative fashion, and is parametrized by

$$\alpha_r=4.9, \quad \beta_r=56, \quad \gamma_r=1450, \quad \text{and} \quad b=0.55.$$

(13.55)

Here b is the cooperativity parameter that effectively reduces the rate of calcium unbinding as more Ca^{2+} ions are bound to the vesicle. These parameters were chosen to fit the response in Figure 13.22A.

One way of discerning the contribution of synaptotagmin-1 to vesicle release, is to conduct experiments in chromaffin cells of both wild type (WT) mice and mice that carry a mutation (R233Q) in the calcium-dependent phospholipid binding domain of synaptotagmin-1. As illustrated in Figure 13.22, this mutation causes a delay in exocytosis (vertical dashed lines) that suggests a higher Ca^{2+} threshold for the release sensor. In addition, overall change in membrane capacitance is reduced in the mutants, suggesting that synaptotagmin-1 may also have an effect on the priming and unpriming of vesicles.

To investigate whether model parameter changes can reproduce the experimental results, we apply the law of mass action to Eq. (13.53) to arrive at the linear system of ordinary differential equations

$$\mathbf{x}'(t) = ([Ca^{2+}](t)\mathbf{A}+\mathbf{B})\mathbf{x}(t)+k_2([Ca^{2+}](t))\mathbf{e}_1$$

(13.56)

for $\mathbf{x} = (SRP_0 \; SRP_1 \; SRP_2 \; SRP_3 \; E_{SRP} \; RRP_0 \; RRP_1 \; RRP_2 \; RRP_3 \; RRP_4 \; E_{RRP})^T$ where $\mathbf{A}$ and $\mathbf{B}$ are two constant matrices and $\mathbf{e}_1$ is the first column of the identity matrix. We have coded this system in `exocytosis.m`, under the assumption that Ca^{2+} is uncaged in the ramplike fashion (as in Figure 13.22)

$$Ca^{2+}(t) = \min\{\exp((t-1.5)\log(10)/2.5), 20\}$$

(13.57)

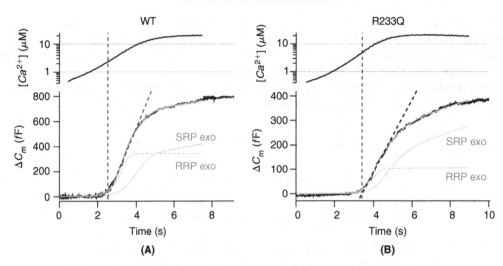

FIGURE 13.22 Capacitance change during an increase in intracellular calcium in both (**A**) wild type and (**B**) mutant chromaffin cells. The calcium ramp was delivered via flash photolysis. The dashed black lines are fits to the slope of the experimental curves and permit us to determine the activation delay. The corresponding vertical dashed lines determine the Ca^{2+} concentration threshold. The solid gray line is the fit from the model in Eq. (13.53), while the dashed gray lines show the time course of exocytosis from the SRP and RRP. Adapted from Sørensen et al. (2003).

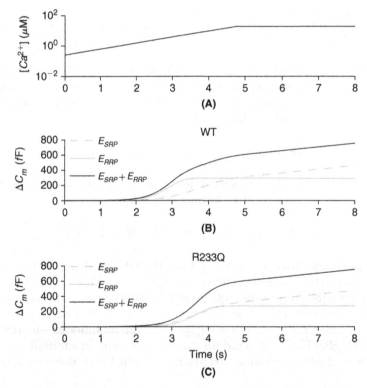

FIGURE 13.23 **A.** The Ca^{2+} ramp stimulus of Eq. (13.57) and the predicted response in both the wild type (**B**) and mutant (**C**) cells. Panel **B** was achieved with the parameter set Eqs. (13.54) and (13.55). Its red traces correspond to the dashed and dotted traces of Figure 13.22A. The mutant simulation in panel **C** required modification of the single model parameter, α_r, the rate at which Ca^{2+} binds to vesicles in the RRP. The change from $\alpha_r = 4.9$ in wild type to $\alpha_r = 2.4$ in the mutant serves to quantify the role of synaptotagmin-1 as a link between intracellular Ca^{2+} and the SNARE apparatus leading to exocytosis. (exocytosis.m)

and illustrate its use in Figure 13.23 for both wild type and mutant cells. The model shows that a single modification to the calcium binding rate of the rapidly releasable pool (α_r) is sufficient to explain the experimental results. This modification also corresponds to a higher threshold for the calcium sensor since the Ca^{2+} dissociation constant is equal to $K_D = \beta_r/\alpha_r$.

13.6 SUMMARY AND SOURCES

We have pursued the notion, championed by Berridge (1998), that the ER comprises a "neuron within a neuron," where the calcium gradient across the ER membrane is analogous to the voltage gradient across the plasma membrane. The section on voltage-gated calcium channels is drawn from Jaffe et al. (1994). For more on pumps and exchangers see Chapter 3 in Fall et al. (2005). The factor of 2 in the two voltage terms of Eq. (13.7) for the sodium–calcium exchanger stems from a symmetry assumption in the underlying barrier model, see Keener and Sneyd (1998) for details. Hudspeth and Lewis (1988a,b) argue that the interplay of calcium and calcium activated potassium currents underlies the "electrical tuning" displayed by hair cells in the auditory and vestibular systems. We reproduce their model in Exercise 3. The most relevant calcium buffers are surveyed in Baimbridge et al. (1992). The design of fluorescent buffers as calcium indicators is discussed in Grynkiewicz et al. (1985). Exercise 8 is derived from this work. Shimomura, Chalfie, and Tsien shared the 2008 Nobel Prize in Chemistry for the discovery and development of such fluorescent indicators. See http://nobelprize.org. The rapid buffer approximation of Exercise 9 is due to Wagner and Keizer (1994). The ryanodine receptor model and the constants characterizing it, Eq. (13.21), are due to Keizer and Levine (1996).

The model of the metabotropic glutamate receptor is built along the lines of the metabotropic GABA receptor in Destexhe et al. (1998). For an alternate treatment see Fiala et al. (1996). The IP_3 receptor model is due to Young and Keizer (1992). Intracellular calcium waves in neurons were first observed by Jaffe and Brown (1994). For a careful study of the initiation and propagation of such waves see Peercy (2008). The CaMKII model is due to Zhabotinsky (2000). The two pool model of exocytosis is due to Sørensen et al. (2003). See Rizo and Rosenmund (2008) for a recent overview of the structural complexity of the synaptic release machinery.

13.7 EXERCISES

1. Drive `hyEcabCa3.m` with a periodic train and show, as in Figure 13.24, that the calcium-dependent potassium current can alter the spike rate.

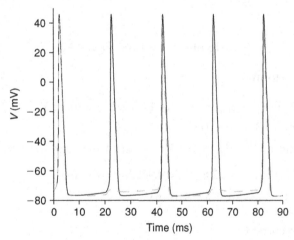

FIGURE 13.24 The calcium-dependent potassium current leads to spike skipping when the cable of §13.2 is driven by a 50 Hz train of 1 ms current injections, at $x_2 = \ell/4$, and of amplitude 300 pA. We here plot the response at midcable. The black trace corresponds to $\overline{g}_{KCa} = 0$ and the red trace to $\overline{g}_{KCa} = 10$ mS/cm^2. The latter exhibits a long period of "after-hyperpolarization" that serves to decrease the spike rate.

2. [†]Closer examination of the L-type calcium channel has determined that it inactivates through a process that is dependent on the concentration of cytosolic calcium. Modify `hyEcabCa3.m` to incorporate calcium-dependent inactivation, via

$$g_{Ca,L} = \overline{g}_{Ca,L} m_L^2 h_L, \qquad h_L = \frac{k_L}{k_L + c} \tag{13.58}$$

and experiment, as in Figure 13.25, with the regulatory parameter, k_L.

3. Sound is detected by the deflection of hair bundles attached to mechanosensitive ion channels in so-called "hair cells." The differentiation of sound into its frequency components is accomplished via mechanical filtering in the

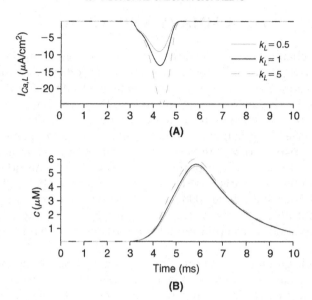

FIGURE 13.25 The effect of calcium-dependent inactivation of the L-type calcium channel on the cable of §13.2. Here $I_{Ca,L}$ and c are midcable traces stemming from a 1 ms, 300 pA current injection at $\ell/4$. (hyEcabCa3Ldrive.m)

inner ear and electrical filtering in individual hair cells. We here reconstruct a model of a bullfrog hair cell in which the interaction of calcium currents and calcium activated potassium currents are seen to explain the cell's frequency response. The potential, V, in the (isopotential) hair cell obeys

$$C_m V' + g_L(V - E_L) + I_{Ca} + I_{KCa} = I_{stim},$$

where

$$C_m = 15 \text{ pF}, \quad g_L = 1 \text{ nS}, \ E_L = -30 \text{ mV}$$

and the calcium current is of the form

$$I_{Ca} = \bar{g}_{Ca} m^3 (V - E_{Ca}), \quad \bar{g}_{Ca} = 4.14 \text{ nS}, \ E_{Ca} = 100 \text{ mV},$$
$$m' = \alpha_m(V)(1 - m) - \beta_m(V),$$
$$\alpha_m(V) = \alpha_0 \exp((V + V_0)/V_A) + K_A, \quad \beta_m(V) = \beta_0 \exp(-(V + V_0)/V_B) + K_B$$
$$\alpha_0 = 0.00097, \ \beta_0 = 22.8, \ K_A = 0.94, \ K_B = 0.51 \text{ ms}^{-1},$$
$$V_A = 6.17, \ V_0 = 70, \ V_B = 8.01 \text{ mV}.$$

and a calcium-gated potassium current

$$I_{KCa} = \bar{g}_{KCa}(O_2 + O_3)(V - E_K), \quad \bar{g}_{KCa} = 16.8 \text{ nS}, \ E_K = -80 \text{ mV}$$

where O_2 and O_3 are the two open states in the five-state scheme

$$C_0 \underset{k_{-1}}{\overset{k_1 c}{\rightleftharpoons}} C_1 \underset{k_{-2}}{\overset{k_2 c}{\rightleftharpoons}} C_2 \underset{\alpha_C}{\overset{\beta_C}{\rightleftharpoons}} O_2 \underset{k_{-3}}{\overset{k_3 c}{\rightleftharpoons}} O_3$$

$$k_{-1} = 0.3, \ k_{-2} = 5, \ k_{-3} = 1.5 \text{ ms}^{-1},$$
$$k_j = k_{-j}/K_j(V), \quad K_j(V) = K_j(0) \exp(\delta_j z V/V_T), \quad V_T = 25.8 \text{ mV}$$
$$K_1(0) = 0.006, \ K_2(0) = 0.045, \ K_3(0) = 0.02 \text{ mM}, \quad \delta_1 = 0.2, \ \delta_2 = 0, \ \delta_3 = 0.2,$$
$$\alpha_C(V) = \alpha_C(0) \exp(-V/V_a), \ \beta_C = 1, \alpha_C(0) = 0.45 \text{ ms}^{-1}, \ V_a = 33 \text{ mV}.$$

Here c denotes the intracellular calcium concentration, in mM, and is presumed to obey

$$c' = \gamma I_{Ca} - K_s c, \quad \gamma = 0.0024 \text{ M/pC}, \ K_S = 2.8 \text{ ms}^{-1}.$$

Apply the law of mass action to the five-state scheme and arrive at a system of ordinary differential equations for $(V, C_0, C_1, C_2, O_2, O_3, c)$. Solve this system using two classes of inputs and reproduce the results in Figure 13.26. In the first case, use a simple 50 ms current pulse of amplitude I_0,

$$I_{stim}(t) = I_0 \mathbb{1}_{(0,50)}(t). \tag{13.59}$$

In the second case, we mimic the transduction of the mechanosensitive hair receptor by supposing that the periodic deflection of the hair bundle

$$x(t;f) = x_0 \sin(2\pi f t), \quad x_0 = 20 \text{ nm}$$

generates the associated current

$$I_{stim}(t,f) = \frac{-\bar{g}_T V}{1 + \exp(a_1 - a_2 x(t;f))(1 + \exp(a_3 - a_4 x(t;f)))} \tag{13.60}$$

with $\bar{g}_T = 3$ nS, $a_1 = 1.2674$, $a_2 = 0.0169$ nm^{-1}, $a_3 = 0.4238$, and $a_4 = 0.0034$ nm^{-1}. We capture the resonant nature of the cell by computing, for each frequency, f, the maximal peak-to-peak response

$$P(f) \equiv \max_{t > t_0} V(t;f) - \min_{t > t_0} V(t;f)$$

where t_0 denotes the duration of the transient, see Figure 13.26B.

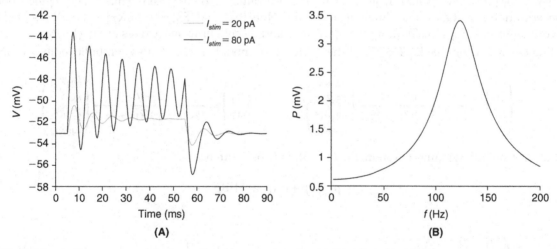

FIGURE 13.26 **A.** The response of the hair cell to current pulses, Eq. (13.59), of amplitude 20 and 80 pA. Note that the frequency of the depolarization increases with the size of the stimulus. (haircell1.m) **B.** The resonant peak associated with the transduced deflection, Eq. (13.60). (haircell2.m)

4. Apply the law of mass action to the reaction scheme, Figure 13.10, of the ryanodine receptor in your derivation of

$$\begin{aligned}
C_1' &= -k_a^+ c^4 C_1 + k_a^- O_1 \\
O_1' &= k_a^+ c^4 C_1 - (k_a^- + k_b^+ c^3 + k_c^+) O_1 + k_b^- O_2 + k_c^- C_2 \\
O_2' &= k_b^+ c^3 O_1 - k_b^- O_2 \\
1 &= O_1 + O_2 + C_1 + C_2.
\end{aligned} \tag{13.61}$$

If the a and b transitions are fast compared to c argue why

$$O_1 = (c/K_a)^4 C_1 \quad \text{and} \quad O_2 = (c/K_b)^3 O_1 = (c/K_b)^3 (c/K_a)^4 C_1. \tag{13.62}$$

Next define $O \equiv O_1 + O_2$ and $w \equiv 1 - C_2$ and show that $C_1 = w - O$ and

$$O = O_1 + O_2 = (c/K_a)^4 (1 + (c/K_b)^3) C_1 = (c/K_a)^4 (1 + (c/K_b)^3)(w - O), \tag{13.63}$$

and so

$$O = w \frac{1 + (c/K_b)^3}{1 + (K_a/c)^4 + (c/K_b)^3}. \tag{13.64}$$

Similarly, show that $w' = -C_2' = k_c^- C_2 - k_c^+ O_1$ and proceed to confirm that w obeys Eq. (13.19) where w_∞ is given by Eq. (13.20).

5. †Apply the law of mass action to Eq. (13.25) to find

$$[mgluR_A]' = \alpha_1[glu][mgluR_0] + \beta_2[mgluR_I] - (\beta_1 + \alpha_2)[mgluR_A]$$
$$- \alpha_3[mgluR_A][G_0] + (\beta_3 + \alpha_4)[mgluR_A G_0]$$

$$[mgluR_I]' = \alpha_2[mgluR_A] - \beta_2[mgluR_I] \tag{13.65}$$

$$[G]' = \alpha_4[mgluR_A G_0] - \alpha_5[G] - \alpha_6[G][PIP_2] + (\beta_6 + \alpha_7)[PIP_2 G]$$

$$[IP_3]' = \alpha_7[PIP_2 G] - \alpha_8[IP_3]$$

while the complices obey

$$[mgluR_A G_0]' = \alpha_3[G_0][mgluR_A] - (\beta_3 + \alpha_4)[mgluR_A G_0]$$
$$[PIP_2 G]' = \alpha_6[G][PIP_2] - (\beta_6 + \alpha_7)[PIP_2 G]. \tag{13.66}$$

We now suppose that Eq. (13.66) is steady with respect to Eq. (13.65). In particular, set the derivatives in Eq. (13.66) to zero, solve for $[mgluR_A G_0]$ and $[PIP_2 G]$ and insert these values into Eq. (13.65). Finally, let $[mgluR_T]$ denote the total concentration of metabotropic glutamate receptors. Note that $[mgluR_0] = [mgluR_T] - [mgluR_A] - [mgluR_I]$ and divide your simplified Eq. (13.65) through by $[mgluR_T]$ and discuss how one arrives at Eq. (13.26).

6. †Regarding our reduction, see Eq. (13.33), of the IP$_3$ receptor model, use MATLAB's symbolic toolbox to show that

$$\begin{pmatrix} x_1 \\ x_2 \\ x_5 \\ x_6 \end{pmatrix} = \frac{y}{(k_{15} + k_{51})(k_{12} + k_{21})} \begin{pmatrix} k_{21}k_{51} \\ k_{51}k_{12} \\ k_{21}k_{15} \\ k_{15}k_{12} \end{pmatrix} \quad \text{and} \quad \begin{pmatrix} x_3 \\ x_4 \\ x_7 \\ x_8 \end{pmatrix} = \frac{1 - y}{(k_{84} + k_{48})(k_{12} + k_{21})} \begin{pmatrix} k_{21}k_{84} \\ k_{84}k_{12} \\ k_{21}k_{48} \\ k_{48}k_{12} \end{pmatrix}.$$

7. Show that the CaMKII dynamical system, Eq. (13.45), may be written

$$\mathbf{p}' = \mathbf{F}\mathbf{p} + b_1([Ca^{2+}])\mathbf{B}\mathbf{p}$$

where

$$\mathbf{F} = \begin{pmatrix} -f_1 & 0 & & & & & \\ f_1 & -f_2 & 0 & & & & \\ 0 & f_2 & -f_3 & 0 & & & \\ & & & \cdots & & & \\ & & 0 & f_8 & -f_9 & 0 & \\ & & & 0 & f_9 & -f_{10} & 0 \\ & & & & 0 & f_{10} & 0 \end{pmatrix} \quad \text{and} \quad \mathbf{B} = \begin{pmatrix} 0 & 1 & & & & & \\ 0 & -1 & 2 & 0 & & & \\ 0 & 0 & -2 & 3 & 0 & & \\ & & & \cdots & & & \\ & & 0 & -8 & 9 & 0 & \\ & & & 0 & -9 & 10 & \\ & & & 0 & 0 & -10 & \end{pmatrix}$$

and that the associated phosphatase/inhibitor system for $\mathbf{q} = ([D]\ [I])^T$, takes the form

$$\mathbf{q}' = \mathbf{C}\mathbf{q} + \mathbf{d}(\mathbf{q}) + \mathbf{g}, \quad \text{where} \quad \mathbf{C} = \begin{pmatrix} -k_4 & 0 \\ -k_4 & -v_{CaN}([Ca^{2+}]) \end{pmatrix}$$

$$\mathbf{d}(\mathbf{q}) = -k_3 q_1 q_2 \begin{pmatrix} 1 \\ 1 \end{pmatrix} \quad \text{and} \quad \mathbf{g} = \begin{pmatrix} k_4[D]_T \\ k_4[D]_T + v_{PKA} I_0 \end{pmatrix}.$$

Code this coupled system, using the model parameters specified in Eq. (13.52), and with a calcium stimulus of the form

$$[Ca^{2+}](t) = 0.1 + 100(\exp(-t) - \exp(-2t)) \quad \mu M, \tag{13.67}$$

arrive at Figure 13.27.

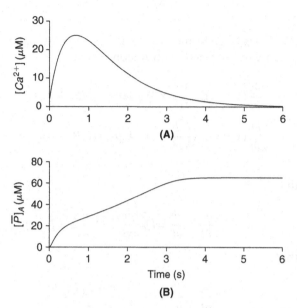

FIGURE 13.27   The dynamic response of the CaMKII system to a transient Ca^{2+} stimulus. (camk2.m)

8. Intracellular calcium concentration is typically inferred from its action on one or more calcium buffers that have been engineered to fluoresce upon the binding of calcium. As in §13.2 we denote calcium concentration by c and use B and b to denote the respective concentrations of free and bound buffer and suppose that

$$c + B \underset{k_2}{\overset{k_1}{\rightleftharpoons}} b. \tag{13.68}$$

We suppose that our buffer, like Fura-2, shifts its excitation spectra with increasing c and that we have measured its fluorescence, F_1 and F_2, at two distinct frequencies. We write each as a linear combination of b and B,

$$F_1 = S_{f_1}B + S_{b_1}b \quad \text{and} \quad F_2 = S_{f_2}B + S_{b_2}b, \tag{13.69}$$

and note that the S coefficients are typically determined via a calibration experiment using known low concentrations of b and B. We now describe how to use Eq. (13.69) to infer c from the ratio $R = F_1/F_2$.

(i) Use the law of mass action in Eq. (13.68) to write a differential equation for b. Set the derivative to zero and confirm that

$$b = cB/K_d \quad \text{where} \quad K_d \equiv k_2/k_1 \tag{13.70}$$

is the dye's dissociation constant. Deduce from Eq. (13.70) that K_d is also the concentration of c at which $b = B$, or, in other words, the concentration of c at which half of the buffer is occupied. The latter interpretation helps explain the frequent use of the word affinity in this context. A buffer is said to have high (low) affinity for calcium if it has a small (large) dissociation constant where small and large are to be interpreted with respect to the resting level $c_r \approx 0.05 \mu M$ of Eq. (13.12). For example, among the native (or endogenous) buffers, calmodulin ($K_d \approx 1\mu M$) is low affinity while parvalbumin ($K_d \approx 0.4$ nM) is high affinity, while among the engineered Ca^{2+} indicators, Fura-2 ($K_d \approx 0.4 \mu M$) and Ca^{2+} Green–1 ($K_d \approx 0.2 \mu M$), are each low affinity.

(ii) Substitute Eq. (13.70) into Eq. (13.69) and find

$$c = K_d \frac{R - (S_{f_1}/S_{f_2})}{(S_{b_1}/S_{b_2}) - R} \frac{S_{f_2}}{S_{b_2}}. \tag{13.71}$$

(iii) In the case of very low c argue from Eq. (13.69) that $F_1/F_2 = S_{f_1}/S_{f_2}$ and call this number R_{min}. In the case of very high c argue from Eq. (13.69) that $F_1/F_2 = S_{b_1}/S_{b_2}$ and call this number R_{max}. Combine these findings and conclude that Eq. (13.71) takes the form

$$c = K_d \frac{R - R_{min}}{R_{max} - R} \frac{S_{f_2}}{S_{b_2}}. \tag{13.72}$$

9. †The argument that led to Eq. (13.70) is often termed the *rapid buffer approximation*. We will now show how it may be used to reduce the dimensionality of the reaction–diffusion system

$$\frac{\partial c}{\partial t}(x,t) = D_c \frac{\partial^2 c}{\partial x^2}(x,t) + k_2 b - k_1 c(B_T - b) + J$$

$$\frac{\partial b}{\partial t}(x,t) = D_b \frac{\partial^2 b}{\partial x^2}(x,t) - k_2 b + k_1 c(B_T - b) \tag{13.73}$$

where J is some input flux.

(i) Deduce from Eq. (13.73) that

$$\frac{\partial c}{\partial t} + \frac{\partial b}{\partial t} = D_c \frac{\partial^2 c}{\partial x^2} + D_b \frac{\partial^2 b}{\partial x^2} + J. \tag{13.74}$$

(ii) Deduce from Eq. (13.70) that

$$\frac{\partial c}{\partial t} + \frac{\partial b}{\partial t} = \frac{(K_d + c)^2 + K_d B_T}{(K_d + c)^2} \frac{\partial c}{\partial t} \tag{13.75}$$

and

$$D_c \frac{\partial^2 c}{\partial x^2} + D_b \frac{\partial^2 b}{\partial x^2} = \frac{1}{(K_d + c)^2} \left((D_c (K_d + c)^2 + D_b K_d B_T) \frac{\partial^2 c}{\partial x^2} - \frac{2 D_b K_d B_T}{K_d + c} \left(\frac{\partial c}{\partial x} \right)^2 \right). \tag{13.76}$$

(iii) Conclude that c obeys the nonlinear diffusion equation

$$((K_d + c)^2 + K_d B_T) \frac{\partial c}{\partial t} = (D_c (K_d + c)^2 + D_b K_d B_T) \frac{\partial^2 c}{\partial x^2} - \frac{2 D_b K_d B_T}{K_d + c} \left(\frac{\partial c}{\partial x} \right)^2 + (K_d + c)^2 J. \tag{13.77}$$

(iv) Under the additional assumptions that the buffer is immobile, $D_b = 0$, and low affinity, $K_d \gg c$, conclude that c obeys

$$(1 + B_T/K_d) \frac{\partial c}{\partial t} = D_c \frac{\partial^2 c}{\partial x^2} + J. \tag{13.78}$$

This equation is very similar to the cable equation, Eq. (6.75), and as such may be solved by an eigenfunction expansion. In particular, with sealed ends, Eq. (13.13), a zero rest state, $c(x,0) = 0$, and a point interior stimulus, $J(x,t) = J_{stim}(t)\delta(x - x_s)$, argue that

$$c(x,t) = \frac{1}{1 + B_T/K_d} \sum_{n=0}^{\infty} q_n(x_s) q_n(x) \int_0^t J_{stim}(s) \exp((t - s)\zeta_n)\, ds \tag{13.79}$$

where the rates are

$$\zeta_n = \frac{D_c}{1 + B_T/K_d} \vartheta_n \tag{13.80}$$

and the eigenfunctions, q_n, and eigenvalues, ϑ_n, are precisely those of Eq. (6.39). Argue that the buffer serves to diminish and retard the response, c, to the stimulus, J.

The Singular Value Decomposition and Applications*

OUTLINE

14.1 The Singular Value Decomposition 223

14.2 Principal Component Analysis and Spike Sorting 226

14.3 Synaptic Plasticity and Principal Components 228

14.4 Neuronal Model Reduction via Balanced Truncation 230

14.5 Summary and Sources 233

14.6 Exercises 233

The singular value decomposition (SVD) is a natural matrix factorization that offers one a quantitative means of discerning what is, and what is not, of importance in the underlying data or model. We build this factorization from ingredients we assembled in our study of the eigendecomposition of symmetric matrices in Chapter 6. We apply this factorization, in its guise as principal component analysis (PCA), to data reduction in the context of sorting spikes that reach a single recording electrode from multiple sources. PCA is a technique for choosing coordinates in which the data exhibit maximal variance. We observe that a simple Hebbian learning rule achieves the same outcome. We then demonstrate how the SVD may be used to reduce the dimension of dynamical models. We show that a 400-dimensional quasi-active cable may be accurately simulated with as few as five variables.

14.1 THE SINGULAR VALUE DECOMPOSITION

The SVD is, in a sense, the eigendecomposition of a rectangular matrix. Of course if $\mathbf{A}$ is m-by-n and $m \neq n$ then it does not make sense to speak of the eigenvalues of $\mathbf{A}$. We turn then to two natural square and symmetric relatives of $\mathbf{A}$,

$$\mathbf{A}^T\mathbf{A} \quad \text{and} \quad \mathbf{A}\mathbf{A}^T.$$

We will argue that the eigenvalues of $\mathbf{A}\mathbf{A}^T$ and $\mathbf{A}^T\mathbf{A}$ are nonnegative and that their nonzero eigenvalues coincide. Let us first confirm this for

$$\mathbf{A} = \begin{pmatrix} 1 & 0 & 1 \\ 0 & 1 & 0 \end{pmatrix}. \tag{14.1}$$

The respective products are

$$\mathbf{A}\mathbf{A}^T = \begin{pmatrix} 2 & 0 \\ 0 & 1 \end{pmatrix} \quad \text{and} \quad \mathbf{A}^T\mathbf{A} = \begin{pmatrix} 1 & 0 & 1 \\ 0 & 1 & 0 \\ 1 & 0 & 1 \end{pmatrix}.$$

Analysis of the first is particularly simple. Its eigenpairs are

$$\lambda_1 = 2, \quad \mathbf{y}_1 = (1 \ 0)^T \quad \text{and} \quad \lambda_2 = 1, \quad \mathbf{y}_2 = (0 \ 1)^T.$$

Regarding $\mathbf{A}^T \mathbf{A}$ we note that

$$\det(\mathbf{A}^T \mathbf{A} - \lambda) = (1 - \lambda)^3 - (1 - \lambda) = \lambda(1 - \lambda)(\lambda - 2)$$

and so its eigenvalues are $\lambda_1 = 2$, $\lambda_2 = 1$, and $\lambda_3 = 0$. Upon evaluating $\mathbf{A}^T \mathbf{A} - \lambda_j \mathbf{I}$ you may confirm that the associated eigenvectors are

$$\mathbf{x}_1 = (1 \ 0 \ 1)^T / \sqrt{2}, \quad \mathbf{x}_2 = (0 \ 1 \ 0)^T, \quad \text{and} \quad \mathbf{x}_3 = (-1 \ 0 \ 1)^T / \sqrt{2}.$$

Hence, for this $\mathbf{A}$, the nonzero eigenvalues of $\mathbf{AA}^T$ and $\mathbf{A}^T \mathbf{A}$ indeed coincide. As, however, their eigenvectors have different dimensions it would seem difficult to compare them. In fact they also are intimately related. In particular, please check that

$$\mathbf{y}_j = \frac{\mathbf{A} \mathbf{x}_j}{\sqrt{\lambda_j}}, \quad j = 1, 2.$$

In preparation for the general SVD we will need the full strength of the eigendecomposition in Exercise 6.4. Recall that we argued there that every symmetric matrix has an orthonormal basis of eigenvectors. To apply this we require a bit more notation. We suppose that $\mathbf{B} \in \mathbb{R}^{n \times n}$ is symmetric and that its characteristic polynomial, $p(\lambda) \equiv \det(\mathbf{B} - \lambda \mathbf{I})$, has $h \leq n$ distinct roots, e.g., $\lambda_1 > \lambda_2 > \cdots > \lambda_h$. We say that λ_j is an eigenvalue of multiplicity n_j if p and its first $n_j - 1$ derivatives all vanish at λ_j. It is a deep and beautiful fact that there will then exist precisely n_j mutually orthogonal eigenvectors, $\mathbf{x}_{j,k}$, $k = 1, 2, \ldots, n_j$, associated with λ_j, and that these multiplicities, n_j, sum to the ambient dimension, n.

Proposition 1. We suppose that $\mathbf{A}$ is real and m-by-n. The eigenvalues of $\mathbf{AA}^T$ and $\mathbf{A}^T \mathbf{A}$ are nonnegative. Their nonzero eigenvalues, including multiplicities, coincide.

Proof. If $\mathbf{A}^T \mathbf{A} \mathbf{x} = \lambda \mathbf{x}$ then $\mathbf{x}^T \mathbf{A}^T \mathbf{A} \mathbf{x} = \lambda \mathbf{x}^T \mathbf{x}$, i.e., $\|\mathbf{A}\mathbf{x}\|^2 = \lambda \|\mathbf{x}\|^2$ and so $\lambda \geq 0$. A similar argument works for $\mathbf{AA}^T$.

Now suppose that $\lambda_j > 0$ and $\mathbf{x}_j$, $\|\mathbf{x}_j\|^2 = 1$, constitute an eigenpair of $\mathbf{A}^T \mathbf{A}$, i.e.,

$$\mathbf{A}^T \mathbf{A} \mathbf{x}_j = \lambda_j \mathbf{x}_j. \tag{14.2}$$

We find, on multiplying through (from the left) by $\mathbf{A}$ that

$$\mathbf{AA}^T \mathbf{A} \mathbf{x}_j = \lambda_j \mathbf{A} \mathbf{x}_j,$$

i.e., λ_j is an eigenvalue of $\mathbf{AA}^T$ with eigenvector $\mathbf{A}\mathbf{x}_j$, so long as $\mathbf{A}\mathbf{x}_j \neq 0$. It follows from the first paragraph of this proof that $\|\mathbf{A}\mathbf{x}_j\| = \sqrt{\lambda_j}$, which, by hypothesis, is nonzero. Hence,

$$\mathbf{y}_j \equiv \frac{\mathbf{A} \mathbf{x}_j}{\sqrt{\lambda_j}}, \tag{14.3}$$

is a unit eigenvector of $\mathbf{AA}^T$ associated with λ_j. In general, if λ_j was an eigenvalue of $\mathbf{A}^T \mathbf{A}$ of multiplicity n_j then for each $\mathbf{x}_{j,k}$ in an orthonormal basis for the associated eigenspace of $\mathbf{A}^T \mathbf{A}$ the above procedure will generate n_j eigenvectors, $\mathbf{y}_{j,k}$, of $\mathbf{AA}^T$. Let us now show that these vectors are indeed orthonormal for fixed j.

$$\mathbf{y}_{j,i}^T \mathbf{y}_{j,k} = \frac{1}{\lambda_j} \mathbf{x}_{j,i}^T \mathbf{A}^T \mathbf{A} \mathbf{x}_{j,k} = \mathbf{x}_{j,i}^T \mathbf{x}_{j,k} = 0.$$

We have now demonstrated that if $\lambda_j > 0$ is an eigenvalue of $\mathbf{A}^T \mathbf{A}$ of multiplicity n_j then it is an eigenvalue of $\mathbf{AA}^T$ of multiplicity at least n_j. Reversing the argument, i.e., generating eigenvectors of $\mathbf{A}^T \mathbf{A}$ from those of $\mathbf{AA}^T$ we find that the multiplicities must indeed coincide. $\qquad \square$

Let us now gather together some of the separate pieces of the proof. For starters, we order the eigenvalues of $\mathbf{A}^T\mathbf{A}$ from high to low,

$$\lambda_1 > \lambda_2 > \cdots > \lambda_h$$

and write

$$\mathbf{A}^T\mathbf{A} = \mathbf{X}\mathbf{\Lambda}_n\mathbf{X}^T \tag{14.4}$$

where

$$\mathbf{X} = (\mathbf{X}_1 \cdots \mathbf{X}_h), \quad \text{and} \quad \mathbf{X}_j = (\mathbf{x}_{j,1} \cdots \mathbf{x}_{j,n_j})$$

and $\mathbf{\Lambda}_n$ is the n-by-n diagonal matrix with λ_1 in the first n_1 slots, λ_2 in the next n_2 slots, etc. Similarly

$$\mathbf{A}\mathbf{A}^T = \mathbf{Y}\mathbf{\Lambda}_m\mathbf{Y}^T \tag{14.5}$$

where

$$\mathbf{Y} = (\mathbf{Y}_1 \cdots \mathbf{Y}_h), \quad \text{and} \quad \mathbf{Y}_j = (\mathbf{y}_{j,1} \cdots \mathbf{y}_{j,n_j})$$

and $\mathbf{\Lambda}_m$ is the m-by-m diagonal matrix with λ_1 in the first n_1 slots, λ_2 in the next n_2 slots, etc. The $\mathbf{y}_{j,k}$ were defined in Eq. (14.3) under the assumption that $\lambda_j > 0$. If $\lambda_j = 0$ let $\mathbf{Y}_j$ denote an orthonormal basis for the associated null space, $\{\mathbf{y} \in \mathbb{R}^m : \mathbf{A}\mathbf{A}^T\mathbf{y} = 0\}$. Finally, call

$$\sigma_j = \sqrt{\lambda_j}$$

and let $\mathbf{\Sigma}$ denote the m-by-n diagonal matrix with σ_1 in the first n_1 slots and σ_2 in the next n_2 slots, etc. Notice that

$$\mathbf{\Sigma}^T\mathbf{\Sigma} = \mathbf{\Lambda}_n \quad \text{and} \quad \mathbf{\Sigma}\mathbf{\Sigma}^T = \mathbf{\Lambda}_m. \tag{14.6}$$

Now recognize that Eq. (14.3) may be written

$$\mathbf{A}\mathbf{x}_{j,k} = \sigma_j\mathbf{y}_{j,k}$$

and that this is simply the column by column rendition of

$$\mathbf{A}\mathbf{X} = \mathbf{Y}\mathbf{\Sigma}.$$

As $\mathbf{X}\mathbf{X}^T = \mathbf{I}$ we may multiply through (from the right) by $\mathbf{X}^T$ and arrive at the **SVD** of $\mathbf{A}$,

$$\boxed{\mathbf{A} = \mathbf{Y}\mathbf{\Sigma}\mathbf{X}^T.} \tag{14.7}$$

Let us confirm this on the $\mathbf{A}$ matrix in Eq. (14.1). We have

$$\mathbf{X} = \frac{1}{\sqrt{2}}\begin{pmatrix} 1 & 0 & -1 \\ 0 & \sqrt{2} & 0 \\ 1 & 0 & 1 \end{pmatrix}, \quad \mathbf{Y} = \begin{pmatrix} 1 & 0 \\ 0 & 1 \end{pmatrix}, \quad \text{and} \quad \mathbf{\Sigma} = \begin{pmatrix} \sqrt{2} & 0 & 0 \\ 0 & 1 & 0 \end{pmatrix}$$

and so $\mathbf{A} = \mathbf{Y}\mathbf{\Sigma}\mathbf{X}^T$. It also agrees with what one receives upon typing [Y,SIG,X] = svd(A) in MATLAB, where SIG = $\mathbf{\Sigma}$.

As a second example, we suppose that $\mathbf{A} = \mathbf{a} \in \mathbb{R}^n$ is a single column. In that case, the inner product, $\mathbf{a}^T\mathbf{a}$ is a scalar, while the outer product, $\mathbf{a}\mathbf{a}^T$ is n-by-n. Regarding the former we note that the nontrivial solution to

$$\mathbf{a}^T\mathbf{a}x = \lambda x \quad \text{is} \quad x = 1 \quad \text{and} \quad \lambda_1 = \mathbf{a}^T\mathbf{a}$$

while a solution to

$$\mathbf{a}\mathbf{a}^T\mathbf{y} = \lambda\mathbf{y} \quad \text{is} \quad \mathbf{y} = \mathbf{a} \quad \text{and} \quad \lambda_1 = \mathbf{a}^T\mathbf{a}.$$

The remaining $n-1$ eigenvalues of $\mathbf{a}\mathbf{a}^T$ are zeros and the eigenvectors may be chosen to be any orthonormal basis for, $\mathbf{a}^\perp$, the orthogonal complement of $\mathbf{a}$,

$$\mathbf{a}^\perp \equiv \{\mathbf{y} \in \mathbb{R}^n : \mathbf{a}^T\mathbf{y} = 0\}.$$

For example, if $\mathbf{a} = (1\ 0\ -1)^T$ then $\mathbf{y}_2 = (0\ 1\ 0)^T$ and $\mathbf{y}_3 = (1\ 0\ 1)^T/\sqrt{2}$ comprise an orthonormal basis for $\mathbf{a}^\perp$. As such

$$\mathbf{Y} = \frac{1}{\sqrt{2}}\begin{pmatrix} 1 & 0 & 1 \\ 0 & \sqrt{2} & 0 \\ -1 & 0 & 1 \end{pmatrix}, \quad \mathbf{X} = 1, \quad \text{and} \quad \mathbf{\Sigma} = \begin{pmatrix} \sqrt{2} \\ 0 \\ 0 \end{pmatrix}$$

are the ingredients in the SVD of $\mathbf{a}$.

14.2 PRINCIPAL COMPONENT ANALYSIS AND SPIKE SORTING

In the processing of high dimensional noisy data the SVD is often used to automatically select prominent features. In one important case, this is done via transforming to coordinates in which the data exhibits extreme variances. To begin, we suppose that we have n observations $\mathbf{a}_1, \mathbf{a}_2, \ldots, \mathbf{a}_n$ of an m-dimensional process. We compute the sample mean

$$\breve{\mathbf{a}} = \frac{1}{n}\sum_{j=1}^n \mathbf{a}_j, \tag{14.8}$$

and construct the *empirical covariance matrix*

$$\breve{\mathbf{C}} = \frac{1}{n}\mathbf{A}\mathbf{A}^T \quad \text{where} \quad \mathbf{A} \equiv (\tilde{\mathbf{a}}_1\ \tilde{\mathbf{a}}_2\ \cdots\ \tilde{\mathbf{a}}_n), \quad \tilde{\mathbf{a}}_j = \mathbf{a}_j - \breve{\mathbf{a}} \tag{14.9}$$

(recall Exercise 11.19). This $\breve{\mathbf{C}} \in \mathbb{R}^{m \times m}$ and we search for the unit vector $\mathbf{u} \in \mathbb{R}^m$ that maximizes the variance

$$\text{var}(\mathbf{u}) \equiv \mathbf{u}^T\breve{\mathbf{C}}\mathbf{u}.$$

We attack this problem by writing $\mathbf{u}$ as a linear combination of the eigenvectors of $\breve{\mathbf{C}}$. In particular, from

$$\breve{\mathbf{C}}\mathbf{y}_j = \lambda_j\mathbf{y}_j, \quad \mathbf{u} = \sum_{j=1}^n u_j\mathbf{y}_j, \quad \text{and} \quad \sum_{j=1}^n u_j^2 = 1$$

we find

$$\text{var}(\mathbf{u}) = \sum_{j=1}^n u_j\mathbf{y}_j^T \sum_{j=1}^n u_j\breve{\mathbf{C}}\mathbf{y}_j = \sum_{j=1}^n u_j\mathbf{y}_j^T \sum_{j=1}^n u_j\lambda_j\mathbf{y}_j = \sum_{j=1}^n \lambda_j u_j^2. \tag{14.10}$$

Recalling that the λ_j are ordered in a decreasing fashion we find that $\text{var}(\mathbf{u}) \leq \lambda_1$ and that this maximum is attained by choosing $\mathbf{u} = \mathbf{y}_1$, the leading eigenvector of $\breve{\mathbf{C}}$. We call $\mathbf{y}_1$ the first **principal component** and call the jth element of $\mathbf{s}_1 \equiv \mathbf{A}^T\mathbf{y}_1$ the **score** for the jth observation on the first principal component.

We next seek that unit vector $\mathbf{u}$ that maximizes $\text{var}(\mathbf{u})$ subject to the additional constraint that it be uncorrelated with the first principal component. We measure correlation via the covariance

$$\text{cov}(\mathbf{u}, \mathbf{y}_1) \equiv \mathbf{u}^T\breve{\mathbf{C}}\mathbf{y}_1 = \lambda_1\mathbf{u}^T\mathbf{y}_1$$

and so uncorrelated means orthogonal, i.e., $\mathbf{u}^T \mathbf{y}_1 = 0$. Inserting this into Eq. (14.10) we find that

$$\max_{\mathbf{u}^T \mathbf{y}_1 = 0} \text{var}(\mathbf{u}) \leq \lambda_2,$$

with equality when $\mathbf{u} = \mathbf{y}_2$. As such, the second principal component is the second eigenvector of $\check{\mathbf{C}}$ and the score for jth observation on the second principal component is the jth element of $\mathbf{s}_2 \equiv \mathbf{A}^T \mathbf{y}_2$.

We now apply this method to the problem of distinguishing the spikes of individual cells within a population from knowledge only of their cumulative impact. This problem occurs when one places an electrode into the extracellular space, common to several adjacent neurons, and records the so-called multi-unit activity over time. The large transmembrane action potentials of the neighboring cells are attenuated by the attending glia and extracellular fluid to the degree that one typically only receives a noisy echo of a spike. As this low amplitude oscillatory echo resembles (recall Chapter 5) the quasi-active response to intracellular excitation we synthesize such records by distorting the sum of the quasi-active responses of three distinct trains of stimuli. In particular, we suppose the cells to have distinct conductances and we suppose each to be driven by a periodic current of the form

$$I(t) = I_0(\exp(-t/\tau_1) - \exp(-t/\tau_2)), \quad I(t) = I(t + T).$$

The precise values of the conductance and current parameters may be found in Table 14.1. We have coded these cells and illustrated our findings in Figure 14.1. Each of the 98 spikelets in Figure 14.1B contains 601 samples. We consider each trace to be a column $\mathbf{a}_j \in \mathbb{R}^{601}$. We next remove the sample mean and construct the data matrix $\mathbf{A}$ per Eq. (14.9). We need not physically construct $\check{\mathbf{C}}$, for [Y,Sig,X]=svd(A) will return the desired principal components in Y. The singular value decomposition of Y, see Figure 14.2, indeed permits us to cluster the spikes emanating from distinct cells.

TABLE 14.1   The conductance and current parameters of the three synthetic cells.

Cell	$\bar{g}_K$	$\bar{g}_{Na}$	g_{Cl}	I_0	τ_1	τ_2	T
1	36	140	2	0.95	0.6	0.5	50
2	38	120	1	0.9	0.5	0.4	90
3	40	100	0.3	0.7	0.7	0.6	70

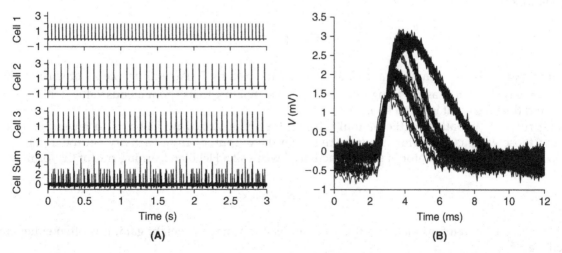

FIGURE 14.1   **A.** The three spike trains and their tainted sum, corrupted by additive Gaussian noise of zero mean and standard deviation equal to 0.1 mV. The experimentalist only has access to the latter. **B.** The spikelets are excised from the long train and aligned. The challenge is to determine both how many cells are firing and to identify which spike belongs to which cell. The eye detects at least five potentially distinct clusters. (spikepca.m)

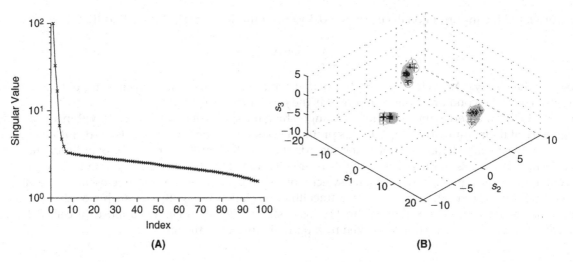

FIGURE 14.2   **A.** The singular values of the data matrix exhibit very rapid decay. This suggests that the greatest variance in the traces is captured by the first three, and possibly four, associated singular vectors, $\mathbf{y}_j$. **B.** We compute the three score vectors, $\mathbf{s}_j = \mathbf{A}^T \mathbf{y}_j$, $j = 1, 2, 3$, and plot (black +) their triples, $(\mathbf{s}_{1,k}, \mathbf{s}_{2,k}, \mathbf{s}_{3,k})$ for the traces $k = 1, \ldots, 98$. As we generated the spikes we know which cell gave rise to which spike. In red we used circles to mark the spikes from cell 1, squares to mark the spikes from cell 2, and diamonds to mark the spikes from cell 3. We note that these fall into easily separated clusters in the space of score coordinates. (spikepca.m)

14.3 SYNAPTIC PLASTICITY AND PRINCIPAL COMPONENTS

In §12.6 we learned that synapses can undergo long-term potentiation (LTP), a strengthening based on coincident presynaptic and postsynaptic activity. LTP and the opposite change, long-term depression (LTD), are thought to be one of the biophysical mechanisms by which learning may be implemented in neuronal networks. In this section, we illustrate how LTP and LTD may be involved in learning associations about external inputs. We focus on the learning stage in the simplest context. We suppose the neuron is linear and that time is discrete. In particular, v_j, the neuron's scalar output at "time" j is assumed to be a weighted sum of its n inputs, $\mathbf{x}_j \in \mathbb{R}^n$. If we denote these weights by $\mathbf{w} \in \mathbb{R}^n$ we find

$$v_j = \mathbf{w}^T \mathbf{x}_j. \tag{14.11}$$

We suppose that the inputs, $\{\mathbf{x}_1, \mathbf{x}_2, \ldots\}$, are independent zero mean and identically distributed, and denote the common correlation matrix by

$$\mathbf{C} \equiv E[\mathbf{x}_j \mathbf{x}_j^T]. \tag{14.12}$$

The collection, $\{\mathbf{x}_j\}_{j=1}^{\infty}$, is an example of a *stochastic process*, indexed by j. (We will devote all of Chapter 16 to such processes). We may think of v_j as the firing rate of the neuron, relative to its spontaneous value, within a short time interval around the time point indexed by j.

Regarding rules for updating $\mathbf{w}$, the natural scheme, first popularized by Hebb, is to reward cooperation by incrementing those weights that bring about "activity" in the output, v_j, from "activity" in the input, $\mathbf{x}_j$. As their product, $v_j \mathbf{x}_j$, is the simplest indicator of such "coactivity," we posit a Hebbian learning rule of the form

$$\mathbf{w}_{j+1} = \mathbf{w}_j + \gamma_j v_j \mathbf{x}_j, \tag{14.13}$$

where γ_j is the degree of reinforcement. As this rule can lead to runaway weight gain, it is often either clipped or normalized via

$$\mathbf{w}_{j+1} = \frac{\mathbf{w}_j + \gamma_j v_j \mathbf{x}_j}{\|\mathbf{w}_j + \gamma_j v_j \mathbf{x}_j\|}. \tag{14.14}$$

For small γ_j this rule takes the form (see Exercise 5)

$$\mathbf{w}_{j+1} = \mathbf{w}_j + \gamma_j v_j(\mathbf{x}_j - v_j \mathbf{w}_j) + O(\gamma_j^2)$$

$$= \mathbf{w}_j + \gamma_j(\mathbf{x}_j \mathbf{x}_j^T - \mathbf{w}_j^T \mathbf{x}_j \mathbf{x}_j^T \mathbf{w}_j \mathbf{I})\mathbf{w}_j + O(\gamma_j^2).$$

(14.15)

With Eq. (14.12) and

$$\boldsymbol{\xi}_j \equiv (\mathbf{x}_j \mathbf{x}_j^T - \mathbf{C})\mathbf{w}_j - \mathbf{w}_j^T(\mathbf{x}_j \mathbf{x}_j^T - \mathbf{C})\mathbf{w}_j \mathbf{w}_j$$

(14.16)

Eq. (14.15) takes the form

$$\mathbf{w}_{j+1} = \mathbf{w}_j + \gamma_j(\mathbf{C} - \mathbf{w}_j^T \mathbf{C} \mathbf{w}_j \mathbf{I})\mathbf{w}_j + \gamma_j \boldsymbol{\xi}_j + O(\gamma_j^2).$$

(14.17)

There is a sizable literature on *Stochastic Approximation Methods* devoted to showing that the solution to such a stochastic difference equation is well approximated by an associated deterministic differential equation (see §14.5). In our case, the independence of $\{\mathbf{x}_j\}_{j=1,2...}$ ensures that if $\gamma_j \to 0$ like $1/j$ then solutions to the difference equation (14.17) converge to solutions to the differential equation

$$\mathbf{w}'(t) = (\mathbf{C} - \mathbf{w}(t)^T \mathbf{C} \mathbf{w}(t)\mathbf{I})\mathbf{w}(t).$$

(14.18)

We first show that solutions to Eq. (14.18) remain bounded. On multiplying each side by $\mathbf{w}^T$ we find

$$\frac{d}{dt}\|\mathbf{w}(t)\|^2 = 2\mathbf{w}(t)^T \mathbf{C} \mathbf{w}(t)(1 - \|\mathbf{w}(t)\|^2).$$

As $\mathbf{C}$ is positive semidefinite this states that $\|\mathbf{w}(t)\|$ is decreasing whenever $\|\mathbf{w}(t)\| > 1$. To investigate the asymptotic behavior we recall the eigendecomposition $\mathbf{C}\mathbf{Q} = \mathbf{Q}\boldsymbol{\Lambda}$ and express $\mathbf{w}(t) = \mathbf{Q}\mathbf{u}(t)$. It follows that $\mathbf{u}$ obeys

$$\mathbf{u}'(t) = \boldsymbol{\Lambda}\mathbf{u}(t) - (\mathbf{u}(t)^T \boldsymbol{\Lambda}\mathbf{u}(t))\mathbf{u}(t)$$

(14.19)

and so $\mathbf{v} \equiv \mathbf{u}/u_1$ obeys

$$\mathbf{v}'(t) = (\boldsymbol{\Lambda} - \lambda_1 \mathbf{I})\mathbf{v}$$

(14.20)

and so, if $\lambda_1 > \lambda_2$ then $u_i/u_1 \to 0$ for each $i > 1$. As the terms are also bounded we have shown that $\mathbf{u}(t) \to \mathbf{e}_1$ and so $\mathbf{w}(t) \to \mathbf{q}_1$. In other words, the normalized Hebbian rule Eq. (14.14) produces a synaptic weight vector that approaches the principal eigenvector of the correlation matrix of the cell's stochastic input.

The previous arguments do not rely on $\{\mathbf{x}_j\}_{j=1,2...}$ being zero mean or equivalently on $\mathbf{C}$ being the covariance matrix of $\{\mathbf{x}_j\}_{j=1,2...}$. For example, we note that if $\mathbf{x}_j = \mathbf{s} + \mathbf{n}_j$ where $\mathbf{s}$ is a fixed unit vector and the $\mathbf{n}_j$ are independently drawn from a zero mean distribution with covariance $\sigma^2 \mathbf{I}$, then

$$\mathbf{C} = E[\mathbf{x}_j \mathbf{x}_j^T] = \mathbf{s}\mathbf{s}^T + E[\mathbf{n}_j \mathbf{n}_j^T] = \mathbf{s}\mathbf{s}^T + \sigma^2 \mathbf{I}$$

and the largest eigenvalue of $\mathbf{C}$ is $1 + \sigma^2$ with $\mathbf{s}$ the associated eigenvector. As $\mathbf{C}^{-1}\mathbf{s} = \mathbf{s}/(1 + \sigma^2)$ we recognize that this neuron behaves like the classical *matched filter* of Exercise 7.

For a slightly richer example, we sample $y_{j,1} \in \mathcal{N}(0,1)$ and $y_{j,2} \in \mathcal{N}(0,16)$ and then stack and rotate by $\pi/6$ to obtain

$$\mathbf{x}_j = \begin{pmatrix} \cos(\pi/6) & \sin(\pi/6) \\ -\sin(\pi/6) & \cos(\pi/6) \end{pmatrix}\begin{pmatrix} y_{j,1} \\ y_{j,2} \end{pmatrix}.$$

(14.21)

We have plotted these points in Figure 14.3A for three distinct trials, each of length 500. For each trial we construct the 2-by-2 *empirical correlation matrix*

$$\check{\mathbf{C}} = \frac{1}{499}(\mathbf{x}_1 \ \mathbf{x}_2 \ \cdots \ \mathbf{x}_{500})(\mathbf{x}_1 \ \mathbf{x}_2 \ \cdots \ \mathbf{x}_{500})^T$$

(14.22)

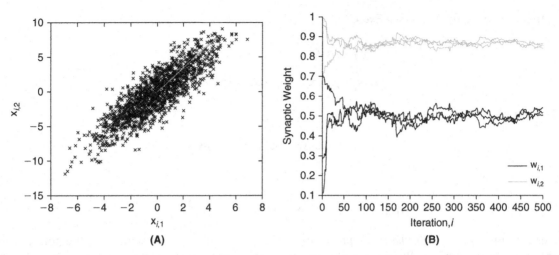

FIGURE 14.3   **A.** Three data trials, black x points, and the associated leading eigenvectors (stretched for better visibility), in red, of the empirical correlation matrix, Eq. (14.22). **B.** The associated trajectories of $\mathbf{w}_j$, per Eq. (14.15), for each of the three trials. The trajectories indeed converge to the leading eigenvector of their respective empirical correlation matrices. (ojasim.m)

and plot its leading eigenvector in red. Figure 14.3B shows the convergence of the weights towards (a scaled version of) the leading eigenvector under the update rule of Eq. (14.15).

14.4 NEURONAL MODEL REDUCTION VIA BALANCED TRUNCATION

We start from the general linear autonomous dynamical system (i.e., with time-independent coefficients $\mathbf{B}$ and $\mathbf{C}$),

$$\mathbf{x}'(t) = \mathbf{B}\mathbf{x}(t) + \mathbf{C}\mathbf{u}(t), \quad \mathbf{x}(0) = \mathbf{x}_0, \quad \mathbf{y}(t) = \mathbf{D}\mathbf{x}(t), \tag{14.23}$$

where $\mathbf{x}(t) \in \mathbb{R}^n$ is the state of the system, $\mathbf{u}(t) \in \mathbb{R}^m$ is the control or stimulus variable, and $\mathbf{y}(t) \in \mathbb{R}^p$ represent observations. In the example to be treated below, $\mathbf{x}$ will be the membrane potential and conductance state variables in the compartments of the quasi-active cable of §9.4, $\mathbf{u}$ the current injected in the cable, and $\mathbf{y}$ the membrane potential observed in one of the cable compartments. We recall two classical results of Modern Control Theory regarding the control and observation of the solution, $\mathbf{x}$. Namely, one can find a stimulus $\mathbf{u}$ that drives the initial disturbance, $\mathbf{x}(0)$, to zero so long as the Controllability Gramian

$$\mathbf{P} \equiv \int_0^\infty \exp(t\mathbf{B}) \mathbf{C}\mathbf{C}^T \exp(t\mathbf{B}^T) \, dt \tag{14.24}$$

is invertible. In a similar fashion, the initial disturbance may be recovered from the observation, $\mathbf{y}$, so long as the Observability Gramian

$$\mathbf{Q} \equiv \int_0^\infty \exp(t\mathbf{B}^T) \mathbf{D}^T \mathbf{D} \exp(t\mathbf{B}) \, dt \tag{14.25}$$

is invertible. Recall that the matrix exponential, $\exp(t\mathbf{B})$, was defined in Eq. (5.30). As $\mathbf{P}$ and $\mathbf{Q}$ will be central to our reduction we pause to develop a number of their key properties. To begin we note that they are both symmetric and positive semidefinite. Next, we note that the integrand of $\mathbf{P}$,

$$\mathbf{E}(t) \equiv \exp(t\mathbf{B}) \mathbf{C}\mathbf{C}^T \exp(t\mathbf{B}^T) \tag{14.26}$$

satisfies the matrix differential equation

$$\mathbf{E}'(t) = \mathbf{B}\mathbf{E}(t) + \mathbf{E}(t)\mathbf{B}^T, \quad \mathbf{E}(0) = \mathbf{C}\mathbf{C}^T \tag{14.27}$$

(Exercise 8). If we now integrate each side we find

$$\mathbf{E}(\infty) - \mathbf{E}(0) = \mathbf{B} \left(\int_0^\infty \mathbf{E}(t)\,dt \right) + \left(\int_0^\infty \mathbf{E}(t)\,dt \right) \mathbf{B}^T.$$

If the eigenvalues of $\mathbf{B}$ are in the left half plane, i.e., have negative real parts, then $\exp(t\mathbf{B}) \to 0$ as $t \to \infty$ and hence $\mathbf{E}(\infty) = 0$. Therefore $\mathbf{P}$ must obey

$$\boxed{\mathbf{BP} + \mathbf{PB}^T + \mathbf{CC}^T = 0.} \tag{14.28}$$

In a similar fashion, we note that the integrand of $\mathbf{Q}$,

$$\mathbf{F}(t) \equiv \exp(t\mathbf{B}^T)\mathbf{D}^T\mathbf{D}\exp(t\mathbf{B}) \tag{14.29}$$

satisfies

$$\mathbf{F}'(t) = \mathbf{B}^T\mathbf{F}(t) + \mathbf{F}(t)\mathbf{B}, \quad \mathbf{F}(0) = \mathbf{D}^T\mathbf{D}. \tag{14.30}$$

If we now integrate each side we find

$$\mathbf{F}(\infty) - \mathbf{F}(0) = \mathbf{B}^T \left(\int_0^\infty \mathbf{F}(t)\,dt \right) + \left(\int_0^\infty \mathbf{F}(t)\,dt \right) \mathbf{B}.$$

Arguing as above, we find $\mathbf{F}(\infty) = 0$, and so conclude that $\mathbf{Q}$ must obey

$$\boxed{\mathbf{B}^T\mathbf{Q} + \mathbf{QB} + \mathbf{D}^T\mathbf{D} = 0.} \tag{14.31}$$

These linear systems for $\mathbf{P}$, Eq. (14.28), and $\mathbf{Q}$, Eq. (14.31), are referred to as Lyapunov equations.

The balancing act in balanced truncation is achieved by a transformation, $\mathbf{\Phi}$, that reduces both $\mathbf{P}$ and $\mathbf{Q}$ to a common diagonal matrix. To begin, we gather the Cholesky factors (recall Exercise 6.7)

$$\mathbf{P} = \mathbf{UU}^T \quad \text{and} \quad \mathbf{Q} = \mathbf{LL}^T \tag{14.32}$$

and compute the SVD of the mixed product

$$\mathbf{U}^T\mathbf{L} = \mathbf{Y}\mathbf{\Sigma}\mathbf{X}^T. \tag{14.33}$$

Here $\mathbf{\Sigma}$ is a diagonal matrix whose entries are the eigenvalues of $\mathbf{U}^T\mathbf{Q}\mathbf{U}$, $\mathbf{Y}$ is an orthogonal matrix whose columns are the eigenvectors of $\mathbf{U}^T\mathbf{Q}\mathbf{U}$, and $\mathbf{X}$ is an orthogonal matrix whose columns are the eigenvectors of $\mathbf{L}^T\mathbf{P}\mathbf{L}$. The diagonal elements of $\mathbf{\Sigma}$ are nonnegative and in descending order and are known as the **Hankel Singular Values** of system Eq. (14.23). We now compose

$$\mathbf{\Phi} = \mathbf{\Sigma}^{-1/2}\mathbf{X}^T\mathbf{L}^T \quad \text{and} \quad \mathbf{\Phi}^{-1} = \mathbf{UY}\mathbf{\Sigma}^{-1/2},$$

and note that the transformed gramians

$$\tilde{\mathbf{P}} \equiv \mathbf{\Phi}\mathbf{P}\mathbf{\Phi}^T \quad \text{and} \quad \tilde{\mathbf{Q}} = \mathbf{\Phi}^{-T}\mathbf{Q}\mathbf{\Phi}^{-1}$$

are balanced and diagonal in the sense that

$$\tilde{\mathbf{P}} = \tilde{\mathbf{Q}} = \mathbf{\Sigma} \tag{14.34}$$

(Exercise 11). Moreover they are the gramians of the transformed state, $\tilde{x} \equiv \Phi x$, which itself is governed by the transformed dynamical system as

$$\tilde{x}'(t) = \widetilde{B}\tilde{x}(t) + \widetilde{C}u(t), \qquad y(t) = \widetilde{D}\tilde{x}(t) \tag{14.35}$$

where $\widetilde{B} = \Phi B \Phi^{-1}$, $\widetilde{C} = \Phi C$, and $\widetilde{D} = D\Phi^{-1}$ (Exercise 12). Based on the decay of the singular values in Σ, we can construct a reduced model by using only the k largest singular values. This corresponds to approximating Eq. (14.35) with

$$x_b'(t) = B_b x_b(t) + C_b u(t) \qquad y_b(t) = D_b x_b(t), \tag{14.36}$$

where B_b is the initial $k \times k$ submatrix of $\widetilde{B}$, C_b is the first k rows of $\widetilde{C}$, and D_b is the first k columns of $\widetilde{D}$.

Let us now put this method into practice on the quasi-active cable of §9.4. The matrix B is a discrete version (with S for ∂_{xx}) of Eq. (9.23) while C, the matrix that marks the equations and compartments that may receive input, is the identity on the current equations coordinates and zero elsewhere. In particular, with reference to the block structure in Eq. (9.23),

$$C = \begin{pmatrix} 0 & 0 & 0 & 0 \\ 0 & 0 & 0 & 0 \\ 0 & 0 & 0 & 0 \\ 0 & 0 & 0 & I \end{pmatrix}.$$

Here each block is N-by-N where N is the number of compartments. The identity in the bottom right block will permit independent current injection into each compartment. Finally, if our output variable of interest is the potential at $x = \ell/10$ then D is the 1-by-$4N$ vector of zeros save for a one in the associated voltage compartment, i.e., at index $3N + N/10$. We have coded the full and reduced systems in stEQcabBT.m and illustrate its use in Figure 14.4.

We stress that the remarkable fit in Figure 14.4(B) of the response to two such widely different systems is **not** dependent on our choice of stimulus. As the reduction was built solely from the associated (B, C, D) system its performance is not affected by the choice of input, u. It is, however, limited to reproducing the response only at those sites specified in the D matrix. We will pursue this limitation in the exercises. Regarding implementation, we note that other than the SVD of Eq. (14.33) we must compute the Cholesky factors of the solution to the two Lyapunov equations, (14.28) and (14.31). MATLAB's control toolbox contains a function lyapchol that delivers exactly what we need.

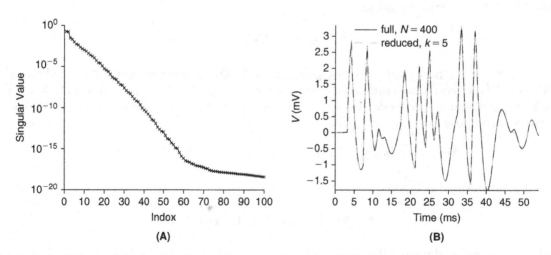

FIGURE 14.4 A. Rapid decay of the singular values of the quasi-active cable of §9.4 with $N = 100$ compartments. **B.** Response of the full, 400-dimensional, and reduced, five-dimensional, quasi-active cable subjected to 50 randomly distributed (in space and time) current injections, each of 1 ms duration and 10 nA amplitude. (stEQcabBT.m)

14.5 SUMMARY AND SOURCES

We have established the SVD and discussed its importance to three central problems of Computational Neuroscience: Spike Sorting, Synaptic Plasticity, and Neuronal Model Reduction. For more on this decomposition, as well as the Schur decomposition of Exercise 9, see Golub and van Loan (1996). Goldman (2009) has exploited the Schur decomposition to build a class of functionally feedforward networks that achieve sustained, memory-like, behavior without positive feedback. The challenges of spike sorting are well documented in Buzsáki (2004) and the connection to PCA is surveyed in Lewicki (1998). Eq. (14.18) is known as the Oja Rule after Oja (1982). The proof that solutions of the difference equation (14.17) converge to solutions of the differential equation (14.18) relies on Theorem 2.3.1 of Kushner and Clark (1978). In our case, the independence of $\{x_j\}_{j=1,2...}$ ensures that $E[\xi_j|\xi_i, i<j, w_i, i\leq j]=0$, and it follows from Theorem 2.3.1 that if $\gamma_j \to 0$ like $1/j$ then solutions to the difference equation (14.17) converge to solutions to the differential equation (14.18). The concept of a matched filter will be encountered again in §24.4, when we study the detection of multidimensional Gaussian signals. Model reduction via balanced truncation goes back to Moore (1981). The results in §14.4 are drawn from Kellems et al. (2009).

14.6 EXERCISES

1. Let us construct, by hand, the SVD of

$$A=\begin{pmatrix} 1 & 0 & 1 & 0 \\ 0 & 1 & 0 & 1 \end{pmatrix}. \tag{14.37}$$

As AA^T is simply twice the 2-by-2 identity matrix argue that

$$\lambda_1=\lambda_2=2 \quad \text{and} \quad y_1=(1\ 0)^T \quad \text{and} \quad y_2=(0\ 1)^T.$$

Turning to A^TA we find

$$A^TA=\begin{pmatrix} 1 & 0 & 1 & 0 \\ 0 & 1 & 0 & 1 \\ 1 & 0 & 1 & 0 \\ 0 & 1 & 0 & 1 \end{pmatrix}.$$

We know from Proposition 1 that its eigenvalues are 2, 2, 0, and 0. The latter two are apparent from the fact that A^TA possesses only two linearly independent rows. For $j=1$ and 2 use Eq. (14.3) to find x_1 and x_2. Solve $A^TAx=0$ to find an orthonormal pair, x_3 and x_4. Please complete the triad by specifying Σ and confirming that $A=Y\Sigma X^T$.

2. The SVD suggests a simple procedure for addressing equations of the form $Ax=b$ in situations where either the solution x does not exist or the solution is not unique. The idea is to construct a pseudoinverse of $A \in \mathbb{R}^{m\times n}$ by reciprocating its nonzero singular values. Because m is not necessarily n we must also be careful with dimensions. To be precise, let Σ^+ denote the n-by-m matrix whose first n_1 diagonal elements are $1/\sigma_1$, whose next n_2 diagonal elements are $1/\sigma_2$ and so on. In the case that $\sigma_h=0$, set the final n_h diagonal elements of Σ^+ to zero. Now, one defines the pseudoinverse of A to be

$$A^+ \equiv X\Sigma^+Y^T. \tag{14.38}$$

Our pseudosolution to $Ax=b$ is naturally A^+b. Though it is too much to hope that $AA^+b=b$ we shall see that our pseudosolution is in fact the actual solution to a related linear system. Please justify each of the following steps

$$(A^TA)A^+b=X\Lambda_nX^TX\Sigma^+Y^Tb$$
$$=X\Lambda_n\Sigma^+Y^Tb$$
$$=X\Sigma^T\Sigma\Sigma^+Y^Tb$$
$$=X\Sigma^TY^Tb$$
$$=A^Tb.$$

We have shown that $x = A^+b$ is a solution to $A^TAx = A^Tb$. This latter system is typically called the set of normal equations. They arise in searching for that x that yields the least squared error, $\|Ax - b\|^2$.

3. †Use Eq. (14.38) to compute, by hand, the pseudoinverse of the A in Eq. (14.37). Confirm that your answer agrees with what `pinv` returns in MATLAB. Use your pseudoinverse to pseudosolve $Ax = (1\ 1)^T$. Show in fact that it is a true solution, but note that it is not unique by finding a second solution, z. Please confirm that $\|x\| \leq \|z\|$.

4. †Show that $x_{LS} = A^+b$ is the vector that minimizes $\|Ax - b\|^2$ with the smallest norm. First, suppose that the first k singular values are nonzero and justify the following steps:

$$\|Ax - b\|^2 = \|Y^T(Ax - b)\|^2$$
$$= \|\Sigma X^Tx - Y^Tb\|^2$$
$$= \sum_{i=1}^{k}(\sigma_i(X^Tx)_i - (Y^Tb)_i)^2 + \sum_{i=k+1}^{m}((Y^Tb)_i)^2.$$

Deduce from this last equation that $(X^Tx)_i = (Y^Tb)_i/\sigma_i$ for $i \leq k$. For $i > k$, X^Tx will have smallest norm if $(X^Tx)_i = 0$. Show that this endows x with smallest norm by arguing that $\|X^Tx\| = \|x\|$. Argue that the resulting x is indeed A^+b.

5. Given Eq. (14.11), assume that γ_j is small and argue that

$$\frac{1}{\|w_j + \gamma_j v_j x_j\|} = \frac{1}{\|w_j\|} - \gamma_j \frac{v_j^2}{\|w_j\|^3} + O(\gamma_j^2).$$

Now argue that this yields Eq. (14.15) when $\|w_j\| = 1$.

6. †Show that if w obeys Eq. (14.18) and $w = Qu$ where $CQ = Q\Lambda$ then u must satisfy Eq. (14.19). Furthermore, show that if $v = u/u_1$ then v must satisfy Eq. (14.20). Finally, deduce from this that $u(t) \to e_1$.

7. †We consider a signal, $s \in \mathbb{R}^m$, corrupted by additive noise, $n \in \mathbb{R}^m$. The *matched filter* is that choice of $w \in \mathbb{R}^m$ that maximizes the signal-to-noise ratio,

$$SNR(w) \equiv \frac{(w^Ts)^2}{E[(w^Tn)^2]}.$$

(i) Argue that if $C = E[nn^T]$ then

$$SNR(w) = \frac{(w^Ts)^2}{w^TCw}.$$

(ii) Now factor $C = UU^T$ per Cholesky (Exercise 6.7) and arrive at

$$SNR(w) = \frac{((U^Tw)^TU^{-1}s)^2}{w^TUU^Tw}.$$

(iii) Next apply the Schwarz inequality, Eq. (1.2), to the numerator to find

$$SNR(w) \leq s^TC^{-1}s,$$

and argue that this bound is achieved when $w = \alpha C^{-1}s$, for any $\alpha \neq 0$. The scale, α, is often chosen to render $E[(w^Tn)^2] = 1$. Show that

$$\alpha = \frac{1}{\sqrt{s^TC^{-1}s}}$$

does the job.

8. Use Eq. (5.29) to confirm that E and F as defined in Eqs. (14.26) and (14.29) satisfy the stated differential equations, (14.27) and (14.30).

9. There is another matrix decomposition, due to Schur, with wide application. It states that for each $\mathbf{B} \in \mathbb{C}^{N \times N}$ there exists a unitary matrix $\mathbf{X} \in \mathbb{C}^{N \times N}$ and an upper triangular matrix $\mathbf{U} \in \mathbb{C}^{N \times N}$ for which

$$\mathbf{B} = \mathbf{XUX}^H. \tag{14.39}$$

We are working here with complex matrices because, lacking any symmetry, real matrices have complex eigenvalues. Here $\mathbf{X}^H$ denotes conjugate transpose of $\mathbf{X}$ and to say $\mathbf{X}$ is unitary is to say that $\mathbf{X}^H \mathbf{X} = \mathbf{I}$.

We now establish Eq. (14.39) by induction. We note that it is trivially true when $N = 1$. We must then deduce that if it is true for matrices of size $N - 1$ then it is true for matrices of size N. To make this step suppose that $\mathbf{y}_1$ is a unit eigenvector of $\mathbf{B}$ with eigenvalue λ and that $\{\mathbf{y}_n\}_{n=2}^N$ comprises an orthonormal basis for $\mathbf{y}^\perp \equiv \{\mathbf{x} \in \mathbb{C}^N : \mathbf{x}^H \mathbf{y} = 0\}$. Lay these $\mathbf{y}_n$ into the columns of the matrix $\mathbf{Y}$ and argue that the product $\mathbf{BY}$ may be decomposed like

$$\mathbf{BY} = (\mathbf{By}_1 \ \mathbf{By}_2 \ \cdots \ \mathbf{By}_N) = \mathbf{Y} \begin{pmatrix} \lambda & \mathbf{v} \\ 0 & \mathbf{V} \end{pmatrix} \tag{14.40}$$

for some $\mathbf{v} \in \mathbb{C}^{1 \times N-1}$ and $\mathbf{V} \in \mathbb{C}^{N-1 \times N-1}$. These are simply names for pieces of the matrix. The crucial piece, for you to justify, is the set of $N - 1$ zeros in the first column. For this is the step that permits induction. In particular, as $\mathbf{V} \in \mathbb{C}^{N-1 \times N-1}$ and the Schur decomposition is assumed to hold in dimension $N - 1$ there exists a unitary $\mathbf{Z}$ and an upper triangular $\mathbf{W}$ for which $\mathbf{V} = \mathbf{ZWZ}^H$. From here argue that

$$\mathbf{X} \equiv \mathbf{Y} \begin{pmatrix} 1 & 0 \\ 0 & \mathbf{Z} \end{pmatrix}$$

is unitary and that $\mathbf{X}^H \mathbf{BX}$ is indeed upper triangular.

10. †We use the Schur decomposition to simplify the Lyapunov equation, (14.28). Substitute $\mathbf{B} = \mathbf{XUX}^H$ into Eq. (14.28), multiply the result on the left by $\mathbf{X}^H$ and on the right by $\mathbf{X}$ and arrive at the simple system

$$\mathbf{U}\mathcal{P} + \mathcal{P}\mathbf{U}^H + \mathcal{C}\mathcal{C}^H = 0. \tag{14.41}$$

How do $\mathcal{P}$ and $\mathcal{C}$ relate to $\mathbf{P}$ and $\mathbf{C}$? Use the triangular nature of $\mathbf{U}$ to show that Eq. (14.41) may be solved by back substitution. In particular, if $\mathbf{B} \in \mathbb{R}^{n \times n}$ give exact formulas for $\mathcal{P}_{n,n}$ and $\mathcal{P}_{n,n-1}$ and sketch an algorithm for the rest.

11. †Confirm the key balance identity, Eq. (14.34).

12. †Confirm that the transformed state, $\tilde{\mathbf{x}}$, indeed obeys Eq. (14.35).

13. Modify `stEQcabBT.m` to accommodate observation of the potential at both $x = \ell/10$ and $x = 9\ell/10$. The $\mathbf{D}$ matrix will now be 2-by-4N. Reproduce Figure 14.5.

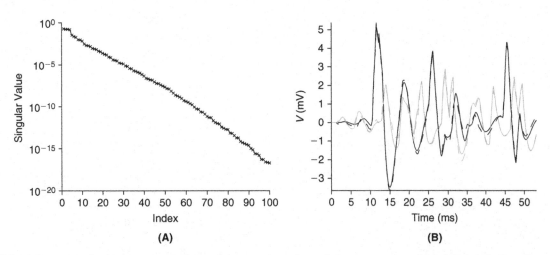

(A)

(B)

FIGURE 14.5 **A.** Significantly less rapid decay of the singular values of the quasi-active cable of §9.4 with $N = 100$ compartments. **B.** Response (at $\ell/10$ in black and at $9\ell/10$ in red) of the full (solid), 400-dimensional, and reduced (dashed), five-dimensional, quasi-active cable subjected to 50 randomly distributed (in space and time) current injections, each of 1 ms duration and 10 nA amplitude. (`stEQcabBT2.m`)

Quantification of Spike Train Variability

OUTLINE

15.1 Interspike Interval Histograms and
Coefficient of Variation   238

15.2 Refractory Period   239

15.3 Spike Count Distribution and Fano Factor 240

15.4 Renewal Processes   240

15.5 Return Maps and Empirical Correlation
Coefficient   243

15.6 Summary and Sources   245

15.7 Exercises   246

Many sensory neurons are spontaneously active when recorded *in vivo* or *in vitro*, i.e., they generate action potentials at random intervals in time. For sensory neurons, spontaneous activity is usually defined as that activity recorded in the absence of any experimental sensory stimulation. Spontaneous activity is in part due to the random release of neurotransmitter at synapses, but other mechanisms presumably also contribute. In sensory receptor cells, the random activation of the transduction machinery such as isomerization of light-sensitive pigments in photoreceptors will cause the activation of downstream neurons. Similarly, ion channels in the membrane of nerve cells spontaneously open and close and thus probably also contribute to fluctuations in membrane potential that could sometimes elicit spontaneous action potentials.

Spontaneous activity and the ensuing spike train variability is important for several reasons.

1. Spontaneous activity can be thought of as *noise* that will limit the reliability at which neural signals can be transmitted. For example, if a photoreceptor spontaneously generates signals in the absence of light, these signals can be confused with a true (faint) light change. Thus, this noise poses a fundamental limit to the ability of an animal to detect light. Similarly, if a sensory neuron is spontaneously active, its action potentials could be a source of "noise" for downstream neurons processing its output. In the case of central neurons the situation is a bit less clear than at the receptor level, since what we characterize as spontaneous activity or "noise" could be of significance to a downstream neuron in a manner that we do not appreciate.

2. Spontaneous activity most probably contributes to the development of neuronal circuits and to the maintenance and regulation of synaptic connections between neurons in mature circuits.

3. Different neurons exhibit different patterns of spontaneous activity. Thus spontaneous activity must be related to the characteristics of neurons such as their morphology, ion channel distribution, and their pattern of synaptic connections. Spontaneous activity therefore offers a way to gain information about neuronal characteristics.

We first introduce the methods used to describe spike train variability of nerve cells and present examples of spontaneous activity patterns encountered in neurons. As we will see, these methods also help describe the variability of neuronal spike trains in responses to external stimuli.

Mathematics for Neuroscientists. DOI: 10.1016/B978-0-12-374882-9.00015-0

15.1 INTERSPIKE INTERVAL HISTOGRAMS AND COEFFICIENT OF VARIATION

The simplest way to describe the variability in spontaneous activity of neurons is to plot a histogram of the time intervals separating two action potentials. That is, if t_i is the time of occurrence of the i-th action potential recorded in the sequence $t_1, \ldots, t_{n+1}$, one defines the i-th *interspike interval* (ISI) as $\Delta t_i = t_{i+1} - t_i, i = 1, \ldots, n$ and plots the relative frequency of occurrence of ISIs in small time interval bins (equally separated bins of 1 or 0.5 ms length, for example). Such a plot is an approximation to the probability density distribution of the ISIs, $p(\Delta t)$. The distribution $p(\Delta t)$ is often called the *ISI distribution*.

When ISI probability densities are determined experimentally, one usually finds a large range of distributions among different types of neurons and even within a single class of neurons thought to be functionally equivalent (Figure 15.1). A distribution that is often observed experimentally is a high probability for short intervals with an exponential decay for longer intervals, as in the case of unit 259-2 in Figure 15.1. Such a distribution resembles the *exponential distribution* introduced in §11.10. As explained in Eq. (11.25), the parameter ϱ of the exponential distribution is the reciprocal of the mean ISI, or the mean rate of discharge (in spikes/s). Thus, the exponential distribution can be fit to experimental data by determining its mean ISI. The exponential distribution has been shown to fit accurately the distribution of time intervals between spontaneous releases at the frog neuromuscular junction (Figure 15.2). We will see shortly that it has to be slightly modified when describing neuronal firing to take into account an important property of spike generation: the *refractory period* (see §15.4). The exponential distribution is the ISI distribution of the *homogeneous Poisson process* introduced in §11.11, which is a simple model for spontaneous activity in neurons or spontaneous release of neurotransmitter at synaptic release sites. In other neurons such as units R-4-10 and 240-1 in Figure 15.1, the ISI distribution is better fit by a *gamma distribution* with parameters ϱ and n (Figure 11.6). Such ISI distributions are more regular with lower coefficients of variation. On the other hand, an example of neurons that have very irregular spike trains are *bursting neurons* whose biophysical characteristics have been discussed in §§10.2 and 10.3. Such cells will typically fire a short "burst" of a few action potentials separated by much longer intervals. ISI distributions of bursting neurons therefore often have two peaks, one corresponding to the typical ISI during the burst (also called the intraburst interval) and a second peak corresponding to the typical interval between two different bursts (also called the interburst interval). An example is provided by unit 261-1 in Figure 15.1. The C_V of the ISI distribution of such bursting neurons can be quite high, up to two or more.

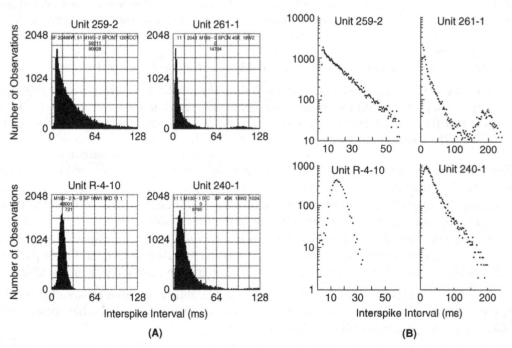

FIGURE 15.1 **A.** ISI histograms for the spontaneous activity of four auditory nerve units recorded in the cat. **B.** Same data plotted in logarithmic units, showing that the decay of the ISI distribution for unit 259-2, and to a lesser extent unit 240-1, is closely approximated by an exponential. Adapted from Rodieck et al. (1962).

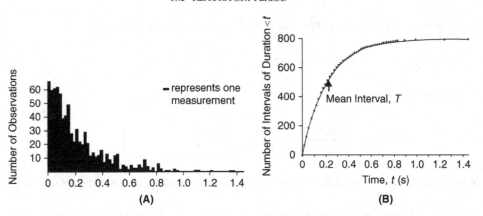

FIGURE 15.2   **A.** Distribution of intervals between two successive miniature end-plate potentials at the frog neuromuscular junction ($n_s = 800$ samples). **B.** Cumulative distribution of intervals fitted to an exponential function $n_s(1 - \exp(-t/T))$, where T is the mean interval. Adapted from Fatt and Katz (1952).

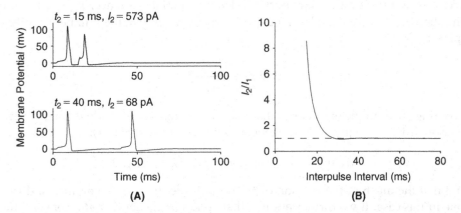

FIGURE 15.3   Relative refractory period in the Hodgkin–Huxley model. **A.** A 1 ms long pulse of 67 pA at time $t_1 = 2$ ms elicits an action potential in the Hodgkin–Huxley model of Chapter 4 (Exercise 4.2). A second, identical pulse at $t_2 = 15$ ms requires at least 573 pA to generate an action potential, while at $t_2 = 40$ ms the minimal required current is 68 pA. **B.** Ratio, I_2/I_1, of the minimal current (I_2) at time t_2 required to generate an action potential relative to I_1 at time $t_1 = 2$ ms as a function of $t_2 - t_1$. The dashed line corresponds to $I_2/I_1 = 1$. (ref_period2.m)

15.2 REFRACTORY PERIOD

The exponential distribution discussed in §15.1 assumes a high probability density for very short ISIs. Neurons, however, cannot fire immediately after an action potential because the sodium channels responsible for the fast membrane potential depolarization need first to recover from inactivation, a process that requires some time. Thus, all nerve cells possess a *refractory period* during which they are hardly excitable (recall Exercise 4.2). When firing is elicited by injecting current close to the spike initiation zone of a neuron, the refractory period can usually be divided into an *absolute refractory period*, during which it is impossible to obtain any action potential with physiological current injections and a *relative refractory period*, during which the threshold current eliciting spikes is increased (Figure 15.3). Both the length of the absolute and relative refractory period depend on the nerve cell under consideration, but typical values in the central nervous system are $0.5 - 1$ ms and ≈ 10 ms, respectively.

The exponential distribution can be easily modified to take into account the (absolute) refractory period of a neuron by assuming that the probability of firing is equal to zero for $\Delta t < t_{ref}$ and follows an exponential distribution for larger values of t:

$$p_{1\,ref}(\Delta t) = \mathbb{1}(\Delta t - t_{ref})\varrho \exp(-\varrho(\Delta t - t_{ref})).$$

An important effect of the refractory period is that it *regularizes* the spike train: i.e., a neuron having a refractory period but otherwise the same mean ISI as a neuron without refractory period will have a more regular spike train. This can be seen in the case of the exponential distribution by computing the coefficient of variation of $p_{1\,ref}$ from the mean and variance. Because the probability density function $p_{1\,ref}$ is simply a translation of p_1 along the time axis

$(p_{1\,ref}(\Delta t) = p_1(\Delta t - t_{ref}))$ it is easy to see that the mean shifts accordingly and the variance is unchanged:

$$m_{\Delta t, t_{ref}} = m_{\Delta t} + t_{ref} \quad \text{and} \quad \sigma^2_{\Delta t, t_{ref}} = \sigma^2_{\Delta t}.$$

This means that in term of the original C_V,

$$C_{V_{ref}} = \frac{\sigma_{\Delta t, t_{ref}}}{m_{\Delta t, t_{ref}}} = \frac{m_{\Delta t}}{m_{\Delta t} + t_{ref}} \frac{\sigma_{\Delta t}}{m_{\Delta t}} = \left(1 - \frac{t_{ref}}{m_{\Delta t, t_{ref}}}\right) C_V.$$

Thus, the closer the mean ISI, $m_{\Delta t, t_{ref}}$, is to the refractory period, the smaller the coefficient of variation.

15.3 SPIKE COUNT DISTRIBUTION AND FANO FACTOR

Another method to characterize the spontaneous activity of a neuron and its variability is to compute the mean number of spikes, $m_{N(0,T)}$, occurring during an interval of length T and its variance, $\sigma^2_{N(0,T)}$. The ratio of the variance to the mean is often called the *Fano factor* and is a measure of the variability in the number of spikes in relation to the mean number of spikes:

$$\mathcal{F}(T) \equiv \frac{\sigma^2_{N(0,T)}}{m_{N(0,T)}}.$$

Let us start by considering the example of a neuron that fires on average n independent spikes in an interval of length T according to a Poisson distribution (e.g., a homogeneous Poisson process, §11.11):

$$P(N(0,T) = k) = \exp(-n)n^k/k!, \quad k = 0,\ldots,\infty.$$

We know from §11.3 that the mean of the Poisson distribution is identical to its variance and thus the Fano factor $\mathcal{F}(T)$ is equal to one in this case. If we further assume that spikes are generated at a constant mean rate ϱ so that $n = \varrho T$, then we see that the Fano factor is equal to 1 for each value of T:

$$\mathcal{F}(T) = 1 \quad \textit{independent of } T \textit{ for a homogeneous Poisson process.}$$

What happens if spikes are generated at a mean rate ϱ but a refractory period is added after each spike? As we saw in the previous section, the mean ISI $m_{\Delta t, ref}$ increases and thus the effective rate decreases: $\varrho_{ref} = \varrho/(1 + \varrho t_{ref})$. The variance in the spike number during an interval of length T also decreases and it turns out that the Fano factor is less than 1. Thus the regularizing effect of the refractory period is also seen in the Fano factor.

Experimentally, the mean and variance of spike counts have been described in a number of systems. In general, there is a considerable heterogeneity between the Fano factors reported in different brain regions. In cortical neurons of the visual system, Fano factors are often above 1, and are thus more variable than expected from a Poisson process with or without refractory period (Figure 15.4).

15.4 RENEWAL PROCESSES

The homogeneous Poisson process is very useful as a basic model of spontaneous activity, but it relies on assumptions that are unlikely to be satisfied by nerve cells and that therefore need to be discussed in more detail. One of these assumptions is that spikes are generated independently of each other. This is of course not very plausible: we have already seen that nerve cells possess a refractory period and therefore will not fire for a certain amount of time following an action potential. Thus, as soon as a refractory period is introduced, the time of the next spike will depend on the time of the preceding spike since it cannot occur before the refractory period has passed. We have also seen that this refractory period can significantly alter the properties of the spike train.

The simplest way to relax the assumption of independence is to assume that the time of occurrence of a spike only depends on the time of occurrence of the previous spike. When this is the case, the ISI histogram fully characterizes the process of spike generation and such a process is called a *renewal process*. A simple way of obtaining a renewal process is to use the following model neuron:

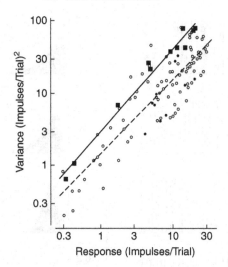

FIGURE 15.4 Plot of response variance as a function of mean response for a cat visual cortical neuron (a simple cell, Chapter 21) stimulated with a drifting sinusoidal grating (2 Hz temporal frequency, see §20.4). The black squares were obtained by averaging 100 trials (500 ms long) at 11 different contrast values. The solid line represents the best fit, with a slope of 1.11 and a variance about 2.8 times the mean (for a mean of 1 spike/trial). The circles break down the hundred trials at each contrast level in subsets of ten trials closest in time, thus minimizing long-term fluctuations in the variance. In this case, the variance is about 1.5 times the mean. The dashed line is the best fit, with a slope of 1. The black circles illustrate the trial-to-trial variability for ten individual trials at a fixed contrast level. Adapted from Tolhurst et al. (1983).

1. The neuron receives random inputs according to a Poisson process.
2. The neuron "counts" or integrates n of these inputs and fires a spike when n inputs have arrived.
3. Immediately after the spike, the memory of the n inputs is reset to zero.

This model is very simple. It is not entirely realistic, because as we know, neurons integrate inputs with a leaky time constant over an extended dendritic tree. It will, however, allow us to make several interesting observations. First, note that this model is a renewal process, because it counts the number of inputs arriving since the last action potential (and only the last one). What is its ISI distribution? It can be computed in exactly the same way as we computed the ISI distribution of the homogeneous Poisson process in §11.11. Namely observe that for the interval (a,b) of length Δt,

$$P_n(\Delta t_0 > \Delta t) = P(N(a,b) < n).$$

Therefore, as the events $\{N(a,b) = k\}$ are mutually exclusive,

$$P_n(\Delta t_0 \leq \Delta t) = 1 - P(N(a,b) < n) = 1 - \sum_{k=0}^{n-1} P(N(a,b) = k) = 1 - \sum_{k=0}^{n-1} \exp(-\varrho \Delta t) \frac{(\varrho \Delta t)^k}{k!} \tag{15.1}$$

for $n \geq 1$ and $\Delta t > 0$. The probability density is obtained by differentiating:

$$p_n(\Delta t) = \frac{\varrho(\varrho \Delta t)^{n-1}}{(n-1)!} \exp(-\varrho \Delta t) \quad \text{for } \Delta t > 0. \tag{15.2}$$

Therefore the ISI distribution of a neuron that sums n Poisson inputs before generating a spike is a gamma process of order n. This result also shows that the spike train variability as measured by the C_V of such a neuron is much reduced compared to a Poisson neuron. This is due to the temporal averaging of the inputs that effectively takes place and reduces variability by a factor $\sqrt{n}$ (Figure 15.5).

Typically, neurons receive several thousand excitatory inputs. If their spike trains were generated by integrating or summing many of these inputs, as described above, one would expect their spike trains to be very regular, even if their inputs were highly irregular, like homogeneous Poisson spike trains. Yet, this is typically not the case. For example, pyramidal neurons in visual cortex typically receive 10,000 excitatory inputs, but recordings *in vivo* in response to visual stimulation possess coefficients of variation about as high as could be expected from a homogeneous Poisson process (Figures 15.4 and 15.6). Thus, we are led to the conclusion that neurons are far from functioning as simple integrators of excitatory inputs.

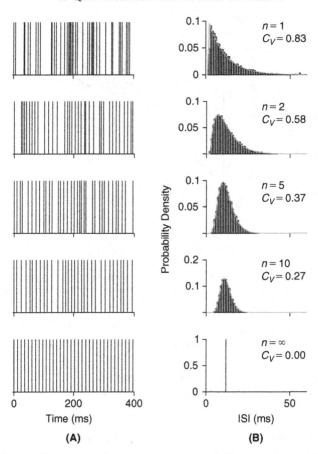

FIGURE 15.5   **A.** Example spike trains corresponding to renewal processes of order n for $n = 1, 2, 5,$ and 10 with a refractory period of 2 ms. In each case, the mean ISI is 12 ms. The bottom example is a perfectly regular spike train (limit of $n \to \infty$). **B.** Corresponding ISI probability density distributions and C_Vs. The red lines are curves obtained from the probability density distribution of gamma distributed random variables and the blue histograms from simulations of 10,000 ISIs. The probability density of the perfectly regular spike train is a delta function, δ. (gamma_spks.m)

What about variability measured by the Fano factor? Since a renewal process is completely determined by its ISI distribution, we would expect the variability computed from the Fano factor to be entirely determined by the ISI variability. This turns out to be the case (see §15.6), although the proof of this result would take us too far afield. We can, however, make a simple argument based on the assumption that the time interval T on which we observe the spike count is much larger than the mean ISI $m_{\Delta t}$. In this case, we expect approximately $m_{N(0,T)} \approx T/m_{\Delta t}$ action potentials. The variance of the time interval during which these $m_{N(0,T)}$ action potentials arrive is given by $\sigma^2 \approx m_{N(0,T)}\sigma^2_{\Delta t}$, since the ISIs are independent. Equivalently, $\sigma = \sqrt{m_{N(0,T)}}\sigma_{\Delta t}$. In this time interval, the average number of action potentials we expect to see is equal to $\sigma/m_{\Delta t}$. Therefore the variability in the number of action potentials is given by $\sigma^2_{N(0,T)} \approx \sigma^2/m^2_{\Delta t} = m_{N(0,T)}\sigma^2_{\Delta t}/m^2_{\Delta t}$. We can now combine these results:

$$\frac{\sigma^2_{N(0,T)}}{m_{N(0,T)}} \approx \frac{m_{N(0,T)}\sigma^2_{\Delta t}}{m^2_{\Delta t}} \cdot \frac{1}{m_{N(0,T)}} = \frac{\sigma^2_{\Delta t}}{m^2_{\Delta t}}.$$

In other words, for large time intervals the Fano factor of a renewal process is equal to the squared coefficient of variation of the ISI distribution:

$$\mathcal{F}(T) \approx C^2_V.$$

This result actually gives us one method of testing if the action potentials of a neuron form a renewal process: pick the ISI sequence generated by the neuron, reshuffle them at random, and compute the Fano factor for large T. This Fano factor will be constant and equal to C^2_V, since after reshuffling the ISI are independent. If the original Fano factor differs from a constant C^2_V value, the original spike train cannot be a renewal process. This also shows that the Fano factor

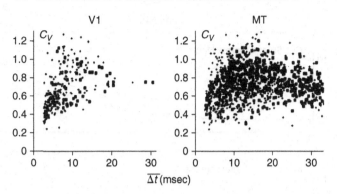

$$\overline{\Delta t}\,(\text{msec})$$

FIGURE 15.6 Coefficient of variation as a function of mean ISI for visual neurons in area V1 and MT of the monkey visual cortex responding to various types of stimuli. Adapted from Softky and Koch (1993).

measures variability over long time scales whereas the C_V captures variability over short time scales on the order of a single ISI. The Fano factor often increases with time, exhibiting long-term correlations that cannot be described by a renewal process (Figure 15.7).

15.5 RETURN MAPS AND EMPIRICAL CORRELATION COEFFICIENT

As seen above, in many cases the assumption of independent ISIs is inadequate to describe the firing pattern of a neuron. This can, e.g., result from membrane currents that are slowly activated and inactivated over a time span comprising several action potentials. The ionic mechanisms that underlie bursting in neurons represent such an example. A simple geometrical way to detect dependencies between successive ISIs is to make a two-dimensional plot of pairs of successive ISIs, $(\Delta t_i, \Delta t_{i+1})$, $i = 1, \ldots, n$. Such plots, see Figure 15.8C and D, are called *return maps*. If the successive ISIs are independent, the probability distribution of the pairs will be symmetric around the 45 degree line because

$$P(\Delta t_i, \Delta t_{i+1}) = P(\Delta t_i)P(\Delta t_{i+1}).$$

A quantitative way of assessing the relation between successive ISIs is to compute their *correlation coefficient*. We introduced the correlation coefficient of two random variables in §11.9. We now give an empirical definition directly based on pairs of experimental observations of two random variables. We then show how the empirical correlation coefficient can be interpreted geometrically and derive its relation to the definition of §11.9. Finally, we apply this concept to ISIs. Let us consider pairs of measurements (x_i, y_i), $i = 1, \ldots, n$, of two random variables X and Y. The means of X and Y, m_X, m_Y and their standard deviations σ_X, σ_Y can be approximated by:

$$\breve{m}_X = \frac{1}{n}\sum_{i=1}^{n} x_i, \quad \breve{m}_Y = \frac{1}{n}\sum_{i=1}^{n} y_i,$$

$$\breve{\sigma}_X = \left(\frac{1}{n}\sum_{i=1}^{n}(x_i - \breve{m}_X)^2\right)^{1/2}, \quad \breve{\sigma}_Y = \left(\frac{1}{n}\sum_{i=1}^{n}(y_i - \breve{m}_Y)^2\right)^{1/2}.$$

We define the *empirical correlation coefficient* between $\mathbf{x} = (x_1, \ldots, x_n)^T$ and $\mathbf{y} = (y_1, \ldots, y_n)^T$ as

$$\breve{\rho}_n \equiv \frac{\frac{1}{n}\sum_{i=1}^{n}(x_i - \breve{m}_X)(y_i - \breve{m}_Y)}{\breve{\sigma}_X \breve{\sigma}_Y}. \tag{15.3}$$

In this equation, the numerator is the empirical covariance of X and Y (see Exercise 11.19). To appreciate the geometrical significance of the empirical correlation coefficient, note that if we define the vectors $\mathbf{x}_0 = \mathbf{x} - \breve{m}_X$ and $\mathbf{y}_0 = \mathbf{y} - \breve{m}_Y$ then the previous equation is none other than the scalar product of $\mathbf{x}_0$ and $\mathbf{y}_0$ divided by their lengths,

$$\breve{\rho}_n = \frac{\mathbf{x}_0^T \mathbf{y}_0}{\|\mathbf{x}_0\| \|\mathbf{y}_0\|}.$$

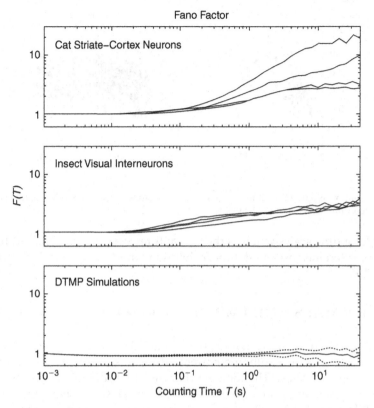

FIGURE 15.7   Fano factor computed from the spontaneous activity of four cells in the primary visual cortex of cats (top), four insect neurons (middle; descending contralateral movement detector neuron of the locust), and a Poisson process with refractory period (dead time modified Poisson or DTMP process, bottom). Note that the Fano factor of the DTMP process is less than 1 and independent of time, as expected from a renewal process. In contrast the Fano factor of both cortical and insect neurons increases with time, suggesting long-term correlations between the spikes that cannot be described by a renewal process. Adapted from Teich et al. (1996).

But the scalar product of two vectors is equal to the product of their lengths and their relative angle: $\mathbf{x}_0^T \mathbf{y}_0 = \cos(\sphericalangle_{\mathbf{x}_0,\mathbf{y}_0})\|\mathbf{x}_0\|\|\mathbf{y}_0\|$. Therefore the empirical correlation coefficient $\check{\rho}_n = \cos(\sphericalangle_{\mathbf{x}_0,\mathbf{y}_0})$ is a number between -1 and 1 that indicates the relative alignment between the two vectors. It is equal to 1 if the two vectors are perfectly aligned or perfectly correlated, $\mathbf{x}_0 = \mathbf{y}_0$ and -1 if $\mathbf{x}_0 = -\mathbf{y}_0$. The correlation coefficient is equal to zero if the two vectors are orthogonal.

Of course, this geometrical interpretation of the empirical correlation coefficient is in agreement with the definition of §11.9 since as the number of observations increases,

$$\check{\rho}_n \to \rho = \frac{E\left[(X - m_X)(Y - m_Y)\right]}{\sigma_X \sigma_Y} = \frac{E\left[XY\right] - m_X m_Y}{\sigma_X \sigma_Y} \quad (n \to \infty).$$

If $\rho = 0$ we say that X and Y are *uncorrelated*. This holds in particular when the random variables X and Y are independent since then $E[XY] = E[X]E[Y]$, but the opposite is not true (i.e., uncorrelated does not necessarily mean independent, see §11.9).

Let us now apply this to ISIs. If we measure a sequence of ISIs $\Delta t_1, \ldots, \Delta t_{n+1}$, we can look at pairs of measurements $(\Delta t_i, \Delta t_{i+1})$ and define the empirical correlation coefficient exactly as in Eq. (15.3):

$$\check{\rho}_n = \frac{\frac{1}{n}\sum_{i=1}^n (\Delta t_i - \check{m}_{1-n})(\Delta t_{i+1} - \check{m}_{2-(n+1)})}{\check{\sigma}_{1-n}\check{\sigma}_{2-(n+1)}}$$

where $\check{m}_{1-n}$ ($\check{\sigma}_{1-n}$) is the mean (standard deviation) over the first n ISIs and $\check{m}_{2-(n+1)}$ ($\check{\sigma}_{2-(n+1)}$) is the mean (standard deviation) over the last n ISIs, respectively. Of course, for a large number of intervals, we can simply replace these means and standard deviations by those of the entire ISI sequence,

$$\breve{m}_{\Delta t} = \frac{1}{n+1}\sum_{i=1}^{n+1}\Delta t_i, \quad \breve{\sigma}_{\Delta t} = \left(\frac{1}{n+1}\sum_{i=1}^{n+1}(\Delta t_i - \breve{m}_{\Delta t})^2\right)^{1/2},$$

since they will be almost identical. We therefore obtain the following definition for the *ISI correlation coefficient at lag 1*,

$$\breve{\rho}_{L1} = \frac{\frac{1}{n}\sum_{i=1}^{n}(\Delta t_i - \breve{m}_{\Delta t})(\Delta t_{i+1} - \breve{m}_{\Delta t})}{\breve{\sigma}_{\Delta t}^2}.$$

Correlation coefficients for higher lags (2,..., etc) are defined accordingly. An example of ISIs yielding a negative serial correlation coefficient is illustrated in Figure 15.8.

15.6 SUMMARY AND SOURCES

This chapter introduced the basic methods used to quantify spike train variability. Spike train variability has long intrigued experimental and theoretical neuroscientists alike. Certainly, whether variability is "pure noise" or a "hidden neural code," has important implications for the way the nervous system processes information. To this day, the issue remains unresolved, with most neurophysiologists believing that, at least in the visual system, spike train variability represents noise, e.g., Shadlen and Newsome (1998). On the other side of the debate, see Butts et al. (2007) for a study of spike train precision in the visual system and its potential role in coding. This article contains references to many earlier articles on the subject. In the auditory or in auditory-like sensory systems like the electrosensory

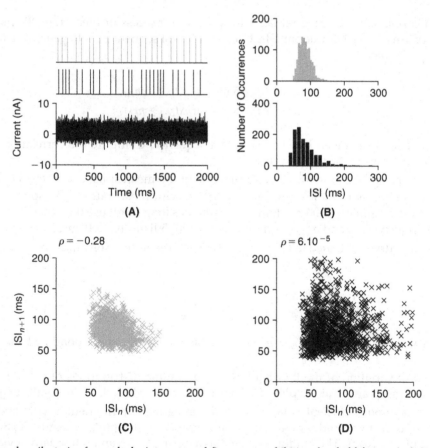

FIGURE 15.8 **A.** Example spike trains from a leaky integrate-and-fire neuron exhibiting threshold fatigue (red, §10.1) and a fixed threshold (black) driven by a random current stimulus (bottom panel). **B.** ISI distribution for both models. **C, D.** Plots of the $n+1$st interspike as a function of the n-th one. The corresponding correlation coefficients are -0.28 and 0, respectively. (neg_corr.m)

system of weakly electric fish, spike train variability can be exceptionally low and is used to convey precise timing information, see Kawasaki (1997). Chapter 15 of Koch (1999) provides an introduction to the subject of spike train variability, see also Gabbiani and Koch (1998). The general relation between the Fano factor and the coefficient of variation of the ISI distribution alluded to in §15.4 is given by

$$\lim_{T \to \infty} \mathcal{F}(T) = C_V^2 \left(1 + 2 \sum_{j=1}^{\infty} \rho_{Lj} \right),$$

(15.4)

where ρ_{Lj} is the correlation coefficient at lag j. Thus, spike trains exhibiting long-range negative ISI correlations will have Fano factors that may be considerably lower than expected from the coefficient of variation of the ISI distribution. Such long-range correlations have been observed in weakly electric fish. Ratnam and Nelson (2000) and Chacron et al. (2001) study their implications for the coding of information in neuronal spike trains. For a proof of Eq. (15.4), see Cox and Lewis (1966, Chapter 4, §6). This reference also contains a good discussion of the subtleties related to the analysis of sequences of events in the stationary case (§16.1). Exercises 5–15 below are based on Cox (1962), which is a basic and practical introduction to renewal processes. In §15.1 and Figure 15.2 spontaneous vesicular release has been described as a homogeneous Poisson process. There is, however, more recent evidence pointing to long-term correlations in spontaneous release, see Lowen et al. (1997). Regarding the role of spontaneous activity in the development of visual neural circuits alluded to in the introduction: we note that it is thought to be involved in conjunction with synaptic plasticity mechanisms, but that molecular cues play an important role as well. For reviews see McLaughlin and O'Leary (2005) and Shah and Crair (2008). We will address the impact of spike train variability on various aspects of sensory and psychophysical performance in Chapters 22–26.

15.7 EXERCISES

1. †Compute the ISI correlation coefficient at lag 1 for a Poisson process of mean rate 40 spk/s and an absolute refractory period of 2 ms. Use 1000 random ISIs. Use the same ISI sequence Δt_i to generate a new sequence of ISIs $\Delta t_i'$ as follows: $\Delta t_1' = \Delta t_1$ and

$$\Delta t_i' = \begin{cases} \Delta t_i + 5 \text{ ms} & \text{if } \Delta t_{i-1} < m_{\Delta t}, \\ \Delta t_i - 5 \text{ ms} & \text{if } \Delta t_{i-1} \geq m_{\Delta t}, \end{cases}$$

for $i > 1$ and where $m_{\Delta t}$ is the mean ISI of the original sequence. Compute the correlation coefficient at lag 1. Explain the difference between the two results.

2. †Plot the variance in the spike count, $\sigma_{N(0,T)}^2$, as a function of the mean spike count, $m_{N(0,T)}$, for a homogeneous Poisson process and a gamma renewal process of order 2 with mean rates of 40 spk/s starting at $t = 0$ (see Figure 15.9). Specifically, simulate 1000 random spike trains 1 s long (hint: use the functions exprnd, gamrnd, and cumsum). Then compute $m_{N(0,T)}$ and $\sigma_{N(0,T)}^2$ on the intervals (0, 50] ms, (0, 100] ms, ... up to (0, 1000] ms, in steps of 50 ms. Compare the curves obtained in this manner with the theoretical formulas, $m_{N(0,T)} = \sigma_{N(0,T)}^2 = T/m_{\Delta t}$ for the Poisson process and

$$m_{N(0,T)} = \frac{1}{2}\varrho T - \frac{1}{4} + \frac{1}{4}e^{-2\varrho T}, \quad \sigma_{N(0,T)}^2 = \frac{1}{4}\varrho T + \frac{1}{16} - \frac{1}{2}\varrho T e^{-2\varrho T} - \frac{1}{16}e^{-4\varrho T}$$

(15.5)

for the gamma renewal process, where $m_{\Delta t} = n/\varrho$ is the mean ISI. Plot the corresponding Fano factors as a function of time.

3. †Plot the coefficient of variation of the ISI distribution for gamma distributions of order 1, 2, 5, and 10 with a refractory period of 2 ms to arrive at the plot of Figure 15.10 below. Hint: Use the results of §15.4.

4. Compute the ISI correlation coefficient at lag 1 of a leaky integrate and fire neuron with and without threshold fatigue firing in response to a random current input. Reproduce the plots of Figure 15.8. Use the following parameters: $C_m = 2$ nF, $\tau = 20$ ms. The random current has a mean of 1 nA and a standard deviation of 1.5 nA, with new samples selected each $dt = 0.1$ ms from a normal distribution. The threshold parameters for the model with threshold fatigue are $v_{thres0} = 8$ mV, $\delta v_{thres} = 4$ mV, and $\tau_{v_{thres}} = 80$ ms (see Eq. (10.6)). The model without threshold

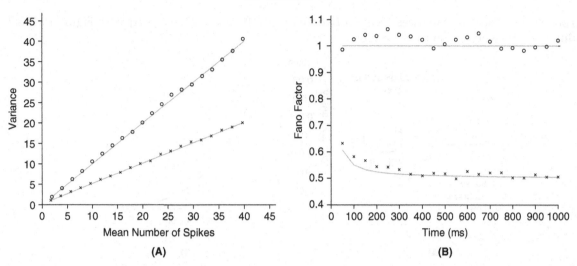

FIGURE 15.9 **A.** Spike count variance as a function of spike count mean for a Poisson (circles) and renewal gamma process of order 2 (crosses). The red lines are the corresponding theoretical formulas. **B.** Fano factor as a function of the time window length. (gamma2_ex1.m)

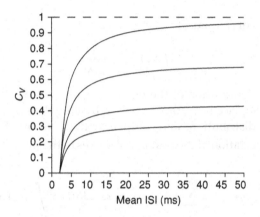

FIGURE 15.10 Coefficient of variation of the ISI distribution for gamma processes of order 1 (Poisson), 2, 5, and 10 with a refractory period of 2 ms as a function of the mean ISI. (cv_ref_ex.m)

fatigue has a fixed threshold of 10.4 mV. Total simulation time: 100 s in both cases (yielding approximately 1200 spikes); number of bins for the ISI distributions in B: 20. Hint: Use a simple forward Euler integration scheme with a time step of $dt = 0.1$ ms.

5. Consider the situation in which we observe beginning at time $t = 0$ the spikes associated with a stationary process that started a long time ago ($t_{start} \to -\infty$). The time interval between the observation start time, $t = 0$ (no spike is assumed to occur at that time), and the next spike is called the *forward recurrence time* (Figure 15.11A). Its probability density, $f_1(t)$, can be computed by the following argument for a renewal process. First note that if the probability density of the ISI distribution is $f(\Delta t)$ with mean $m_{\Delta t}$ then the probability density of a spike occurring in a given small interval is $\chi = 1/m_{\Delta t}$ where $m_{\Delta t}$ is the mean of $f(\Delta t)$. Next, if a spike occurred u ms before $t = 0$ then the probability density of observing the next spike x ms after $t = 0$ is $(1/m_{\Delta t})f(u + x)$. Finally, we need to integrate this expression over all possible times u for the previous spike to occur:

$$f_1(x) = \int_0^\infty \frac{1}{m_{\Delta t}} f(u + x)\, du = \frac{1}{m_{\Delta t}} \int_x^\infty f(y)\, dy = \frac{1 - F(x)}{m_{\Delta t}}, \tag{15.6}$$

where $F(\Delta t)$ is the cumulative distribution associated with $f(\Delta t)$. Show that if the renewal process is a homogeneous Poisson process, $f_1(x) = f(x)$. Show that for a gamma process of order 2, $f_1(x) = (\varrho/2)(\varrho x + 1)\exp(-\varrho x)$. Plot

$f_1(x)$ and $f(x)$ for the gamma process of order two for a mean ISI $m_{\Delta t} = 25\,\text{ms}$, to arrive at Figure 15.11B. Interpret the difference between the two distributions.

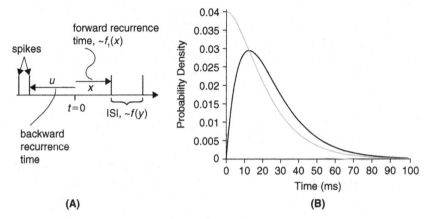

FIGURE 15.11   **A.** Definition of the forward recurrence time, x (distributed as $f_1(x)$), and the backward recurrence time, u. The ISI probability density is $f(y)$. **B.** Plot of $f(x)$ (black) and $f_1(x)$ (red) for a stationary gamma process of order two with a mean ISI of 25 ms. (gamma_frect.m)

6. Show that the Laplace transform of f_1 in Eq. (15.6) is given by

$$\mathcal{L}(f_1)(s) = \frac{1 - \mathcal{L}(f)(s)}{m_{\Delta t}}.$$

7. †Derive the probability density distribution of the ISIs for a gamma renewal process, Eq. (15.2), using Laplace transforms. Hint: Compute the Laplace transform of the probability density function for $Y = X_1 + \cdots + X_n$, where X_i are independent exponential distributions and compare with the result of Exercise 3.7.

8. Let $m_{N(0,t)} = E[N(0,t)]$ be the expectation of the number of spikes in the interval $(0, t]$ for a gamma renewal process starting at time $t = 0$. Show that

$$m_{N(0,t)} = \sum_{l=1}^{\infty} K_l(t), \quad \text{where} \quad K_l(t) = \int_0^t k_l(x)\,\mathrm{d}x \qquad (15.7)$$

is the cumulative distribution function of the l-th interval, $S_l = X_1 + \cdots + X_l$. Hint: By definition, $m_{N(0,t)} = \sum_{l=1}^{\infty} l P(N(0,t) = l)$. Show using arguments similar to those of §15.4 that $P(N(0,t) = l) = K_l(t) - K_{l+1}(t)$ and insert this result into the above definition.

9. Use Eq. (15.7) to show that for a gamma renewal process of order n starting at time $t = 0$

$$\mathcal{L}(m_{N(0,T)})(s) = \frac{1}{s} \frac{\mathcal{L}(p_n)(s)}{1 - \mathcal{L}(p_n)(s)}, \qquad (15.8)$$

where $p_n(\Delta t)$ is the ISI distribution of the process. Hint: Apply the Laplace transform term by term to Eq. (15.7). Since $k_l(x)$ is the probability density of the sum of independent random variables, its Laplace transform is the product of the Laplace transforms of the respective densities (Exercise 11.20). Finally, use the identity $\sum_{l=1}^{\infty} x^l = x/(1-x)$ for $|x| < 1$.

10. Use Eq. (15.8) to show that for $n = 2$, $m_{N(0,t)}$ is given by Eq. (15.5). Hint: Show that

$$\mathcal{L}(m_{N(0,T)})(s) = \frac{\varrho^2}{s^2(s + 2\varrho)}$$

and split this expression in partial fractions. That is, find constants A, B, and C so that

$$\mathcal{L}(m_{N(0,T)})(s) = \frac{A}{s^2} + \frac{B}{s} + \frac{C}{s + \varrho^2}.$$

Then use the results of Exercises 3.3–3.8 to arrive at the result.

11. Let $m_{N(0,t)} = E[N(0,t)]$ be the mean spike count of a renewal process starting at $t=0$. Show that

$$\sigma_{N(0,t)}^2 = E[(N(0,t) - E[N(0,t)])^2] = \xi(t) - m_{N(0,t)} - m_{N(0,t)}^2,$$

with $\xi(t) = E[N(0,t)(N(0,t)+1)]$.

12. Show that for a renewal process of order n,

$$\mathcal{L}(\xi)(s) = \frac{2}{s} \sum_{l=1}^{\infty} l\mathcal{L}(k_l)(s) = \frac{2}{s} \frac{\mathcal{L}(p_n)}{(1 - \mathcal{L}(p_n)(s))^2}.$$

Hint: Adopt the same strategy as in Exercises 8 and 9. Derive an infinite series for $\xi(t)$ in terms of the cumulative distribution functions $K_l(t)$ and take the term by term Laplace transform, using the fact that $\mathcal{L}(K_l)(s) = (1/s)\mathcal{L}(k_l)(s)$ since $K_l(0) = 0$. To sum the series use $\sum_{l=1}^{\infty} lx^l = x/(1-x)^2$.

13. †Show that if the renewal process is gamma of order 2,

$$\mathcal{L}(\xi)(s) = \frac{2\varrho^2(s+\varrho)^2}{s^3(s+2\varrho)^2}$$

and, by carrying out a partial fraction expansion,

$$\mathcal{L}(\xi)(s) = \frac{\varrho^2}{2s^3} + \frac{\varrho}{2s^2} - \frac{1}{8s} + \frac{1}{8(s+2\varrho)} - \frac{\varrho}{4(s+2\varrho)^2}. \tag{15.9}$$

Use this result in combination with those of Exercises 10 and 11 to derive Eq. (15.5) for $\sigma_{N(0,T)}^2$.

14. Show that for a stationary renewal process, $m_{N(0,t)} = t/m_{\Delta t}$ where $m_{\Delta t}$ is the mean ISI. Hint: Compute the Laplace transform of $m_{N(0,t)}$ as in Exercise 9. The difference with Eq. (15.8) is that for a stationary process observed from time $t=0$, the interval to the first spike is given by the forward recurrence time (Exercise 5). This leads to a slightly different expression for the Laplace transform of $k_l(x)$ and application of the identity $\sum_{l=0}^{\infty} x^l = 1/(1-x)$ for $|x| < 1$.

15. Show that for a stationary gamma process of order n

$$\mathcal{L}(\xi)(s) = \frac{2}{m_{\Delta t}s^2} \frac{1}{1 - \mathcal{L}(p_n)(s)}.$$

Hint: Proceed as in Exercise 12, using the Laplace transform for k_l obtained in the previous exercise.

16. Show that for a stationary gamma process of order 2

$$\xi(t) = \frac{\varrho^2 t^2}{4} + \frac{3\varrho t}{4} + \frac{1}{8} - \frac{1}{8}e^{-2\varrho t}$$

and consequently

$$\sigma_{N(0,t)}^2 = \frac{\varrho t}{4} + \frac{1}{8} - \frac{1}{8}e^{-2\varrho t}. \tag{15.10}$$

Hint: Apply the result of the previous exercise and carry out a partial fraction expansion to invert the Laplace transform term by term.

17. Compare the mean vs. variance curve of a stationary process of order 2 (Exercises 14 and 16) with those of a gamma process starting at $t=0$ (Exercise 2) by plotting them on the same graph. Use a mean ISI of 25 ms. Interpret the result.

16

Stochastic Processes

16.1	Definition and General Properties	251	16.5	Spectral Analysis	259
16.2	Gaussian Processes	252	16.6	Summary and Sources	262
16.3	Point Processes	254	16.7	Exercises	262
16.4	The Inhomogeneous Poisson Process	257			

OUTLINE

In analyzing neural data, we often have to deal with quantities that fluctuate randomly in time, like the intracellular membrane potential of a neuron recorded *in vivo* or a sequence of extracellular action potentials. Variables that fluctuate randomly in time are called *stochastic processes* or *random functions*. In this chapter, we define two types of stochastic processes that are used, respectively, to describe continuous variables, such as random potential fluctuations, and events, like random sequences of action potentials. We have already encountered the simplest such processes in previous chapters in the form of the homogeneous Poisson and gamma renewal processes. We delve into the characteristics of stochastic processes and introduce several examples that will subsequently play a central role in the analysis of random fluctuations of continuous variables and discrete spike trains: the Wiener process, white noise and the inhomogeneous Poisson process. Finally, we study the application of Fourier transforms to stochastic processes, which will allow us to characterize their frequency content, a topic called spectral analysis. The subjects covered in this chapter are further generalized in the exercises.

16.1 DEFINITION AND GENERAL PROPERTIES

A stochastic process is a collection or ensemble of random variables indexed by a variable t, usually representing time. For example, random membrane potential fluctuations (e.g., Figure 10.2) correspond to a collection of random variables $X(t)$, for each time point t. This may be made explicit by specifying an event space Ω for the ensemble and for each event $\mu \in \Omega$ writing $X(\mu, t)$ for the value taken by X at time t given the event μ. Thus, when the event μ is fixed and t is varied $X(\mu, t)$ is a random function. Conversely, at each fixed time point t, $X(\mu, t)$ spans the range of all possible values of X as the event $\mu \in \Omega$ varies and is thus a random variable. In practice, a random process is characterized by the set of its *joint distributions* $p(X(\mu, t_1), \ldots, X(\mu, t_n))$ of values taken at fixed times $t_1, \ldots, t_n$.

Stochastic processes are thus a direct generalization of random vectors as defined in §11.9. Indeed, we will see a close parallel in the next section, when we consider Gaussian stochastic processes in more detail. Several of the tools used to characterize random vectors can be extended to stochastic processes. For example, the mean value of a stochastic process and its "covariance" are defined by

$$m_X(t) \equiv E[X(t)] \quad \text{and} \quad C_X(t_1, t_2) \equiv E[(X(t_1) - m_X(t_1))(X(t_2) - m_X(t_2))].$$

Usually, for a stochastic process X, C_X is called the *autocovariance function* of the process and the term covariance is reserved for the correlation between two different stochastic processes. The term "autocorrelation" is also often used

Mathematics for Neuroscientists. DOI: 10.1016/B978-0-12-374882-9.00016-2

instead of autocovariance, but a more consistent approach is to define the *autocorrelation function* as the autocovariance normalized by the respective standard deviations,

$$R_X(t_1, t_2) = \frac{C_X(t_1, t_2)}{C_X(t_1, t_1)^{1/2} C_X(t_2, t_2)^{1/2}}.$$

Stationarity. A large number of stochastic processes have the property that their average statistical properties are independent of where they are formed along the time axis. Such stochastic processes are said to have various types of *stationary properties*. For example, the mean $m_X(t) = E[X(t)]$ can be independent of t. When in addition the autocovariance function $C_X(t_1, t_2) = E[(X(t_1) - m_X)(X(t_2) - m_X)]$ depends only on the time difference, $\tau = t_2 - t_1$, a stochastic process is called *weakly stationary*. In this case, the autocovariance function is usually written as

$$C_X(\tau) = E[(X(t) - m_X)(X(t + \tau) - m_X)].$$

Note that the right hand side of this equation is independent of t and this implies that C_X is symmetric, i.e., $C_X(\tau) = C_X(-\tau)$ (Exercise 1). More generally, X is said to be *stationary* if $p(X(t_1), \ldots, X(t_n)) = p(X(t_1 + \tau), \ldots, X(t_n + \tau))$ for all τ, i.e., the joint probabilities of X at different times are independent of the reference point τ. This implies in particular that both the mean and autocovariance functions are independent of the reference time point. Thus, a stationary process is also weakly stationary.

Ergodicity. Another important property of certain stochastic processes is that averages over the ensemble of values taken at a fixed time, e.g., $E[X(t)]$, can be replaced by an average over time on *any* sample function $X(\mu_0, t)$ from the stochastic ensemble (with μ_0 fixed). Let us denote by $X_0(t) = X(\mu_0, t)$ a particular sample random function from the stochastic process X. If X is ergodic then

$$E[X(t)] = \lim_{T \to \infty} \frac{1}{T} \int_{-T/2}^{T/2} X_0(s)\, ds. \tag{16.1}$$

Of course, this implies that $E[X(t)] = m_X$ is independent of t since this is the case for the right hand side of Eq. (16.1). For the autocovariance function, $C_X(\tau)$, ergodicity means that:

$$C_X(\tau) = \lim_{T \to \infty} \frac{1}{T} \int_{-T/2}^{T/2} X_0(s) X_0(s + \tau)\, ds. \tag{16.2}$$

Intuitively, ergodicity means that each sample function is "sufficiently diverse" over long time periods to be representative of the variability that is encountered locally across the whole sample of functions belonging to the stochastic ensemble. In the case of neurophysiological experiments, the validity of the ergodicity assumption, i.e., replacing ensemble averages by time averages, is often implicitly assumed. This is very convenient since it permits one to use a single stimulus presentation instead of repeated presentations of stimuli from the same ensemble. As is clear from Eqs. (16.1) and (16.2), ergodicity can only hold in the case of stationary (time-invariant) processes and is likely to be at best only a (useful) approximation in the case of neurophysiological experiments.

16.2 GAUSSIAN PROCESSES

A stochastic process $X(\mu, t)$ is called *Gaussian* if for each subset of time points $t_1, \ldots, t_n$ (with n arbitrary) the random vector $(X(t_1), \ldots, X(t_n))^T$ is Gaussian. Thus, a Gaussian stochastic process is a direct generalization of the Gaussian random vectors introduced in §11.9. Just as for Gaussian random vectors, Gaussian processes have several special properties. For example, a Gaussian process is entirely determined by its mean $m_X(t)$ and its autocovariance function $C_X(t, s)$.

The Wiener process is a Gaussian process that was first used to describe the random, or "Brownian," motion of particles in a fluid. The Wiener process $W(t)$ is defined for $t \geq 0$ and has the following properties:

1. $W(0) = 0$ with probability 1.
2. For $0 \leq s < t$ the random variable $W(t) - W(s)$, also called the *increment* of W between s and t, is normally distributed with mean zero and variance $t - s$.
3. For $0 \leq s < t < u < v$ the increments $W(t) - W(s)$ and $W(v) - W(u)$ are independent.

Note that by setting $s=0$ in property 2 and using property 1, we immediately see that $W(t)$ is a Gaussian random variable with zero mean and variance t. Thus, although the mean of W is independent of t, its variance is not: it increases linearly with t. In particular, W is not (weakly) stationary, according to the definition of §16.1. It also follows from property 3 that for $0 = t_0 < t_1 < t_2 \cdots < t_n$ the vector $(W(t_1), W(t_2) - W(t_1), \ldots, W(t_n) - W(t_{n-1}))^T$ is Gaussian with probability density,

$$p(dW_1, dW_2, \ldots, dW_n) = \frac{1}{(2\pi)^{n/2}} \frac{1}{\sqrt{dt_1 dt_2 \cdots dt_n}} \exp\left(-\frac{dW_1^2}{2dt_1} - \frac{dW_2^2}{2dt_2} - \cdots - \frac{dW_n^2}{2dt_n}\right), \tag{16.3}$$

where $dW_j = W(t_j) - W(t_{j-1})$ and $dt_j = t_j - t_{j-1}$. The function

$$f : (x_1, x_2, \ldots, x_n) \to (x_1, x_1 + x_2, x_2 + x_3, \ldots, x_{n-1} + x_n)$$

transforms

$$(W(t_1), W(t_2) - W(t_1), \ldots, W(t_n) - W(t_{n-1}))^T \to (W(t_1), W(t_2), \ldots, W(t_n))^T.$$

Thus, by applying the transformation law described in §11.9, it follows that the random vector $(W(t_1), \ldots, W(t_n))^T$ is Gaussian with density

$$p(w_1, \ldots, w_n) = \frac{1}{(2\pi)^{n/2}} \frac{1}{\sqrt{dt_1 dt_2 \cdots dt_n}} \exp\left(-\frac{w_1^2}{2dt_1} - \frac{(w_2 - w_1)^2}{2dt_2} - \cdots - \frac{(w_n - w_{n-1})^2}{2dt_n}\right). \tag{16.4}$$

This shows that the Wiener process is indeed a Gaussian stochastic process.

What does a typical sample path of Brownian motion look like over the interval $[0, T]$? We can take advantage of the fact that the increments of W are independent (or, equivalently, of Eq. (16.3)) to answer this question numerically. First, select a small interval Δt and equally spaced points $(\Delta t, 2\Delta t, \ldots, n\Delta t = T)$. For each i, set $W_i = W(i\Delta t)$ and select a Gaussian random number $\Delta W_i = W_i - W_{i-1}$ with zero mean and variance Δt. Then, as explained above,

$$W_n = W_0 + \sum_{i=1}^{n} \Delta W_i. \tag{16.5}$$

This equation permits the computation of a sample path at each time point $i\Delta t$. Some example sample paths as well as sample means and variances are illustrated in Figure 16.1A and B.

White noise. According to Eq. (16.5), the sample paths of Brownian motion can be approximated numerically by considering the increments, ΔW_i, of the Wiener process. A natural question that arises is whether it is possible to define the derivative of the Wiener process through the limit $Z(t_i) = \lim_{\Delta t \to 0} \Delta W_i / \Delta t$. If this were at all possible, we would expect the stochastic process $Z(t)$ to derive several of its properties from those of $W(t)$. In particular, since ΔW_i is a Gaussian stochastic process with zero mean, we expect $Z(t)$ to be one as well. Furthermore,

$$E[\Delta W_i \Delta W_j] = 0$$

implies that $Z(t_i)$ should be independent of $Z(t_j)$ for $t_i \neq t_j$ (remember from §11.9 that two uncorrelated, jointly Gaussian random variables are independent). Finally, the variance of $Z(t)$ should be increasingly well approximated by

$$E\left[\frac{(\Delta W_i)^2}{\Delta t^2}\right] = \frac{1}{\Delta t}.$$

However, this expression becomes infinite as $\Delta t \to 0$, and therefore $Z(t)$ cannot be a stochastic process in the usual sense. It is nonetheless possible to make sense of the last two equations by noting that they represent the discrete approximation to a δ-function (recall §3.1 and Exercise 7.20). We can therefore interpret them as implying that the autocovariance function of the white noise process is given by

$$E[Z(t_1)Z(t_2)] = \delta(t_1 - t_2). \tag{16.6}$$

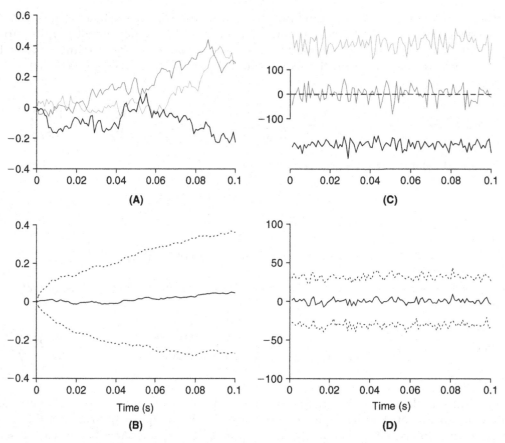

FIGURE 16.1 **A.** Three sample paths of a Wiener process. These paths were obtained by summing up and scaling by Δt the white noise paths in C. **B.** Sample mean and mean $\pm$ one standard deviation of 100 Wiener sample paths. Note the time dependence of the standard deviation, implying that the Wiener process is not stationary. **C.** Three sample paths of white noise sampled at a time step $\Delta t = 1$ ms. For clarity, two of the paths have been shifted above and below the horizontal zero line (dashed). **D.** Mean and mean $\pm$ one standard deviation of 100 white noise samples (solid and dotted lines, respectively). (rand_fig2.m)

Thus, we can think of white noise as being a stationary, zero mean Gaussian stochastic process whose autocovariance function is given by Eq. (16.6). Although this represents only a formal construction, it will prove useful for analytical calculations. In practice, white noise can always be approximated numerically by the procedure outlined above, through independent increments ΔW_i of the Wiener process for a sufficiently small time step Δt.

Autocovariance function of the Wiener process. The computation of the autocovariance function of white noise raises the question of what the autocovariance function of the Wiener process is. To answer this question, we use Eq. (16.4): for $t_1 < t_2$ we know that

$$E[W(t_1)W(t_2)] = \iint\limits_{-\infty}^{\infty} p(w_1, w_2)w_1 w_2 dw_1 dw_2.$$

This integral can easily be computed to yield $E[W(t_1)W(t_2)] = t_1$ (Exercise 3). Since we assumed $t_1 < t_2$, this implies that $E[W(t_1)W(t_2)] = \min(t_1, t_2)$ if t_1, t_2 are arbitrary. Note that since the Wiener process is not stationary, the autocovariance function is not a function of $t_2 - t_1$.

16.3 POINT PROCESSES

Another important class of stochastic processes arises when we want to describe random discrete events in time. For example, consider the action potentials generated by a neuron whose spontaneous activity is recorded *in vivo*. Each action potential is associated with a specific point in time, e.g., the peak of the membrane potential depolarization, so that in a given observation interval we obtain a sequence $\{t_1, \ldots, t_n\}$ of time points. If we were to repeat the measurement over the same interval we would obtain a different set of spike occurrence times, $\{t'_1, \ldots, t'_m\}$. In other words, the spike occurrence times are random. There are several possible ways to describe the properties of such point processes. We can consider the sample paths associated with each sequence of action potentials, similar to those considered for Brownian motion in the previous paragraph. The sample paths are obtained from the sequence of action potential occurrence times by defining a function $l(t)$ equal to zero at $t = 0$ and such that it is incremented by 1 at each action potential, i.e., $l(t) = 0$ for $0 \leq t < t_1$, $l(t) = 1$ for $t_1 \leq t < t_2$, and so forth. Some example sample paths are illustrated in Figure 16.2. Note that in contrast to the sample paths of Brownian motion, the sample paths of a point process are *discontinuous* since they possess discrete jump points associated with each event occurrence time. The function $l(t)$ is called the *counting function* associated with a sequence of occurrence times. If we denote by $L(t)$ the associated stochastic process, then by definition $L(t) = N(0, t)$, where $N(0, t)$ is the number of spikes in the interval $(0, T]$. Thus, just as Gaussian stochastic processes can be described by their distribution of values taken at time points $(t_1, \ldots, t_n)$, a point process can be described by the distribution of the number of events occurring in any time interval $(0, T]$. We introduced the simplest type of point process, the homogeneous Poisson process, in this way (§11.11).

Formally, the derivative of $l(t)$ is given by a sum of δ-functions, since the derivative of a step function is the δ-function (Exercise 7.21):

$$\frac{dl}{dt} = \sum_{i=1}^{n} \delta(t - t_i). \tag{16.7}$$

This is the *spike train*, $m(t)$, associated with the sequence of occurrence times. By extension, we denote by $M(t) = \sum_{i=1}^{n} \delta(t - t_i)$ the spike trains associated with a point process, where both n and $\{t_i\}$ are now random variables, and $M(t) = dL/dt$.

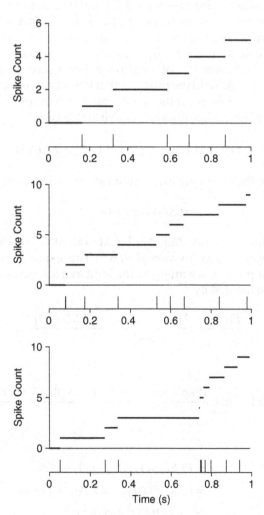

FIGURE 16.2 Three sample paths of a homogeneous Poisson process. Below each path the jump times are indicated by spikes. (rand_fig3.m)

Autocovariance function of the homogeneous Poisson process. If we denote by $M_P(t) = \sum_{i=1}^{n} \delta(t-t_i)$ the spike trains associated with a homogeneous Poisson process ($M_P(t) = 0$ if $n = 0$), we can formally compute $E[M_P(t_a)M_P(t_b)]$ using Eqs. (11.26) and (11.27) (Exercise 4). We find $E[M_P(t_a)M_P(t_b)] = \varrho\delta(t_b - t_a) + \varrho^2$. It is also easy to see that $E[M_P(t)] = \varrho$ and the autocovariance function of the Poisson process spike train is therefore given by

$$E[(M_P(t_a) - \varrho)(M_P(t_b) - \varrho)] = \varrho\delta(t_b - t_a). \tag{16.8}$$

Note that this autocovariance function is equal to that of white noise when $\varrho = 1$. Just as in the case of white noise, this results from the fact that two events in a Poisson process are independent, regardless of how close they are. Thus, we expect on average zero correlation between events occurring at two different times t_a and t_b. This calculation also shows that two stochastic processes with widely different sample functions can have identical correlation functions.

Stationarity. An important assumption that was made in formulating the homogeneous Poisson process (§11.11) and renewal processes (§15.4) is that the rate at which action potentials are generated does not change over time. In the case of a point process, stationarity means that for any intervals $(a_1, b_1), \ldots, (a_n, b_n)$ the probability distribution of spikes in these intervals is identical to the one obtained after translating the intervals by a fixed time t_0:

$$P(N(a_1, b_1), \ldots, N(a_n, b_n)) = P(N(a_1 + t_0, b_1 + t_0), \ldots, N(a_n + t_0, b_n + t_0)),$$

for all t_0. In practice this is of course impossible to verify. What can be checked, e.g., is that the mean number of spikes in different intervals remains the same over the course of time. Furthermore, the assumption of stationarity is not always realistic since neurons often have firing rates that evolve over time. This is the case, e.g., when a stimulus is presented and *adaptation* reduces neuronal activity.

Autocovariance function of a stationary point process. In general, the autocovariance function of the spike train associated with a stationary point process also contains a δ-function, just as that of the homogeneous Poisson process. To illustrate this point, first note that the rate of events of a stationary point process is constant and its probability is given by $\chi \Delta t$ for a sufficiently small interval Δt, just as for the homogeneous Poisson process. More precisely, if we denote by $\Delta L_t = L(t + \Delta t) - L(t)$ the increments of a stationary point process, then $P(\Delta L_t = 1) = \chi \Delta t + o(\Delta t)$. The second term, $o(\Delta t)$, denotes a function of Δt with the property that it tends to zero faster than Δt: $\lim_{\Delta t \to 0} o(\Delta t)/\Delta t = 0$. This condition ensures that no two events occur at the same time. Furthermore, if ΔL_t takes only the values 0 and 1 then $(\Delta L_t)^2 = \Delta L_t$. This is expected when Δt is sufficiently small and hence,

$$E[\Delta L_t] = P(\Delta L_t = 1) = \chi \Delta t + o(\Delta t), \quad E\left[(\Delta L_t)^2\right] = \chi \Delta t + o(\Delta t) \quad (\Delta t \to 0). \tag{16.9}$$

From these two equations we derive the following expression for the variance of ΔL_t:

$$\mathrm{var}(\Delta L_t) = \chi \Delta t + o(\Delta t).$$

Since the spike train is formally obtained by dividing ΔL_t by Δt and taking the limit $\Delta t \to 0$ (Eq. (16.7)), its autocovariance function at time zero is approximated by $\mathrm{var}(\Delta L_t)/\Delta t^2$. This expression diverges like $\chi/\Delta t$ as Δt tends to zero. Just as in the case of the Wiener process, we interpret the limit as a δ-function, $\chi\delta(\tau)$. At times greater than zero, the autocovariance function is approximated by

$$\frac{E[(\Delta L_t - E[\Delta L_t])(\Delta L_{t+\tau} - E[\Delta L_{t+\tau}])]}{\Delta t^2}. \tag{16.10}$$

If we define the conditional density

$$\chi_c(\tau) = \lim_{\Delta t \to 0} \frac{P(\text{spike in } (t+\tau, t+\tau+\Delta t)|\text{spike at } t)}{\Delta t}, \tag{16.11}$$

we can write

$$\begin{aligned}
E[\Delta L_t \Delta L_{t+\tau}] &= P(\Delta L_t = 1, \Delta L_{t+\tau} = 1) + o(\Delta t^2) \\
&= (\chi \Delta t)P(\Delta L_{t+\tau} = 1|\Delta L_t = 1) + o(\Delta t^2) \\
&= \chi\chi_c(\tau)(\Delta t)^2 + o(\Delta t^2).
\end{aligned}$$

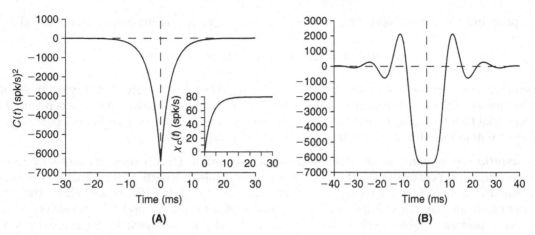

FIGURE 16.3   **A.** Autocovariance function of a gamma renewal process of order 2, with a mean rate of 80 spk/s. The delta function spike at time 0 is not illustrated. Inset: χ_c for the same process. **B.** Autocovariance function of a gamma process of order 10. (gamma_corr.m)

Substituting this result and Eq. (16.9) in Eq. (16.10) and taking the limit $\Delta t \to 0$ yields $\chi(\chi_c(\tau) - \chi)$ so that the autocovariance function of the spike train is given by

$$C_M(\tau) = E[(M(t) - \chi)(M(t+\tau) - \chi)] = \chi \delta(\tau) + \chi(\chi_c(|\tau|) - \chi), \tag{16.12}$$

since $C_M(\tau) = C_M(-\tau)$. By definition, $\chi_c(\tau)\Delta t$ is the probability of observing a spike (any, not only the first one) in the interval Δt starting at a time τ following a spike. Thus, values of $\chi_c(\tau) < \chi$ or equivalently $C_M(\tau) < 0$ for $\tau \neq 0$ correspond to a suppressed probability of spiking as compared to the mean χ, while values of $\chi_c(\tau) > \chi$ or $C_M(\tau) > 0$ correspond to an increased probability of spiking.

We illustrate two examples of autocovariance functions for stationary renewal gamma processes of orders 2 and 10 in Figure 16.3. The interspike interval distribution of the gamma process of order 2 has a reduced probability for short intervals compared to a Poisson process (Figure 15.5B). This translates into a reduced probability of firing following a spike and thus $\chi_c < \chi$ at short values of τ. Consequently the autocovariance function is <0 at short time intervals (Figure 16.3A). The gamma process of order 10 has a very regular spike train. This leads to positive correlations at multiples of the firing period (Figure 16.3B).

16.4 THE INHOMOGENEOUS POISSON PROCESS

The homogeneous Poisson process is based on a constant rate of events, ϱ. We generalize this model by assuming a time-dependent event rate, $\varrho(t)$. Formally the definition of the inhomogeneous Poisson process is identical to the one given in §11.11, except for the replacement of ϱ by $\varrho(t)$. In particular, this means that for each interval $(a, b]$ the number of events has a mean given by

$$\kappa \equiv \int_a^b \varrho(t)\,dt$$

and follows the Poisson distribution,

$$P(N(a,b) = k) = e^{-\kappa} \frac{\kappa^k}{k!}.$$

Repeating exactly the same calculation presented in §11.11 and using the fact that for Δt sufficiently small,

$$\int_{a - \Delta t/2}^{a + \Delta t/2} \varrho(t)\,dt \approx \varrho(a)\Delta t$$

we obtain the probability density of observing spikes at times $t_1, \ldots, t_n$ during the observation interval $(0, T]$:

$$p_{(0,T]}(t_1, \ldots, t_n) = \varrho(t_1) \cdots \varrho(t_n) \exp(-\kappa). \qquad (16.13)$$

This equation reflects the fact that at each time point $t_1, \ldots, t_n$ the probability density of observing an event is proportional to the instantaneous rate and these probabilities are to be multiplied since they are independent of each other. The final exponential factor is again a normalization constant ensuring that the probability of observing an arbitrary number of events within the interval at arbitrary times sums to 1 (Eq. (11.27)).

Numerical simulation of inhomogeneous Poisson processes. Equation (16.13) suggests one way to simulate an inhomogeneous Poisson process: split the time axis in small intervals of length Δt such that $\varrho(t)$ is approximately constant and the probability of encountering two or more events in each interval is negligible. The probability of an event occurring in the interval will then be well approximated by $\varrho(t)\Delta t$, and the probability of no event by $1 - \varrho(t)\Delta t$. Draw a random number, $r \in (0,1)$, for each interval and place an event in the interval when $r \leq \varrho(t)\Delta t$. This method is inefficient because it requires the use of a random number generator for each interval Δt. We now describe a more accurate and efficient method based on the probability distribution of successive interevent times.

Assume that an event occurs at time a. Just as in §11.11, the probability density of the interval up to the next event is obtained from

$$P(\Delta t_0 < (b-a)) = 1 - P(\Delta t_0 \geq (b-a)) = 1 - P(N(a,b) = 0)$$
$$= 1 - e^{-\kappa} = 1 - e^{-\int_0^{b-a} \varrho(t+a)\,dt}.$$

Setting again $b - a = \Delta t$ and taking the derivative we obtain

$$p_a(\Delta t) = \varrho(a + \Delta t)e^{-\int_0^{\Delta t} \varrho(t+a)\,dt}.$$

This equation directly generalizes the formula derived in §11.11 for the homogeneous Poisson process. To make effective use of this formula, we define

$$y = y(\Delta t) = \int_0^{\Delta t} \varrho(t+a)\,dt.$$

The probability density of y is obtained from the probability density of Δt and the transformation law for probability densities under a smooth variable change,

$$p(y) = p_a(\Delta t) \left(\frac{dy}{d\Delta t} \right)^{-1} = \exp(-y)$$

(see §11.8). This equation tells us that y is an exponentially distributed random variable with rate 1.

We can thus simulate a sequence of events corresponding to the inhomogeneous Poisson process with rate $\varrho(t)$ using the following procedure:

1. Set $a = 0$.
2. Select an exponentially distributed random threshold value y_i, for the starting index $i = 0$.
3. Integrate

$$Y(t) = \int_0^t \varrho(a+s)\,ds$$

until the threshold $Y(t) = y_i$ ($i = 0$) is reached. Call this time point t_i ($i = 0$).
4. Generate an event at t_i, set $a = t_i$ ($i = 0$), and repeat this recipe from point 2 on for index $i = i + 1$ (i.e., $1, 2, 3, \ldots$, and so forth).

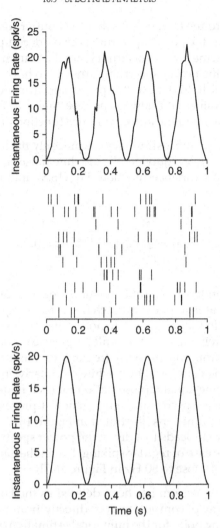

FIGURE 16.4 Simulation of an inhomogeneous Poisson process whose instantaneous rate is given in the bottom panel. The middle panel shows 10 spike trains obtained using the algorithm described above. On top is the mean instantaneous firing rate computed over 10 ms bins by simulating 1000 spike trains. (rand_fig3.m)

Note that we have implicitly assumed in the previous algorithm that an event occurs at time point zero by setting $a = 0$ as a starting value. Note also that the algorithm presented in steps 1–4 is identical to that used to simulate a perfect integrate-and-fire neuron satisfying the differential equation $v'(t) = \varrho(t)$ and a threshold v_{thres} that is updated randomly according to an exponential distribution after each spike (see §10.1). Figure 16.4 illustrates the simulation of an inhomogeneous Poisson process with a sinusoidal time-varying rate using this method.

16.5 SPECTRAL ANALYSIS

The autocovariance function of a stochastic process $C_V(t_1, t_2)$ defined in §16.1 is a measure of the statistical dependence of the random values taken by a stochastic process at two time points. We have seen two examples (white noise and the Poisson process) for which no dependence exists between random values taken at different time points. Most processes encountered in reality will have a more complex structure, as illustrated, e.g., by the Wiener process. Another measure equivalent to the autocovariance function can be defined in the case of weakly stationary stochastic processes, i.e., those for which the autocovariance function, $C(\tau)$, depends only on the time difference, $\tau = t_2 - t_1$. This measure is called the *power spectrum* and is defined as the Fourier transform of the autocovariance function,

$$S(\omega) \equiv \hat{C}(\omega) = \int\limits_{-\infty}^{\infty} C(\tau) e^{-2\pi i \omega \tau} \, d\tau. \tag{16.14}$$

We know from Fourier analysis of deterministic functions that the Fourier transform decomposes a function into its frequency components (Chapter 7). Thus, the power spectrum is also a decomposition of the autocovariance function into its frequency components. However, the power spectrum is not the Fourier transform of just any function: because of the definition of the autocovariance, the power spectrum turns out to have very special properties. First, note that since $C(\tau)$ is real and symmetric, the same holds true for the power spectrum $S(\omega)$ (Exercise 7). We will shortly see that the power spectrum is even more constrained: it is always *positive*, $S(\omega) \geq 0$. Thus, the power spectrum is a measure of the *strength* of each frequency component in the autocovariance function of the stochastic process.

Power spectrum of the Poisson process. Before justifying more precisely the last statement, let us start by computing the power spectrum of the Poisson process or, equivalently, of white noise since they have the same autocovariance function. We simply substitute the autocovariance function, Eq. (16.8), into the definition of the power spectrum, Eq. (16.14):

$$S(\omega) = \int\limits_{-\infty}^{\infty} \varrho \delta(\tau) e^{-2\pi\omega\tau}\, d\tau = \varrho. \tag{16.15}$$

Thus, the power spectrum is equal to ϱ independent of frequency. Note that $S(\omega) \geq 0$, as promised. The fact that each frequency has the same power spectral value implies that each frequency is equally represented in the autocovariance function. This is intuitively reasonable. In the case of white noise, changes in the value of a sample white noise path can occur at any time scale with equal probability and thus all frequencies should be equally represented. Indeed, the term "white" in white noise originates from this property (remember that if all frequencies are equally represented in an electromagnetic wave, the resulting color of light is white). Similarly, in the case of the Poisson process a new event can occur at any time scale, implying equal representation for each frequency.

Figure 16.5 below illustrates the power spectra of gamma renewal processes of orders 2 and 10, which are the Fourier transforms of the autocovariance functions illustrated in Figure 16.5. For the process of order 2, the reduced probability of spiking at short time intervals leads to a dip in the power spectrum at low frequencies, a characteristic manifestation of refractory effects. In the case of regular spiking, like in the gamma process of order 10, we observe a peak at the firing frequency of the model (close to 80 Hz in Figure 16.5B).

Wiener–Khinchin theorem.* The power spectrum has been defined as the Fourier transform of the autocovariance function. We now give an alternative way of computing $S(\omega)$ directly from the sample functions of the underlying stochastic process. This will be the starting point for the numerical estimation of the power spectrum in §18.3 and will also show as a byproduct that $S(\omega)$ is positive at all frequencies. For simplicity we assume the stochastic process to have zero mean and it must of course be at least weakly stationary. Let $X(\mu, t)$ be a sample path of a stochastic process indexed by $\mu \in \Omega$ and set

$$X_T(\mu, t) = X(\mu, t)\mathbb{1}_{[-T/2, T/2]}(t). \tag{16.16}$$

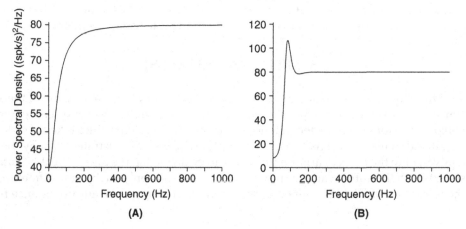

FIGURE 16.5   **A.** Power spectrum of a gamma renewal process of order 2, with a mean rate of 80 spk/s. **B.** Power spectrum of a gamma process of order 10. (`gamma_powersp.m`)

Let us denote by $\hat{X}_T(\mu,\omega)$ the Fourier transform of $X_T(\mu,t)$. The Fourier transform always exists, because X_T is nonzero only over a finite time interval. Each sample path yields a different Fourier transform and thus $\hat{X}_T(\cdot,\omega)$ is a random variable for each frequency ω. Now define

$$S_T(\omega) = \frac{E[|\hat{X}_T(\omega)|^2]}{T},$$

i.e., the average square modulus of the frequency component $\hat{X}_T(\omega)$, normalized by interval length. The Wiener–Khinchin theorem states that in the limit of long intervals T,

$$\boxed{\lim_{T\to\infty} S_T(\omega) = S(\omega).}$$

Note that $S_T(\omega)$ is always nonnegative and thus the same is true of $S(\omega)$.

Proof. We show that

$$S_T(\omega) = \int_{-T}^{T} (1-|\tau|/T)C(\tau)e^{-2\pi i\omega\tau}\,d\tau$$

$$= \int_{-\infty}^{\infty} g_T(\tau)C(\tau)e^{-2\pi i\omega\tau}\,d\tau,$$

(16.17)

with $g_T(\tau) = (1-|\tau|/T)\mathbb{1}_{[-T,T]}$. Since $0 \le g_T(\tau) \le 1$ and $g_T(\tau) \to 1$ as $T \to \infty$ this in turn implies that

$$S_T(\omega) \to \int_{-\infty}^{+\infty} C(\tau)e^{-2\pi i\omega\tau}\,d\tau \quad \text{as} \quad T\to\infty,$$

provided $C(\tau)$ decays sufficiently fast as $\tau \to \infty$. First,

$$\hat{X}_T(\mu,\omega)^* = \int_{-T/2}^{T/2} X_T(\mu,t_1)e^{2\pi i\omega t_1}dt_1, \quad \hat{X}_T(\mu,\omega) = \int_{-T/2}^{T/2} X_T(\mu,t_2)e^{-2\pi i\omega t_2}dt_2,$$

so that

$$|\hat{X}_T(\mu,\omega)|^2 = \hat{X}_T(\mu,\omega)^*\hat{X}_T(\mu,\omega)$$

$$= \int_{-T/2}^{T/2}\int_{-T/2}^{T/2} X_T(\mu,t_1)X_T(\mu,t_2)e^{-2\pi i\omega(t_2-t_1)}\,dt_2dt_1$$

$$= \int_B f(t_1,t_2)\,dt_1dt_2,$$

where $f(t_1,t_2) = X_T(\mu,t_1)X_T(\mu,t_2)e^{-2\pi i\omega(t_2-t_1)}$ and B is a two-dimensional square, as sketched in Figure 16.6A. We now perform the change of variables $\{t_1,t_2\} \to \{t_1, \tau=t_2-t_1\}$ which converts B into a parallelogram with upper and lower boundaries determined by the lines $(\alpha, \pm T/2 - \alpha)$ with $\alpha \in [-T/2, T/2]$, respectively, as illustrated in Figure 16.6B. Therefore,

$$\int_B f(t_1,t_2)\,dt_1dt_2 = \int_{-T}^{0}\int_{-T/2-\tau}^{T/2} f(t_1,t_1+\tau)\,dt_1d\tau + \int_{0}^{T}\int_{-T/2}^{T/2-\tau} f(t_1,t_1+\tau)\,dt_1d\tau$$

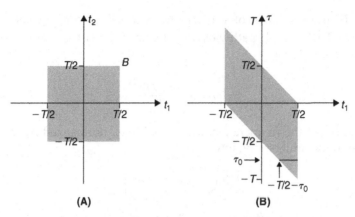

FIGURE 16.6   **A.** Integration boundaries of the square B in $\{t_1, t_2\}$ coordinates. **B.** Integration boundaries after the transformation $\{t_1, t_2\} \to \{t_1, \tau\}$.

and if we now substitute into the definition of f,

$$|X_T(\mu, \omega)|^2 = \int\limits_{-T}^{0} \int\limits_{-T/2-\tau}^{T/2} X_T(\mu, t_1) X_T(\mu, t_1 + \tau) e^{-2\pi i \omega \tau} \, dt_1 d\tau$$

$$+ \int\limits_{0}^{T} \int\limits_{-T/2}^{T/2-\tau} X_T(\mu, t_1) X_T(\mu, t_1 + \tau) e^{-2\pi i \omega \tau} \, dt_1 d\tau.$$

Taking expectations on both sides and using $E[X_T(t_1) X_T(t_1 + \tau)] = C(\tau)$ we obtain

$$E[|X_T(\omega)|^2] = \int\limits_{-T}^{0} \int\limits_{-T/2-\tau}^{T/2} C(\tau) e^{-2\pi i \omega \tau} \, dt_1 d\tau + \int\limits_{0}^{T} \int\limits_{-T/2}^{T/2-\tau} C(\tau) e^{-2\pi i \omega \tau} \, dt_1 d\tau$$

$$= \int\limits_{-T}^{T} (T - |\tau|) C(\tau) e^{-2\pi i \omega \tau} \, d\tau,$$

and after division by T we arrive at Eq. (16.17).   □

16.6 SUMMARY AND SOURCES

This chapter offers a basic introduction to stochastic processes. In the next two chapters, we will encounter additional examples of relevance to neuroscience and tackle the problem of estimating numerically the power spectrum of a stochastic process. In addition to the references given in §11.12, Doob (1953) is a classical reference for the mathematically inclined. We like the first two chapters of Goodman (1985). Cox and Isham (1980) provide an accessible introduction to point processes and Tuckwell (1988) surveys the application of stochastic processes to theoretical neuroscience up to its publication. Our derivation of the autocovariance function of a stationary point process is similar to that of Cox and Lewis (1966, Chapter 4, §4). The proof of the Wiener–Khinchin theorem follows Bendat and Piersol (2000, §5.2.2). For a more rigorous treatment, see Priestley (1981, Chapter 4) and Percival and Walden (1993, Chapter 4). The time rescaling theorem introduced in Exercise 24 is often used to test the adequacy of models for the discharge (conditional intensity) of a given neuron. See Johnson (1996) and Brown et al. (2002) for further relevant information.

16.7 EXERCISES

1. Show that for a weakly stationary stochastic process, $C_X(\tau) = C_X(-\tau)$.
2. Generate 100 sample paths of the discrete approximation to white noise, 100 ms long, with a sampling step $\Delta t = 1$ ms and a standard deviation $1/\sqrt{\Delta t}$. Plot three of them to reproduce Figure 16.1C. Compute the sample

mean and standard deviation and replicate Figure 16.1D. Sum the samples after multiplying them by Δt to obtain 100 sample paths of the discrete approximation to the Wiener process. Compute the sample mean and standard deviation and reproduce Figure 16.1A and B.

3. Compute the autocovariance function of the Wiener process.

4. Compute the autocovariance function of the homogeneous Poisson process. Hint: Use the formal identity

$$\int_0^T \delta(t_a - t)\delta(t_b - t)\,dt = \delta(t_a - t_b) \quad (= \delta(t_b - t_a))$$

for $t_a, t_b \in (0, T)$.

5. Reproduce the plots of Figure 16.3 for the autocovariance function of the stationary gamma renewal process of orders $n = 2$ and $n = 10$, respectively. Assume a mean rate $\chi = 80$ spk/s and use the formula

$$\chi_c(\tau) = \frac{\varrho}{n}\left(1 + \sum_{k=1}^{n-1} z_k e^{\varrho(z_k - 1)}\right) \tag{16.18}$$

with $z_k = \exp(2\pi i k/n)$ for $k = 1, \ldots, n-1$.

6. Simulate 1000 sample spike trains from an inhomogeneous Poisson process with rate

$$\varrho_s(t) = 10(\sin(2\pi f_s t - \pi/2) + 1)$$

with $f_s = 4$ Hz and $t \in (0, 1]$ s. Use the algorithm described in §16.4 and forward Euler integration with a time step $dt = 0.1$ ms. Compute the average instantaneous firing rate by dividing the interval $(0, 1]$ in 100 bins 10 ms long and averaging the number of spikes in each bin. Use this to reproduce Figure 16.4.

7. Show that the power spectrum is a real symmetric function. Hint: Combine the results of Exercises 7.13 and 7.14.

8. Reproduce the plots of Figure 16.5 for the power spectrum of the stationary gamma renewal processes of order $n = 2$ and $n = 10$, respectively. Assume a mean rate $\chi = 80$ spk/s and use the formula

$$S(\omega) = \chi\left(1 - 2\chi \sum_{k=1}^{n-1} \frac{\varrho(z_k - 1)z_k}{(2\pi\omega)^2 + (\varrho(z_k - 1))^2}\right) \tag{16.19}$$

with $z_k = \exp(2\pi i k/n)$ for $k = 1, \ldots, n-1$.

9. Argue, starting from the definition of χ_c, Eq. (16.11), that

$$\chi_c(\tau) = \frac{d}{d\tau} E[N(0, \tau)],$$

where $N(0, \tau)$ is the spike count of the same process, but with time shifted so that a spike occurs at time $t = 0$. Hint: Start from the equation

$$P(\text{spike in } (t + \tau, t + \tau + \Delta t)|\text{spike at } t) = E[N(t + \tau + \Delta t, t) - N(t + \tau, t)] + o(\Delta t^2). \tag{16.20}$$

10. Show that for a gamma renewal process of order n the Laplace transform of χ_c is given by

$$\mathcal{L}(\chi)(s) = \frac{\mathcal{L}(p_n)(s)}{1 - \mathcal{L}(p_n)(s)},$$

where p_n is the probability density of the ISI distribution. Hint: Use the results of Exercises 9 and 15.9 and Eq. (3.16).

11. Show that the roots, s_k, of $1 - \mathcal{L}(p_n)(s)$ are given by $s_k = \varrho(z_k - 1)$, where $z_k = \exp(2\pi i k/n)$ for $k = 0, \ldots, n-1$.

12. With the notation $g(s) = \mathcal{L}(p_n)(s)$, $\mathcal{L}(\chi_c)(s) = g(s)/(1 - g(s))$, show that

$$\frac{g(s)}{1 - g(s)} = \frac{1}{n} \sum_{i=0}^{n-1} \frac{\varrho z_i}{s - s_i}.$$

Hint: First convince yourself that the roots of $1 - g(s)$ derived in the previous exercise are simple so that the following partial fraction expansion holds

$$\frac{g(s)}{1 - g(s)} = \sum_{i=0}^{n-1} \frac{\alpha_i}{s - s_i}. \tag{16.21}$$

Next show that $\alpha_i = -1/g'(s_i)$. For this purpose, multiply both sides of Eq. (16.21) by $(s - s_i)$ and let $s \to s_i$. Use L'Hôpital's rule to compute the left hand side. Finally, show that $g'(s_i) = -n/(\varrho + s_i)$ and use the value of s_i derived in the previous exercise.

13. Show that $\chi_c(\tau)$ is given by Eq. (16.18). Hint: Compute the inverse Laplace transform based on the result of Exercise 10. Treat separately the root s_0 from the roots s_i, $i = 1, \ldots, n-1$.

14. [†]Show that if $C(\tau) = \chi \delta(\tau) + \chi(\chi_c(|\tau|) - \chi)$ is the autocovariance function of a stationary point process, then its power spectrum is given by

$$S(\omega) = \chi + \chi \left(\mathcal{L}(\phi_c)(2\pi i\omega) + \mathcal{L}(\phi_c)(-2\pi i\omega) \right), \tag{16.22}$$

where $\phi_c(|\tau|) = \chi_c(|\tau|) - \chi$.

15. [†]Show that for a stationary, gamma renewal process of order n, the power spectrum, $S(\omega)$, is given by Eq. (16.19). Hint: Compute the Laplace transform of ϕ_c using the results of Exercise 12 and insert this in Eq. (16.22).

16. [†]Modify the code written for Exercise 6 to use a threshold that is not exponentially distributed. Instead, use a random threshold distributed as a gamma random variable with orders 1–10 and a mean of 1. Plot a figure similar to Figure 16.4 but for the gamma order 10 threshold. Compute and plot the Fano factor for the spike count over the entire 1 s interval as a function of the gamma order to arrive at Figure 16.7.

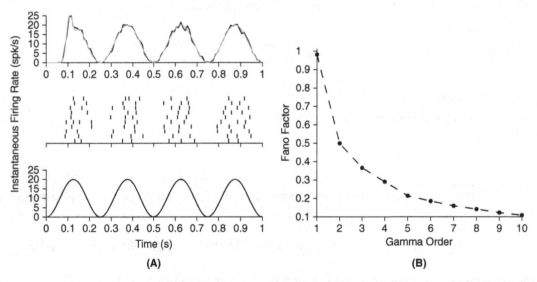

(A) **(B)**

FIGURE 16.7   **A.** Simulation of an integrate-and-fire neuron with random, gamma distributed threshold of order 10 stimulated with a sinusoidal current as in Exercise 6. Top: instantaneous firing rate estimated using 1000 trials. The red curve is a theoretical fit derived in Exercise 17. Middle: 10 sample spike trains. Bottom: stimulus. **B.** Fano factor as a function of the gamma order of the threshold. (rand_gamma.m)

17. Let $N_s(0, t)$ be the spike count of the integrate-and-fire neuron with gamma random threshold stimulated with the sinusoidal input

$$\varrho_s(t) = 10(\sin(2\pi f_s t - \pi/2) + 1).$$

Let $\chi_{sc}(t) = dE[N_s(0,t)]/dt$ be its instantaneous rate, as plotted in Exercise 16. Show that

$$\chi_{sc}(t) = \frac{d}{dt}E[N_s(0,t)] = \chi_c(s(t))\varrho_s(t), \tag{16.23}$$

where $\chi_c(t)$ is the instantaneous rate of the corresponding unmodulated process (Eq. (16.18)) and $s(t)$ is the transformed time variable

$$s(t) = \int_0^t \varrho_s(y)\,dy.$$

Hint: The random threshold values $x_1,\ldots,x_l$ determine the spike times $t_1,\ldots,t_l$ through the equations

$$x_i = \int_{t_{i-1}}^{t_i} \varrho_s(y)\,dy \quad i=1,\ldots,l, \tag{16.24}$$

with $t_0 = 0$. Therefore, the following equation holds for the transformed time variable $s(t)$:

$$s(t_l) = x_1 + \cdots + x_l.$$

Now argue as in Exercise 15.8 that $E[N_s(0,t)] = \sum_{l=1}^{\infty} K_l(s(t))$.

18. Plot the prediction, Eq. (16.23), to arrive at the red curve in Figure 16.7.

19. Argue that if the integrate-and-fire neuron with gamma distributed random threshold of Exercise 17 has started in the infinite past ($t_{start} \to -\infty$), then its instantaneous rate $\chi_{sc}(t)$ is proportional to the stimulus $\varrho_s(t)$. Hint: Prove the claim in two different ways. First by using directly Eq. (16.23). Second, from the distribution of transformed spike times $s(t_i)$ and using the conservation of probabilities, $\chi \Delta s = \chi_{sc} \Delta t$.

20. †Generalize the result of Exercise 4 to compute the autocovariance function of the inhomogeneous Poisson process.

21. If the rate of an inhomogeneous Poisson process is itself a stationary random variable, the resulting point process is called a *doubly stochastic* Poisson process. We will encounter such processes when we describe the spike trains of neurons in response to random stimuli in Chapter 23. If $E_\varrho[\varrho(t)] = \bar{\varrho}$ and $N(0,t)$ is the number of spikes of such a process in the interval $(0,t]$, show that

$$E[N(0,t)] = \bar{\varrho}t, \quad E\left[(N(0,t) - E[N(0,t)])^2\right] = \bar{\varrho}t + 2\int_0^t (t-u)C_\varrho(u)\,du,$$

where $C_\varrho(t)$ is the autocovariance function of $\varrho(t)$. Conclude from this equation that the Fano factor of a doubly stochastic point process is always greater than one. Hint: Compute the expectation in two steps, first for a fixed rate and then over the ensemble of rates:

$$E[N(0,t)] = E_\varrho[E[N(0,t)|\varrho(t)]].$$

22. Show that if X is a stochastic process with a white power spectrum up to a cut-off frequency f_N its power spectral density and autocovariance function are given by

$$S(\omega) = \frac{\sigma^2}{2f_N}\mathbb{1}_{(-f_N,f_N)}(\omega), \quad \text{and} \quad C(\tau) = \sigma^2\frac{\sin 2\pi f_N\tau}{2\pi f_N\tau},$$

respectively. Hint: By definition, the spectral power density is constant over the interval $[-f_N;f_N]$ and $\sigma^2 = C(0)$.

23. We define for a renewal process the *hazard function* as the probability rate of the next spike occurring at interval t given that the interval is at least that long,

$$h(t) = \frac{p(t)}{\int_t^\infty p(s)\,ds} \tag{16.25}$$

where $p(t)$ is the interspike interval distribution. Show that for a gamma renewal process of order 2 with rate parameter ϱ,

$$h(t) = \frac{\varrho^2 t}{1 + \varrho t}. \tag{16.26}$$

24. The arguments of Exercises 17 and 19 can be generalized as follows. Remember from §16.3 that $L(t) = N(0, t)$ denotes the number of spikes in the interval $(0, T]$ and assume that we are given the entire *history* of the process up to time t, $\mathcal{H}_t = \{0 < t_1 < t_2 \cdots t_n < t\}$, i.e., the exact spike times t_i, $i = 1, \ldots, n$, preceding t and up to it. Define the *conditional intensity* of the point process as

$$\varrho_i(t|\mathcal{H}_t) \equiv \frac{\mathrm{d}}{\mathrm{d}t} E[L(t|\mathcal{H}_t)] = \lim_{\Delta t \to 0} \frac{P(\Delta L_t|\mathcal{H}_t)}{\Delta t}.$$

The *time rescaling theorem* states that given spike times t_j, $j = 1, \ldots, m$, and the conditional intensity, $\varrho_i(t|\mathcal{H}_t)$, from which they originate, the transformation

$$s(t_j) = \int_0^{t_j} \varrho_i(t|\mathcal{H}_t) \, \mathrm{d}t \tag{16.27}$$

results in $s_j = s(t_j)$ being a homogeneous Poisson process with unit rate. For a stationary renewal process, the conditional intensity at time t depends only on the previous spike time, t_{last}, and is given by the hazard function, Eq. (16.25),

$$\varrho_i(t|t_{last}) = h(t - t_{last}).$$

(i) Show that for a stationary gamma process of order 2 with parameter ϱ

$$s(t_j) = s(t_{j-1}) + \varrho(t_j - t_{j-1}) - \log\big(1 + \varrho(t_j - t_{j-1})\big). \tag{16.28}$$

Hint: Use Eq. (16.26).

(ii) Check that Eq. (16.26) indeed yields a Poisson process with unit rate by generating a gamma order 2 spike train with parameter $\varrho = 40$. Then compute the transformed spike times and estimate numerically the resulting interspike interval distribution. Superpose on your plot the expected exponential distribution with unit rate. Hint: Generate 100,000 gamma distributed intervals using `gamrnd`. Use `hist` with 100 bins to estimate the ISI distribution.

17

Membrane Noise*

OUTLINE

17.1 Two-State Channel Model   267   17.4 Synaptic Noise   272

17.2 Multistate Channel Models   270   17.5 Summary and Sources   275

17.3 The Ornstein–Uhlenbeck Process   271   17.6 Exercises   275

The electrical current flowing through voltage-activated or synaptic conductances is generated by channels inserted across the lipid bilayer membrane of neurons (Figure 2.2). The current passing through *single* channels can be resolved by means of the *patch-clamp* technique, in which a fairly blunt ($\approx 1 \, \mu$m diameter) electrode is sealed onto the cell's membrane allowing it to sense directly the current developing across one or a few channels immediately below it (Figure 17.1A, B).

Such recordings show that single channels behave in a stochastic manner, randomly transitioning between two or more different states (Figure 17.1C). In this chapter, we start by introducing a new class of stochastic processes called *Markov processes* which capture the random properties of single channels. We then introduce a simple and efficient algorithm to simulate numerically one or more such channels. In §17.3 we define the simplest *continuous* Markov process called the *Ornstein–Uhlenbeck*, or *OU process*. We show in §17.4 how the OU process can be used to model random synaptic inputs impinging over extended dendritic trees in simplified neuron models. This allows us in turn to investigate how random background synaptic activity affects the properties of single neurons under conditions resembling those they experience *in vivo*.

17.1 TWO-STATE CHANNEL MODEL

We consider a simple channel with open and closed states and transition probabilities α, $\beta \neq 0$ (Figure 17.1C). Specifically, let $X(t) = 0$ or 1 if the channel is closed or open, respectively. We assume channel transitions between states to be independent of time, t, and for Δt sufficiently small (i.e., in the limit $\Delta t \to 0$),

$$p_{12}(\Delta t) = P(X(t + \Delta t) = 1 \mid X(t) = 0) = \alpha \Delta t, \quad p_{11}(\Delta t) = 1 - \alpha \Delta t$$
$$p_{21}(\Delta t) = P(X(t + \Delta t) = 0 \mid X(t) = 1) = \beta \Delta t, \quad p_{22}(\Delta t) = 1 - \beta \Delta t.$$

Note that $p_{11} + p_{12} = p_{21} + p_{22} = 1$.

Markov property. We assume that the future state of the channel is independent of its past states up to the last known state. For $t_3 > t_2 > t_1$,

$$P(X(t_3) = S_3 \mid X(t_2) = S_2, X(t_1) = S_1) = P(X(t_3) = S_3 \mid X(t_2) = S_2)$$

with $S_i = 0, 1$, for $i = 1, 2, 3$. This property generalizes to arbitrary sequences $t_{n+1} > t_n > \cdots > t_1$.

17. MEMBRANE NOISE*

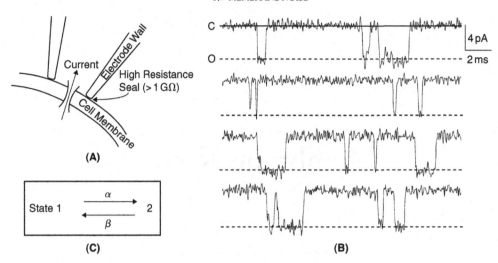

FIGURE 17.1 **A.** Schematic illustration of the patch-clamp technique. An electrode with a large ($\approx 1\,\mu$m) tip diameter (see Figure 13.20) is brought in close contact with the cell membrane so as to form a high resistance seal. This permits one to measure single channel currents flowing in and out of the patch. **B.** Single channel recording of an NMDA receptor. Adapted from Dravid et al. (2008). **C.** Simple two-state channel model (state 1: closed; state 2: open).

The Markov property allows us to derive a differential equation for p_{11}. Namely,

$$p_{11}(t_1 + \Delta t) = P(X(t_1 + \Delta t) = 0 \mid X(t_1) = 0)p_{11}(t_1) + P(X(t_1 + \Delta t) = 0 \mid X(t_1) = 1)p_{12}(t_1)$$
$$= (1 - \alpha \Delta t)p_{11}(t_1) + \beta \Delta t p_{12}(t_1),$$

or with $\Delta t \to 0$,

$$p_{11}' = -\alpha p_{11} + \beta p_{12}.$$

Similarly, $p_{22}' = -\beta p_{22} + \alpha p_{21}$, $p_{12}' = \alpha p_{11} - \beta p_{12}$, and $p_{21}' = \beta p_{22} - \alpha p_{21}$, with the initial conditions $p_{11}(0) = 1$, $p_{12} = 0$, $p_{21}(0) = 0$, and $p_{22}(0) = 1$. Define $\tau = 1/(\alpha + \beta)$, $p_\infty = \alpha/(\alpha + \beta)$, and $q_\infty = \beta/(\alpha + \beta)$. The solutions to these equations are, Exercise 1,

$$p_{11}(t) = q_\infty + p_\infty e^{-t/\tau}, \quad p_{12}(t) = 1 - p_{11}(t) = p_\infty - p_\infty e^{-t/\tau},$$
$$p_{22}(t) = p_\infty + q_\infty e^{-t/\tau}, \quad p_{21}(t) = 1 - p_{22}(t) = q_\infty - q_\infty e^{-t/\tau}. \tag{17.1}$$

These transition probabilities allow us to compute the time evolution of the open and closed channel probabilities from an arbitrary initial state. If $P(X(0) = 0) = \pi_0$ and $P(X(1) = 1) = \pi_1$, $\pi_0 + \pi_1 = 1$, then

$$P(X(t) = 0) = P(X(0) = 0)p_{11}(t) + P(X(0) = 1)p_{21}(t)$$
$$= q_\infty + (\pi_0 p_\infty - \pi_1 q_\infty)e^{-t/\tau},$$
$$P(X(t) = 1) = P(X(0) = 0)p_{12}(t) + P(X(0) = 1)p_{22}(t)$$
$$= p_\infty + (\pi_1 q_\infty - \pi_0 p_\infty)e^{-t/\tau}.$$

Therefore, any initial distribution (π_0, π_1) converges exponentially towards the steady-state distribution (q_∞, p_∞).

Matrix formulation. If we set

$$\mathbf{Q} = \begin{pmatrix} q_{11} & q_{12} \\ q_{21} & q_{22} \end{pmatrix} = \begin{pmatrix} -\alpha & \alpha \\ \beta & -\beta \end{pmatrix} \quad \text{and} \quad \mathbf{P} = \begin{pmatrix} p_{11} & p_{12} \\ p_{21} & p_{22} \end{pmatrix} \tag{17.2}$$

the differential equation and initial conditions for p_{ij}, $i, j = 1, 2$ can be written more compactly as $\mathbf{P}' = \mathbf{PQ}$, $\mathbf{P}(0) = \mathbf{I}$. In addition, $\mathbf{PQ} = \mathbf{QP}$ (Exercise 2). If $\mathbf{P}(t)$ and $\mathbf{Q}$ were scalars then the solution of this differential equation would be

$P(t) = \exp(t\mathbf{Q})$. This analogy, recall Eq. (5.30), carries over to matrices. In particular

$$\mathbf{P}(t) = \exp(t\mathbf{Q}) \equiv \mathbf{U} \exp(t\mathbf{Z}) \mathbf{U}^{-1} \tag{17.3}$$

where $\mathbf{Z}$ is the diagonal matrix of eigenvalues of $\mathbf{Q}$ and $\mathbf{U}$ is the corresponding matrix of eigenvectors. Because $\mathbf{Q}$ in Eq. (17.2) is two dimensional we can compute, by hand, its exponential (Exercise 3). Looking back, however, we recognize that Eq. (17.1) reveals

$$\exp(t\mathbf{Q}) = \begin{pmatrix} q_\infty & p_\infty \\ q_\infty & p_\infty \end{pmatrix} + \begin{pmatrix} p_\infty & -p_\infty \\ -q_\infty & q_\infty \end{pmatrix} e^{-t/\tau}. \tag{17.4}$$

Steady-state vector. In matrix notation, if $\boldsymbol{\pi}^T(0) = (\pi_0 \; \pi_1)$ is the initial probability distribution of channels, then $\boldsymbol{\pi}^T(t) = \boldsymbol{\pi}^T(0)\mathbf{P}(t)$ and $\boldsymbol{\pi}^T(t)$ satisfies the differential equation $d\boldsymbol{\pi}^T/dt = \boldsymbol{\pi}^T\mathbf{Q}$. At steady-state $d\boldsymbol{\pi}_{ss}^T/dt = 0$ or equivalently $\boldsymbol{\pi}_{ss}^T\mathbf{Q} = 0$. Therefore the steady-state distribution $\boldsymbol{\pi}_{ss}^T = (q_\infty \; p_\infty)$ is a *left* eigenvector of $\mathbf{Q}$ with eigenvalue zero. By transposing this last equation, $\mathbf{Q}^T\boldsymbol{\pi}_{ss} = 0$, we see that, equivalently, $\boldsymbol{\pi}_{ss}$ is an eigenvector of $\mathbf{Q}^T$ with eigenvalue zero.

Distribution of open and closed states. Let $F_2(t)$ be the probability that the time spent by the channel in the open state is less than or equal to t and $p_2(t)$ the corresponding probability density so that

$$F_2(t) = \int\limits_0^t p_2(s)\,\mathrm{d}s.$$

Thus $R_2(t) = 1 - F_2(t)$ is the probability that the time spent in the open state is larger than t. We can now derive a differential equation for R_2 in a similar manner as for p_{ij} above:

$$R_2(t + \Delta t) = R_2(t)P(X(t + \Delta t) = 1 \mid X(t) = 1) = R_2(t)(1 - \beta\Delta t).$$

Hence, as $\Delta t \to 0$, $R_2' = -\beta R_2$, and $R_2(t) = \exp(-\beta t)$, since $R_2(0) = 1$. This implies $F_2(t) = 1 - \exp(-\beta t)$ and $p_2(t) = \beta \exp(-\beta t)$. Since this is an exponential distribution, the mean open state duration equals $1/\beta$. Similarly, the distribution of closed states is $f_1(t) = \alpha \exp(-\alpha t)$ and the mean closed state duration is $1/\alpha$. The probability distributions of open and closed states permit one to simulate the sample trajectory of a single channel. The algorithm can be extended to efficiently simulate multiple independent single channels (Figure 17.2, Exercise 4).

Current noise. We now assume that a single open channel passes current $i = \gamma(V - V_{rev})$ where γ is the single channel conductance and V_{rev} the channel equilibrium potential. The membrane potential is assumed to be clamped at V. At equilibrium, the mean current through a single channel will thus be ip_∞. Many properties of the channel can be derived by observing the current fluctuations of a channel population. For n independent channels at equilibrium, the current

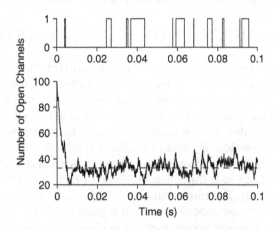

FIGURE 17.2   Top: simulation of a single channel transitioning between closed and open states with rates $\alpha = 100\,1/\mathrm{s}$ and $\beta = 500\,1/\mathrm{s}$. Bottom: simulation of 200 identical channels with 100 of them initially open. The dashed line indicates the average number of open channels at steady state. (twostatechan.m)

is $I(t) = i \sum_{j=1}^{n} X_j(t)$, where $X_j(t)$ tracks the closed/open state of channel j. The mean current is $\bar{I} = E[I(t)] = nip_\infty$. Since the channels' openings and closings are independent of one another, they are uncorrelated, $E[(X_j(t) - p_\infty)(X_k(t+h) - p_\infty)] = 0$ for $j \neq k$. If we define the current autocovariance function $C(h) = E[(I(t) - \bar{I})(I(t+h) - \bar{I})]$, then

$$
\begin{aligned}
C(h) &= i^2 E\left[\sum_{j=1}^{n} (X_j(t) - p_\infty) \sum_{k=1}^{n} (X_k(t+h) - p_\infty) \right] \\
&= i^2 \sum_{j,k=1}^{n} E[(X_j(t) - p_\infty)(X_k(t+h) - p_\infty)] \\
&= i^2 \sum_{j=1}^{n} E[(X_j(t) - p_\infty)(X_j(t+h) - p_\infty)] \\
&= ni^2 (E[X_1(t)X_1(t+h)] - p_\infty^2).
\end{aligned}
\tag{17.5}
$$

We have used the fact that distinct channels are uncorrelated to derive the third line from the second and the fact that all channels are identical to obtain the fourth line. Since X_1 takes only values 0 or 1, we have, for $h > 0$

$$
\begin{aligned}
E[X_1(t)X_1(t+h)] &= P(X_1(t) = 1, X_1(t+h) = 1) \\
&= P(X_1(t) = 1)P(X_1(t+h) = 1 \mid X_1(t) = 1) \\
&= p_\infty p_{22}(h).
\end{aligned}
$$

Similarly, for $h < 0$, $E[X_1(t)X_1(t+h)] = p_\infty p_{22}(-h)$. Substituting these results into Eq. (17.5) and using Eq. (17.1),

$$
C(h) = ni^2 p_\infty q_\infty e^{-|h|/\tau}.
$$

This equation shows that we can compute the channel's time constant τ of relaxation to steady state by recording current noise and fitting its autocovariance function to an exponential. Equivalently, the Fourier transform of $C(h)$ is

$$
\hat{C}(\omega) = ni^2 p_\infty q_\infty \frac{2\tau}{1 + (2\pi\tau\omega)^2}
\tag{17.6}
$$

(Exercise 5) and can be fit to a *Lorentzian* $\propto 1/(1 + (2\pi\tau\omega)^2)$.

The current variance is equal to $\sigma_I^2 = C(0) = ni^2 p_\infty(1 - p_\infty)$. This is expected since at each time point the channels' open and closed states will be binomially distributed (§11.2). If the recording conditions are such that $p_\infty \ll 1$, e.g., low V for a voltage-activated channel, then $\sigma_I^2 \approx ni^2 p_\infty$ and $\gamma = \sigma_I^2 / \bar{I}(V - V_{rev})$, allowing one to compute the single channel conductance from the mean and variance of the current fluctuations (Exercise 6).

17.2 MULTISTATE CHANNEL MODELS

In the previous chapters, we encountered several kinetic models similar to the simple two-state model of §17.1. For example, the synaptic model of §2.5, the Hodgkin–Huxley sodium and potassium conductance models of §4.2 or the kinetic models of Chapter 13. Their stochastic properties can be simulated with the methods introduced in §17.1. We use the Hodgkin–Huxley sodium channel as an example. In §4.2 we learned that the open channel probability is given by the product m^3h of three activation gates and one inactivation gate. Each of these gates behaves as an independent two-state subunit, as in the previous section. Instead of tracking each subunit separately, we consider states $m_i h_j$, $i = 0, 1, 2, 3$ and $j = 0, 1$ characterized by the total number of open activation and inactivation subunits. Thus, the state $m_3 h_1$ is the open state of the channel. Each state transition involves a single gate. Hence a state like $m_2 h_0$ can transition to the adjacent states $m_1 h_0$, $m_3 h_0$, or $m_2 h_1$. The transition rate to $m_3 h_0$ is equal to α_m, since the only closed m gate has to open for the transition to occur. In contrast, one of two open m gates has to close to transition to $m_1 h_0$ and therefore the transition rate is $2\beta_m$. The resulting model is summarized in Figure 17.3. We number the different states, S, from 1 to 8 and define q_{ij} for $i \neq j$ as the transition rate from state i to j. In addition let $q_i = \sum_{j \neq i} q_{ij}$ which is the total escape rate from state i (transition rate to another state, $P(S(t + \Delta t) \neq i \mid S(t) = i)/\Delta t$ as $\Delta t \to 0$), and $q_{ii} = -q_i$. Just as in the

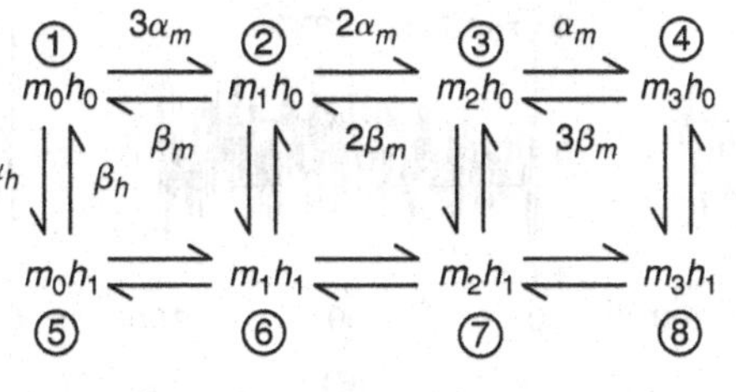

FIGURE 17.3 Equivalent eight states kinetic model of the Hodgkin–Huxley sodium channel.

two-state model, the resulting matrix $\mathbf{Q} = (q_{ij})$ determines the evolution of the transition probabilities: $\mathbf{P}' = \mathbf{Q}\mathbf{P}$ so that $\mathbf{P}(t) = \exp(t\mathbf{Q})$. Direct computation of $\mathbf{P}(t)$ is illustrated in Exercise 7.

Numerical simulations: Gillespie's algorithm. Just as in the previous section, the distribution of times in state i is given by $f_i(t) = q_i \exp(-q_i t)$, where q_i is the total escape rate from state i. In addition, once a transition out of state i occurs, the probability of transitioning to state j is:

$$\frac{P(S(t+\Delta t) = j \mid S(t) = i)}{P(S(t+\Delta t) \neq j \mid S(t) = j)} = \frac{q_{ij}\Delta t}{q_i \Delta t} = \frac{q_{ij}}{q_i}.$$

Therefore, starting from state i, the simulation of a single channel trajectory proceeds by drawing first an exponentially distributed random number according to f_i to determine the time of the next transition. To determine which transition occurred, a random number, r uniformly distributed between zero and one is then drawn. The state j that satisfies

$$\sum_{k=1}^{j-1} q_{ij}/q_i < r \leq \sum_{k=1}^{j} q_{ij}/q_i$$

is the new updated state. This algorithm can be extended to efficiently simulate multiple independent channels (Exercise 14).

17.3 THE ORNSTEIN–UHLENBECK PROCESS

We now introduce a stochastic process that will allow us to efficiently simulate random synaptic noise. The OU process, X, is a generalization of the Wiener process described in §16.2. If dt represents an infinitesimal time step, we know from Eq. (16.4) that the value of $W(t + dt)$ is given by $W(t + dt) = W(t) + dW(t)$ where $dW(t)$ is a Gaussian random variable independent of $W(t)$ with variance dt. Equivalently, since $dW(t) \sim \mathcal{N}(0, dt)$ we may write $dW(t) = N(t)(dt)^{1/2}$, where $N(t) \sim \mathcal{N}(0,1)$. We now generalize this equation by assuming that the stochastic variable X satisfies the stochastic differential equation

$$X(t+dt) = X(t) - \frac{1}{\tau}X(t)\,dt + c^{1/2}N(t)(dt)^{1/2} \tag{17.7}$$

and $X(t_0) = x_0$. To understand the meaning of this equation, first note that if $c^{1/2} = 0$ it has the solution $X(t) = x_0 \exp(-(t - t_0)/\tau)$ and therefore $X(t)$ relaxes exponentially towards x_0. When $c^{1/2} \neq 0$ and $\tau \to \infty$ the last term is the same random drift as for the Wiener process, up to a constant scaling. Therefore, in general, $X(t)$ will fluctuate randomly, with the last term driving it away from zero, while the second term acts as a damping factor tending to bring X back towards zero.

It follows from Eq. (17.7) that $X(t)$ is a Markov process, since its value at $t + dt$ depends only on its value at t. Furthermore $X(t + dt)$ will be Gaussian, provided $X(t)$ is, since it is the sum of two Gaussian, independent variables. This is certainly the case for $X(t_0) = x_0 \sim \mathcal{N}(x_0, 0)$ and therefore for any $t \geq t_0$.

Distribution of X(t). Although it is possible to simulate $X(t)$ by discretizing Eq. (17.7) (i.e., replace dt by Δt, a small, but finite time step) we can also solve exactly for the distribution of $X(t)$, which then yields an exact update for $X(t + \Delta t)$ from $X(t)$. Since $X(t)$ is Gaussian, we need only compute its mean $m(t) = E[X(t)]$, $m(t_0) = x_0$ and its variance

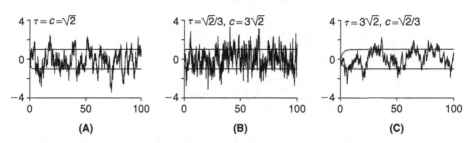

FIGURE 17.4   Simulations of three OU processes with the steady-state variance $c\tau/2 = 1$, but different ratios for c/τ (1, 9, and 1/9, respectively). The solid lines denote $\pm$ one standard deviation of $X(t)$ (i.e., $\sqrt{v(t)}$). (ou_f1.m)

$v(t) = E[(X(t) - m(t))^2]$, $v(t_0) = 0$. Taking means on both sides of Eq. (17.7) yields

$$E[X(t + dt)] = E[X(t)] - \frac{1}{\tau} E[X(t)]\, dt$$

or $m' = -m(t)/\tau$ and so $m(t) = x_0 \exp(-(t - t_0)/\tau)$. Similarly, $v(t) = (c\tau/2)(1 - \exp(-2(t - t_0)/\tau))$ (Exercise 15). Hence, $X(t) \sim \mathcal{N}(m(t), v(t))$. Note that the mean converges to zero and the variance to $c\tau/2$ when $t \gg t_0$. We now use the Markov property to compute $X(t + \Delta t)$: replace t by $t + \Delta t$, t_0 by t, and x_0 by $X(t)$ to obtain

$$X(t + \Delta t) \sim \mathcal{N}(X(t)e^{-\Delta t/\tau},\ c\tau \left(1 - e^{-2\Delta t/\tau}\right)/2)$$

or, equivalently, if n is a sample from a unit Gaussian distribution,

$$X(t + \Delta t) = X(t)e^{-\Delta t/\tau} + n\sqrt{c\tau(1 - e^{-2\Delta t/\tau})/2}.$$

Simulations of the OU process using this update formula are illustrated in Figure 17.4.

Autocovariance and power spectrum. The autocovariance of $X(t)$ can be computed analytically,

$$C(t_1, t_2) = E[X(t_1)X(t_2)] - m(t_1)m(t_2) = \frac{c\tau}{2}e^{-(t_2 - t_1)/\tau}\left(1 - e^{-2(t_1 - t_0)/\tau}\right)$$

for $t_0 \le t_1 \le t_2$, Exercise 17. As $t_0 \to \infty$, C depends only on $h = t_2 - t_1$: $C(h) = (c\tau/2)\exp(-|h|/\tau)$. Thus, as was the case for the two-state channel, Eq. (17.6), the power spectrum is a Lorentzian: $\hat{C}(\omega) = (c\tau/2) \cdot 2\tau/(1 + (2\pi\tau\omega)^2)$.

17.4 SYNAPTIC NOISE

We can now use the OU process to approximate the random synaptic input fluctuations experienced by extended neurons like neocortical pyramidal cells *in vivo*. Recall from Exercise 9.6 that we can replace the random synaptic bombardment experienced by a neuron across its dendritic tree by two effective synaptic conductances localized at the soma, one being excitatory and the other one inhibitory. These effective conductances are derived by voltage clamping the soma at two different membrane potentials (Figure 9.27) and solving a pair of linear equations, Eq. (9.31), in terms of the clamp currents. Figure 17.5 illustrates the properties of the effective excitatory and inhibitory conductances obtained by simulating the synaptic bombardment impinging onto a neocortical pyramidal neuron as it receives random spontaneous inputs over its entire dendritic tree. Specifically, the model neuron received $\approx 16,500$ fast excitatory (AMPA) and 3400 fast inhibitory (GABA) synaptic inputs randomly activated at a rate of 1 and 5.5 events/s, respectively. Each input was modeled as a homogeneous Poisson process and any two excitatory or inhibitory inputs were weakly correlated with each other to mimic *in vivo* experimental observations (we will learn how to generate pairwise correlated homogeneous Poisson processes in Exercise 18.10). Both the excitatory and inhibitory conductances can be approximated by OU processes plus a constant $(X(t) + C)$. The constant value corresponds to the mean excitatory (g_{e0}) and inhibitory (g_{i0}) conductance produced at the soma by the synapses distributed over the dendritic tree. The time

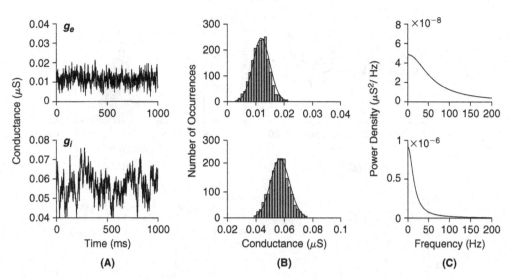

FIGURE 17.5 Properties of two OU processes that reproduce well the excitatory and inhibitory conductances measured at the soma of a neocortical pyramidal neuron and resulting from spontaneous activation of synapses over its entire dendritic tree. **A.** Time course of excitatory (top) and inhibitory (bottom) conductances. **B.** Corresponding histograms of conductance values. **C.** Corresponding power spectra. Note that these properties differ from those illustrated in Figures 9.27 and 9.28 for the model studied in Exercise 9.6. The parameters of the processes are: $g_{e0} = 0.012 \, \mu S$, $\tau_e = 2.7$ ms, and $\sigma_e = 0.003 \, \mu S$ for the excitatory process; $g_{i0} = 0.057 \, \mu S$, $\tau_i = 10.5$ ms, and $\sigma_i = 0.0066 \, \mu S$ for the inhibitory process. (ou_f2.m)

constants of the two OU processes (τ_e and τ_i) depend on the time constant of the individual excitatory and inhibitory synapses. Typically, the excitatory events are faster and thus have a shorter time constant. The standard deviation of the OU processes (σ_e and σ_i) mainly depends on the correlation level between individual excitatory and inhibitory inputs.

Subthreshold properties. We now study the impact of spontaneous background activity by simulating its effect in a single-compartment model of a pyramidal neuron described by the following differential equation (Exercise 19):

$$C_m \frac{dV}{dt} = -g_L(V - E_L) - I_{Na} - I_{Kdr} - I_M - \frac{1}{a} I_{syn},$$ (17.8)

where I_{Na} and I_{Kdr} are the fast sodium and delayed rectifier currents generating action potentials, and I_M is a voltage-dependent potassium current that generates spike frequency adaptation. The synaptic currents, $I_{syn} = I_e + I_i$ are scaled by the total surface area of the neuron, a. The excitatory synaptic current is $I_e = (g_{e0} + X_e(t))(V - V_e)$, where X_e is an OU process with parameters τ_e, σ_e, and V_e is the synaptic reversal potential. The inhibitory synaptic current is defined analogously. Spontaneous activity has several sizable effects on the subthreshold membrane properties of the model. First, it shifts the resting membrane potential from −80 mV to a mean value of approximately −65 mV and causes the membrane potential to fluctuate randomly around that value (Figure 17.6A and B). It also considerably modifies the input resistance of the membrane and its time constant (Figure 17.6C and D). These changes are a result of the constant synaptic bombardment experienced by neurons *in vivo*, which increases membrane conductance, rendering them more "leaky" and thus less prone to depolarize or hyperpolarize in response to current or synaptic inputs. In addition, their responses to such stimuli tend to be much faster since the membrane time constant is decreased at higher conductances, an observation familiar from earlier, simpler models (Exercise 2.3).

Suprathreshold properties. When the cell fires in response to a depolarizing current pulse, the random background activity generates variability in the spike occurrence times and the interspike interval distribution (Figure 17.7A). This variability depends on how strong the current is relative to that generated by spontaneous synaptic activity. Thus, as the injected current increases and the mean interspike interval decreases, the coefficient of variation of the interspike intervals decreases as well (Figure 17.7B). In addition, changing the parameters of the spontaneous conductances changes the firing frequency *vs.* injected current (f-I) curve of the model. If the mean background inhibitory conductance is changed, the f-I curve typically shifts horizontally (Figure 17.7C). This effect is quite different from that of inhibition seen in the subthreshold regime, as in Exercise 2.6, for example. Roughly

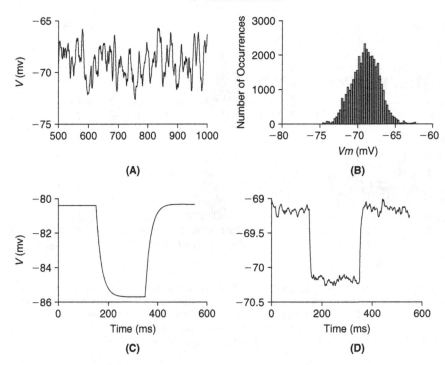

FIGURE 17.6 Impact of spontaneous synaptic activity on membrane potential. **A.** Membrane noise generated by spontaneous synaptic activity. **B.** Histogram of membrane potential values (mean: −69 mV, standard deviation: 1.81 mV). **C.** Response to a −0.25 μA/cm^2 pulse. The membrane potential hyperpolarizes from −80.8 to −86 mV for a difference of 5.2 mV. **D.** Response to the same pulse in the presence of background activity (average over 1000 repetitions). The mean membrane potential before and during the pulse is approx. −69 and −70 mV, respectively, for a mean difference of 1 mV. (`destex_f1.m`)

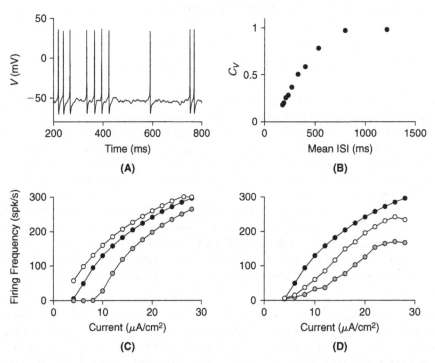

FIGURE 17.7 Suprathreshold effects of spontaneous synaptic activity. **A.** Irregular firing elicited by a 5 μA/cm^2 current in the presence of spontaneous activity. **B.** Coefficient of variation as a function of mean interspike interval in response to currents ranging from 4 to 9 μA/cm^2. As current increases, the mean interspike interval and the C_V decrease. **C.** Changes in the mean inhibitory conductance to twice (red circles) or half (white circles) their standard value shift the current firing frequency curve along the horizontal axis. **D.** Simultaneous changes in the mean and standard deviation of the excitatory and inhibitory conductances change the gain of the firing frequency curve. (`destex_f2.m`)

speaking, it results from the fact that during spiking the membrane potential is mainly controlled by the cell's intrinsic conductances. This causes the change in inhibitory conductance to effectively act like a constant current change. In contrast, changing both the mean and standard deviations of the excitatory and inhibitory currents leads to changes in the slope of the f-I curve (Figure 17.7D). This effect mainly arises from a broadening of the distribution of membrane potential fluctuations when the standard deviations are increased, which tends to smooth out the f-I curve. Thus changes in spontaneous activity can dynamically change the input–output characteristics of a neuron.

17.5 SUMMARY AND SOURCES

This chapter has provided an introduction to membrane noise, starting from single channels and up to the noise experienced *in vivo* by neurons due to embedding in large networks of neurons. In particular, we have seen that membrane noise is central to the biophysics of single ion channels and that it affects the integrative properties of single neurons. The patch-clamp technique played a crucial role in the study of membrane noise and was pioneered by Neher and Sakmann who were awarded the 1991 Nobel Prize in Medicine (http://nobelprize.org). The theory of Markov processes developed in this chapter has allowed us to elegantly characterize the stochastic properties of single ion channels. In addition, the simple algorithm of Gillespie (1977) enables one to efficiently simulate many such channels simultaneously. Taken together, this makes Markov processes an invaluable tool to model many random phenomena in neuroscience. Hawkes (2004) contains additional information on the stochastic modeling of single ion channels and many useful references. See Hille (2001) for further experimental examples. We also recommend the review of White et al. (2000). The potential impact of channel noise on single neuron computation has been investigated in Steinmetz et al. (2000) and its effects on axons in Faisal et al. (2005). Section 17.3 follows the presentation of Gillespie (1996). Section 17.4 is based on Destexhe et al. (2001) and Fellous et al. (2003), which should be consulted for further details. For a biophysical explanation of the results presented in Figure 17.7, see Holt and Koch (1997) and Doiron et al. (2001). The review by Destexhe et al. (2003) contains further references to much of the relevant literature.

17.6 EXERCISES

1. Compute the solutions of the differential equations for p_{11}, p_{12}, p_{21}, and p_{22}, as given in Eq. (17.1). Hint: Use the fact that $p_{11} + p_{12} = 1$ and $p_{21} + p_{22} = 1$.

2. Show that $\mathbf{PQ} = \mathbf{QP}$, where $\mathbf{P}$ and $\mathbf{Q}$ are defined in Eq. (17.2). Hint: Show that $\mathbf{I} + \Delta t \mathbf{Q} = \mathbf{P}(\Delta t)$, then use the Markov property to compute $\mathbf{P}(t)(\mathbf{I} + \Delta t \mathbf{Q})$ and $(\mathbf{I} + \Delta t \mathbf{Q})\mathbf{P}(t)$.

3. [†]Compute, by hand, the eigenvalues and eigenvectors of the $\mathbf{Q}$ matrix of Eq. (17.2). Assemble $\exp(t\mathbf{Q})$ per Eq. (17.3) and confirm that it agrees with Eq. (17.4). Hint: Use the results of Exercise 5.3 to compute $\mathbf{U}^{-1}$.

4. Simulate the sample time course history of a single two-state channel with $\alpha = 100$ 1/s and $\beta = 500$ 1/s. Carry out the same simulation for 200 channels, starting with 100 open channels to reproduce Figure 17.2. Hint: You don't need to keep track of each channel individually, only the number of open and closed ones. If N_c channels are closed and N_o are open, the total rate of transition is $\lambda = N_c \alpha + N_o \beta$. Compute the time of the next transition by selecting an exponentially distributed random variable with mean $1/\lambda$. If a transition occurs, the probabilities of $C \to O$ and $O \to C$ are, respectively

$$\lambda_1 = \frac{N_c \alpha}{\lambda} \quad \text{and} \quad \lambda_2 = \frac{N_o \beta}{\lambda}.$$

Therefore, for each transition you need to draw a second random number r between zero and one and decide on a $C \to O$ transition if $r \le \lambda_1$ and $O \to C$ otherwise. Update N_c and N_o accordingly and proceed to compute the random time of the next transition.

5. [†]Show by a direct calculation that the Fourier transform of $C(h)$ is given by Eq. (17.6).

6. [†]Show that to first order in p_∞, $\sigma_I^2 \approx n i^2 p_\infty$ and use this approximation to derive the formula $\gamma = \sigma_I^2 / \bar{I}(V - V_{rev})$.

7. **Detailed balance.** Let $\mathbf{Q} = (q_{nm})$ be the transition matrix of a multistate model and $\boldsymbol{\pi}_e$ the corresponding equilibrium vector: $\mathbf{Q}^T \boldsymbol{\pi}_e = 0$. Assume that the following equation holds for all n, m:

$$\pi_{en} q_{nm} = \pi_{em} q_{mn}$$

(detailed balance). Define $\mathbf{C} = \operatorname{diag}\left(\pi_{e1}^{1/2}, \ldots \pi_{en}^{1/2}\right)$. Show that $\mathbf{R} = \mathbf{CQC}^{-1}$ is symmetric. Express the eigenvalues and eigenvectors of $\mathbf{Q}$ in terms of those of $\mathbf{R}$. Compute from this $\exp(t\mathbf{Q})$. This exercise is a direct analog of our proof, in §8.2, of the fact that the Hines matrix was similar to a symmetric matrix.

8. [†]Compute the equilibrium vector for the two-state channel of §17.1, verify detailed balance and compute the associated matrix $\mathbf{R}$.

9. Compute numerically the maximal steady-state open probability of the Hodgkin–Huxley sodium channel and the corresponding membrane potential. Show that they are equal to 0.0077 and −37.94 mV, respectively.

10. At $V = -37.94$ mV, compute the mean open and closed times of the "activation" gate, m, of the sodium channel, as well as the mean time between transitions. Carry out the same calculation for the "inactivation" gate, h.

11. Compute numerically the equilibrium vector of the m gate at $V = -37.94$ mV and verify detailed balance within numerical error by computing its relative deviation from zero,

$$(\pi_{e1}q_{12} - \pi_{e2}q_{21})/(0.5(\pi_{e1}q_{12} + \pi_{e2}q_{21})).$$

Repeat for the h gate.

12. Using the results of the previous exercise, predict the equilibrium vector for the eight-state sodium channel model of Figure 17.3 at $V = -37.94$ mV. Compute numerically the transition matrix for the eight-state model of the sodium channel as well as the associated equilibrium vector; compare with your prediction.

13. Simulate a single sodium channel at $V = -37.94$ mV using the following two methods.
   (i) Simulate three independent m gates and one h gate. Then use the gate states to compute the state of the associated sodium channel.
   (ii) Use the transition matrix computed in Exercise 12 and the Gillespie algorithm of §17.3. Arrive at a figure similar to Figure 17.8.

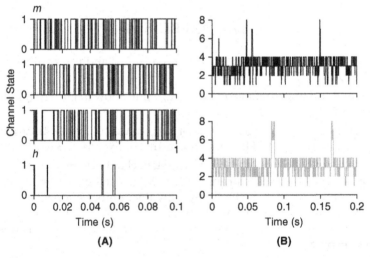

FIGURE 17.8 Simulations of a single sodium channel. **A.** Sample random openings (state 1) and closings (state 0) of three independent m gates and an h gate. **B.** Top: resulting derived state of the corresponding sodium channel. Bottom: direct simulation of the eight-state model. (na_chan.m)

14. [†]Simulate 200 sodium channels, all starting in the open state at a membrane potential of −37.94 mV. Generate a figure similar to Figure 17.9. Hint: Just as in the case of the two-state channel, you do not need to keep track of each channel individually. The transition matrix of the sodium channel has 20 distinct nonzero transitions, q_{12}, q_{15}, etc... Renumber them from 1 to 20 and call the corresponding rates r_i, $i = 1, \ldots, 20$, e.g., $r_1 = q_{12}$, $r_2 = q_{15}$, etc... For each transition, let $i(j)$, $j = 1, \ldots, 20$ be the corresponding start state and N_i the number of channels in state i, $i = 1, \ldots, 8$. Following a transition, compute:

$$\lambda = \sum_{j=1}^{20} N_{i(j)}r_j \quad \text{and} \quad \lambda_j = N_{i(j)}r_j/\lambda.$$

Draw a random number x_1 uniformly distributed between 0 and 1 and set the time to the next transition as $(1/\lambda)\log(1/x_1)$. Then draw a random number x_2 uniformly distributed between 0 and 1 and determine the transition l such that

$$\sum_{k=1}^{l-1}\lambda_k < x_2 \le \sum_{k=1}^{l}\lambda_k.$$

Decrease the number of channels in state $i(l)$ by one and increment the final state accordingly. Repeat the iteration.

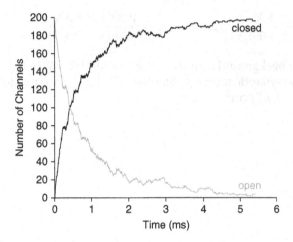

FIGURE 17.9   Simulations of 200 sodium channels, all starting in the open state at $t=0$. (multnachan.m)

15. Show that the variance of the OU process is given by

$$v(t) = (c\tau/2)(1 - \exp(-2(t-t_0)/\tau)).$$

Hint: Square Eq. (17.7) and keep terms of order dt or lower. Show that, with $f(t) = E[X^2(t)]$, the following differential equation holds: $f'(t) = (-2/\tau)f(t) + c$ with $f(t_0) = x_0$. Solve this differential equation and use the solution to compute $v(t)$.

16. Simulate three OU processes with the parameters given in the legend of Figure 17.4 and reproduce the plots of that figure.

17. Compute analytically the autocovariance function of the OU process. Hint: Define $h(t_1,t_2) = E[X(t_1)X(t_2)]$. Compute $h(t_1,t_2+dt_2)$ using Eq. (17.7) and show that h satisfies the following differential equation:

$$\frac{d}{dt_2}h(t_1,t_2) = -\frac{1}{\tau}h(t_1,t_2)$$

with the boundary condition $h(t_1,t_1) = f(t_1)$. Solve this differential equation and use the solution to compute the autocovariance function of X.

18. Simulate two OU processes with the parameters given in the legend of Figure 17.5 and reproduce the plots of that figure.

19. Simulate the model of Eq. (17.8) and reproduce Figures 17.6 and 17.7. The various currents are given by

$$I_K = \bar{g}_K n^4 (V - V_K),\quad \bar{g}_K = 10,\quad V_K = -90,$$
$$I_{Na} = \bar{g}_{Na} m^3 h (V - V_{Na}),\quad \bar{g}_{Na} = 51.6,\quad V_{Na} = 50,$$
$$I_M = \bar{g}_M p (V - V_K),\quad \bar{g}_M = 0.5,$$
$$I_L = g_L (V - V_L),\quad g_L = 0.045,\quad V_L = -80$$

with conductances in mS/cm^2 and reversal potentials in mV. The associated gating variables n, m, h, and p are governed by the following forward and backward rate functions

$$\alpha_n = \frac{-0.032(V - V_T - 15)}{\exp(-(V - V_T - 15)/5) - 1} \quad \text{and} \quad \beta_n = 0.5\exp(-(V - V_T - 10)/40), \quad V_T = -58,$$

$$\alpha_m = \frac{-0.32(V - V_T - 13)}{\exp(-(V - V_T - 13)/4) - 1} \quad \text{and} \quad \beta_m = \frac{0.28(V - V_T - 40)}{\exp((V - V_T - 40)/5) - 1}$$

$$\alpha_h = 0.128\exp(-(V - V_T - V_S - 17)/18) \quad \text{and} \quad \beta_h = \frac{4}{1 + \exp(-(V - V_T - V_S - 40)/5)}$$

$$\alpha_p = \frac{0.0001(V + 30)}{1 - \exp(-(V + 30)/9)} \quad \text{and} \quad \beta_p = \frac{-0.0001(V + 30)}{1 - \exp((V + 30)/9)}, \quad V_S = -10.$$

Steady state, without synaptic background activity is at $V = -80.3935$ mV. In Eq. (17.8), the total dendritic area a is equal to 34636×10^{-8} cm^2. The synaptic reversal potentials V_e and V_i are equal to 0 and -80 mV, respectively. The membrane capacitance is $C_m = 1$ μF/cm^2.

Power and Cross Spectra

OUTLINE

18.1 Cross Correlation and Coherence   279   18.4 Summary and Sources   286

18.2 Estimator Bias and Variance   280   18.5 Exercises   286

18.3 Numerical Estimate of the Power Spectrum*   282

The last chapter has illustrated the usefulness of power spectra to describe the frequency characteristics of stochastic processes. In this chapter, we generalize the power spectrum to characterize the frequency-dependent relation between *two* stochastic processes. This leads us to define first the cross spectrum of two stochastic processes and then their coherence. Next, we tackle the problem of estimating numerically power and cross spectra from experimental data. §18.2 makes some basic preliminary observations on the properties of estimates arising from random data samples. §18.3 then tackles the numerical power spectrum estimation problem. As we will see in the forthcoming chapters, the tools introduced here are basic workhorses that play a central role in the analysis of neural data.

18.1 CROSS CORRELATION AND COHERENCE

If X and Y are two stochastic processes, the covariance of X and Y is defined as

$$C_{XY}(t_1, t_2) = E[(X(t_1) - m_X(t_1))(Y(t_2) - m_Y(t_2))]$$

and is a measure of the degree of dependence between $X(t_1)$ and $Y(t_2)$ since its normalized value,

$$\gamma(t_1, t_2) = \frac{C_{XY}(t_1, t_2)}{\sqrt{C_{XX}(t_1, t_1)}\sqrt{C_{YY}(t_2, t_2)}}$$

is the correlation coefficient between $X(t_1)$ and $Y(t_2)$, with $-1 \leq \gamma \leq 1$.

We now define an analogous quantity in the frequency domain for two jointly stationary processes X and Y. For notational simplicity we will assume that X and Y have zero mean, or equivalently consider the centered processes $X - m_X$, $Y - m_Y$. If $t_2 = t_1 + \tau$, stationarity implies that the covariance and autocovariance of X and Y depend only on τ:

$$C_{XY}(\tau) = C_{XY}(t_1, t_1 + \tau) = E[X(t_1)Y(t_1 + \tau)]$$

and similarly for C_{XX}, C_{YY}. The Fourier transforms of $C_{XY}(\tau)$, $C_{XX}(\tau)$, and $C_{YY}(\tau)$ (which we assume to exist) are the cross spectrum $S_{XY}(\omega)$ and the power spectra $S_{XX}(\omega)$, $S_{YY}(\omega)$. Define the *coherence function* as

$$\gamma(\omega) = \frac{S_{XY}(\omega)}{\sqrt{S_{XX}(\omega)}\sqrt{S_{YY}(\omega)}}.$$

Note that in general the coherence function is a complex function (with nonzero imaginary part) since $C_{XY}(\tau) \neq C_{XY}(-\tau)$. The mean squared coherence $M_{XY}(\omega) = |\gamma(\omega)|^2$ lies in the range $0 \leq M_{XY}(\omega) \leq 1$ (Exercise 3).

The coherence is a measure of the relative linearity of two stochastic processes at each frequency. In particular, let Y be obtained from X by convolution,

$$Y(t) = h \star X(t) = \int h(t - t_0) X(t_0) \, dt_0,$$

then,

$$C_{XY}(\tau) = h \star C_{XX}(\tau), \quad C_{YY}(\tau) = (h \star \tilde{h}) \star C_{XX}(\tau) \tag{18.1}$$

where $\tilde{h}(t) = h(-t)$ (Exercise 4). From Eq. (18.1) we conclude that

$$S_{XY}(\omega) = \hat{h}(\omega) S_{XX}(\omega), \quad S_{YY}(\omega) = |\hat{h}(\omega)|^2 S_{XX}(\omega)$$

and therefore when $S_{XX}(\omega) \neq 0$,

$$\gamma(\omega) = \frac{\hat{h}(\omega)}{|\hat{h}(\omega)|} = e^{i\phi}, \quad \phi \in [0, 2\pi).$$

Therefore the mean squared coherence is equal to 1 when X and Y are linearly related.

Conversely, if X and Y are not linearly related, we may approximate Y by $h \star X$, where the filter h is selected so as to minimize the mean square error between Y and $h \star X$, $e(t) = Y - h \star X(t)$. Equivalently, we minimize the power spectrum of e since it integrates to the mean square error, or variance of $e(t)$. The autocovariance of e can be computed to yield

$$E[e(t_1)e(t_1 + \tau)] = C_{YY}(\tau) - \tilde{h} \star C_{XY}(\tau) - h \star C_{YX}(\tau) + (h \star \tilde{h}) \star C_{XX}(\tau) \tag{18.2}$$

(Exercise 5). Fourier transforming, we obtain the power spectrum of the error,

$$S_{ee}(\omega) = S_{YY}(\omega) - \hat{h}^*(\omega) S_{XY}(\omega) - \hat{h}(\omega) S_{XY}^*(\omega) + |\hat{h}(\omega)|^2 S_{XX}(\omega).$$

If we add and subtract $|S_{XY}|^2 / S_{XX}$ we can complete the square contained in the above expression and obtain

$$\boxed{S_{ee}(\omega) = S_{XX}(\omega) \left| \hat{h}(\omega) - \frac{S_{XY}(\omega)}{S_{XX}(\omega)} \right|^2 + S_{YY}(\omega)(1 - M_{XY}(\omega)),}$$

where $M_{XY}(\omega) = |\gamma(\omega)|^2$. Hence, the optimal filter is $\hat{h}_{opt}(\omega) = S_{XY}(\omega) / S_{XX}(\omega)$. Furthermore, if we define $Y_{lin} = h_{opt} \star X$, it is not difficult to see that when the error is minimized

$$S_{YY} = S_{ee} + S_{YY} M_{XY} \quad \text{and} \quad S_{YY} = S_{Y_{lin} Y_{lin}} + S_{ee}.$$

Therefore the mean squared coherence, M_{XY}, is the fraction of the power spectrum of Y that can be accounted for by the linear approximation provided by Y_{lin}.

Figure 18.1B shows the mean square coherence between an OU process and the same process with broad band white noise added to it (Figure 18.1A). In Figure 18.1C, a narrower band white noise, W, is mapped nonlinearly through a sigmoid function g (Figure 18.1D, top right inset). The coherence between W and $g(W)$ is depicted in the main panel of Figure 18.1D.

18.2 ESTIMATOR BIAS AND VARIANCE

In the next section we will want to estimate numerically the power spectrum of a stochastic process given a long sample function. This will raise two questions about the *bias* and *variance* of the estimate. We introduce these concepts in a much simpler setting.

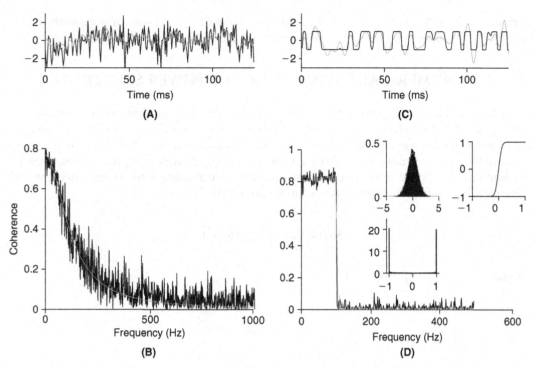

FIGURE 18.1   **A**. Sample path of an OU process, X_{OU}, illustrated in red and with white noise added to it, $X_{OU} + W$, in black (cut-off frequency: 1000 Hz). **B**. Mean squared coherence between X_{OU} and $X_{OU} + W$. The black trace is computed numerically (Welch method, see §18.3) and the red curve is obtained analytically. **C**. White noise, W, in red (cut-off frequency: 100 Hz) and the same white noise passed through a static nonlinearity, $g(W)$, in black. **D**. Mean squared coherence between W and $g(W)$ computed numerically (black) or analytically (red). The three insets illustrate the probability distribution of the white noise (top, left), the static nonlinearity (top, right), and the probability distribution of $g(W)$ (bottom, left), respectively. (coherence_est.m)

Suppose that we want to estimate the mean, μ, of a Gaussian random variable, X, and that we are given only n samples from its distribution, $x_1, \ldots, x_n$. We could of course use any sample x_i as our estimate, discarding the other ones, but this would not be a wise strategy. Instead, we form the *sample mean*, $\check{m}_X = (1/n) \sum_{i=1}^{n} x_i$. The average value of the sample mean (assume we are given several distinct sets $x_1, \ldots, x_n$) can easily be computed

$$E[\check{m}_X] = \frac{1}{n} \sum_{i=1}^{n} E[x_i] = \frac{1}{n} n\mu = \mu.$$

Thus, the sample mean is an *unbiased* estimator of the mean, since on average its value equals μ. This is a desirable property for an estimator based on random variables. Since each sample x_i is assumed to be given independently, we can also compute the variance of $\check{m}_X$, also called the standard error of the mean,

$$\mathrm{var}(\check{m}_X) = E[(\check{m}_X - \mu)^2] = \frac{1}{n^2} \sum_{i=1}^{n} E[(x_i - \mu)^2] = \frac{\sigma^2}{n}.$$

Therefore $\check{m}_X$ has the desirable property that its variability decreases as the number of samples increases.

Let us now define a second, slightly different estimator of the mean,

$$\tilde{m}_X = \frac{1}{n+1} \sum_{i=1}^{n} x_i = \frac{n}{n+1} \check{m}_X.$$

This estimator is clearly biased: $E[\tilde{m}_X] = (n\mu/(n+1))$ and its variance is given by

$$\mathrm{var}(\tilde{m}_X) = \frac{n^2}{(n+1)^2} E[(\check{m}_X - \mu)^2] = \frac{n}{(n+1)^2} \sigma^2.$$

Clearly, the variance of $\tilde{m}_X$ is lower than that of $\check{m}_X$. Thus, we have decreased the variance at the expense of bias, a common trade-off when considering different estimators of the same quantity.

18.3 NUMERICAL ESTIMATE OF THE POWER SPECTRUM*

We would now like to estimate the power spectrum of a random process $X(t)$ from discrete samples, $x_j = x(-T/2 + t_j)$, $t_j = j\Delta t$, $j = 0, \ldots, N-1$, where $x(t)$ is a sample of X. In this section, we will use $-T/2$ as the reference time point since this allows us to transition more easily from continuous to discrete time. Estimating the power spectrum also yields an estimate of the autocovariance function by Fourier transform. Additionally, the cross spectrum or coherence function is estimated in exactly the same manner. For simplicity, we assume X to be zero mean, weakly stationary and ergodic. Our starting point is the Wiener–Khinchin theorem (§16.5),

$$S(\omega) = \lim_{T \to \infty} \frac{1}{T} E[|\hat{x}_T(\omega)|^2]. \tag{18.3}$$

This formula suggests the initial approximation

$$S(\omega) \approx \frac{1}{T} \left| \int_{-T/2}^{T/2} x(t) e^{-2\pi i \omega t} \, dt \right|^2. \tag{18.4}$$

With $\Delta\omega = 1/(N\Delta t)$, $\omega_k = k\Delta\omega$, $k = 0, \ldots, N-1$,

$$S(\omega_k) \approx \frac{\Delta t}{N} \left| \sum_{j=0}^{N-1} x_j e^{-2\pi i k j/N} \right|^2.$$

If the units of x are, e.g., meters, then $S(\omega_k)$ has units of m^2/Hz. Note that the factor $\Delta t/N$ ensures the normalization

$$\int_{-\infty}^{\infty} S(\omega) \, d\omega \approx \sum_{k=0}^{N-1} \Delta\omega S(\omega_k) = \frac{1}{N} \sum_{j=0}^{N-1} |x_j|^2 \approx E[X(t)^2]. \tag{18.5}$$

The middle equality follows by Parseval's identity (Eq. (7.10) and Exercise 7). Next, we drop the factor Δt and consider the *periodogram* estimate of the power spectrum,

$$\check{S}_k^{(p)} = \frac{1}{N} \left| \sum_{j=0}^{N-1} x_j e^{-2\pi i k j/N} \right|^2 \tag{18.6}$$

so that $S(\omega_k) \approx S_k^{(p)} \Delta t$. One naturally inquires about the bias and variance of this estimator. Although detailed answers to both of these questions are known, a full exposition would require material beyond the scope of this chapter. We therefore only present a summary of the most salient points.

Bias. In general, the estimator $\check{S}_k^{(p)}$ turns out to be biased when T is finite. However, the bias is typically not very significant, unless the signal has a high dynamic range. This can be understood in terms of Eq. (18.4) which states that we approximate the Fourier transform by multiplying the infinitely long sequence $x(t)$ with a window function

$$p_T(t) = \mathbb{1}_{[-T/2, T/2]}(t).$$

Because this function abruptly turns on and off at $\pm T/2$ it contains high frequency components. Since in the frequency domain $(\hat{p}_T \star \hat{x})(\omega) = \hat{x}_T(\omega)$ the frequency content of $\hat{x}(\omega)$ could likely be spread over many frequency bins after convolution with $\hat{p}_T$. To make this argument rigorous, consider the continuous estimate of the power spectrum before discretizing, i.e., the right hand side of Eq. (18.4),

$$S_{Tx}(\omega) = \left| \int_{-T/2}^{T/2} x(t)e^{-2\pi i\omega t}\,dt \right|^2.$$

The bias of $S_{Tx}(\omega)$ is

$$E[S_{Tx}(\omega)] = S_T(\omega) = \int_{-T}^{T} (1-|\tau|/T)C(\tau)e^{-2\pi i\omega\tau}\,d\tau = \int_{-\infty}^{\infty} g_T(\tau)C(\tau)e^{-2\pi i\omega\tau}\,d\tau$$

where we used Eq. (18.4) to derive the second equality and $g_T(\tau) = (1-|\tau|/T)p_{2T}(\tau)$. On recalling the definition of the Fourier transforms of g and C we obtain

$$E[S_{Tx}(\omega)] = \int_{-\infty}^{+\infty} \hat{g}_T(\omega_1)S(\omega-\omega_1)\,d\omega_1.$$

Thus, the true power spectrum is convolved with $\hat{g}_T$. A simple calculation shows that

$$\hat{g}_T(\omega) = \frac{\sin^2(\pi\omega T)}{T\pi^2\omega^2} \tag{18.7}$$

(Exercise 8). Since $g_T(\tau) \to 1$ as $T \to \infty$ it follows that $\hat{g}_T \to \delta$ as $T \to \infty$. Therefore the periodogram estimate is unbiased as $T \to \infty$. For a finite T, this is, however, not the case. Figure 18.2A plots $\hat{g}_T$ when $T = 32$ on a logarithmic scale. After convolution, $S(\omega)$ will usually spread across a broad frequency range, corresponding to the side lobes of $\hat{g}_T$. This phenomenon is illustrated in Figure 18.2B and C for two cosine waves discretely sampled over the interval $[0, T]$ with $\Delta t = 1$ and $N = 32$. The first example (Figure 18.2B) illustrates the exceptional case were the bias is exactly equal

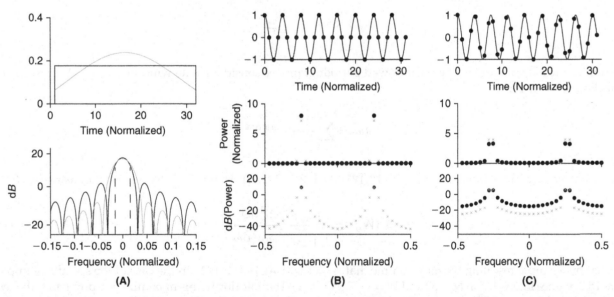

FIGURE 18.2 **A.** The top panel depicts a rectangular window, g_T, of length $N = 32$ (black) and the window corresponding to the discrete prolate spheroidal sequence (dpss) of order zero with $N = 32$ and $NW = 1$ (red). The bottom panel illustrates the Fourier transform of $\hat{g}_T$ and of the discrete spheroidal sequence shown on top, on a logarithmic scale (i.e., $dB(x) = 10\log_{10}(x)$). **B.** The top panel shows the time domain representation of $\cos(2\pi ft)$ at integer sampling points $t = 0, 1, \ldots, 31$, $f = 1/4$. The power spectrum (black squares, middle, and bottom panels) computed from Eq. (18.6) has two nonzero peaks at $\pm f$, as expected. The middle panel is on a linear scale and the bottom one on a logarithmic scale. The red crosses illustrate the windowed periodogram computed with the zeroth order dpss of A. In the middle panel only the three largest values are shown for clarity. **C.** Same as B for $\omega = 1/4 + 0.5\Delta\omega$. (fleak.m)

to zero. The top panel shows a cosine wave and its sample points with an oscillation frequency $\omega_0 = 1/4 = 8/32$ that corresponds to a multiple of the sampling frequency interval $\Delta\omega = 1/N = 1/32$. The bias contributed by frequency ω_0 to frequency bin k is equal to zero, since it is weighted by $\hat{g}_T(8 - k/32) = 0$. Accordingly, the periodogram illustrated in the middle and bottom panels of Figure 18.2B has only two nonzero components at $\pm\omega_0$. The frequency of the cosine wave illustrated in Figure 18.2C is increased by half of $\Delta\omega$. Accordingly, the power is equally divided between the two immediately adjacent frequency bins, as illustrated in the middle panel. This *local* bias corresponds to multiplication with the value of $\hat{g}_T$ at $\pm 0.5/N$ on the main lobe of the function (dashed lines in the bottom panel of Figure 18.2A). However, the power is not exclusively distributed over these two bins: as illustrated in the bottom panel of Figure 18.2C, there is a long range bias that affects *all* the other bins. It is most visible on a logarithmic scale as it is much smaller than the peak value of the periodogram. This bias is often called *leakage* because power "leaks" to adjacent bins.

To reduce the long range bias, we multiply x by a *data window* function, h, and obtain a *windowed* estimate of the power spectrum,

$$S_{hx}(\omega) = \left| \int_{-\infty}^{\infty} h(t)x(t)e^{-2\pi i\omega t}\,dt \right|^2,$$

with the following bias,

$$E[S_{hx}] = \int_{-\infty}^{\infty} |\hat{h}(\omega_1)|^2 S(\omega - \omega_1)\,d\omega_1 \tag{18.8}$$

(Exercise 9). The corresponding discrete windowed periodogram is

$$\check{S}_k^{(w)} = \frac{1}{N} \left| \sum_{l=0}^{N-1} x_l h_l e^{-2\pi ikl/N} \right|^2.$$

We impose the normalization $\sum_{k=0}^{N-1} |h_k|^2 = 1$ which ensures that on average the integrated power is equal to the variance of x:

$$E\left[\sum_{k=0}^{N-1} \check{S}_k^{(w)} \right] = \sigma^2.$$

To minimize the long range bias of the windowed periodogram, we consider a data window, $v_{k,0}, k = 0, \ldots, N-1$, such that its Fourier transform

$$\hat{v}_0(\omega) = \sum_{k=0}^{N-1} v_{k,0} e^{-2\pi ik\Delta t\omega}$$

has maximal energy in the frequency band $[-W, W] \subset [-1/2\Delta t, 1/2\Delta t]$. That is, $\hat{v}_0$ maximizes, with respect to $\hat{f}$

$$\beta^2(W, \hat{f}) = \frac{\int_{-W}^{W} |\hat{f}(\omega)|^2\,d\omega}{\int_{-1/2\Delta t}^{1/2\Delta t} |\hat{f}(\omega)|^2\,d\omega} \tag{18.9}$$

Note that by a simple rescaling we may assume that $\Delta t = 1$ and $\omega \in [-1/2, 1/2]$. In the case of the specific example of Figure 18.2, we are interested in $N = 32$ and $W = 1/32$ ($NW = 1$). The solution to this maximization problem is the *zeroth order discrete prolate spheroidal sequence*, or dpss, illustrated on the top panel of Figure 18.2A (Exercise 15). Multiplying x_k by $v_{k,0}$ causes the resulting values to smoothly taper towards the boundaries of the interval $[0, T)$, therefore limiting the high frequency leakage attributed to the rectangular window. The Fourier transform of $v_{k,0}$ is illustrated on the bottom panel of Figure 18.2A. Indeed, we see that the side lobes are reduced compared to those of the rectangular window. Accordingly, the long range leakage is decreased in Figure 18.2C (bottom panel, red crosses). Note, however, that some leakage is introduced in the case of the frequencies coinciding with multiples of $\Delta\omega$ (Figure 18.2B, bottom).

This is due to the fact that minimizing the long-range leakage of $v_{k,0}$ causes the main lobe of $\hat{v}_0$ to slightly broaden (Figure 18.2A, bottom). As a consequence, the sampling points k/N do not coincide with the zeros of $\hat{v}_0$ any more. This broadening means that by windowing with $v_{k,0}$ we lose some of the fine resolution in the estimate of the power spectrum: this is the trade-off incurred by imposing minimal long-range leakage.

Higher order dpss. The maximization problem of Eq. (18.9) can be considered on the $N-1$ dimensional space orthogonal to $(v_{0,0}, \ldots, v_{N-1,0})^T$. This yields the first order dpss, $v_{k,1}, k = 0, \ldots, N-1$, which, by definition, has a concentration smaller than that of $v_{k,0}$: $\beta^2(W, \hat{v}_0) > \beta^2(W, \hat{v}_1)$. Proceeding in the same way, we can generate a sequence of N dpss with decreasing concentration that together span $\mathbb{R}^N$. Typically, n_{NW} of these sequences have a concentration $\beta^2(W)$ close to 1, where n_{NW} is the largest integer smaller than $2NW - 1$ (with $W < 1/2$). We will put these additional sequences to use in the multitaper method of power spectrum estimation described below.

Variance. The variance of $\check{S}_k^{(p)}$ turns out to be on the order of $S(\omega_k)^2$, independent of N. This severe problem is not entirely surprising: when N is increased, it generates additional frequency samples in Eq. (18.6) and therefore a finer frequency grid, not a better estimate of a fixed number of frequency samples. In addition, we have dropped the averaging operation when transitioning from Eqs. (18.3) to (18.4). There are two simple solutions to this problem: the first one, the Welch method, consists in splitting the interval T in m subintervals $[0, T/m), [T/m, 2T/m), \ldots$ and computing an estimate $\check{S}_k^{(p)l}, l = 1, \ldots, m$ on each subinterval separately followed by averaging,

$$\check{S}_k^{(w)} = \frac{1}{m} \sum_{l=1}^{m} \check{S}_k^{(p)l}.$$

This will reduce the variance by approximately $1/m$. Since $\check{S}_k^{(p)}$ is typically replaced by the windowed periodogram which smoothly tapers the sample values towards the boundaries of each subinterval, this estimate can be improved by *overlapping* the segments, i.e., by adding the intervals $[T/(m/2), T/(3m/2))$, etc. The second method consists in averaging directly $\check{S}_k^{(p)}$ over several frequency bins by convolving with an appropriate window function G in the frequency domain, $\check{S}^{(c)} = \check{S}^{(p)} \star G$. Such a window G is called a *smoothing* or *spectral* window. Many different types of spectral windows have been proposed, with various trade-offs depending on the particular situation considered. The simplest example of a spectral window consists in averaging over n adjacent frequency values, e.g., for $n = 3$,

$$\check{S}_k^{(c)} = (\check{S}_{k-1}^{(p)} + \check{S}_k^{(p)} + S_{k+1}^{(p)})/3,$$

corresponding to $G = (1/3, 1/3, 0, \ldots, 0, 1/3)^T$. Of course, both methods sacrifice frequency resolution for a decrease in variance. Figure 18.3A and B depict the periodogram and Welch power spectrum estimates of the OU process describing the excitatory synaptic conductance in §17.4, respectively.

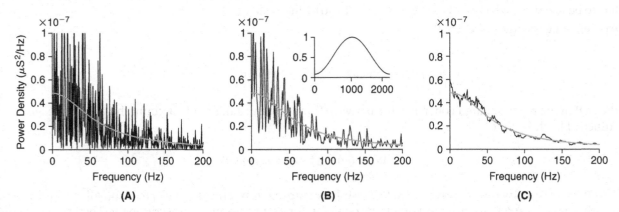

FIGURE 18.3   Numerical estimation of the power spectrum of the OU process illustrated in Figure 17.5, top. **A.** Periodogram estimate (4096 sample points, $dt = 0.5$ ms). The red line is the analytical value derived in §17.3. Note the decrease in variance as the analytical value decreases with frequency. **B.** Welch estimate with a Hamming data window (inset, default window used by MATLAB) based on 2048 sample long subsegments. **C.** Multitaper estimate with $N = 4096$, $NW = 14$. (`power_spec.m`)

Multitaper method. The multitaper method is computationally more intensive, but often yields more accurate results than those described above, particularly when the available data are short. It relies on the simultaneous use of multiple independent data windows, also called *tapers*, hence the name. These data windows are the n_{NW} discrete prolate spheroidal sequences of length N that have high concentration, $\beta^2(W)$, on the frequency interval W, as discussed above. We obtain in this way nearly independent estimates of the power spectrum,

$$\check{S}_k^{(mt)l} = \left| \sum_{j=0}^{N-1} x_j v_{j,l} e^{-2\pi ikj/N} \right|^2, \quad l=0,\ldots,n_{NW}-1.$$

These estimates are then combined either by simple averaging, $\check{S}_k^{(mt)} = (1/n_{NW})\sum_{l=0}^{m-1} \check{S}_k^{(mt)l}$ or by using more sophisticated, nonlinear combinations to obtain an estimate $\check{S}_k^{(mt)}$ that simultaneously minimizes bias and variance. The number n_{NW} of dpss increases with W (and N). For example, if $NW=4$ then $l=0,\ldots,6$. This allows for additional averaging and decreases the variance of the estimate $S_k^{(mt)}$. On the other hand, it also smoothes out details of the spectrum, as explained above. A multitaper power spectrum estimate of the OU process describing the excitatory synaptic conductance in §17.4 is illustrated in Figure 18.3C.

18.4 SUMMARY AND SOURCES

The techniques developed in this chapter to compute power spectra, cross spectra, and coherence are basic workhorses that play a fundamental role in the analysis of neural data from the level of single ion channels up to the behavior of whole organisms. The properties of the coherence function derived in §18.1 make it for instance the method of choice to characterize the relation between two stochastic processes. We will encounter several concrete applications of these tools in subsequent chapters. Section 18.1 is based on Carter (1987, §1). The material in §18.3 is classical and has been covered in many books and review articles. A comprehensive reference is Percival and Walden (1993). See in particular their §3.9, Chapters 6–8 for further details on the dpss defined by Eq. (18.9) and in Exercise 15.

18.5 EXERCISES

1. Show that the following inequality holds:

$$|C_{XY}(\tau)| \leq C_{XX}(0)C_{YY}(0). \tag{18.10}$$

   Hint: Clearly, the following inequality holds independent of the value of $a \in \mathbb{R}$: $E[(aX(t)+Y(t+\tau))^2] \geq 0$. Argue that equality holds when $Y(t+\tau) = -aX(t)$ with probability 1, in which case equality also holds in Eq. (18.10). In the ">" case, derive a quadratic equation for a (i.e., $a^2x + ay + z > 0$) and conclude that its discriminant, $\Delta = y^2 - 4xz$, has to be negative, which leads to Eq. (18.10) with strict inequality ($<$).

2. Argue, along the lines of §16.5, that

$$\lim_{T\to\infty} S_{XYT}(\omega) = S_{XY}(\omega) \quad \text{where} \quad S_{XYT}(\omega) = \frac{E[\hat{X}_T(\omega)^* \hat{Y}_T(\omega)]}{T}.$$

3. Prove that the mean squared coherence lies between 0 and 1. Hint: Taking into account the previous exercise, it is sufficient to show that

$$|S_{XYT}(\omega)|^2 \leq S_{XXT}(\omega)S_{YYT}(\omega). \tag{18.11}$$

   This latter inequality can be proven as in Exercise 1, by starting from $E[|\hat{X}_T(\omega) + u\hat{Y}_T(\omega)\exp(i\phi)|^2] \geq 0$ for $a \in \mathbb{R}$ and an arbitrary phase ϕ. Derive again a quadratic equation for a and compute its discriminant. Then select the phase ϕ appropriately to obtain Eq. (18.11).

4. Prove Eq. (18.1).

5. Compute the autocovariance of the error, Eq. (18.2).

6. †Under the same assumptions as in §18.2, show that

$$\check{\sigma}^2 = \frac{1}{n-1} \sum_{i=1}^{n} (x_i - \check{x})^2$$

is an unbiased estimator of the variance, σ^2.

7. †Prove Eq. (18.5).

8. Derive Eq. (18.7).

9. Compute the bias of the windowed periodogram, Eq. (18.8). Hint: First write

$$S_{hx}(\omega) = \int\limits_{-\infty}^{\infty} h(t_1)x(t_1)e^{-2\pi i \omega t_1}\, dt_1 \int\limits_{-\infty}^{\infty} h(t_2)x(t_2)e^{2\pi i \omega t_2}\, dt_2. \qquad (18.12)$$

Taking the expectation leads to a double integral with the product of the covariance of X and h (twice) in the integrand. By Fourier transforming C and h the integral can be simplified to the form given in Eq. (18.8).

10. One method to generate correlated Poisson spike trains is to "thin" a "mother" spike train. If the sample mother spike train, x_m, has rate ϱ_m, we generate a new spike train by keeping each spike with probability β. Clearly, the new spike train is again Poisson and has rate $\varrho = \beta \varrho_m$. If this process is repeated N times, we obtain Poisson spike trains $x_1, \ldots, x_N$ with pairwise covariance $C_{x_i x_j}(\tau) = \varrho\beta\delta(\tau)$ or, equivalently, with correlation coefficient β $(i,j=1,\ldots,N, i \neq j)$. Generate 10 such spike trains from a mother spike train with rate $\varrho_m = 200$ spk/s, $\beta = 0.1$ and plot them together with the mother spike train to arrive at a plot similar to Figure 18.4A. Compute numerically the covariance between the two spike trains, normalized by their standard deviations to arrive at a plot similar to Figure 18.4B, with a peak at time zero whose numerical value is $\approx \beta$. Hint: Generate two correlated spike trains with the above method, $32768\,(=2^{15})$ ms long with a sampling step $dt = 0.5$ ms, and compute their cross spectral density with the MATLAB function cpsd. Use the default Hamming window, 2048 samples long and an overlap of 1024 samples. Compute the inverse Fourier transform of the result, correct for the time shift and divide by the standard deviations of the spike trains.

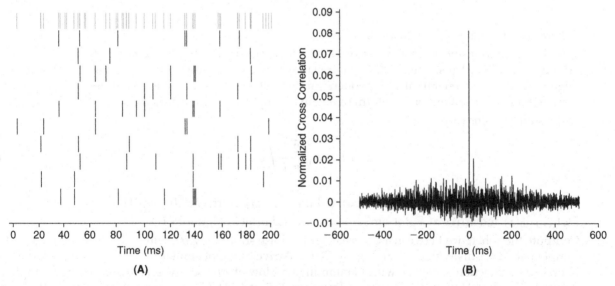

FIGURE 18.4   **A.** The mother spike train is plotted in red on top and 10 derived spike trains, $\varrho_m = 200$ spk/s and $\beta = 0.1$. **B.** Cross correlation between two derived spike trains, computed numerically. (cross_poiss.m)

11. Compute analytically the coherence between an OU process, X and $Z = X + Y$, where Y is an independent white Gaussian noise, up to a cut-off frequency f_N. The OU process is assumed to have parameters σ_{OU} and τ, while the white noise is assumed to have variance σ_w^2. Compare this theoretical result with the numerical one, and reproduce Figure 18.1A and B. Use the following parameters for the OU process: $\sigma_{OU} = 0.55\ \mu$S and $\tau = 2.7$ ms. Use a sampling step $dt = 0.5$ ms, corresponding to a cut-off frequency $f_N = 1000$ Hz for the white noise and $\sigma_w = 1\ \mu$S.

Hint: Use 65536 (2^{16}) samples and the function mscohere with a standard Hamming window of 2048 samples and an overlap of 1024 samples.

12. In this exercise, we develop a method to generate Gaussian random noise samples that are white up to a cut-off frequency f_N, but that are sampled at a frequency higher than $2f_N$. For this purpose consider first N Gaussian random variables $x_0,\ldots,x_N$ of zero mean, identical variance and such that $E[x_n x_m] = C_{n-m} \pmod N$, with $C_k = C_{-k} \pmod N$. Set

$$\hat{x}_j = \sum_{k=0}^{N-1} x_k e^{-2\pi i k j/N} \quad \text{and} \quad \hat{x}_{jr} = \Re(\hat{x}_j),\ \hat{x}_{ji} = \Im(\hat{x}_j).$$

(i) Show that $\hat{x}_{-j} = \hat{x}_j^* = \hat{x}_{jr} - i\hat{x}_{ji}$. Hint: This is the discrete version of Exercise 7.13.

(ii) Show that both $\hat{x}_{jr}$ and $\hat{x}_{ji}$ are Gaussian random variables with zero mean.

(iii) Show that $E[\hat{x}_j \hat{x}_l] = \delta_{j-l} N S_j$, where δ is the Kronecker delta of Eq. (1.4) and

$$S_j = \sum_{k=0}^{N-1} C_k e^{-2\pi i k j/N}.$$

(iv) Show that $\hat{x}_{ji}$ is independent of $\hat{x}_{jr}$ and that

$$E[\hat{x}_{jr}^2] = E[\hat{x}_{ji}^2] = \frac{1}{2}E[|\hat{x}_j|^2].$$

Hint: It is sufficient to show that $E[\hat{x}_{jr}\hat{x}_{ji}] = 0$. Use the result derived in (iii) with $l=j$ and $l=-j$.

(v) Show that $\hat{x}_{jr}, \hat{x}_{ji}$ are independent of $\hat{x}_{lr}, \hat{x}_{li}$ for $l \neq j$. Hint: Proceed as in (iv) by considering the result derived in (iii) for j and $\pm l(\neq j)$.

(vi) Show that to approximate the power spectrum of white noise with variance σ^2 between $-f_N$ and f_N (Exercise 16.22) requires

$$E[|\hat{x}_j|^2] = \frac{N\sigma^2}{2f_N \Delta t},$$

where Δt is the time domain discretization step.

(vii) Use the previous results to generate Gaussian white noise with a cut-off frequency of $f_N = 100$ Hz, $\sigma = 1$, and a sampling step of 1 ms. The resulting Gaussian white noise sample should be similar to that depicted in Figure 18.1C. Hint: Generate at each frequency independent Gaussian random samples with the appropriate variance and inverse Fourier transform to obtain a sample in the time domain.

13. Define the static nonlinearity

$$g_{\alpha,l}(x) = \alpha\sqrt{\frac{2}{\pi}}\frac{1}{l}\int_0^x e^{-t^2/2l^2}\,dt. \tag{18.13}$$

(i) Show that $g_{\alpha,l}(x) \in (-\alpha,\alpha)$ for $x \in (-\infty,\infty)$ and that $g_{\alpha,l}(x) = \alpha\,\mathrm{erf}(x/\sqrt{2}l)$ (see §11.5).

(ii) Plot $g_{1,1/10}(x)$ and arrive at a plot similar to the second inset in Figure 18.1D.

(iii) Compute the coherence between a Gaussian white noise stimulus, $X(t)$, with cut-off frequency $f_N = 100$ Hz sampled at $\Delta t = 1$ ms with $\sigma = 1$ and $g_{1,1/10}(X(t))$. Arrive at a plot similar to that depicted in Figure 18.1D. Hint: Use the function mscohere with a Hamming window of 1024 samples, an overlap of 512 samples and a sample, $x(t)$, of total length 32768 ms. (See Exercises 22.7 and 22.8 for further results relevant to this exercise.)

14. †Compute numerically the power spectra and the autocovariance functions of gamma renewal processes of orders 2 and 10 to arrive at Figure 18.5. Assume a mean firing rate of 80 spk/s and compare the results to Figures 16.5 and 16.3. Hint: Use a time step $dt = 0.5$ ms and approximate the δ-function for each spike by $1/dt$. Use a data stretch 32768 ms long. To estimate the power spectrum, use pswelch with a Hamming window 2048 samples long and an overlap of 1024. To estimate the autocovariance function, compute the inverse Fourier transform of the power spectrum. Compare the value of the autocovariance function at zero lag with the discretized prediction, χ/dt, obtained from Eq. (16.11).

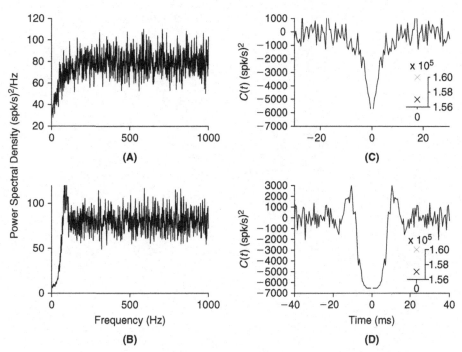

FIGURE 18.5   **A.** Numerical estimate of the power spectrum of a gamma order 2 process with mean rate of 80 spk/s. **B.** Numerical estimate of the power spectrum of a gamma order 10 process with mean rate of 80 spk/s. **C.** Autocovariance function of the gamma order 2 process. The inset compares the theoretical prediction for $C(0)$ (red cross) with the numerical estimate (black cross). **D.** Same as C, but for a gamma order 10 process. (power_auto_g2_g10.m)

15.   (i) Set $\Delta t = 1$ in Eq. (18.9) and show that it may be rewritten as

$$\beta^2(W,\hat{f}) = \frac{\sum_{j,k=0}^{N-1} f_j A_{jk} f_k}{\sum_{j=0}^{N-1} f_j^2} = \frac{\mathbf{f}^T \mathbf{A} \mathbf{f}}{\mathbf{f}^T \mathbf{f}} \tag{18.14}$$

with $\mathbf{f} = (f_0, \ldots, f_{N-1})^T$.

(ii) Show that $\mathbf{A}$ is symmetric positive semidefinite and that its largest eigenvalue is ≤ 1. Thus, $\mathbf{A}$ has a complete set of orthogonal eigenvectors with eigenvalues in $[0,1]$. Hint: Use Exercises 6.1 and 6.8 and use Parseval's identity, Eq. (7.10).

(iii) Show that the vector $\mathbf{f}$ that achieves the maximum in Eq. (18.14) is an eigenvector associated with the largest eigenvalue of $\mathbf{A}$. Hint: The gradient with respect to $\mathbf{f}$ of β^2 vanishes at the maximum.

19

Natural Light Signals and Phototransduction

O U T L I N E

19.1 Wavelength and Intensity   291   19.4 A Model of Phototransduction   294

19.2 Spatial Properties of Natural Light Signals   293   19.5 Summary and Sources   297

19.3 Temporal Properties of Natural Light Signals 293   19.6 Exercises   298

The first step in processing signals from the outer world is to transduce them into membrane potential changes in receptor cells at the periphery of the nervous system. In the case of light, this process is called *phototransduction*. Light is absorbed in photoreceptors by specialized molecules called *rhodopsins* that initiate a biochemical cascade of reactions resulting in a photocurrent across the membrane of the photoreceptor that leads either to depolarization or hyperpolarization of the membrane potential (depending on the photoreceptor type) and synaptic release of neurotransmitter onto postsynaptic cells. Before describing in more detail these mechanisms, we need to describe the most salient properties of light in the natural world as this has an important impact on its processing by the visual system.

19.1 WAVELENGTH AND INTENSITY

Light is electromagnetic radiation with a wavelength between 360 and 830 nm (Figure 19.1A). Phototransduction depends on the wavelength of light because rhodopsin molecules have specific absorption spectra. An example is illustrated in Figure 19.2A.

Irradiance and illuminance. Phototransduction also depends on the intensity of light impinging on a photoreceptor. This can be measured by the number of photons crossing a unit surface per unit time (Figure 19.3A). This number corresponds to the amount of energy crossing the unit surface per unit time, since at a given wavelength λ or equivalently, frequency $\nu = c/\lambda$, the energy of a photon is $E(\nu) = h\nu$, where h is Planck's constant ($\approx 6.63 \times 10^{-34}$ joule·s) and c is the speed of light. Thus, if the flux of photons per unit surface and unit time is N_{ph}, then the equivalent energy flux (per unit area and time) is $W(\lambda) = N_{ph}E(\nu)$. The international units for $W(\lambda)$ are joule/(s·m^2) or watt/m^2 since power is given in joule/s = watt. $W(\lambda)$ is called the *irradiance* impinging on the surface. A corresponding quantity that is more directly related to human vision is called the *illuminance* and is obtained by scaling $W(\lambda)$ by the normalized absorption characteristics of the human eye, $V(\lambda)$ (Figure 19.2B). Illuminance is measured in lumen/m^2 or lux. The peak value of $V(\lambda)$ (at $\lambda = 555$ nm) is normalized to one and a scaling constant $C = 683$ lumen/watt converts from watt/m^2 to lumen/m^2. Thus, illuminance is obtained from irradiance by scaling light power according to the absorption properties of the human visual system. This procedure converts *radiometric* (physical) quantities into *photometric* ones, subjectively adapted to the human visual system.

Mathematics for Neuroscientists. DOI: 10.1016/B978-0-12-374882-9.00019-8

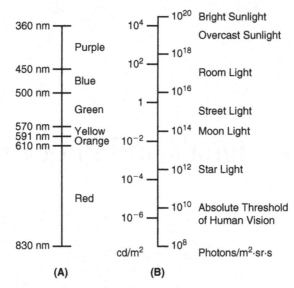

(A)   **(B)**

FIGURE 19.1   **A.** Wavelength range (left) of the principal colors in the visible spectrum (right). **B.** The values on the left (in cd/m^2) are typical luminances of a white card under increasing illumination (top to bottom: from starlight to bright sunlight as indicated on the right). The radiance values given on the left (in photons/m^2·sr·s, where sr is the abbreviation for steradians) are computed under the assumption that the light wavelength is 555 nm. Adapted from Land and Nilsson (2002).

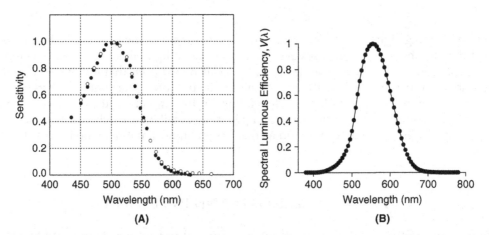

(A)   **(B)**

FIGURE 19.2   **A.** Spectral sensitivity of human rod photoreceptors and spectral sensitivity of human subjects at low light levels (adapted from Wandell, 1995). **B.** Standardized spectral luminous efficiency $V(\lambda)$ of human subjects at daylight levels. CIE (1931). (`stdobs_plot.m`)

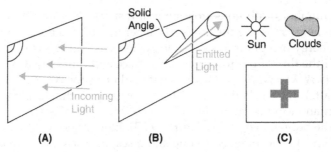

(A)   **(B)**   **(C)**

FIGURE 19.3   **A.** The irradiance and the corresponding spectrally corrected photometric quantity, the illuminance, characterize the power and luminous flux, impinging on a unit surface, respectively. **B.** Radiance and luminance characterize the light power and luminous flux emitted by an object per unit solid angle and per unit surface of the emitter. **C.** The luminance of a gray cross on a white background can change by an order of magnitude or more depending on the ambient light conditions (e.g., sunny vs. cloudy day; or indoors vs. outdoors). Yet, we perceive it as unchanged because our visual system encodes primarily the contrast or relative luminance change between the white background and the gray cross.

Radiance and luminance. Typically, light that enters photoreceptors originates from objects in the environment that partially reflect sunlight impinging on them. The light intensity emanating from an object is given by the amount of power radiated per unit of emitting surface and per unit of solid angle, so that its units are in watt/m^2· sr (Figure 19.3B). It is a radiometric quantity called the *radiance*. The corresponding photometric quantity is obtained by scaling the light power according to the properties of the visual system, i.e., multiplying by $CV(\lambda)$. This is called the *luminance* and has units of lumen/m^2· steradians, or candela/m^2, where the candela (= lumen/steradian) characterizes the luminous flux of a point source per unit solid angle. Typical values of object luminances under various illumination conditions are given in Figure 19.1B. As may be seen from the figure, one of the most challenging aspects of phototransduction is that the light intensity, or more precisely the luminance of objects in the environment, can vary by 10 orders of magnitude. This means that photoreceptors need to change their operating point or *adapt* to the ambient lighting conditions. In vertebrates, the entire dynamic range of light is covered by two types of photoreceptors, rods, and cones, with rods used at low light levels (approximately from night up to room light levels) and cones at high light levels (from room to daylight levels). In invertebrates, a single photoreceptor type can typically cover the entire range.

Contrast constancy. An important characteristic of the visual system is that at high illumination levels, it is usually more sensitive to *relative* changes in luminance than absolute ones. Consider, e.g., a white card with a gray cross at its center (Figure 19.3C). The luminance of the gray cross can be described in terms of the background luminance of the white card as $I_0 + cI_0$, where $-1 < c < 0$ and I_0 is the background luminance. Although we will encounter several ways of defining contrast depending on the stimuli used, the quantity c is the contrast of the cross relative to the background in the present context. If the card is viewed under a bright sun, both the luminance of the white card and the cross will be much stronger than if the card is viewed under a cloudy sky. Yet, we perceive the gray cross in the same way, irrespective of the illuminance. This is due to the fact that our visual system codes for the contrast of the cross, i.e., how much light it reflects relative to the white background irrespective of the absolute luminance level. In the above description, a change in lighting conditions would change I_0 and thus the luminance of the white background and gray cross identically, whereas the contrast remains unchanged.

19.2 SPATIAL PROPERTIES OF NATURAL LIGHT SIGNALS

By studying the characteristics of natural images (i.e., images encountered in day-to-day life), we can gain a better understanding of the tasks that the visual system faces in transducing light signals into electrical ones. Figure 19.4A shows a typical image from a natural outdoor scene in daylight. The distribution of luminances derived from 10 similar images is illustrated in Figure 19.4B, after shifting the mean luminance to zero. The distribution covers more than three orders of magnitude and is quite skewed with a long tail at large luminance values. Typically, contrast varies over a much smaller range than luminance, since even the darkest black object will reflect about 2 percent of the light compared to 100 percent for a white one, or a 50-fold range. As illustrated in Figure 19.4C, taking the logarithm of the luminance results in a considerably more symmetric distribution that is also more compact. Figure 19.4D illustrates the power spectrum as a function of spatial frequency. The power spectrum decays rapidly and approximately as a second power of spatial frequency, ω_s^{-2}, over two logarithmic units, as illustrated in Figure 19.4E. Therefore, in contrast to images that are fully random representing spatial white noise, natural images possess substantial correlations across pixels, with higher frequencies largely suppressed compared to lower ones. This is due to the fact that luminance varies only slowly over extended objects, leading to long-range correlations.

19.3 TEMPORAL PROPERTIES OF NATURAL LIGHT SIGNALS

In principle, the time series of luminance values registered by a single photoreceptor in a natural environment could be derived from its velocity distribution, due to body, head, and eye movements and the spatial properties of natural images described in the previous section. Such time series can also be measured directly as illustrated in Figure 19.5A. As in the case of natural images, they are heavily skewed with long tails towards large luminance values (Figure 19.5B). Taking the logarithm leads again to a much more compact and symmetric distribution (Figure 19.5C). The power spectrum is illustrated in Figure 19.5D and E, and is approximately inversely related to frequency (ω_t^{-1}). Therefore, time series of luminance values also possess strong correlations.

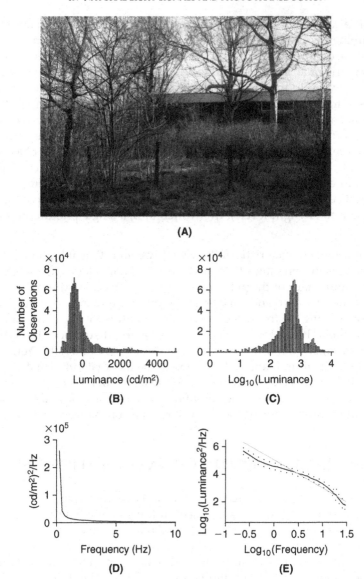

(A)

(B)

(C)

(D)

(E)

FIGURE 19.4   **A.** A natural image obtained from van Hateren's image database (1998). **B.** Average distribution of luminance over 10 similar natural images. Note the skew and long tail at high luminances. **C.** The same mean distribution plotted in logarithmic units is more symmetric. **D.** Mean power spectrum along horizontal and vertical directions in 10 natural images. **E.** Mean ± standard deviation of the same power spectrum plotted on a double logarithmic scale (solid and dotted black lines, respectively). The red line is a linear fit to the data, and has a slope of −2.04. (`disp_hist.m`, `disp_im.m`, `scene_2d.m`)

19.4 A MODEL OF PHOTOTRANSDUCTION

The previous two sections show that at high light levels, photoreceptors face the challenging task of transducing highly skewed and broad distributions of luminance. As illustrated in Figures 19.4C and 19.5C, a logarithmic mapping of light intensity into membrane potential would result in a compressed and symmetric distribution and therefore a good use of the photoreceptor dynamic range. It turns out that, to a first approximation, this is the case in fly photoreceptors, as illustrated in Figure 19.6. Similar results also hold for vertebrate cones at high light levels. Rods and cones hyperpolarize in response to light increments and depolarize in response to light decrements. In contrast, insect photoreceptors depolarize in response to light increments and hyperpolarize in response to light decrements. Just as with rods and cones, insect photoreceptors are *graded potential* neurons that usually lack spike generating conductances. In both vertebrate and invertebrate photoreceptors, a strong compression of light signals is characteristic of high light levels, but the situation is reversed at low light levels, when photoreceptors need to amplify weak light signals instead of compressing them (§25.1).

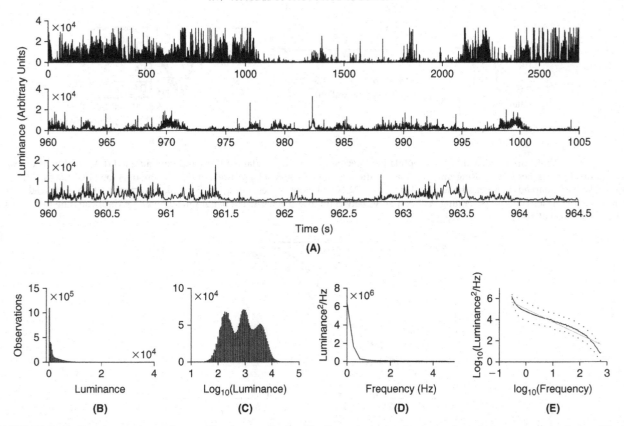

FIGURE 19.5 **A.** Top: A time series of natural luminances lasting 45 minutes is depicted at increasingly high temporal resolution. Obtained from van Hateren's time series database (1997). **B.** Histogram of luminance values for the time series depicted in A. **C.** Histogram of the logarithm of luminance values. **D.** Power spectrum of the time series. **E.** Power spectrum plotted on a double logarithmic scale (mean ± sd; solid and dotted lines, respectively). The red line is a linear fit to the data, and has a slope of −1.21. (`disp_ts2.m`)

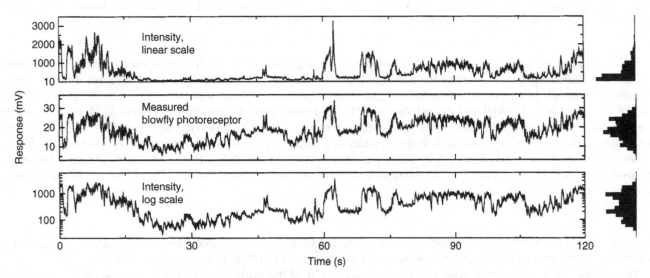

FIGURE 19.6   Top: Time series of natural light intensity. Middle: Recording from a fly photoreceptor in response to the stimulus on top. Bottom: Logarithm of the time series, illustrating the similarity with the fly photoreceptor membrane potential. The histograms on the right plot from top to bottom the distribution of light intensity, membrane potential, and the logarithm of light intensity, respectively. Adapted from van Hateren and Snippe (2006).

A logarithmic mapping of luminance into the membrane potential of photoreceptors represents a simple method of implementing contrast constancy at high light levels. If luminance is encoded logarithmically relative to a reference background luminance I_0 and an object has contrast c, then the response will be proportional to $\log(I_0 + cI_0) − \log(I_0) = \log(1 + c)$ which is independent of I_0.

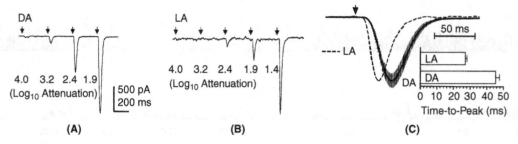

FIGURE 19.7 Photocurrent elicited in a Drosophila photoreceptor under dark adapted (DA) and light adapted (LA) conditions in response to brief (5 ms) light flashes of increasing intensities ($\log_{10}$ attenuation indicated; a $\log_{10}$ attenuation of 0 amounts to $\approx 10^5$ effectively absorbed photons). **A**. Dark adapted. **B**. Light adapted (background: $\approx 22{,}000$ photons/s, generating a 175 pA plateau current). **C**. Normalized averaged responses to brief flashes (arrow) generating peak responses between 150 and 500 pA. The bar graph summarizes the mean time-to-peak values. Adapted from Gu et al. (2005).

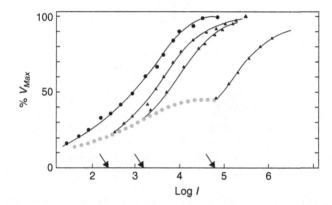

FIGURE 19.8 Response of blowfly photoreceptors to light pulses delivered in the dark (black dots) or from different background luminance values (black triangles). The corresponding background luminances are indicated by the arrows on the abscissa. The red dots correspond to the steady-state adaptation of the membrane potential to varying background intensities. The abscissa is the logarithm of the light intensity (background or background plus pulse) relative to a fixed reference level. The ordinate is the membrane potential deflection normalized relative to the maximal deflection, V_{Max}, that could be elicited by a light pulse. Adapted from Laughlin and Hardie (1978).

Photoreceptors do not only logarithmically compress light signals. They also adjust their mean membrane potential, the gain of their response as well as their integration time depending on the light level (Figures 19.7 and 19.8). In particular, longer integration times at lower light levels counter the effects of noise in the photoreceptor response. Figure 19.9 illustrates a model that reproduces well the response of fly photoreceptors at high light levels. A model with a similar structure reproduces vertebrate cone responses as well. The incoming light intensity, $I(t)$, is first low-pass filtered (LP_1). Next, two feedback loops dynamically adjust the gain of the response. The first feedback loop divides the output, $x(t)$, of the filter LP_1 by a low-pass filtered version of it (LP_2). In response to light steps, this causes the initial decrease of the response after a delay since LP_2 has a slower dynamics than LP_1 (Figure 19.9B, solid arrow). At steady state, the output satisfies

$$y(t) = x(t)/y(t) \quad \text{or} \quad y(t) = \sqrt{x(t)}.$$

A similar quadratic dependence of visual sensitivity on light intensity is typically observed at low light levels (De Vries–Rose law), in contrast to the logarithmic dependence observed at high light intensities (Weber's law).

The second feedback loop divides $y(t)$ by an exponential of the output of the third low-pass filter, LP_3. Thus, at steady state,

$$z(t) = y(t)/\exp z(t) \quad \text{or} \quad \log z(t) + z(t) = \log y(t).$$

When $z(t) \gg \log z(t)$, the second term on the left hand side dominates and $z(t) \approx \log y(t)$. In contrast, at small values of z, the first term dominates and the gain control mechanism is inactivated: $z(t) \approx y(t)$. The low-pass filter LP_3 decays slowly, on a time scale matched to the correlations observed in natural scenes, thus adjusting the gain control mechanism over the natural range of temporal luminance fluctuations. This causes the slow decay of the response to light intensity steps in Figure 19.9B (dashed arrow). The final nonlinearity NL_1 is given by $P(t) = z(t)/(1 + z(t))$ and

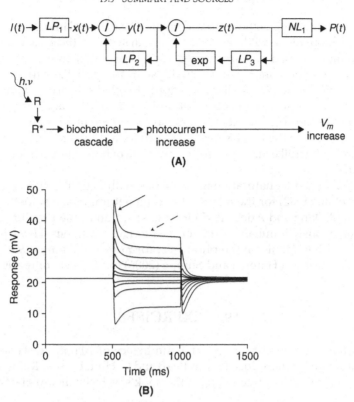

(A)

(B)

FIGURE 19.9   **A**. Schematic of the photoreceptor model. The lower diagram illustrates a rough match to the various steps involved in phototransduction. R and R* denote rhodopsin molecules before and after light absorption, respectively. V_m denotes the photoreceptor membrane potential. **B**. Response of the model to light intensity steps. Note the fast adaptation (solid arrow), caused by the first gain control loop and the slower one, caused by the second gain control loop (dashed arrow). (`photoreceptor_model.m`)

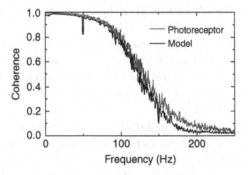

FIGURE 19.10   Mean squared coherence between model and measured photoreceptor response. The thin gray line labeled 'photoreceptor' is the theoretical maximum that may be achieved, showing that the model is close to it. Adapted from van Hateren and Snippe (2001).

implements the saturation of the photoreceptor response. $P(t)$ is convolved with a final, linear filter to fit its values to experimental photoreceptor responses (not shown in Figure 19.9A).

The performance of the model is quantified in Figure 19.10, which shows the mean squared coherence between the model output and an experimentally measured photoreceptor response. The thin gray line is obtained by computing the photoreceptor mean squared coherence between different responses to the same stimulus and therefore sets an upper limit to the coherence determined by the trial-to-trial variability of the response.

19.5 SUMMARY AND SOURCES

In this chapter, we have introduced the basic characteristics of natural light. Because all visual systems initially have to cope with the same light signals, they have often evolved very similar algorithms to process these stimuli at early stages of their visual systems, such as those described in §19.4. We will study an example of how the properties of natural light inform our understanding of the temporal processing of visual information in the next chapter (§20.6). As visual processing becomes more refined at later stages of visual systems, these basic properties progressively lose their importance relative to more refined and specialized aspects of visual scenes that are specific to the animal's natural environment. For example, some areas of our visual system are specialized to process faces, while honey bees need to recognize the flowers they pollinate. Similar rules apply to other sensory systems, like audition for instance. Neuroscientists have often debated how useful natural stimuli are to understand early vision. Indeed, much of the research and results described in the subsequent chapters have been obtained with artificial visual stimuli such as those described in §§20.2 and 21.1. See Rust and Movshon (2005) for a critical review of these issues in the context of the monkey visual system and O'Carroll et al. (1996) for an example of how natural light signals are related to motion detection across insect species.

Many papers have been published on natural image statistics, with Laughlin (1981) being one of the earliest. We also recommend Srinivasan et al. (1982) for the relation between natural image statistics and neural processing, as well as van Hateren (1997) and Dong and Atick (1995) for a description of the properties of natural images. Mante et al. (2005) considers simultaneously luminance and contrast in natural scenes. Hyvärinen et al. (2009) is a recent book surveying the subject. Further details on the photoreceptor model of Figures 19.9 and 19.10 may be found in van Hateren and Snippe (2001). See van Hateren and Snippe (2006) for a direct comparison of phototransduction in blowflies and primate cones.

19.6 EXERCISES

1. Compute a mean subtracted, average histogram of the luminance of 10 natural scene images both in linear and logarithmic (base 10) coordinates to reproduce Figure 19.4B and C. Hint: Use the following code to read each of the images (imk00001.iml − imk00010.iml, obtained from the book's web site or van Hateren's time series database):

```
f1=fopen('filename', 'rb', 'ieee-be');
w=1536;h=1024;
buf=fread(f1, [w,h],'uint16');
fclose(f1);
```

Use 101 bins equally spaced between −1200 and 5000 in linear coordinates and −0.5 and 4 in logarithmic coordinates. For each bin, average the bin values over the 10 images.

2. Compute, for each image of Exercise 1, the power spectra along vertical and horizontal dimensions, respectively. Average the resulting 20 power spectra to arrive at Figure 19.4D and E. Fit the power spectrum in logarithmic coordinates to a straight line. Hint: Use the central 1024 bins from each horizontal line of each image. Use pwelch with a window size of 256 and an overlap of 128 pixels, respectively. The maximal (two-sided) frequency is 60 cycle/deg as each pixel represents 1 min of arc.

3. Compute a histogram of luminance values in linear and logarithmic coordinates for the time series ts001.bin (obtained from the book's web site or van Hateren's time series database) to arrive at plots similar to Figure 19.5B and C. Hint: Do not subtract the mean, use 100 bins.

4. Compute an estimate of the power spectral density of luminance values for the same time series as in Exercise 3. Hint: The sampling rate is 1200 sample/s and the time series is 45 mins long or 3,240,000 samples. Split the data in 4.5 min data chunks, 324,000 samples long. Compute the power spectrum on each data chunk using pwelch with a 4096 samples long window and an overlap of 2048. After taking the logarithm, resample in 100 equally spaced bins between the smallest and largest positive frequency values using spline. Average over the 10 data chunks.

20

Firing Rate Codes and Early Vision

O U T L I N E

20.1 Definition of Mean Instantaneous Firing Rate 299

20.2 Visual System and Visual Stimuli 300

20.3 Spatial Receptive Field of Retinal Ganglion Cells 301

20.4 Characterization of Receptive Field Structure 303

20.5 Spatio-Temporal Receptive Fields 306

20.6 Static Nonlinearities* 308

20.7 Summary and Sources 308

20.8 Exercises 309

In many cases, neuronal responses at early stages of sensory systems can be described as linear transformations of their inputs. This makes it possible to characterize their properties in terms of the frequency content of the stimulus by use of Fourier transforms. In the following, we will concentrate on single cells in the visual system of higher vertebrates such as cats and monkeys that have been extensively studied. However, similar methods have been applied to the visual system of invertebrates and to other sensory modalities like audition. As will be clear from a comparison of the predictions made by the models described in this chapter and the figures illustrating experimental data, the following description of neuronal responses is in many respects schematic. Nerve cells recorded experimentally rarely fit unambiguously or perfectly in simple categories.

20.1 DEFINITION OF MEAN INSTANTANEOUS FIRING RATE

When stimuli are repeatedly presented to the eye of an animal such as a fly, a cat, or a monkey, the responses recorded from visual neurons are usually variable from trial to trial. We have learned in Chapter 15 some methods to characterize variability of neuronal spike trains. The origin of variable neuronal responses to identical stimuli is not well understood. A simple explanation is that noise at the level of the photoreceptors and ion channels is responsible for it. This would be consistent with variability in spontaneous activity that is observed in the same neurons. It could also be that part of the variability observed in response to sensory stimuli is due to specific causes that we do not understand, reflecting the processing of sensory information by neurons. Neurophysiologists usually average out this variability by repeating the same stimulus and computing the resulting mean instantaneous firing rate. The most common procedure consists in taking a spike train in response to the stimulus and to convolve it with a smoothing filter such as a Gaussian profile, $\phi(t) = \exp(-t^2/2\tau^2)/\sqrt{2\pi\tau^2}$. In this equation, τ represents the time window over which spike times are averaged. There is no fixed rule to choose τ and usually its value is set in relation to the typical interspike interval observed during stimulus presentation so as to average over a few spikes. For interspike intervals of 10–20 ms, τ would be chosen to be around 20–50 ms. Of course longer time windows will average over more spikes at the expense of temporal resolution. Let $j = 1, 2, \ldots$ denote the index for the trial number and let $\delta(t - t_i^j)$, $i = 1, \ldots, N_j$ denote the ith spike of trial j so that the jth response to the stimulus is given by $r_j(t) = \sum_{i=1}^{N_j} \delta(t - t_i^j)$. We define an

Mathematics for Neuroscientists. DOI: 10.1016/B978-0-12-374882-9.00020-4

estimate of the instantaneous firing rate during trial j via the convolution

$$f_j(t) = r_j(t) \star \phi(t) = \int_{-\infty}^{\infty} r_j(s)\phi(t-s)\,\mathrm{d}s = \sum_{i=1}^{N_j} \phi(t - t_i^j). \tag{20.1}$$

This simply corresponds to placing a filter function $\phi(s)$ around each spike. The convolution in Eq. (20.1) can be computed efficiently using the fast Fourier transform algorithm (Chapter 7). The estimated instantaneous firing rate is then obtained by averaging across trials:

$$f(t) = \frac{1}{N} \sum_{j=1}^{N} f_j(t).$$

20.2 VISUAL SYSTEM AND VISUAL STIMULI

We will focus on describing the responses of a subset of nerve cells belonging to the first three visual processing stations of the cat or monkey visual system to a simplified set of visual stimuli.

Early visual processing. The first three visual processing stations and the cells of interest in each one of them may be briefly described as follows (Figure 20.1A).

1. At the back of the eye, visual signals are transduced into electrical signals by photoreceptor cells (Chapter 19) and processed by a complex multilayered circuitry called *the retina*. The output neurons of the retina are called *retinal ganglion cells*. They are the first spiking neurons in the light processing pathway and their axons form *the optic nerve*.

2. Retinal ganglion cells project to the lateral geniculate nucleus (LGN) of the thalamus. There, they make synaptic contacts with *LGN relay neurons*. We have already encountered these cells during our investigation of bursting neurons (§10.3).

3. LGN relay neurons in turn send their axons to the intermediate layers of the first cortical visual area (denoted by V1 in monkeys and sometimes by area 17 in cats).

From V1, visual information is sent to many different areas that are organized in a hierarchical manner (Figure 20.1B). These areas are connected by hundreds of feedforward and feedback pathways. Two of the best studied cortical areas are V1 and MT, which will be the only ones mentioned in this book. All of these visual stations are organized in a two-dimensional array perpendicular to the depth of the neural tissue. Neurons at each position in this array process signals from a specific position in the visual field that varies smoothly across the array. Thus, the

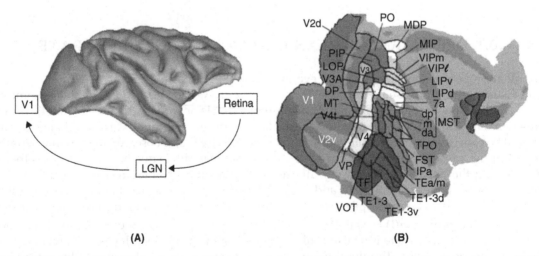

(A)   (B)

FIGURE 20.1   **A**. Side view of the right hemisphere of the macaque cortex. Visual information originates in the retina and is first sent to the LGN of the thalamus by the axons of retinal ganglion cells. The LGN is a deep brain structure not visible in the picture. From there information is sent to area V1 of visual cortex, located close to the occipital pole. **B**. A flattened view of the cortex with the approximate boundary of visual areas denoted in black. Each area has its own abbreviation. Shades of gray correspond to the depth of the tissue within the foldings of the brain (called sulci). Adapted from VanEssen (2005).

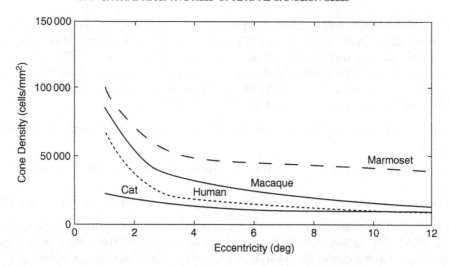

FIGURE 20.2   Spatial density of cone photoreceptors as a function of the angular distance to the center of the fovea (eccentricity) in four species. The peak density is thought to be on the order 200,000 cells/mm^2 for all three primates. Adapted from Goodchild et al. (1996).

retina, the LGN, V1, and MT all form *maps* of the two-dimensional visual space (§27.7). In the following we will ignore the fact that both eyes provide slightly different viewpoints and that this information can be used by neurons in V1 to retrieve depth information. The density of photoreceptors and the coverage of visual space is typically highest at the *fovea* in the retina and decreases towards the periphery (Figure 20.2). Our visual system generates the illusion of a large, high resolution field of view by moving the fovea rapidly (several times per second, §26.6) at different positions in the visual field, thus providing a patchy, high resolution map. In the following, we will ignore eye movements and assume that the eyes remain steady in their orbits. Experimentally, this assumption holds true during experiments in anesthetized animals. It holds approximately in awake subjects that are required to fixate on a specific point in the visual field during an experiment.

Visual stimuli. We restrict our attention to the processing of gray scale visual stimuli and ignore the fact that neurons respond to color as well. Thus, a visual stimulus at a given point in space and time can be described by a single number, the *intensity* of light (or *luminance*) ranging between 0 (dark, black), and a maximal intensity i_{max} (bright, white). An important aspect of visual processing is that neurons in general modulate their firing rate mainly in response to changes in the *contrast* of a stimulus rather than light intensity (§19.1). Of course, information about light intensity is required and transmitted as well along visual pathways, since otherwise we could not distinguish an outdoor scene from an indoor one for example. Let $i(x,y,t)$ be the spatio-temporal distribution of light intensity of a stimulus. If the stimulus is a stationary sinusoidal wave of intensity in the x direction, then $i(x,y,t) = i(x)$ and

$$i(x) = i_{mean}\big(1 + c_{max}\cos(2\pi\omega_x x)\big). \tag{20.2}$$

We denote by i_{mean} the mean light intensity and by $c_{max}\cos(2\pi\omega_x x)$ the fluctuation around the mean, or contrast variation. The (maximal) contrast of the pattern is c_{max}. In experimental situations, the contrast is often defined as $(i_{max} - i_{min})/(i_{max} + i_{min})$, which is equal to c_{max} for the stimulus of Eq. (20.2). The encoding mainly in terms of contrast is a necessity for visual neurons because light intensity varies by more than seven orders of magnitude from dim night light to bright outdoor light (Figure 19.1) while the dynamic firing range of neurons comprises at most two orders of magnitude. Relative variations around the mean, i.e., contrast variations, are typically much smaller (§§19.2, 19.3). In the following we will therefore almost always assume a fixed mean intensity and only specify the contrast of the stimulus.

20.3   SPATIAL RECEPTIVE FIELD OF RETINAL GANGLION CELLS

The definition of receptive fields. The response properties of mammalian visual neurons have been investigated since the 1950s starting with retinal ganglion cells. Such recordings typically reveal that only changes in contrast in a restricted portion of visual space affects the firing of a neuron. The area that directly affects the firing rate of a retinal ganglion cell (or of other visual neurons) is called its (classical) *receptive field*. For retinal ganglion cells, receptive field sizes are smallest at the fovea, where photoreceptors are most densely packed and their size increases with the eccentricity, i.e., the distance from the fovea. Both the size of receptive fields and their eccentricity are measured in degrees of visual angle and in minutes of arc (1 arc min = 1/60 of a degree). At the fovea, receptive field sizes can be estimated to be on the order of a few minutes of arc, based on anatomical data and the acuity thresholds of experimental subjects. The size increases to a few degrees at higher eccentricities (i.e., at 20–40 degrees from the fovea center). These numbers refer to the center region of the receptive field defined below.

Center-surround organization. The receptive fields of retinal ganglion cells are circular in shape and can be subdivided into two distinct regions:

1. a circular *center* region where an increase in luminosity causes an increase of the firing rate above its spontaneous level.
2. a circular *annulus* surrounding the center region where an increase in luminosity causes a decrease in firing rate.

Such a receptive field is said to possess a *center-surround* organization and retinal ganglion cells that respond as described above are called ON ganglion cells. OFF retinal ganglion cells have the same center-surround organization but an increase of luminosity in the center causes a decrease in firing rate and *vice-versa* for the surround annulus as illustrated in Figure 20.3.

Superposition and homogeneity. For a subclass of retinal ganglion cells called X-cells, the presentation of two different contrast patterns at different positions in the receptive field (e.g., two bars or two spots) causes a response that is approximately the algebraic sum of the responses to the two patterns presented in isolation. This property is called the superposition property and can be summarized by the following equation:

$$R_{c_1+c_2}(t) = R_{c_1}(t) + R_{c_2}(t), \tag{20.3}$$

where $R_c(t)$ denotes the change in firing rate as a function of time relative to spontaneous activity. In other words, the firing rate is $R_{spont} + R_c(t)$ in response to pattern c. Pattern $c_1 + c_2$ is simply the sum (superposition) of the two patterns c_1 and c_2.

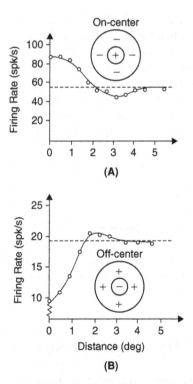

FIGURE 20.3   Average firing rate in response to a spot of light for an ON-center (**A**) and OFF-center (**B**) retinal ganglion cell of the cat as a function of the distance from the center of the receptive field. The dashed line represents the spontaneous activity level. Note that inhibitory regions do not exactly counterbalance excitatory ones. Therefore these neurons convey some information about the average luminance of stimuli in their receptive fields, in addition to their spatial contrast. Adapted from Maffei (1968).

Similarly, if the contrast of a pattern is doubled then the response of the cell is also doubled. This property is called homogeneity and typically holds for a restricted range of contrast values (typically for contrasts less than 0.45). We may write this in an equation as follows:

$$R_{\lambda c}(t) = \lambda R_c(t).$$ (20.4)

The response of a neuron possessing these two properties for arbitrary patterns can be described by a linear filtering operation:

$$R_c(t) = \iint\limits_{-\infty}^{\infty} w(x,y)c(x,y,t)\,dxdy,$$ (20.5)

where $c(x,y,t)$ is the stimulus contrast pattern and $w(x,y)$ is a weighting function that fully characterizes the spatial receptive field of the cell. Since the receptive fields and their weighting functions are effectively localized and different from zero only on a small area of the visual field, we can use integration boundaries of $\pm\infty$ in Eq. (20.5) without affecting any of the following arguments. Clearly a neuron whose responses are described by Eq. (20.5) will satisfy the homogeneity and superposition equations above. Conversely, the two equations (20.3) and (20.4) imply that a representation of the type of Eq. (20.5) exists, as may be seen by using Eq. (20.6) below to define $w(x,y)$. In Eq. (20.5) we have assumed that the cell's response follows perfectly the temporal modulations of the contrast pattern (after weighting with the spatial receptive field function $w(x,y)$). This is of course an idealization that will be addressed in §20.5.

20.4 CHARACTERIZATION OF RECEPTIVE FIELD STRUCTURE

Two methods have classically been used to determine experimentally the structure of neuronal receptive fields, i.e., the function $w(x,y)$ characterizing the linear filtering performed by the cell. The two methods are complementary and based on the equivalence of the spatial and frequency characterization of linear transformations.

Spatial domain stimuli. The first method consists in flashing small dots or bars at various positions in the visual field and recording the response of the neuron. If we approximate the brief flashing of a dot stimulus by a δ-function in space,

$$c_{dot}(x,y,t) = \delta(x-x_0)\delta(y-y_0)c_{dot}(t),$$

where $c_{dot}(t)$ is the time course of contrast activation of the dot, then the response of the cell is given by

$$R_{c_{dot}}(t) = \iint w(x,y)c_{dot}(x,y,t)\,dxdy = w(x_0,y_0)c_{dot}(t).$$ (20.6)

For simplicity, in this and subsequent equations we drop the integration boundaries whenever they equal $\pm\infty$. Thus, the response to a localized stimulus such as a dot will be directly proportional to the spatial receptive field weighting function $w(x,y)$ at the point where the dot is presented.

Receptive field symmetry. In the case of retinal ganglion cells, the spatial structure of the receptive field is well described by a difference of Gaussians, or "Mexican hat," model (Figure 20.3),

$$w(x,y) = k_c \exp(-(r/r_c)^2) - k_s \exp(-(r/r_s)^2), \quad \text{with} \quad r^2 = x^2 + y^2.$$ (20.7)

In this equation, the factors k_c and k_s determine the gain and relative weighting of the center and surround, whereas r_c and r_s control the extent of the center and surround regions, respectively. Such receptive fields are of course radially symmetric. Thus, if we present a stimulus whose contrast varies only along one dimension, e.g., a sinusoidal grating, the response of the neuron will be independent of the orientation of the grating. In the case of a one-dimensional pattern oriented along the x-axis, we can replace Eq. (20.5) by a one-dimensional equation:

$$R_c(t) = \int u(x)c(x,t)\,dx \quad \text{where} \quad u(x) \equiv \int w(x,y)\,dy.$$ (20.8)

For the receptive field of Eq. (20.7) we obtain

$$u(x) = k_c r_c \sqrt{\pi} \exp(-(x/r_c)^2) - k_s r_s \sqrt{\pi} \exp(-(x/r_s)^2) \qquad (20.9)$$

(Exercise 1). Note that in the case of a stationary, flashed sinusoidal grating, the response depends on the grating *phase* with respect to the center of the receptive field. By symmetry, a grating of the type $\sin(2\pi\omega_x x)$ will cause a zero response when placed in Eq. (20.8), whereas a grating shifted 90 degrees in phase, $\cos(2\pi\omega_x x) = \sin(2\pi\omega_x x + \pi/2)$ will cause a nonvanishing response. This point is illustrated in Figure 20.4.

Frequency properties of spatial receptive fields. Let us consider a one-dimensional spatial receptive field $u(x)$ as in Eq. (20.8). The spatial Fourier transform of the receptive field is given by,

$$\hat{u}(\omega_x) = \int e^{-2\pi i \omega_x x} u(x)\, dx.$$

For each frequency, ω_x, the spatial Fourier transform is a complex number and can be written as

$$\hat{u}(\omega_x) = \eta(\omega_x) e^{2\pi i \psi(\omega_x)} = \eta(\omega_x)(\cos(2\pi\psi(\omega_x)) + i\sin(2\pi\psi(\omega_x))), \qquad (20.10)$$

with modulus $\eta(\omega_x) \geq 0$ and phase $\psi(\omega_x)$. The value of the modulus and phase at different frequencies are not all independent. They are constrained by the properties of $u(x)$. First, because $u(x)$ is real, $\hat{u}(-\omega_x)^* = \hat{u}(\omega_x)$, where * denotes complex conjugation (Exercise 7.13). Thus,

$$\eta(\omega_x) = \eta(-\omega_x) \quad \text{and} \quad \psi(\omega_x) = -\psi(-\omega_x). \qquad (20.11)$$

If, in addition, the spatial receptive field is symmetric about the x-axis, $u(x) = u(-x)$, the Fourier transform also satisfies $\hat{u}(\omega_x) = \hat{u}(-\omega_x)$ (Exercise 7.14). Combining these two results, we obtain $\hat{u}(\omega_x) = u(\omega_x)^*$, i.e., the Fourier transform is real and $\psi(\omega_x) = 0$. This last property can be directly verified in the case of the Mexican hat model of retinal ganglion

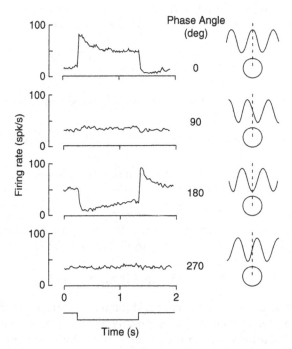

FIGURE 20.4 Response of an OFF-center X-cell in the cat to the introduction and withdrawal of a stationary sinusoidal grating pattern. The pattern had a contrast of 0.32 and its spatial frequency was 0.13 cycle/degree. The angular position (in degrees) of the cosine grating, relative to the midpoint of the receptive field center, is given at the right of the figure and is illustrated by the sketches. The downward deflection in the lowest trace indicates withdrawal of the stimulus (contrast turned off, the screen returns to uniform mean luminance) whereas the upward deflection indicates introduction of the pattern (contrast turned on). Note background activity level at 90 and 270 deg. Adapted from Enroth-Cugell and Robson (1966).

cell receptive fields by computing the Fourier transform from Eq. (20.9):

$$\hat{u}(\omega_x) = k_c r_c^2 \pi e^{-(r_c \pi \omega_x)^2} - k_s r_s^2 \pi e^{-(r_s \pi \omega_x)^2} \tag{20.12}$$

(Exercise 3).

Frequency domain stimuli. The second type of stimuli used to study neuronal receptive fields are drifting sinusoidal gratings, such as

$$c_{drift}(x,t) = c_{max} \cos\big(2\pi(\omega_x x - \omega_t t - \phi_x)\big).$$

At time $t=0$ this represents a grating with spatial frequency ω_x and phase ϕ_x with respect to the origin. For $t>0$ the grating drifts in such a way that for a fixed spatial point the time frequency of contrast change is ω_t. The speed of the drifting grating is $v=\omega_t/\omega_x$ as may be seen by rewriting

$$c_{drift}(x,t) = c_{max} \cos\big(2\pi(\omega_x(x-vt) - \phi_x)\big).$$

The reason behind the use of such stimuli is that they provide a characterization of the spatial frequency response of the neuron: for a sinusoidal grating of spatial frequency ω_x drifting at frequency ω_t the response after neuronal filtering will be characterized by a gain $\eta(\omega_x)$ and a phase shift $\psi(\omega_x)$, as in Eq. (20.10). To see this, we compute the response to such a drifting grating,

$$R_{drift}(t) = \int u(x)c_{drift}(x,t)\,dx = c_{max} \int u(x)\cos\big(2\pi(\omega_x x - \omega_t t - \phi_x)\big)\,dx.$$

Since the receptive field $u(x)$ is a real function and since $\cos\big(2\pi(\omega_x x - \omega_t t - \phi_x)\big) = \Re\big(e^{-2\pi i(\omega_x x - \omega_t t - \phi_x)}\big)$, we may rewrite,

$$
\begin{aligned}
R_{drift}(t) &= c_{max}\Re\int u(x)e^{-2\pi i(\omega_x x - \omega_t t - \phi_x)}\,dx\\
&= c_{max}\Re\big(e^{2\pi i(\omega_t t + \phi_x)}\hat{u}(\omega_x)\big)\\
&= c_{max}\eta(\omega_x)\cos\big(2\pi(\omega_t t + \phi_x + \psi(\omega_x))\big).
\end{aligned}
\tag{20.13}
$$

For a "Mexican hat" ganglion cell model, $\psi(\omega_x)$ will be zero and we see that the response is modulated in time just as the stimulus is, with a peak amplitude determined by $c_{max}\eta(\omega_x)$. The responses of a retinal ganglion cell to drifting sinusoidal gratings are shown in Figure 20.5. On the left side the spatial frequency (ω_x) of the drifting sinusoidal grating was varied, while on the right hand side the contrast (c_{max}) was varied.

Contrast sensitivity. According to Eq. (20.13), the peak modulation in firing rate elicited by a drifting grating is given by $R_{peak} = c_{max}\eta(\omega_x)$. Thus, $\eta(\omega_x) = R_{peak}/c_{max}$ may be measured by two different methods:

1. Measure the peak rate modulation (R_{peak}) elicited by drifting gratings of fixed contrast (c_{max}) and varying spatial frequency (ω_x).
2. Determine for each spatial frequency (ω_x) the contrast value c_{max}^0 needed to elicit a fixed target peak firing rate modulation R_{peak}^0. The inverse, $1/c_{max}^0$, is proportional to $\eta(\omega_x)$ and is called the *contrast sensitivity*. This method is expected to be accurate over a wider range of spatial frequencies if $\eta(\omega_x)$ varies by several orders of magnitude. The target peak modulation R_{peak}^0 is usually chosen to be relatively small (e.g., $R_{peak}^0 = 10$ spk/s) so as to guarantee a linear contrast response.

The left panel of Figure 20.6 plots the contrast sensitivity of a retinal ganglion cell measured with horizontal and vertical drifting gratings (filled and open circles, respectively). As expected from the rotational symmetry of the receptive field, contrast sensitivity is independent of motion direction. The solid line is a fit with Eq. (20.9).

Dependence on mean luminance. The contrast sensitivity depends on the mean luminance, i_{mean}, of the stimulus (see Eq. (20.2)). This is illustrated on the right panel of Figure 20.6. At low mean luminances the contrast sensitivity resembles more a low-pass filter than at high mean luminances. This may be interpreted from fits with Eq. (20.9) as a decrease in the influence of the surround over the center of the receptive field at low mean luminances.

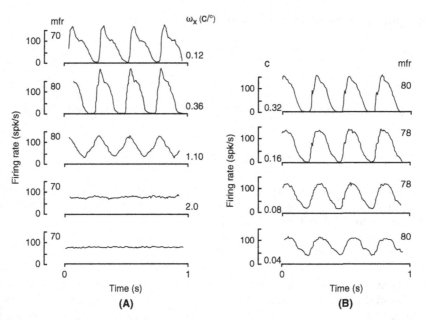

FIGURE 20.5   **A**. Response of an ON-center retinal ganglion X-cell in the cat to sinusoidal gratings of different spatial frequencies (indicated on the right) and constant contrast (0.4) drifting at a constant temporal frequency (4 c/s). The mean firing rate (mfr) is given on the left. **B**. Response of an ON-center retinal ganglion X-cell to sinusoidal gratings of constant spatial frequency (0.36 c/deg) but different contrasts (c, given on the left of each trace) drifting across the receptive field at a constant temporal frequency (4 c/s). The mean firing rate (mfr) is indicated on the right of each trace. Adapted from Enroth-Cugell and Robson (1966).

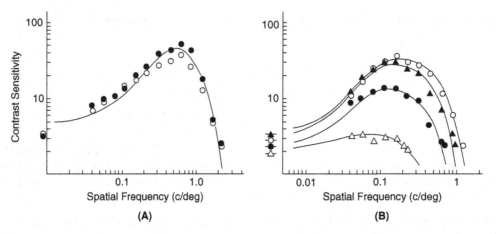

FIGURE 20.6   **A**. Contrast sensitivity in response to vertically (open circles) and horizontally (filled circles) drifting sinusoidal patterns. **B**. Contrast sensitivity at four mean luminance levels of the stimulus screen (16, 0.5, $1.6 \cdot 10^{-2}$, and $5 \cdot 10^{-4}$ cd/m^2). Data from retinal ganglion cells in the cat. Adapted from Enroth-Cugell and Robson (1966).

20.5 SPATIO-TEMPORAL RECEPTIVE FIELDS

Up to now we have assumed that our retinal ganglion cells follow temporal variations in the stimulus perfectly. This is of course not the case. The notion of receptive field therefore needs to be extended to the temporal domain by assuming that the neuron also filters the temporal variations in the stimulus. We therefore generalize Eq. (20.5) as follows:

$$R_c(t) = \iint \int_0^t w(x,y,t_0)c(x,y,t-t_0)\,dt_0 dx dy. \qquad (20.14)$$

This new equation simply states that the response at time t can be influenced by stimuli presented at that time or earlier, since t_0 varies from 0 to t. Stimulation is also assumed to start at time 0 and earlier times are not considered.

Finally, $R_c(t)$ cannot depend on future stimuli (since t_0 is not allowed to be negative). Alternatively, just as in the case of the spatial weighting function, Eq. (20.5), we can replace the time integration boundaries by $\pm\infty$ by defining $w(x,y,t_0) = 0$ for $t_0 < 0$ and assuming the stimulus started much earlier than t, since the weighting function $w(x,y,t_0)$ is effectively localized in time.

Space-time separability. When the spatial and temporal contributions to the receptive field are independent of each other we may write

$$w(x,y,t_0) = w_s(x,y)w_t(t_0).$$

In such a case, the receptive field is said to be *space-time separable* and the spatial weighting is globally modulated by w_t as time evolves. Note that Eq. (20.5) can be recovered from Eq. (20.14) by setting $w(x,y,t_0) = w_s(x,y)\delta(t_0)$, and therefore the space-time receptive field corresponding to Eq. (20.5) is separable and instantaneous at t_0.

A typical temporal response is biphasic in the time domain. We give an example that fits well the responses of X-type LGN relay cells in the cat, the targets of X-type retinal ganglion cells in the lateral geniculate nucleus of the thalamus:

$$w_t(t_0) = t_0(1 - \alpha t_0/2)e^{-\alpha t_0}\mathbb{1}(t_0) \tag{20.15}$$

where $\alpha = 2\pi\nu_c$ and $\nu_c = 5.5$ Hz (Figure 20.7D). To gain insight into the temporal processing implemented by filtering with w_t, we compute the Fourier transform of Eq. (20.15),

$$\hat{w}_t(\omega_t) = \frac{2\pi i \omega_t}{(\alpha + 2\pi i \omega_t)^3} \tag{20.16}$$

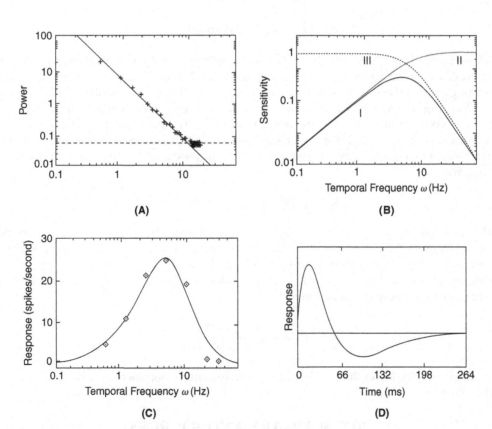

FIGURE 20.7   **A**. Measured temporal power spectrum from natural images at low spatial frequencies. The temporal decay follows a $\approx 1/\omega_t^2$ law. The dotted line indicates the noise floor. **B**. Predicted LGN temporal filter (curve I) which whitens the temporal power spectrum of natural images at low temporal frequencies (curve II) and acts as a low-pass filter at higher frequencies (curve III). **C**. Comparison between predicted temporal tuning curve (solid curve) and experimental cat LGN data. **D**. Temporal impulse response corresponding to the filter shown above. Adapted from Dong and Atick (1995).

(Exercise 4). From this equation, the gain can easily be computed at each temporal frequency,

$$|\hat{w}_t(\omega_t)| = \frac{2\pi\omega_t}{(\alpha^2 + (2\pi\omega_t)^2)^{3/2}}.$$

The gain increases from zero frequency to reach a maximum around 5 Hz and then decreases towards higher frequencies: it therefore represents a *band-pass* filtering of the contrast signal, emphasizing temporal frequencies around 5 Hz and filtering out higher and lower frequencies (Figure 20.7C). Band-pass filtering is also characteristic of the temporal response of retinal ganglion cells, although it is usually less pronounced than in LGN cells. In the cat, peak frequencies are typically around 1–4 cycles/s (or Hz). One explanation for the band-pass properties of LGN cells is illustrated in Figure 20.7. As we noted in §19.3 the temporal power spectrum of natural images decays as a power law of frequency, $\omega_t^{-\alpha}$ (Figure 19.5E). The exponent α typically lies between 1 and 2 and also depends on spatial frequency. At spatial frequencies below 0.5 c/deg its value is $\alpha \approx 2$ (Figure 20.7A). To optimally encode the range of temporal frequencies between 0.1 and 10 Hz thus requires the cell to boost the gain of higher frequencies (curve II in Figure 20.7B) up to the point where noise becomes significant (dotted line in Figure 20.7A) requiring low-pass filtering at higher frequencies (curve III in Figure 20.7B). The resulting filter is the combination of these two operations (curve I in Figure 20.7B) and is compared with experimental data in Figure 20.7C.

While in general the spatio-temporal receptive fields of both retinal and LGN X-cells are separable, a fraction of cells exhibits nonseparable spatio-temporal receptive fields. We will postpone a discussion of nonseparable spatio-temporal receptive fields until the next chapter, as their role is more evident in visual cortex.

20.6 STATIC NONLINEARITIES*

We have up to now assumed that the output of Eqs. (20.5) and (20.14) remain positive when added to the spontaneous firing rate:

$$R(t) = R_{spont} + R_c(t) \geq 0.$$

In some cells such as X-retinal ganglion cells, the spontaneous activity is often high and the changes in firing rate $R_c(t)$ due to changes in contrast remain above $-R_{spont}$ (Figures 20.3–20.5). But this is not always the case, particularly when the spontaneous firing rate is low or null as is often the case in cortical neurons. Similarly, the contrast gain response of a cell is usually linear only over a restricted range of values and tends to saturate at high contrast because firing rates cannot exceed a maximal rate R_{max} set by the refractory period. The usual model used to take into account these two observations consists in passing $R_c(t)$ through a static (i.e., time-independent) nonlinear function. Let us assume for simplicity that the spontaneous activity is equal to zero. The simplest nonlinearity that will ensure a positive firing rate is *half-wave rectification*:

$$R^+(t) = \lfloor R_c(t)\rfloor_+ = R_c(t)\mathbb{1}(R_c(t)). \tag{20.17}$$

Of course this discards half of the information originally present about the contrast modulation. Because usually visual cells come in ON and OFF types we can assume that a second neuron with opposite polarity receptive field encodes the second half of the contrast modulation, i.e., $R^-(t) = \lfloor -R_c(t)\rfloor_+$.

While equation (20.17) takes care of negative firing rates it does not implement saturation of firing rates. A model that fits well the responses of many visual neurons is

$$R^+(t) = R_{max}\frac{\lfloor R_c(t)\rfloor_+^2}{\sigma^2 + \lfloor R_c(t)\rfloor_+^2}. \tag{20.18}$$

Note that if the contrast is much lower than σ, Eq. (20.18) is an expansive nonlinearity while for contrasts much larger than σ it is compressive.

20.7 SUMMARY AND SOURCES

In this chapter, our presentation follows closely Enroth-Cugell and Robson (1966). Because of its simplicity, the description of neurons' receptive fields in terms of linear weighting functions and their Fourier transforms has become a sort of universal language for much of neuroscience research carried out at the level of whole organisms, i.e., Systems Neuroscience. Yet, as emphasized in the introduction to this chapter, not all neurons fit that scheme, even at early stages of the visual system, and much of the interesting visual processing is nonlinear. For example, the Y-cells also described by Enroth-Cugell and Robson (1966) present distinct nonlinear properties. We will encounter another specific example in §21.3, the complex cells of primary visual cortex. In other sensory systems like olfaction, the linear system approach has been fairly unsuccessful thus far, as reviewed in the introduction of French and Meisner (2007).

A good exposition from a computational perspective of the topics covered in this chapter and the next one is given by Abbott and Dayan (2001, Chapters 1 and 2). See Dan et al. (1996) for an experimental test of the results summarized in Figure 20.7. The static nonlinearity of Eq. (20.18) is an example of the Naka–Rushton function which is often used to model the transformation between stimulus contrast and firing rate: $R = R_{max}c^n/(c^n + \sigma^n)$, where n is positive and we assume that the response is equal to zero at zero contrast (i.e., no spontaneous activity). We have reformulated the equation in terms of the firing rate of the neuron since under the assumptions of this chapter it depends linearly on contrast. The article by Duong and Freeman (2008) provides fits of the Naka–Rushton function to LGN neurons as well as references to earlier work. The Naka–Rushton function also fits the contrast–response functions of V1 neurons quite well, see Albrecht and Hamilton (1982). At high contrasts, the saturation in Eq. (20.18) is commonly thought to reflect some sort of inhibitory normalization mechanism implemented at the level of cell networks.

20.8 EXERCISES

1. Show that the two-dimensional receptive field function $w(x,y)$ given in Eq. (20.7) reduces to $u(x)$ as given in Eq. (20.8) after integration over the y variable. Hint: Use the following formula,

$$\int_0^\infty \exp(-q^2 x^2)\, dx = \frac{\sqrt{\pi}}{2q}. \tag{20.19}$$

This latter formula can be derived from Eq. (7.39) by using the symmetry of the integrand around 0 and a change of integration variable.

2. †Show that in general a two-dimensional, rotationally symmetric receptive field $w(x,y) = w(r)$, $r = \sqrt{x^2 + y^2}$ can be reduced to a one-dimensional one given by the following equation:

$$u(x) = 2 \int_{|x|}^\infty \frac{w(r)r}{\sqrt{r^2 - x^2}}\, dr.$$

3. †Compute the Fourier transform of $u(x)$ (Eq. (20.9)). Hint: Use the Fourier transform of a Gaussian computed in Exercise 7.15.

4. Show that the Fourier transform of Eq. (20.15) is given by Eq. (20.16). Hint: Find a function g such that $\hat{w}_t(\omega_t) = \mathcal{L}(g)(s)$, where $s = \alpha + 2\pi i\omega_t$. Then use the result derived in Exercise 3.5.

5. †The contrast sensitivity function depicted in Figure 20.6 belongs to a retinal ganglion cell whose spatial receptive field is described by the following parameters: $r_c = 0.24$ deg, $r_s = 0.96$ deg, $k_s/k_c = 0.06$, $k_c = 1$.

   (i) Plot the Fourier transform of the receptive field in the frequency domain using Eq. (20.12). Scale the Fourier transform so as to have a peak value of 50, as in Figure 20.6A. The result is illustrated in Figure 20.8A. Hint: Use $\Delta f = 0.01$ cycles/deg in the frequency domain and `loglog` to plot in double logarithmic coordinates.

   (ii) Plot the corresponding spatial receptive field using Eq. (20.9) and the scaling factor determined in (i). Hint: Use $\Delta x = 0.006$ deg in the space domain, $N = 2048$ points ($N/2 - 1$ negative spatial positions, $x = 0$ and $N/2$ positive spatial positions).

   (iii) Compute the Fast Fourier transform of the spatial receptive field and verify that it matches the theoretical result by plotting them, as in Figure 20.8A. Hint: The spatial receptive field values at negative positions ($x < 0$) should be placed in *wrap-around order* by exploiting the periodicity of the discrete Fourier transform, $u(x_{-1}) = u(x_{N-1})$. Argue that the imaginary part of the fast Fourier transform should be equal to zero and plot only the real part at positive frequencies.

(iv) Generate three one-dimensional cosine gratings (maximal contrast ± 1) with spatial frequencies $\omega_x = 0.1, 1, 2$ cycles/deg drifting over the receptive field for 1000 ms (sampled at 1 ms resolution) at a temporal frequency $\omega_t = 3$ cycles/s. Compute numerically the response of the LGN cell to the drifting grating from the spatial receptive field using Eq. (20.8). Verify that the maximal amplitude modulation matches the theoretical prediction by plotting it as in Figure 20.8A. What is the translation speed of the three gratings? Hint: Generate the moving gratings by filling an array of 1000×2048 points (the first dimension is time and the second dimension is space). Use MATLAB matrix multiplication to compute the response of the LGN cell.

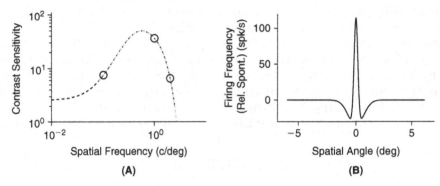

(A)   (B)

FIGURE 20.8   **A.** Receptive field of a retinal ganglion cell computed directly from Eq. (20.12) (black dashed line) or computed numerically by fast Fourier transform of Eq. (20.9) (red dashed line). The three black dots are obtained by computing the peak response of the spatial filter illustrated in B to sinusoidal gratings with spatial frequency $f_x = 0.1$, 1, and 2 c/deg and temporal frequency $f_t = 3$ c/s. **B.** Spatial receptive field of a retinal ganglion cell computed from Eq. (20.9). See Exercise 5 for model parameters. (`rgc_rf1.m`)

6. †(i) Plot the contrast sensitivity as a function of frequency for the retinal ganglion cell model of Exercise 5, together with the following contrast sensitivity model, which is more appropriate for low light conditions. Peak contrast sensitivity value: 30, $r_c \to 1.5 r_c$, $r_s \to 1.5 r_s$, $k_c \to k_c/1.5$, and $k_s \to k_s/1.53$. Plot the two corresponding spatial receptive fields.

(ii) A stationary contrast edge with high contrast to the left ($c = 1$ for $x \le x_0$) and low contrast to the right ($c = 0$ for $x > x_0$) is flashed in the cell's receptive field. Compute and plot the change in firing rate of the retinal ganglion cell model as a function of the position x_0 of the edge in the cell's receptive field both at high and at low light levels.

Models of Simple and Complex Cells

OUTLINE

21.1 Simple Cell Models   311

21.2 Nonseparable Receptive Fields   318

21.3 Receptive Fields of Complex Cells   320

21.4 Motion-Energy Model   321

21.5 Hubel–Wiesel Model   321

21.6 Multiscale Representation of Visual
      Information   322

21.7 Summary and Sources   323

21.8 Exercises   323

The receptive field properties of neurons in the retina and LGN are fairly similar both in their spatial center-surround organization and in their temporal band-pass structure. What happens at the level of primary visual cortex where LGN axons project? The first systematic investigations of cortical visual responses were made by Hubel and Wiesel at the end of the 1950s and early 1960s, taking advantage of newly engineered *tungsten electrodes* that permitted stable extracellular recordings from nerve cells over long periods of time in awake animals. Similar electrodes are still in use today for extracellular recordings in cats and monkeys. Hubel and Wiesel soon discovered that the responses of cortical neurons are much richer than what had been described at earlier stages of visual processing and reported the existence of two major types of cells called *simple* and *complex* in the primary visual cortex of the cat. They went on to characterize many other aspects of the representation of visual information by cortical neurons and cell assemblies in primary visual cortex. We will focus here on describing the linear and nonlinear properties of simple and complex cell receptive fields as well as some aspects of the transformation of neural signals occurring at the cortical level.

21.1 SIMPLE CELL MODELS

Spatial characteristics of simple cell receptive fields. Simple cells are similar to retinal ganglion cells and LGN relay neurons in possessing well-defined ON and OFF regions where increase and decrease in contrast cause an increase and decrease in firing rate, respectively. Furthermore, stimuli presented in these regions show summation of responses, with antagonistic effects of ON and OFF regions, consistent with a linear receptive field structure. Spontaneous activity is typically low and therefore responses are half-wave rectified as explained in §20.6. The main difference with retinal and LGN relay cells is the spatial structure of the ON and OFF regions: instead of being circular they are elongated along a principal axis and therefore the boundary is linear rather than circular (Figure 21.1). One important consequence is that simple cells respond best to elongated bars with an orientation parallel to their boundary. The bars need to be placed at the right position in the receptive field to maximally overlap with the corresponding ON or OFF regions, depending on their contrast. Presentation of moving bars or sinusoidal gratings gives rise to strong responses, provided that the orientation of the grating or the bar matches the receptive field orientation.

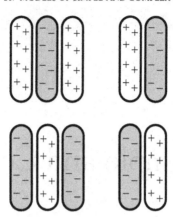

FIGURE 21.1   Typical simple cell receptive fields described by Hubel and Wiesel with even symmetric and odd symmetric spatial profile. Excitatory regions are marked by pluses and inhibitory regions by minuses.

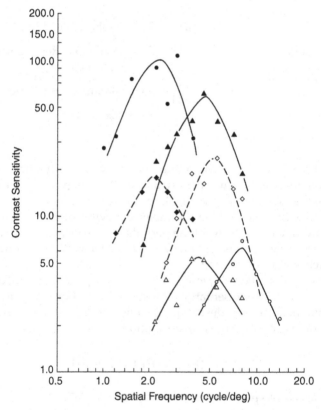

FIGURE 21.2   Contrast sensitivity for six cortical cells of area V1 in the macaque. Note the fairly sharp and symmetrical tuning of the response on both sides of the peak. Adapted from DeValois et al. (1982a).

Thus, the spatial receptive field properties of simple cells can be described by the size of the receptive field and its elongation as well as its orientation with respect to the coordinate axes. A further important characteristic of simple cells is their tuning to the spatial frequency of sinusoidal stimuli. Experiments show that simple cells are typically much more sharply tuned to spatial frequency than retinal or LGN cells. When responses are quantified as a function of spatial frequency, they fall off sharply on each side of a peak value (Figure 21.2; compare with Figure 20.6). In macaque monkeys, the peak spatial frequency tuning is typically located between 0.5 and 20 cycles/deg.

Gabor receptive field model.   To describe the two-dimensional spatial receptive field of simple cells, we will assume that the elongated boundary between ON and OFF regions lies parallel to the y-axis of a two-dimensional Cartesian coordinate system, with the origin $(0,0)$ at the center of the receptive field. With this convention, the spatial receptive fields of simple cells are well described by a *Gabor function*:

$$w(x,y) = \frac{1}{2\pi\sigma_x\sigma_y}\exp\left(-\frac{x^2}{2\sigma_x^2}-\frac{y^2}{2\sigma_y^2}\right)\cos(2\pi(k_x x-\phi_x)). \tag{21.1}$$

Along the x-axis, this function describes a sinusoidal wave that is dampened with distance from the center of the receptive field. The spatial extent in the x-direction is determined by the standard deviation σ_x. Typically $\sigma_x < \sigma_y$ and the oscillatory sinusoidal wave is aligned perpendicular to the elongated axis of the receptive field, with the parameter σ_y controlling the elongation of the receptive field. The number of oscillatory lobes, and therefore the number of positive (ON) and negative (OFF) regions, is determined by the spatial frequency, k_x for a fixed value of σ_x. In general, it is determined by the ratio of k_x and σ_x. The parameter k_x also determines the optimal spatial frequency for which the cell is tuned and ϕ_x is the spatial phase of the receptive field. If $\phi_x = 0$ then the receptive field is symmetric around $x=0$ (an even function of x), whereas for $\phi_x = -1/4$ we have $\cos(2\pi k_x x+\pi/2)=\sin(2\pi k_x x)$ and the receptive field is an odd function of x.

Thus the Gabor function describes a localized spatial frequency filter (Figure 21.3). This can also be seen by inspection of the Fourier transform of the Gabor filter,

$$\hat{w}(\omega_x,\omega_y) = \frac{1}{2}\left(e^{-2\pi i\phi_x}e^{-\sigma_x^2(2\pi)^2(\omega_x-k_x)^2/2}+e^{2\pi i\phi_x}e^{-\sigma_x^2(2\pi)^2(\omega_x+k_x)^2}\right)e^{-\sigma_y^2(2\pi)^2\omega_y^2/2},$$

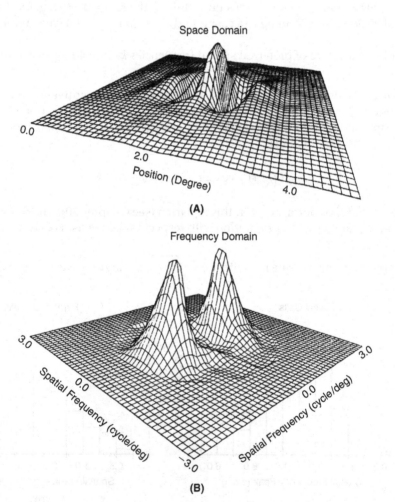

FIGURE 21.3 Receptive field profile in the spatial (**A**) and frequency (**B**) domain of a cat simple cell that is fairly narrowly tuned in frequency. Adapted from Webster and DeValois (1985).

which has two peaks at $(\pm k_x, 0)$ (Exercise 2). Note also that the tuning width in both spatial frequency directions ω_x and ω_y is inversely related to the spatial tuning width in the x and y directions.

Parameters of the Gabor model. The complete Gabor receptive field model depends on nine parameters. We explicitly describe them here and give representative values for some of them. Additional information follows in subsequent sections. Five of the parameters in Eq. (21.1) have been suppressed: three are related to the spatial location of the receptive field and its orientation. We have assumed in Eq. (21.1) that the origin of our coordinate system coincides with the center of the receptive field. Furthermore, we have assumed that the y-axis is parallel to the elongated axis of the receptive field whereas the x-axis lies along the narrow axis of the receptive field. This requires two translational parameters to match receptive field center with the origin of the coordinate system and one rotational parameter to align the coordinate axes with the receptive field axes. Another parameter that is suppressed in Eq. (21.1) is a global scaling factor needed to convert the output $w(x, y)$ into firing rate. The last parameter that has been ignored is the relative orientation of the cosine wave with respect to the main axes of the Gaussian envelope: we have namely assumed that the cosine wave is perfectly aligned with the narrower axis of the receptive field. This turns out to be the case for about 50 percent of the cells encountered, the remaining half typically has a different alignment, within ± 45 degrees of the minor axis.

The spatial size of simple cell receptive fields is controlled by the parameters σ_x and σ_y of the Gabor function. Spatial size varies over a wide range close to the fovea (1:30 range) and receptive field size also typically increases towards the periphery of the visual field. The aspect ratio $\lambda = \sigma_x/\sigma_y$ of the receptive field is much more constrained with a typical value of 0.6. The receptive field in the frequency domain consists of a linear superposition of two Gaussian centered at $(k_x, 0)$ and $(-k_x, 0)$, respectively. The overlap between these two Gaussian envelopes is typically insignificant (Figure 21.3).

The spatial phase ϕ_x of the receptive field ranges uniformly in the range 0–90 deg. Odd and even receptive fields (i.e., phases of 0 deg and 90 deg corresponding to a cosine and a sine in Eq. (21.1)) were among the first ones described by Hubel and Wiesel.

In the macaque monkey, the range of preferred spatial frequencies k_x typically lies between 0.5 and 16 cycles/deg (Figure 21.4).

Parametrization of two-dimensional moving gratings. In contrast to the receptive fields of retina and LGN neurons analyzed in the previous chapter, the receptive field model for simple cells is not rotationally symmetric. We therefore need to consider the response to a two-dimensional grating instead of a one-dimensional one. A two-dimensional moving sinusoidal grating has the functional form

$$c_{drift}(x, y, t) = \cos(2\pi(\eta_x x + \eta_y y - \eta_t t - \eta_0)). \tag{21.2}$$

Note that we have suppressed the contrast c_{max} in this equation (see Chapter 20). The parameters (η_x, η_y) determine the spatial frequency of the grating and its orientation with respect to the x-axis. This is most easily seen by rewriting

$$(\eta_x, \eta_y) = \eta(\cos\xi, \sin\xi), \quad \text{with} \quad \eta = \sqrt{\eta_x^2 + \eta_y^2}, \quad \text{and} \quad \xi = \tan^{-1}(\eta_y/\eta_x).$$

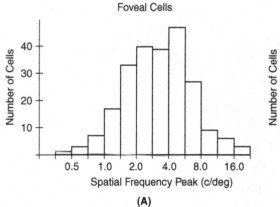
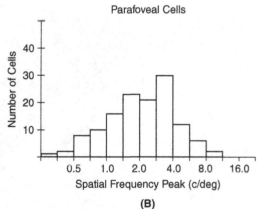

FIGURE 21.4   Peak spatial frequency tuning of foveal (**A**) and parafoveal (**B**) cells in macaque V1 neurons. Adapted from DeValois et al. (1982a).

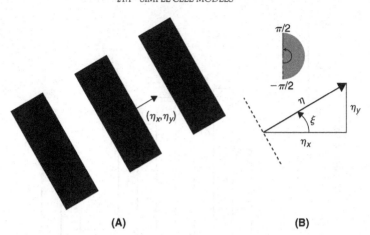

(A)   **(B)**

FIGURE 21.5   **A.** Schematic illustration of a grating and the vector (η_x, η_y) used to characterize it. **B.** The components η_x and η_y determine the angle $\xi = \tan^{-1}(\eta_y/\eta_x)$. The top inset shows how the angle varies (gray shaded area) as the orientation of the grating varies. The length of the vector, η is the spatial frequency of the grating (in cycle/degree). The dashed line illustrates points having the same contrast at any given time.

The parameter η is the spatial frequency of the grating and the unit vector $(\cos\xi, \sin\xi)$, with $\xi \in (-\pi/2, \pi/2]$ or equivalently $\eta_x > 0$, gives the direction of contrast change: at a fixed moment in time contrast is always constant along points joined by a line perpendicular to this vector (Figure 21.5). The factor η_0 determines the phase of the grating at time $t = 0$. The speed of motion is η_t/η, as in the case of the one-dimensional moving grating. Both Gabor filters and sinusoidal gratings are parametrized in terms of spatial and temporal frequencies (k_x, η_x, and η_t).

Response to moving gratings.   The response of a Gabor filter to the sinusoidal grating of Eq. (21.2) is given by

$$
\begin{aligned}
R_{drift}(t) &= \frac{1}{2}\cos\big(2\pi(\eta_t t + \eta_0 - \phi_x)\big)\exp(-\sigma_x^2(2\pi)^2(\eta_x - k_x)^2/2 - \sigma_y^2(2\pi)^2\eta_y^2/2) \\
&\quad + \frac{1}{2}\cos\big(2\pi(\eta_t t - \eta_0 + \phi_x)\big)\exp(-\sigma_x^2(2\pi)^2(\eta_x + k_x)^2/2 - \sigma_y^2(2\pi)^2\eta_y^2/2) \\
&\approx \frac{1}{2}\cos\big(2\pi(\eta_t t + \eta_0 - \phi_x)\big)\exp(-\sigma_x^2(2\pi)^2(\eta_x - k_x)^2/2 - \sigma_y^2(2\pi)^2\eta_y^2/2)
\end{aligned}
\tag{21.3}
$$

(Exercise 3). The last approximation is valid because of the negligible overlap between the two Gaussians (Figure 21.3B) and since η_x is assumed to be positive. Thus, we see that the response oscillates at the same temporal frequency as the moving grating, independent of the direction of motion ($\eta_t > 0$ is rightward motion and $\eta_t < 0$ is leftward motion).

Spatial frequency tuning.   We can rewrite Eq. (21.3) in terms of the spatial frequency η and orientation ξ of the grating:

$$
R_{drift} \approx \frac{1}{2}\cos(2\pi(\eta_t t + \eta_0 - \phi_x))e^{-\sigma_x^2(2\pi)^2(\eta\cos\xi - k_x)^2/2}e^{-\sigma_y^2(2\pi)^2\eta^2\sin\xi^2/2}.
\tag{21.4}
$$

The spatial frequency tuning of the response is obtained by varying the spatial frequency (η) of the drifting grating around the optimum ($\eta = k_x$) positioned in its optimal orientation, i.e., $\xi = 0$. Since the second Gaussian remains equal to 1, the peak response is proportional to $\exp(-\sigma_x^2(2\pi)^2(\eta - k_x)^2/2)$.

The *bandwidth, b,* of the cell is defined as the difference between the highest frequency, η_h, and the lowest frequency, η_l, that yield half of the maximal response in *octaves* (i.e., in base 2 logarithmic units):

$$
b = \log_2 \eta_h - \log_2 \eta_l.
$$

The reason for choosing a logarithmic scale is that the tuning response is fairly symmetrical (Figure 21.2) and therefore

$$
\log_2 \eta_h = \log_2 k_x + \frac{b}{2}, \quad \log_2 \eta_l = \log_2 k_x - \frac{b}{2}
$$

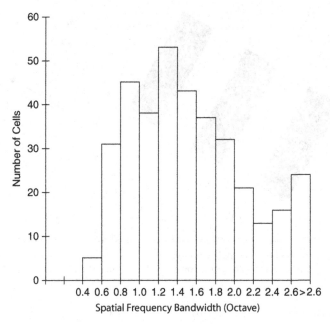

FIGURE 21.6   Distribution of spatial frequency bandwidths for a large sample of cortical V1 neurons in the macaque monkey. Adapted from DeValois et al. (1982a).

or equivalently

$$\eta_h = k_x 2^{b/2}, \quad \eta_l = k_x 2^{-b/2}.$$

Thus a cell that has a peak spatial frequency tuning at 1 cycle/deg and a bandwidth of 1 octave ($b=1$) would have half maximal responses at 0.7 and 1.4 cycle/deg, respectively. A cell with the same bandwidth but peak tuning at 10 cycle/deg would have half-maximal responses at 7 and 14 cycle/deg. The bandwidth of simple cells is fairly constant with a typical value of 1.4 octaves (range: 0.4–2.6; Figure 21.6). The bandwidth can be computed in terms of the product $k_x \sigma_x$ as

$$b = \log_2 \frac{k_x \sigma_x + \sqrt{2 \log 2}}{k_x \sigma_x - \sqrt{2 \log 2}}, \quad k_x \sigma_x = \sqrt{2 \log 2} \frac{2^b + 1}{2^b - 1} \tag{21.5}$$

(Exercise 4). In the case $b=1.4$ we obtain $k_x \sigma_x = 2.614$. A consequence of this equation is that the parameter σ_x tends to be inversely related to k_x (since bandwidths are fairly constant, irrespective of peak frequency tuning).

Orientation tuning. Orientation tuning is usually determined at the optimal spatial frequency ($\eta = k_x$) by changing the angle ξ of the drifting grating. The orientation bandwidth is defined as the difference in orientation $\Delta \xi = \xi_h - \xi_l$ from the peak orientation (which is 0 deg by definition of our coordinate axes) for which the response has declined to half of its peak value. The prediction obtained from Eq. (21.4) is

$$\Delta \xi = 2 \sin^{-1} \lambda \frac{\sqrt{2 \log 2}}{k_x \sigma_x} = 2 \sin^{-1} \lambda \frac{2^b - 1}{2^b + 1}, \tag{21.6}$$

where λ is the aspect ratio of the receptive field (Exercise 5). For an aspect ratio of 0.6 and a bandwidth of 1.4 we obtain $\Delta \xi = 31$ deg (Figure 21.7). This equation predicts a positive correlation between orientation and spatial frequency tuning that is consistent with experimental observations (Figure 21.8).

Response to stationary gratings. Stationary gratings can be obtained by superposing two gratings moving in opposite directions. If we set for simplicity $z = \eta_x x + \eta_y y - \eta_0$, we obtain:

$$\frac{1}{2} \left(\cos(2\pi(z + \eta_t t)) + \cos(2\pi(z - \eta_t t)) \right) = \cos(2\pi z) \cos(2\pi \eta_t t),$$

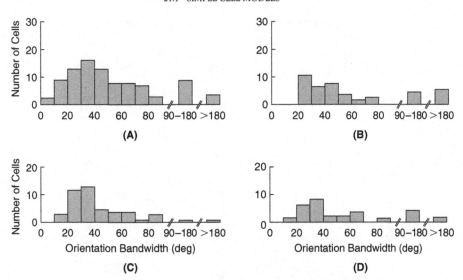

FIGURE 21.7 Distribution of orientation bandwidths for four samples of cortical V1 neurons in the macaque. **A.** Foveal simple cells (n = 92 cells, median orientation bandwith = 42.3). **B.** Foveal complex cells (n = 46, median = 44.5). **C.** Parafoveal simple cells (n = 47, median = 33.8). **D.** Parafoveal complex cells (n = 37, median = 43.8). There are no notable differences between simple or complex cells and between foveal and parafoveal cells. Adapted from DeValois et al. (1982b).

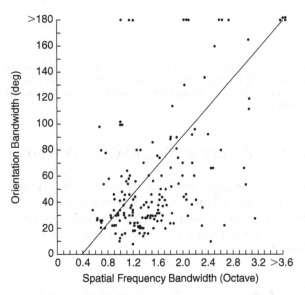

FIGURE 21.8 Scatterplot of orientation bandwidth as a function of spatial frequency bandwidth for 168 cells in V1 of the macaque monkey. There is a positive correlation of 0.5 between the two variables. Adapted from DeValois et al. (1982a).

which is a standing wave. Superposing two such moving stimuli yields

$$R_{stat}(t) \approx \frac{1}{4} \cos(2\pi \eta_t t) \cos(2\pi (\eta_0 - \phi_x)) e^{-\sigma_x^2 (2\pi)^2 (\eta_x - k_x)^2/2} e^{-\sigma_y^2 (2\pi)^2 \eta_y^2/2},$$

where we have used the same approximation as in Eq. (21.3).

Spatial phase dependence. Just as in the case of retinal and LGN cells, the Gabor model predicts a dependence of the response of a simple cell to the spatial phase of a stationary grating, depending on the alignment of ON and OFF regions with the respective oscillatory regions of the grating. This prediction has been verified experimentally (Figure 21.9).

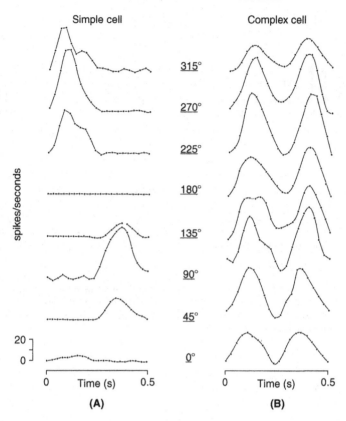

FIGURE 21.9 **A.** Response of a simple cell to a stationary counterphasing grating placed at various phases with respect to the center of its receptive field. Note the spatial dependence of the response with two peaks 180 degrees apart and phase shifted in time by the same phase. **B.** Same experiment for a complex cell. Note the frequency doubling of the response and position independence. Data from area V1 in the macaque monkey. Adapted from DeValois et al. (1982a).

21.2 NONSEPARABLE RECEPTIVE FIELDS

Temporal responses. The temporal impulse response of simple cells is typically biphasic, like the one of LGN neurons described in the previous lecture, but simple cells also exhibit triphasic responses. Thus, it is not surprising that simple cells also act as band-pass filters in the temporal domain. Typically, peak temporal frequency tuning is around 8 Hz, with bandwidths of ≈ 2.5 octaves and thus less sharp than in the spatial domain. To simplify subsequent calculations, we will use the following two-model response functions:

$$
\begin{aligned}
f_{te}(t) &= \frac{1}{\sqrt{2\pi}\,\sigma_t} e^{-(t-t_\Delta)^2/2\sigma_t^2} \cos(2\pi k_t(t-t_\Delta)), \\[2mm]
f_{to}(t) &= \frac{1}{\sqrt{2\pi}\,\sigma_t} e^{-(t-t_\Delta)^2/2\sigma_t^2} \sin(2\pi k_t(t-t_\Delta)),
\end{aligned}
\tag{21.7}
$$

with $k_t = 8$ cycle/s, $\sigma_t = 31$ ms, and $t_\Delta = 86$ ms (Figure 21.10A). In the following, the delay t_Δ will often be set to zero as it simply implies a shift of the time axis.

Nonseparable receptive fields. The receptive fields of simple cells are often nonseparable, i.e., they cannot be described as a product of spatial and temporal responses (Figure 21.11). A simple method to generate nonseparable receptive fields is to add two separable spatio-temporal receptive fields together. If we define even and odd one-dimensional Gabor filters,

$$
g_{se}(x) = \frac{1}{\sqrt{2\pi}\,\sigma_x} e^{-x^2/2\sigma_x^2} \cos(2\pi k_x x) \quad \text{and} \quad g_{so}(x) = \frac{1}{\sqrt{2\pi}\,\sigma_x} e^{-x^2/2\sigma_x^2} \sin(2\pi k_x x),
\tag{21.8}
$$

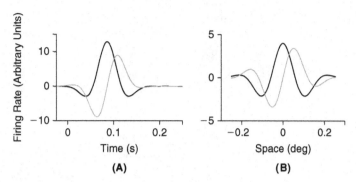

(A)   **(B)**

FIGURE 21.10   **A.** Response functions of the even (black) and odd (red) temporal filters of Eq. (21.7). The firing rate on the abscissa has been rescaled to arbitrary units, with zero representing the mean firing rate. **B.** Response functions of the even (black) and odd (red) spatial filters of Eq. (21.8). The parameters are: $k_x = 4.2$ cycle/deg and $\sigma_x = 0.1$ deg. (`temp_space_rfs.m`)

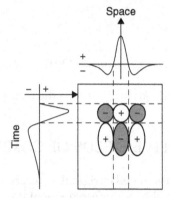

FIGURE 21.11   Sketch of a separable spatio-temporal receptive field. Adapted from Adelson and Bergen (1985).

(Figure 21.10B) we can define two nonseparable receptive fields as follows:

$$g_e^-(x,t) = g_{se}(x)f_{te}(t) + g_{so}(x)f_{to}(t) = \frac{1}{2\pi\sigma_x\sigma_t}e^{-x^2/2\sigma_x^2 - t^2/2\sigma_t^2}\cos(2\pi(k_x x - k_t t)),$$

$$g_o^-(x,t) = g_{so}(x)f_{te}(t) - g_{se}(x)f_{to}(t) = \frac{1}{2\pi\sigma_x\sigma_t}e^{-x^2/2\sigma_x^2 - t^2/2\sigma_t^2}\sin(2\pi(k_x x - k_t t)).$$

An important property of nonseparable receptive fields is that they are selective to the direction of motion of a sinusoidal grating. *Direction selectivity* to moving stimuli is a new property that emerges at the level of visual cortex. To see why nonseparable receptive fields are direction selective, we need to look at the spatio-temporal structure of the receptive field (Figure 21.12). Since it is oriented in space-time it will favor a specific orientation of a stimulus in space-time which corresponds to a specific speed of propagation. In the case of a one-dimensional sinusoidal grating,

$$c(x,t) = \cos(2\pi(\eta_x x - \eta_t t - \phi_x)),$$

we obtain the response of the cell by convolution of the stimulus with the receptive field,

$$R(t) = \iint g_e^-(x,t_0)c(x,t-t_0)\,dt_0 dx = \Re\left\{e^{2\pi i(\eta_t t + \phi_x)}\iint g_e^-(x,t_0)e^{-2\pi i(\eta_x x + \eta_t t_0)}\,dt_0 dx\right\}.$$

In this equation, both the spatial and temporal integration boundaries can be set equal to $\pm\infty$ since g_e^- is effectively localized in space and time. The Fourier transform of g_e^- is real,

$$\hat{g}_e^-(\omega_x,\omega_t) = \frac{1}{2}\left(e^{-\sigma_x^2(2\pi)^2(\omega_x+k_x)^2/2}e^{-\sigma_t^2(2\pi)^2(\omega_t-k_t)^2/2} + e^{-\sigma_x^2(2\pi)^2(\omega_x-k_x)^2/2}e^{-\sigma_t^2(2\pi)^2(\omega_t+k_t)^2/2}\right), \tag{21.9}$$

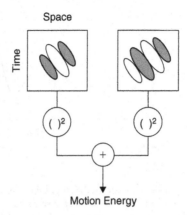

FIGURE 21.12   Schematic illustration of the motion-energy model. Adapted from Adelson and Bergen (1985).

(Exercise 6) and therefore

$$R(t) = \hat{g}_e^-(\eta_x, \eta_t) \cos\left(2\pi(\eta_t t + \phi_x)\right).$$ (21.10)

Because Eq. (21.9) is nonzero only around $(k_x, -k_t)$ and $(-k_x, k_t)$ the response is most sensitive to a negative preferred speed of $-k_t/k_x$.

21.3 RECEPTIVE FIELDS OF COMPLEX CELLS

Complex cells form the second major class of cells originally described by Hubel and Wiesel. Like simple cells, complex cells are selective for bars presented at a preferred orientation in the receptive field and they are tuned for spatial frequency. In contrast to simple cells, they will respond irrespective of the particular position at which a bar is flashed in the receptive field and are largely insensitive to the polarity (ON or OFF) of the stimulus. Two other important differences with simple cells are also observed in response to moving and to counterphase gratings, respectively: (i) the response to moving gratings is sustained and lacks the modulation in time seen in simple cells, (ii) the response to counterphase gratings exhibits *frequency doubling* (Figure 21.9).

These properties can be explained by assuming that the response of complex cells is obtained by squaring and summing the responses of two Gabor receptive fields 90 degrees out of phase, like the ones defined in Eq. (21.8):

$$R_{cc}(t) = R_{se}^2(t) + R_{so}^2(t),$$

where

$$R_{se}(t) = \int g_{se}(x)c(x,t)\,dx, \quad R_{so}(t) = \int g_{so}(x)c(x,t)\,dx,$$

and $c(x,t)$ is the stimulus. Note that we have neglected temporal filtering for simplicity. Because the responses of simple cells are half-wave rectified this squared sum can be implemented only with a minimum of four simple cells,

$$R_{cc}(t) = \lfloor R_{se}(t)\rfloor_+^2 + \lfloor R_{se}^-(t)\rfloor_+^2 + \lfloor R_{so}(t)\rfloor_+^2 + \lfloor R_{so}^-(t)\rfloor_+^2,$$

where the responses R_{se}^- and R_{so}^- are to the same receptive field profile but of opposite polarity: $-g_{se}$ and $-g_{so}$, respectively. The pair of receptive fields g_{se} and g_{so} is called a *quadrature pair* and squaring and summation over such a pair is an efficient way of implementing phase independence of the responses.

Response to moving gratings. We compute the response to a moving grating $c(x,t) = \cos\left(2\pi(\eta_x x - \eta_t t - \eta_0)\right)$. Just as in the case of Eq. (21.10) we know that,

$$R_{se}(t) = \hat{g}_{se}(\eta_x)\cos(2\pi(\eta_t t + \eta_0)) = \frac{1}{2}(\alpha + \beta)\cos(2\pi(\eta_t t + \eta_0)),$$

where we have used the abbreviations $\alpha = \exp(-\sigma_x^2 (2\pi)^2 (\omega_x - k_x)^2/2)$ and $\beta = \exp(-\sigma_x^2 (2\pi)^2 (\omega_x + k_x)^2/2)$. Similarly,

$$R_{so}(t) = \frac{1}{2}(\alpha - \beta)\sin(2\pi(\eta_t t + \eta_0)),$$

and the complex cell response is obtained from

$$R_{cc}(t) = (\alpha^2 + \beta^2)/4 + \alpha\beta\{\cos^2(2\pi(\eta_t t + \eta_0)) - \sin^2(2\pi(\eta_t t + \eta_0))\}/2 \approx \alpha^2/4,$$

where the approximation is valid for a spatial frequency ω_x around the optimal frequency k_x. Thus we see that the response to a moving grating is approximately unmodulated.

Response to stationary gratings. To obtain the response to counterphase gratings we can use the results obtained above for moving gratings and the superposition property

$$\cos(2\pi(\eta_x x - \eta_0))\cos(\eta_t t) = \frac{1}{2}\{\cos(2\pi(\eta_x x - \eta_t t - \eta_0)) + \cos(2\pi(\eta_x x + \eta_t t - \eta_0))\}.$$

This implies that

$$R_{se}(t) = \frac{1}{2}(\alpha + \beta)\cos(2\pi\eta_t t)\cos(2\pi\eta_0), \quad \text{and} \quad R_{so}(t) = \frac{1}{2}(\alpha - \beta)\cos(2\pi\eta_t t)\sin(2\pi\eta_0).$$

Squaring and summing yields

$$R_{cc}(t) = \cos^2(2\pi\eta_t t)\{\alpha^2 + \beta^2 + 2\alpha\beta(\cos^2 2\pi\eta_0 - \sin^2 2\pi\eta_0)\}/4 \approx \cos^2(2\pi\eta_t t)\alpha^2/4.$$

In the last line we have used the same approximation as in the case of a moving grating. This represents a doubling of the frequency since $\cos^2(2\pi\eta_t t) = (\cos(4\pi\eta_t t) + 1)/2$, see Figure 21.9.

21.4 MOTION-ENERGY MODEL

If we apply the quadrature model of the previous section to space-time oriented receptive fields we obtain a complex cell model that is selective for the direction of motion and whose responses are independent of the phase of a drifting sinusoidal grating:

$$R_{me}^-(t) = R_{e-}^2(t) + R_{0-}^2(t)$$

where

$$R_{e-}(t) = \iint g_e^-(x,t_0)c(x,t-t_0)\,\mathrm{d}t_0\mathrm{d}x, \quad R_{0-}(t) = \iint g_0^-(x,t_0)c(x,t-t_0)\,\mathrm{d}t_0\mathrm{d}x,$$

for the stimulus $c(x,t)$. This model is called the *motion-energy model* (Figure 21.12) and resembles the definition of kinetic energy in some physical systems. The motion-energy model is thought to describe the responses of neurons projecting to area MT of macaque monkeys, as well as the responses of a subset of MT neurons (component cells). Area MT is specialized in detecting motion. Formally, the motion-energy model is equivalent to the *Reichardt correlation model* describing the extraction of motion information in insect visual systems.

21.5 HUBEL–WIESEL MODEL

The original work of Hubel and Wiesel proposed a purely feedforward model describing the emergence of simple cell receptive fields from a superposition of LGN receptive fields as well as the generation of phase invariant responses in complex cells by averaging over simple cells with different phases (Figure 21.13).

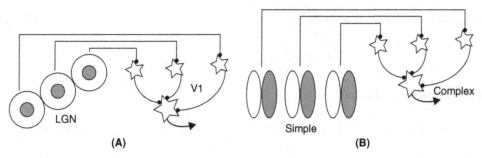

FIGURE 21.13 **A.** Hubel and Wiesel model describing the emergence of simple cell receptive fields from LGN center-surround receptive fields by convergence of responses. **B.** Model for the emergence of complex receptive fields from simple cell receptive fields by summation of several simple cell responses staggered in space. Adapted from Hubel and Wiesel (1962).

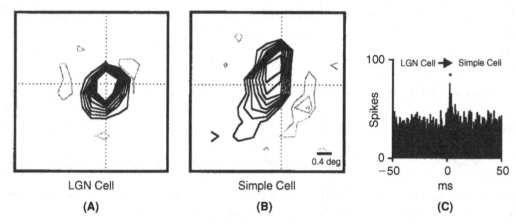

FIGURE 21.14 **A.** Receptive field of an LGN relay neuron with gray lines indicating ON and black lines OFF regions. **B.** Receptive field of a simple cell in V1 recorded simultaneously. **C.** The cross correlation between spontaneous spike trains of the two cells has a peak slightly offset from zero indicating that whenever the LGN cell fires, the V1 simple cell has an increased probability of firing after a short delay of a few milliseconds. This suggests that the two cells are synaptically connected. Adapted from Alonso et al. (2001).

In agreement with this model, the receptive fields of synaptically connected LGN and V1 neurons are indeed spatially in register (Figure 21.14). Yet, details of the model have been surprisingly difficult to confirm at an anatomical and physiological level and are still under debate today. Alternative models explain the emergence of simple cell and complex cell receptive fields based on intracortical connections. These models often rely on anatomical data showing that 95% of the synapses onto cortical neurons are of intracortical origin. It has also been shown theoretically that complex receptive fields can be generated directly from LGN inputs, provided neurons are endowed with active membrane conductances.

21.6 MULTISCALE REPRESENTATION OF VISUAL INFORMATION

The representation of visual information at the level of primary visual cortex appears to have some characteristics of multiscale representations used in image analysis such as *wavelet transforms*. Simple cell receptive fields are localized in space and frequency. Furthermore their receptive fields vary over a range of scales. This analogy has been used both in image analysis as a motivation for investigating multiscale representations and in theoretical work on primary visual cortex to explore how cortical neurons might encode information about natural images (Figure 21.15). There is at present no comprehensive theory that can explain what kind of processing cortical neurons do on visual inputs, but several theories can explain in part the properties of visual cortical neurons based on a multiscale representation of natural images.

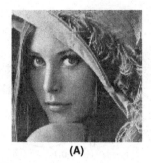 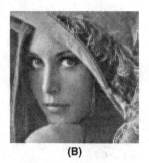

(A)   (B)

FIGURE 21.15   **A**. Original image of "Lena." **B**. Reconstruction of "Lena" based on the activity associated with Gabor receptive field functions sampling visual space at discrete locations over seven different scales (octaves) and with eight different orientations. Adapted from Lee (1996).

21.7 SUMMARY AND SOURCES

This chapter presented the basic receptive field properties of neurons in primary visual cortex. While simple cell receptive fields can be conceived as a fairly straightforward elaboration of the receptive fields encountered at earlier stages of the visual system, complex cells present genuinely different properties. Remarkably, we have learned that a simple combination of linear and static nonlinear operations can account for much of the experimental data. Hubel and Wiesel shared half of the Nobel Prize in Medicine in 1981. Since their original work, the properties of visual neurons in area V1 have been studied in many laboratories. The book by DeValois and DeValois (1990) summarizes results pertinent to this chapter up to its publication. For more recent results, see the reviews of DeAngelis et al. (1995) and Ringach (2004). Our model of simple cell temporal response properties in §21.2 allows us to carry out analytical calculations, but is oversimplified. The temporal profiles of real neurons are typically skewed, as schematically illustrated in Figure 21.11, so that a time domain Gabor does not fit well. We explore a more realistic model in Exercise 12 based on Emerson et al. (1992). See DeAngelis et al. (1999) for a discussion of quadrature pairs and Mel et al. (1998) for further discussion of the Hubel and Wiesel model.

21.8 EXERCISES

1. Compute, by hand, the Fourier transforms of

$$f(x) = \frac{1}{\sqrt{2\pi}\sigma_x} e^{-x^2/2\sigma_x^2} \cos\left(2\pi(k_x x - \phi_x)\right) \quad \text{and} \quad h(x) = \frac{1}{\sqrt{2\pi}\sigma_x} e^{-x^2/2\sigma_x^2} \sin\left(2\pi(k_x x - \phi_x)\right).$$

2. †Compute the Fourier transform of a two-dimensional spatial Gabor filter, Eq. (21.1).

3. Compute the response of the simple cell model to a drifting grating, Eq. (21.3).

4. Compute the bandwidth of the Gabor receptive field model, Eq. (21.5).

5. †Compute the orientation tuning width of the Gabor receptive field model, Eq. (21.6).

6. Compute the Fourier transform of g_e^-, Eq. (21.9), and of g_o^-.

7. Plot the temporal and spatial one-dimensional Gabor functions of Eqs. (21.7) and (21.8) to arrive at Figure 21.10. Hint: For the temporal receptive field, use $dt = 1$ ms and plot over the interval $[-25, 250]$ ms. For the spatial one, use $dx = 0.004$ deg, with 128 points centered at 0.

8. †Plot the three-dimensional spatio-temporal profile of the following two Gabor filters:

$$g_e(x,t) = g_{se}(x)f_{te}(t), \quad \text{and} \quad g_e^-(x,t) = g_{se}(x)f_{te}(t) + g_{so}(x)f_{to}(t).$$

Plot the corresponding Fourier transforms $\hat{g}_e(\omega_x, \omega_t)$ and $\hat{g}_e^-(\omega_x, \omega_t)$ to arrive at Figure 21.16. Hint: For simplicity, set the delay t_Δ equal to zero, use $dt = 2$ ms and 128 points centered at 0. In the frequency domain, consider spatial frequencies between ± 10 c/deg and temporal frequencies between ± 25 c/s evenly sampled at 128 points.

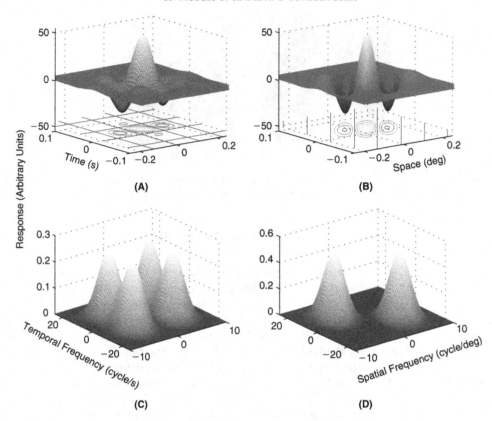

FIGURE 21.16 **A.** Spatio-temporal receptive field profile of g_e. **B.** Spatio-temporal receptive field profile of g_e^-. **C.** Fourier domain profile of $\hat{g}_e$. **D.** Fourier domain profile of $\hat{g}_e^-$. (gabor3dex.m)

9. †Compute numerically (using MATLAB) and plot the responses as a function of time of the filters $g_e(x,t)$ and $g_e^-(x,t)$ (Exercise 8) to a one-dimensional sinusoidal grating drifting in their receptive field. Use a grating moving to the right with spatial frequency $\eta_x = 4$ cycle/deg and temporal frequency $\eta_t = 8$ cycle/s. Simulate 2000 ms with a step $\Delta t = 2$ ms. Compute numerically and plot the response of the same filters to the grating moving to the left to yield Figure 21.17. Interpret the results in relation to the plots of Figure 21.16C and D. Hint: Represent the grating as a matrix with columns and lines corresponding to different space and time values, respectively. Take advantage of the fact that g_e is separable, which allows you to compute the spatial and temporal components of the responses successively. Use matrix multiplication to compute the spatial component first and convolution, i.e., the MATLAB function conv to compute the temporal component.

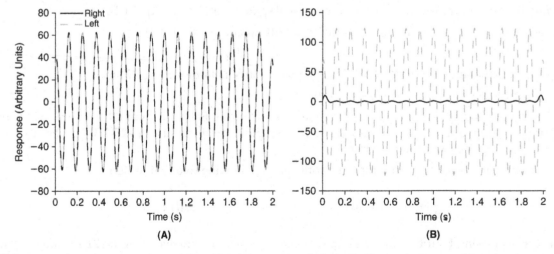

FIGURE 21.17 **A.** Response of $g_e(x,t)$ to left and right moving gratings. **B.** Response of $g_e^-(x,t)$ to left and right moving gratings. (gab3dresp.m)

10. †Compute and plot the responses as a function of time of the following two complex cell models to a one-dimensional sinusoidal grating drifting in their receptive field.

   (i) The response of complex cell 1 is obtained by squaring the response of $g_e(x,t)$ and adding the squared response of the corresponding odd filter $g_o(x,t) = g_{so}(x)f_{to}(t)$ (Exercise 8).

   (ii) The response of complex cell 2 is obtained in the same way, but using $g_e^-(x,t)$ and the corresponding odd filter $g_o^-(x,t) = g_{so}(x)f_{te}(t) - g_{se}(x)f_{to}(t)$. Use the same grating (right or left motion) and simulation parameters as in Exercise 9. Compare the results with those of Exercise 9 and explain the differences.

11. †The response of a directionally selective simple cell to moving gratings is described by

$$R_{rect}(t) = R_{max}\frac{\lfloor R_1(t)\rfloor_+^2}{\sigma^2 + \lfloor R_1(t)\rfloor_+^2} \quad \text{where} \quad \lfloor R\rfloor_+ = R\mathbb{1}(R)$$

and

$$R_1(t) = R_{spont} + R_c(t) \quad \text{with} \quad R_c(t) = \iint g_e^-(x,t_0)c(x,t-t_0)\,dx dt_0.$$

The parameters are: $R_{spont} = 10$ spk/s, $\sigma = 60$ spk/s, and $R_{max} = 120$ spk/s. The spatio-temporal receptive field is given by

$$g_e^-(x,t) = \frac{1}{2\pi\sigma_x\sigma_t}e^{-x^2/2\sigma_x^2 - t^2/2\sigma_t^2}\cos(k_x x - k_t t)$$

with $\sigma_x = 0.1$ deg, $k_x = 4.2$ c/deg, $\sigma_t = 31$ ms, and $k_t = 8$ c/s.

   (i) Plot R_{rect} as a function of R_1. Use values of R_1 between 0 and 150 spk/s.

   (ii) Compute and plot the response $R_{rect}(t)$ for a grating given by $c(x,t) = \cos(\eta_x x \pm \eta_t t)$ moving either to the left or to the right. Use the parameters $\eta_x = 4$ c/deg and $\eta_t = 8$ c/s and a time interval of motion of 2000 ms.

12. †A more realistic model of nonseparable receptive fields assumes the following temporal weighting functions:

$$f_1(t) = \alpha(kt)^{n_1}e^{-kt}\left(\frac{1}{n_1!} - \beta\frac{(kt)^2}{(n_1+2)!}\right)$$

$$f_2(t) = \alpha(kt)^{n_2}e^{-kt}\left(\frac{1}{n_2!} - \beta\frac{(kt)^2}{(n_2+2)!}\right)$$

with $\alpha = 100$ an arbitrary scale factor, $\beta = 0.9$, $n_1 = 6$, $n_2 = 9$, and $k = 120$ s^{-1}. The nonseparable receptive field is given by

$$g(x,t) = g_{se}(x)f_1(t) + g_{so}(x)f_2(t),$$

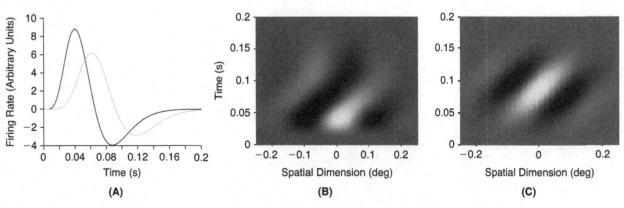

FIGURE 21.18 **A.** Plot of the temporal weighting functions f_1 (black) and f_2 (red). **B.** Spatio-temporal receptive field of $g(x,t)$. Lighter and darker shades of gray indicate firing increase and decrease, respectively (scale arbitrary). **C.** For comparison, spatio-temporal receptive field of the Gabor filter g_e^-. (ts_rfs.m)

where g_{se} and g_{so} are given by Eq. (21.8) with the same parameters as in Exercise 7.

(i) Plot the two temporal weighting functions f_1 and f_2 between 0 and 200 ms to arrive at Figure 21.18A.

(ii) Plot the spatio-temporal receptive field of $g(x,t)$ to arrive at Figure 21.18B. Hint: Use the function `meshc` and a `view` angle of (0,90) as well as a `colormap` set to "gray."

(iii) Plot the nonseparable spatio-temporal filter obtained from Gabor functions (see Exercise 8) in the same way to obtain Figure 21.18C and compare it to the one plotted in (ii).

(iv) Compute the response of the filter $g(x,t)$ to leftward and rightward drifting gratings, with the same parameters as in Exercise 9.

Stochastic Estimation Theory

O U T L I N E

22.1 Minimum Mean Square Error Estimation   327

22.2 Estimation of Gaussian Signals*   329

22.3 Linear Nonlinear (LN) Models*   331

22.4 Summary and Sources   332

22.5 Exercises   332

Although the stimuli used in the previous two chapters to characterize the receptive fields of visual neurons were deterministic, random stimuli can be used as well for this purpose. In this chapter, we derive the general solution to the problem of recovering the mapping between stimulus and firing rate using random stimuli, which is given by the *conditional expectation* or *mean*. We then show how to recover the mapping from stimulus to firing rate when the underlying neuron's receptive field is characterized by a linear weighting function. The linear case turns out to be optimal when the stimuli and firing rates are jointly Gaussian. Finally, we show how simple nonlinear transformations can be recovered using Gaussian random stimuli.

22.1 MINIMUM MEAN SQUARE ERROR ESTIMATION

We consider the situation where we are given the instantaneous firing rate of a neuron, $Y_0(t)$, in response to a random stimulus, $X_0(t)$. Here X and Y are assumed to be two stochastic processes and $X_0(t) = X(\omega_0, t)$, $Y_0(t) = Y(\omega_0, t)$ are two realizations corresponding to an event $\omega_0 \in \Omega$ (see §16.1). Our goal is to describe the relation between $X_0(t)$ and $Y_0(t)$. In other words, we want to find a function g such that $g(X_0(t))$ approximates $Y_0(t)$ as well as possible, independent of ω_0. The function g could be as simple as a convolution of X_0 with a filter h, i.e., $g(X_0(t)) = h \star X_0(t)$, or a static nonlinear transformation, e.g., $g(x) = x^3$ or a combination of several such functions. A natural measure of error is the time-averaged squared error,

$$\varepsilon^2(g) = \lim_{T \to \infty} \frac{1}{2T} \int\limits_{-T}^{T} (Y_0(t) - g(X_0(t)))^2 \, dt.$$

If we assume the pair of stochastic processes (X, Y) to be stationary and ergodic, we can replace the time average by an ensemble average. If, for a fixed $t = t_1$, we set $Y(t_1) = Y_1$, then

$$\varepsilon^2(g) = E[(Y_1 - g(X(t_1)))^2 | X] = \int (y_1 - g(X(t_1)))^2 \, p(y_1 | X) \, dy_1$$

where $p(y_1 | X)$ is the conditional distribution of Y_1 given X and y_1 represents a specific value of Y_1. Note that ε^2 is independent of the particular choice of t_1 by stationarity. If we now formally take the derivative of the quadratic term with respect to g,

$$\frac{\partial \varepsilon^2}{\partial g} = -2 \int (y_1 - g(X(t_1))) p(y_1|X) \, dy_1,$$

and set it equal to zero to obtain a local extremum, g_{opt}, we find that

$$g_{opt}(X(t_1)) = \int y_1 p(y_1|X) \, dy_1 = E[Y(t_1)|X].$$

Furthermore, $\partial^2 \varepsilon^2 / \partial g^2 = 2$ and therefore the optimal estimate of Y (resp. Y_0) given X (resp. X_0) is the conditional mean or expectation of Y given X.

Linear estimate. In practice, the conditional mean is difficult to compute since it requires an estimation of the conditional density of Y given X. A simpler approach consists in constraining the form of the estimator g. For example, we may try to estimate Y linearly from X after subtracting their respective means,

$$Y_{est}(t) - m_Y = \int g(t - t_0)(X(t_0) - m_X) dt_0 = g \star (X(t) - m_X).$$

We computed the optimal g in §18.1 by using Fourier transforms,

$$\hat{g}(\omega) = \frac{S_{XY}(\omega)}{S_{XX}(\omega)}.$$

In particular, if Y is a linear function of X, $Y(t) - m_Y = k \star (X(t) - m_X) + N(t)$ with $k(t) = 0$ for $t < 0$ implementing causality, and the noise $N(t)$ is independent of X, then k can be recovered from the cross correlation between X and Y, and the power spectrum of X.

Figure 22.1A–C illustrates the reconstruction of the LGN filter of Eq. (20.15) from a white noise contrast stimulus and the corresponding firing rate vector obtained by linear convolution. In this case, negative firing rates correspond either to decreases relative to the mean firing rate or to the response of a second neuron characterized by an inverted transfer function (i.e., OFF instead of ON). The red line in Figure 22.1C illustrates the case when the firing rate is passed through a nonlinear function after the convolution, see Figure 22.1D, and will be dealt with in §22.3.

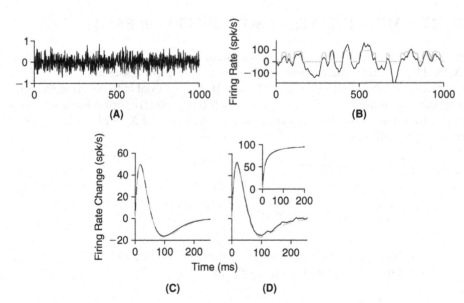

FIGURE 22.1   **A.** Sample path of the white noise stimulus. **B.** Firing rate vector (black) obtained by convolving the stimulus with the LGN filter (illustrated in C or D, dashed red line) and after transformation (red) using the static nonlinearity g illustrated in D (inset, dashed red line, see §22.3). **C.** Reconstruction (black) of the original LGN filter (dashed red line) from the linearly filtered stimulus. **D.** Reconstruction from the nonlinear transform. Inset shows the reconstruction (black) of the nonlinear function g (dashed red line, see §22.3). (`lgn_est3.m`)

22.2 ESTIMATION OF GAUSSIAN SIGNALS*

The results of the last section raise the question of when linear estimation is optimal in the mean square sense. This turns out to be the case for Gaussian random signals. To illustrate this point, we will for simplicity assume the stimulus X to be sampled at discrete times $t_k = k \Delta t$, $k = 1, \ldots, n$, so as to form a random vector $\mathbf{v}_X = (X_1, \ldots, X_n)^T$ and similarly for the firing rate vector $\mathbf{v}_Y = (Y_1, \ldots, Y_p)^T$ (see §11.9). Since the following results hold for vectors $\mathbf{v}_X$ and $\mathbf{v}_Y$ of different length, we allow $n \neq p$. For example, the vector $\mathbf{v}_Y$ could represent the firing rates of two or more neurons in response to the stimulus $\mathbf{v}_X$. A neuron's firing rate will be well approximated by a Gaussian vector if its mean is well above the variance, so that the firing rate will not be negative, or alternatively if we combine the firing rates, f_1, f_2 of two neurons responding to the positive and negative parts of the signal according to $f_1 - f_2$. Next, we assume that $\mathbf{v}_X$ and $\mathbf{v}_Y$ are jointly Gaussian with means $\mathbf{m}_X = (m_{X_1}, \ldots, m_{X_n})^T$, $\mathbf{m}_Y = (m_{Y_1}, \ldots, m_{Y_p})^T$, and covariances $\mathbf{C}_{XX} = E[(\mathbf{v}_X - \mathbf{m}_X)(\mathbf{v}_X - \mathbf{m}_X)^T]$, $\mathbf{C}_{YY} = E[(\mathbf{v}_Y - \mathbf{m}_Y)(\mathbf{v}_Y - \mathbf{m}_Y)^T]$ of dimensions $n \times n$ and $p \times p$, respectively. Let us define $Z_1 = X_1, \ldots, Z_n = X_n, Z_{n+1} = Y_1, \ldots, Z_{n+p} = Y_p$, and form the concatenated vector $\mathbf{v}_Z = (Z_1, \ldots, Z_{n+p})^T$. Clearly, $\mathbf{v}_Z \sim \mathcal{N}(\mathbf{m}_Z, \mathbf{C}_{ZZ})$, where $\mathbf{m}_Z = (m_{X_1}, \ldots, m_{X_n}, m_{Y_1}, \ldots, m_{Y_p})^T$. The covariance, $\mathbf{C}_{ZZ}$, is composed of four submatrices,

$$\mathbf{C}_{ZZ} = \begin{pmatrix} \mathbf{C}_{XX} & \mathbf{C}_{XY} \\ \mathbf{C}_{YX} & \mathbf{C}_{YY} \end{pmatrix}$$

where $\mathbf{C}_{XY} = E[(\mathbf{v}_X - \mathbf{m}_X)(\mathbf{v}_Y - \mathbf{m}_Y)^T] \in \mathbb{R}^{n \times p}$ and $\mathbf{C}_{YX} = E[(\mathbf{v}_Y - \mathbf{m}_Y)(\mathbf{v}_X - \mathbf{m}_X)^T] \in \mathbb{R}^{p \times n}$. By subtracting $\mathbf{m}_Z$ from $\mathbf{v}_Z$, we may assume that $\mathbf{v}_Z$ has zero mean. If $\mathbf{x} = (x_1, \ldots, x_n)^T$ and $\mathbf{y} = (y_1, \ldots, y_p)^T$ are specific instances of the random vectors $\mathbf{v}_X$ and $\mathbf{v}_Y$, and $\mathbf{z} = (\mathbf{x}^T \mathbf{y}^T)^T$ is their concatenation then the conditional density $p(\mathbf{y}|\mathbf{x})$ is given by

$$p(\mathbf{y}|\mathbf{x}) = \frac{p(\mathbf{x}, \mathbf{y})}{p(\mathbf{x})} = \frac{(2\pi)^{p/2} |\det \mathbf{C}_{XX}|^{1/2} \exp(\mathbf{x}^T \mathbf{C}_{XX} \mathbf{x}/2)}{(2\pi)^{(n+p)/2} |\det \mathbf{C}_{ZZ}|^{1/2} \exp(\mathbf{z}^T \mathbf{C}_{ZZ}^{-1} \mathbf{z}/2)}.$$

We now use the following identity for the inverse of $\mathbf{C}_{ZZ}$:

$$\mathbf{C}_{ZZ}^{-1} = \begin{pmatrix} \mathbf{C}_{XX}^{-1} & 0 \\ 0 & 0 \end{pmatrix} + \begin{pmatrix} -\mathbf{C}_{XX}^{-1} \mathbf{C}_{XY} \\ \mathbf{I} \end{pmatrix} \mathbf{Q}^{-1} - \mathbf{C}_{YX} \mathbf{C}_{XX}^{-1} \mathbf{I},$$

where the matrix $\mathbf{I}$ is a $p \times p$ identity matrix and

$$\mathbf{Q} = \mathbf{C}_{YY} - \mathbf{C}_{YX} \mathbf{C}_{XX}^{-1} \mathbf{C}_{XY}$$

(Exercise 1). This implies that

$$\mathbf{z}^T \mathbf{C}_{ZZ}^{-1} \mathbf{z} = \mathbf{x}^T \mathbf{C}_{XX} \mathbf{x} + (\mathbf{y} - \mathbf{C}_{YX} \mathbf{C}_{XX}^{-1} \mathbf{x})^T \mathbf{Q}^{-1} (\mathbf{y} - \mathbf{C}_{YX} \mathbf{C}_{XX}^{-1} \mathbf{x}).$$

Furthermore, since $\det \mathbf{C}_{ZZ} = \det \mathbf{C}_{XX} \det \mathbf{Q}$ (Exercise 2) we can write

$$p(\mathbf{y}|\mathbf{x}) = (2\pi)^{-p/2} |\det \mathbf{Q}|^{-1/2} \exp\left(-(\mathbf{y} - \mathbf{C}_{YX} \mathbf{C}_{XX}^{-1} \mathbf{x})^T \mathbf{Q}^{-1} (\mathbf{y} - \mathbf{C}_{YX} \mathbf{C}_{XX}^{-1} \mathbf{x})/2\right).$$

We therefore infer that $\mathbf{v}_Y$ given $\mathbf{v}_X$ is Gaussian with conditional mean $\mathbf{C}_{YX}\mathbf{C}_{XX}^{-1}\mathbf{v}_X$ and covariance $\mathbf{Q}$. We may hence write

$$\mathbf{v}_Y = \mathbf{H}\mathbf{v}_X + \mathbf{v}_N,$$

with $\mathbf{H} = \mathbf{C}_{YX}\mathbf{C}_{XX}^{-1}$. The noise $\mathbf{v}_N$ has covariance $\mathbf{Q}$ and is uncorrelated and therefore independent of $\mathbf{v}_X$ (Exercise 3). We have thus decomposed $\mathbf{v}_Y$ into a linear component dependent of $\mathbf{v}_X$ and an independent noise term $\mathbf{v}_N = (N_1,\ldots,N_p)^T$, as summarized by the following equations:

$$\begin{pmatrix} \mathbf{v}_X \\ \mathbf{v}_Y \end{pmatrix} = \begin{pmatrix} \mathbf{I} & 0 \\ \mathbf{H} & \mathbf{I} \end{pmatrix} \begin{pmatrix} \mathbf{v}_X \\ \mathbf{v}_N \end{pmatrix}, \quad \begin{pmatrix} \mathbf{v}_X \\ \mathbf{v}_N \end{pmatrix} = \begin{pmatrix} \mathbf{I} & 0 \\ -\mathbf{H} & \mathbf{I} \end{pmatrix} \begin{pmatrix} \mathbf{v}_X \\ \mathbf{v}_Y \end{pmatrix}$$

with

$$E\left[\begin{pmatrix} \mathbf{v}_X \\ \mathbf{v}_N \end{pmatrix} (\mathbf{v}_X \ \mathbf{v}_N) \right] = \begin{pmatrix} \mathbf{C}_{XX} & 0 \\ 0 & \mathbf{Q} \end{pmatrix}. \tag{22.1}$$

Figure 22.2 illustrates an example of this reconstruction method using again a white noise stimulus (panel A) and a firing rate vector obtained by convolution with the LGN filter of Eq. (20.15) (panel B). Note that the matrix $\mathbf{H}$ illustrated in panel C is banded along the main diagonal, as expected from the joint stationarity of the stimulus and firing rate. Taking into account time-invariance allows to recover the LGN filter, as illustrated in panel D.

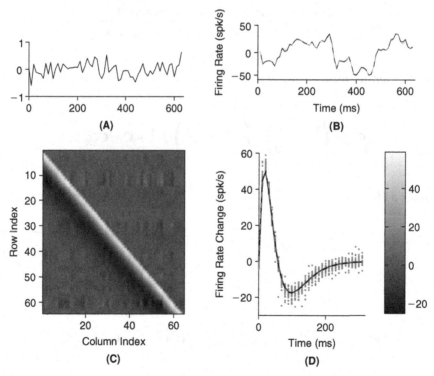

FIGURE 22.2   A. Sample path of the white noise stimulus (sampling interval: 10 ms). **B.** Firing rate vector (black) obtained by convolving the stimulus with the LGN filter (illustrated in D, black line) and prediction obtained by convolving the stimulus with $\mathbf{H}$ (red line). **C.** Matrix $\mathbf{H}$, obtained by computing the cross correlation between firing rate and stimulus and the inverse of the stimulus autocovariance matrix. Gray scale bar to the right of D. **D.** The black line illustrates the LGN filter (sampling interval: 10 ms). The gray dots are the values of $\mathbf{H}$ plotted as a function of their distance to the main diagonal, i.e., matrix element H_{ii+k} is plotted at abscissa $k\Delta t$. The red dashed line is the average of all matrix elements for a fixed abscissa value. (lgn_est5.m)

22.3 LINEAR NONLINEAR (LN) MODELS*

We now consider a simple linear, nonlinear model for the neuron's firing rate in response to the stimulus X:

$$Z(t) = g(Y(t)) + N(t), \quad Y(t) = (k \star X)(t),$$

where g is a static nonlinearity, i.e., a function $g(y)$ independent of t, such as $g(y) = y^2$. The noise term $N(t)$ is assumed to be independent of X and therefore Y. The stochastic process X is assumed to have zero mean. Our goal is to recover k and g from the input X and the firing rate $Z(t)$. First, we note the following result.

Theorem (Bussgang). Let $Y(t)$ be a stationary Gaussian stochastic process with autocovariance function $C_{YY}(\tau)$ and $Z_0(t) = g(Y(t))$ be obtained by passing Y through a static nonlinearity g. Then the cross correlation between Z_0 and Y is given by

$$C_{YZ_0}(\tau) = \alpha C_{YY}(\tau) \quad \text{where} \quad \alpha = \frac{E[Yg(Y)]}{\sigma_Y^2}.$$

Proof. Exercise 4.   □

In other words, the presence of the static nonlinearity cannot be detected in the time dependence of the cross correlation as it is identical to the autocovariance of Y. Only the value of the constant α depends on g. This result allows us to compute the cross correlation between X and Z in two steps. Since N is independent of X and Y, we first note that according to Bussgang's theorem

$$C_{YZ}(\tau) = E[Y(t)Z(t+\tau)] = \alpha C_{YY}(\tau) = \alpha(k \star \tilde{k}) \star C_{XX}(\tau), \tag{22.2}$$

with $\tilde{k}(t) = k(-t)$ (see Exercise 18.4 for the last equality). Second, since $Y(t) = (k \star X)(t)$,

$$C_{YZ}(\tau) = \int k(t-t_0)E[X(t_0)Z(t+\tau)]\,dt_0 = \tilde{k} \star C_{XZ}(\tau). \tag{22.3}$$

Fourier transforming Eqs. (22.2) and (22.3), and equating them yields

$$\hat{k}(\omega) = \frac{1}{\alpha}\frac{S_{XZ}(\omega)}{S_{XX}(\omega)},$$

provided $\alpha \neq 0$ and $\hat{k}(\omega) \neq 0$. Thus, we recover k from the cross correlation of the firing rate with the input stimulus and its power spectrum, just as in the linear case. To recover g, we estimate numerically the cumulative distribution functions

$$F_1(y) = \int_{-\infty}^{y} p_1(y_0)\,dy_0, \quad \text{and} \quad F_2(z) = \int_{-\infty}^{z} p_2(z_0)\,dz_0$$

where p_1 and p_2 are the probability densities of Y and Z, respectively. Clearly, $F_2(g(y)) = F_1(y)$, under the assumption that g is smooth and one-to-one (§11.8). Since X is Gaussian, Y is as well, and its cumulative distribution function is given by

$$F_1(y) = \Phi((y-\mu_Y)/\sigma_Y), \quad \Phi(x) = \int_{-\infty}^{x} e^{-y^2/2}\,dy.$$

The cumulative distribution of Z is obtained by numerically estimating $p_2(z)$ through a histogram and subsequent numerical integration. This yields $g(y)$ numerically through

$$g(y) = F_2^{-1}(\Phi((y-\mu_Y)/\sigma_Y)).$$

The entire reconstruction procedure is illustrated in Figure 22.1A, B, and D for a LGN model neuron endowed with the static nonlinearity illustrated in the inset of Figure 22.1D.

22.4 SUMMARY AND SOURCES

The use of random stimuli to characterize the transformation between stimulus and firing rate as presented in this chapter originates from the engineering field of system identification. Marmarelis and Marmarelis (1978) is a comprehensive reference surveying early applications to neuroscience. More recent applications of these methods usually assume a specific model describing the transformation between stimulus and firing rate, enabling further progress in its identification. See, e.g., Paninski (2004) and Schwartz et al. (2006). In practice, the use of broad band random stimuli works best to characterize neurons close to the sensory periphery. Often, as one progresses deeper within a sensory system, neurons become much more sharply tuned and less responsive to broad band, random stimuli. The application of system identification methods to experimental data should always be coupled with an error analysis to assess how well the derived model captures the data. We illustrate this point in §23.2. The derivation of the optimal linear estimator in the Gaussian case (§22.2) is modeled on Scharf (1991, §7.5). Banded matrices like $\mathbf{H}$ in Figure 22.2 are called *Toeplitz* matrices and generalize the circulant matrices already encountered in Chapter 7. For further details, see Gray (2006). Our proof of Bussgang's theorem in Exercise 4 below follows Bendat (1990, §2.5). The result stated in Eq. (22.4) below is due to Price (1958).

22.5 EXERCISES

1. Let

$$\mathbf{M} = \begin{pmatrix} \mathbf{A} & \mathbf{B} \\ \mathbf{C} & \mathbf{D} \end{pmatrix}$$

with the submatrices $\mathbf{A}, \mathbf{B}, \mathbf{C},$ and $\mathbf{D}$ having, respectively, dimensions equal to $n \times n, n \times p, p \times n,$ and $p \times p$. Assume that there exist matrices $\mathbf{F}, \mathbf{G},$ and $\mathbf{H}$ with

$$\mathbf{AF} = -\mathbf{B}, \quad \mathbf{GA} = -\mathbf{C}, \quad \mathbf{H} = \mathbf{D} - \mathbf{CA}^{-1}\mathbf{B}.$$

Show that

$$\mathbf{M}^{-1} = \begin{pmatrix} \mathbf{A}^{-1} & 0 \\ 0 & 0 \end{pmatrix} + \begin{pmatrix} \mathbf{F} \\ \mathbf{I} \end{pmatrix} \mathbf{H}^{-1} \begin{pmatrix} \mathbf{G} & \mathbf{I} \end{pmatrix},$$

under the assumption that all inverses exist.

2. Verify the following two identities

$$\begin{pmatrix} \mathbf{I} & 0 \\ \mathbf{H} & \mathbf{I} \end{pmatrix} \begin{pmatrix} \mathbf{C}_{XX} & 0 \\ 0 & \mathbf{Q} \end{pmatrix} \begin{pmatrix} \mathbf{I} & \mathbf{H}^T \\ 0 & \mathbf{I} \end{pmatrix} = \mathbf{C}_{ZZ}$$

and

$$\begin{pmatrix} \mathbf{I} & 0 \\ -\mathbf{H} & \mathbf{I} \end{pmatrix} \begin{pmatrix} \mathbf{C}_{XX} & \mathbf{C}_{XY} \\ \mathbf{C}_{YX} & \mathbf{C}_{YY} \end{pmatrix} \begin{pmatrix} \mathbf{I} & -\mathbf{H}^T \\ 0 & \mathbf{I} \end{pmatrix} = \begin{pmatrix} \mathbf{C}_{XX} & 0 \\ 0 & \mathbf{Q} \end{pmatrix}.$$

Hint: Use Exercise 5.4. Conclude that

$$\det \mathbf{C}_{ZZ} = \det \mathbf{C}_{XX} \det \mathbf{Q}.$$

3. Use the identities of Exercise 2 to prove Eq. (22.1).
4. Prove Bussgang's theorem.

(i) Assume for simplicity that Y has zero mean and set $Y_1 = Y(t)$, $Y_2 = Y(t+\tau)$. Show that

$$p(y_1, y_2) = \frac{1}{2\pi\sigma^2\sqrt{1-\rho^2}} e^{-\frac{1}{2\sigma^2}y_2^2} e^{-\frac{1}{2\sigma^2(1-\rho^2)}(y_1-\rho y_2)^2}$$

where $\sigma^2 = C_{YY}(0)$ and $\rho\sigma^2 = C_{YY}(\tau)$. Hint: Use the identity derived in Exercise 1.

(ii) Use this result to compute

$$E[Y_1 g(Y_2)] = \iint\limits_{-\infty}^{\infty} y_1 g(y_2) p(y_1, y_2)\, dy_1 dy_2$$

by integrating first over y_1 and then over y_2.

5. Replicate the results illustrated in Figure 22.1.

   (i) Generate Gaussian white noise with a sampling step of 1 ms and standard deviation of 0.25 over 32768 ms and plot the first 1000 ms (Figure 22.1).

   (ii) Compute the LGN temporal weighting function of Eq. (20.15) and scale it such that it peaks at 50 spk/s. Use `conv` to convolve the stimulus with the temporal weighting function. Plot the resulting model's response as in Figure 22.1B (black trace).

   (iii) Estimate the temporal weighting function from the model's response and the stimulus (Figure 22.1C). Hint: Use the "two-sided" version of `tfestimate` with a window of 1024 points and an overlap of 1/2 the window length to estimate the transfer function in the frequency domain. Then use `ifft` to revert to the time domain.

   (iv) Pass the model's response through the static nonlinearity $y = 100x/(10+x)$ to obtain the modified model's response as in Figure 22.1B (red trace).

   (v) Use the modified model's response to compute the parameter α (§22.3) and recover the temporal weighting function as in (iii). Finally, follow the steps outlined in §22.3 to recover the static nonlinearity (Figure 22.1D).

6. Replicate the results illustrated in Figure 22.2.

   (i) Generate white noise with a time step of 10 ms. Use the same standard deviation as in Exercise 5, 0.25, at each time point and generate $128 \cdot 64$ points (Figure 22.2A).

   (ii) Store these data in a 128 by 64 matrix and convolve each row with the same LGN temporal weighting function as in Exercise 5, but sampled at 10 ms intervals (32 points) to obtain the corresponding firing rate samples (Figure 22.2B).

   (iii) Now compute the inverse of the white noise covariance matrix and the cross covariance with the firing rate to obtain $\mathbf{H}$ (Figure 22.2C).

   (iv) Compute the mean of the elements on the main diagonal and repeat this operation up to the 32nd diagonal below it. Plot these mean values as well as the corresponding individual diagonal elements as a function of the time interval difference associated with the respective diagonals to obtain Figure 22.2D.

   (v) Use $\mathbf{H}$ to estimate the stimulus (Figure 22.2B, red trace).

7. Use Bussgang's theorem to show that the cross correlation between a Gaussian, zero mean, stationary stochastic process X and $Y = g_{\alpha,l}(X)$ is given by

$$C_{XY}(\tau) = \sqrt{\frac{2}{\pi}} \frac{1}{\sigma_X^2} \frac{1}{\sqrt{1+l^2}} C_{XX}(\tau),$$

where the static nonlinearity $g_{\alpha,l}$ is defined in Eq. (18.14).

8. Additionally, the autocovariance of Y is given by

$$C_{YY}(\tau) = \frac{2\alpha^2}{\pi} \sin^{-1}\left(\frac{C_{XX}(\tau)}{\sigma_X^2 + l^2}\right). \tag{22.4}$$

Use this result and Exercise 7 to derive numerically the coherence between X and Y when X is white noise with a cut-off frequency of 100 Hz. Show that this allows you to reproduce the red curve in Figure 18.1D. Hint: Fast Fourier transform C_{XY} and C_{YY} after discretizing with a resolution $dt = 1$ ms and using 256 points centered at zero.

Reverse-Correlation and Spike Train Decoding

OUTLINE

23.1 Reverse-Correlation   335   23.3 Summary and Sources   340

23.2 Stimulus Reconstruction   338   23.4 Exercises   340

We have seen in the previous chapter how random stimuli allow one to characterize the receptive fields of neurons in terms of their instantaneous firing rate. In this chapter, we first extend these results to spike train responses. Next, we quantify the ability of single spike trains to encode sensory stimuli by using them to reconstruct the stimulus. These two related techniques are often called reverse-correlation and spike train decoding, respectively.

23.1 REVERSE-CORRELATION

For simplicity, we will only explain how reverse-correlation allows one to determine the temporal receptive field of a neuron. The fundamental principle remains the same for spatio-temporal receptive fields. Let us first define the firing rate modulation due to the random stimulus $X(t)$ as,

$$f(t) = E[Y(t) - f_{mean} \mid X],$$ (23.1)

where $Y(t) = \sum_{i=1}^{N} \delta(t - t_i)$ represents the spike train in response to a single presentation of the waveform $X(t)$. The average, $E[\cdot \mid X]$, is taken over repeated presentations of the same waveform $X(t)$. The number $f_{mean} = E[Y(t)]$ is the mean firing rate of the cell.

We assume that time-varying stimulus changes are encoded linearly by firing rate changes. In terms of Eq. (23.1) above this means that,

$$E[Y(t) - f_{mean} \mid X] = \int w_t(t - t_0) X(t_0) \, dt_0.$$

If we multiply both sides of this equation by $X(t_1)$ and take expectations with respect to X, we arrive at

$$E[X(t_1)(X(t) - f_{mean})] = \int w_t(t - t_0) E[X(t_1)X(t_0)] \, dt_0.$$

Setting $t = t_1 + \tau$ yields

$$C_{XY}(\tau) = w_t \star C_{XX}(\tau), \quad \text{or} \quad \hat{w}_t(\omega) = \frac{S_{XY}(\omega)}{S_{XX}(\omega)}.$$ (23.2)

This formula is formally identical to that obtained in the previous chapter from the neuron's firing rate.

Mathematics for Neuroscientists. DOI: 10.1016/B978-0-12-374882-9.00023-X

We now assume that the stimulus, X, is Gaussian white noise. Recall from Chapter 16 that Gaussian white noise has an autocovariance function that is a Dirac delta function, Eq. (16.6). Thus, Gaussian white noise is totally uncorrelated in time and each frequency is equally well represented since its power spectrum is constant, independent of frequency, Eq. (16.15). Such stimuli allow us to determine the receptive field weighting function of a neuron directly from the time of occurrence of single spikes. To see how this arises, first note that since $C_{XX}(t) = \sigma^2 \delta(t)$, the right hand side of Eq. (23.2) reduces to $\sigma^2 w_t(\tau)$. To obtain from the left hand side an expression that depends explicitly on the time of spike occurrences, we first observe that

$$E[(Y(t+\tau) - f_{mean})X(t)] = E[Y(t+\tau)X(t)],$$

because $E[X(t)] = 0$. We can now replace the average over the Gaussian white noise ensemble by a time average, assuming that the ergodicity property holds:

$$E[Y(t+\tau)X(t)] = \frac{1}{T} \int_0^T Y(t+\tau)X(t)\, dt.$$

If we evaluate the right hand side when Y is a spike train, we see that

$$\frac{1}{T} \int_0^T Y(t+\tau)X(t)\, dt = \frac{1}{T} \int_0^T \sum_{i=1}^N \delta(t+\tau - t_i)X(t)\, dt = \frac{1}{T} \sum_{i=1}^N X(t_i - \tau) = \frac{f_{mean}}{N} \sum_{i=1}^N X(t_i - \tau).$$

Summing up,

$$w_t(\tau) = \frac{f_{mean}}{\sigma^2} \left(\frac{1}{N} \sum_{i=1}^N X(t_i - \tau) \right). \tag{23.3}$$

In other words, the transfer function w_t at time τ is given by the spike-triggered average of the random stimulus values τ ms prior to each spike. Because of the time reversal between the left and right hand side of Eq. (23.3), this method is called reverse-correlation. In practice, the frequency domain formulation of Eq. (23.2) is more practical to use than Eq. (23.3).

Figure 23.1 illustrates the implementation of the reverse-correlation method using either a broad band white noise stimulus with a cut-off frequency of 500 Hz, or a narrower band one, with a cut-off frequency of 50 Hz (black and red traces in panel A, respectively). The corresponding temporal receptive fields computed by reverse-correlation from the spike trains illustrated in panel B are plotted in panels C and D, respectively.

Generalization and equivalence with other receptive field mapping techniques. The reverse-correlation method can be extended to determine the spatial structure of a neuron's receptive field in addition to its temporal structure. This is accomplished by presenting spatio-temporal white noise and by keeping track of where the stimulus was presented in space as well as in time. The reverse-correlation technique was first developed to characterize the properties of auditory neurons, and has by now been successfully used to estimate the weighting functions of many types of neurons, including retinal, LGN, and cortical simple cell receptive fields, for example. An example of a simple cell receptive field obtained by reverse-correlation is illustrated in Figure 23.2.

Three assumptions have to be kept in mind when reverse-correlation is applied to determine the receptive field of a neuron: (i) ergodicity, (ii) stationarity, and (iii) linearity of the response. If, e.g., the response properties of a neuron depend on the specific frequency content of the stimulus, then the receptive field mapped by presenting sinusoidal stimuli at various frequencies could turn out to be very different from that obtained with white noise, in which all frequencies are presented simultaneously. Of course, this is ruled out by the assumption of linearity. In practice, the receptive fields obtained with different stimuli (e.g., sine waves or white noise) have yielded comparable results in several cell types. One advantage of using white noise is simplicity: only a single stimulus type is used throughout the experiment. The frequency content ($f_{Nyquist}$) of the white noise stimulus should be chosen high enough to exceed the maximal frequency to which a neuron is sensitive. This does not pose substantial problems in the visual system where both spatial and temporal cut-off frequencies are usually low. On the other hand, high cut-off frequencies will increase

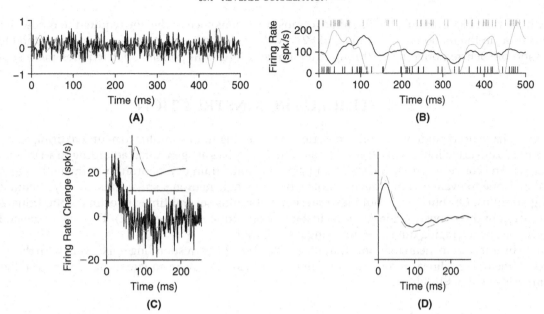

FIGURE 23.1 **A.** Sample path of white noise stimuli with cut-off frequencies of 500 Hz (black) and 50 Hz (red), respectively. **B.** Firing rate vector obtained by convolving the 500 Hz and 50 Hz cut-off frequency stimuli with the LGN filter (black and red lines, respectively). The corresponding spike trains (black and red at bottom and top, respectively) are sample paths of an inhomogeneous Poisson process. **C.** Reverse-correlation between the 500 Hz cut-off frequency stimulus and spike train (black line) and LGN filter (red dashed line). The inset shows the estimate from the firing rate (black line) and the LGN filter (dashed red line). **D.** Reverse-correlation between the 50 Hz cut-off frequency stimulus and spike train (black line). The LGN filter is shown by the dashed red line. (`lgn_revcor_wn3.m`)

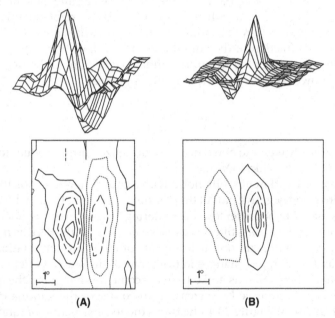

FIGURE 23.2 Two-dimensional spatial response profiles of two different simple cell receptive fields. **A.** This cell had a strong bright (ON) excitatory region and a weaker dark (OFF) inhibitory region with a somewhat longer extent. **B.** In this cell, the bright excitatory region is stronger than the dark inhibitory region but their sizes are comparable. Adapted from Jones and Palmer (1987).

the noise in the estimate of the transfer function, as illustrated in Figure 23.1C and D. However, it should be pointed out that typically as one progresses deeper within the nervous system, white noise mapping works increasingly less well. This is due to the fact that neurons become increasingly specific in their responses the farther they are from the sensory periphery and, accordingly, highly artificial stimuli like white noise become increasingly less effective and relevant.

Just as derived in §22.3 using Bussgang's theorem, Eq. (23.2) can be applied to obtain the linear weighting function of a receptive field even in cases where linear processing is followed by a static nonlinearity, such as those described in Chapter 20. This is, e.g., the case in simple cells, where the firing rate is thought to be described by linear weighting, followed by half-wave rectification. Other nonlinear transformations such as the one required to model the response of complex cells as in the motion-energy model of §21.4 will cause the basic reverse-correlation method to fail. The characterization of such receptive fields through random stimuli is still possible, but requires more sophisticated techniques.

23.2 STIMULUS RECONSTRUCTION

Up to now we have used random stimuli to describe the mapping from stimulus to neuronal firing rate. The firing rate can in turn be converted into a spike train by assuming that spikes are generated according to an inhomogeneous Poisson process. The converse problem consists in using the spike train of a neuron to estimate the stimulus. This technique allows one to evaluate how much "information" a single neuron's spike train conveys about a random, time-varying stimulus. Of course, we could also present a stimulus several times to estimate the firing rate of the neuron and carry out the reconstruction from the instantaneous firing rate (Exercise 2). This will in general improve the reconstructions by averaging out noise from single spike trains.

If we denote by $X(t)$ a zero mean random stimulus and by $Y(t)$ the corresponding spike train with the mean firing rate subtracted, the optimal linear reconstruction filter minimizing the mean square error, ε^2, between the stimulus and its estimate is given in §18.1 by

$$\hat{h}(\omega) = \frac{S_{YX}(\omega)}{S_{YY}(\omega)}.$$

In other words, it is obtained by computing the Fourier transform of the cross correlation between the spike train and the stimulus, as well as its power spectrum. If we define the noise in the reconstructions as the difference between the stimulus and its estimate, $N(t) = X(t) - (h \star Y)(t)$, then the mean square error is equal to the variance of the noise $\varepsilon^2 = E[N(t)^2]$. In the worst case, where the spike train does not provide any information about the time-varying stimulus, the best estimate is the stimulus mean, which is equal to zero. Therefore, in this case the mean squared error is equal to the variance of the stimulus, σ^2. We can thus define the *normalized error*, $\varepsilon_n = \varepsilon/\sigma$, which characterizes the accuracy of the reconstruction as a fraction of the stimulus standard deviation. The *coding fraction* $\gamma = 1 - \varepsilon_n$ is the fraction of the stimulus encoded in units of the stimulus standard deviation. In the frequency domain, the signal-to-noise ratio is defined from the power spectrum of the stimulus and noise as

$$SNR(\omega) = \frac{S_{XX}(\omega)}{S_{NN}(\omega)} \geq 1. \tag{23.4}$$

The signal-to-noise ratio is identically equal to one when the normalized error is equal to 1. The spike train will carry information about any frequency ω for which $SNR(\omega) > 1$.

Figure 23.3 illustrates the reconstruction of white noise with a cut-off frequency of 10 Hz (panel A, top) from two spike trains encoding the positive and negative part of the stimulus, respectively (panel A, bottom). The spike trains are inhomogeneous Poisson processes obtained after low-pass filtering the stimulus. In panel B, the signal-to-noise ratio is illustrated as a function of frequency. Low-pass filtering causes a decrease in the SNR as frequency increases. Typically, the quality of the reconstructions will depend on the firing rate of the neuron in relation to the cut-off frequency of the stimulus, because higher and more rapid changes in firing rate allow one to better encode fast stimulus changes, as illustrated in panel C. Panel D shows that as spike trains become more regular, the quality of the reconstruction increases. This was achieved in this example by increasing the order of the gamma distribution determining the neuron's random threshold (Exercise 3). Figure 23.4 illustrates the reconstruction of random amplitude modulations of an electric field from the spike train of a first order sensory neuron in weakly electric fish. In this case, a very high estimation accuracy is obtained from a single spike train. The neuron can track with high accuracy the stimulus because the typical interspike intervals are much shorter than the time scale of the stimulus fluctuations.

The optimal reconstruction filter can be computed analytically under the following two assumptions. First, we assume that the firing rate and the stimulus are linearly related,

$$E[Y(t) - m_Y \mid X] = \int k(t - t_0) X(t_0) \, dt_0 = (k \star X)(t)$$

meaning that

$$E[(Y(t) - m_Y) X(t + \tau)] = E[k \star X(t) X(t + \tau)] = \tilde{k} \star R_{XX}(\tau).$$

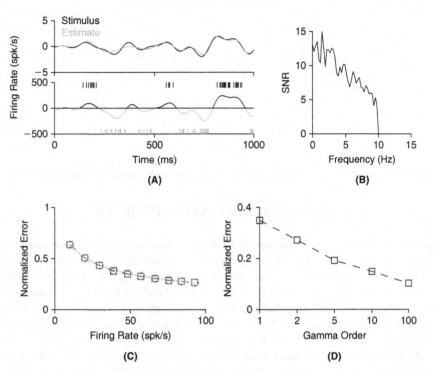

FIGURE 23.3 **A.** The top panel illustrates a sample path of a white noise stimulus with a cut-off frequency of 10 Hz (black) and its estimate (red), obtained from the spike trains of two neurons encoding the stimulus positive and negative parts, respectively (mean firing rate: 50 spk/s). The bottom panel illustrates the instantaneous firing rates of the two neurons, obtained by low-pass filtering the stimulus (exponential filter with a time constant $\tau = 20$ ms). The firing rate of the neuron encoding the negative part of the stimulus has been multiplied by -1 for clarity. The corresponding spike trains above and below the instantaneous firing rates are sample paths of an inhomogeneous Poisson process with the depicted instantaneous firing rates. **B.** Corresponding signal-to-noise ratio as a function of frequency computed from the stimulus and noise power spectra, respectively. **C.** Normalized error as a function of the Poisson neurons' mean firing rate. The black squares are obtained from simulations and red circles analytically. **D.** Normalized error for random spike train models with decreasing spike train variability ($n = 1$ is a Poisson neuron and $n = 100$ approximates an integrate and fire neuron). (`rec_wn8.m`)

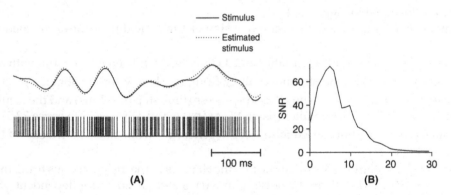

FIGURE 23.4 **A.** Example reconstruction from the spike train of a P-receptor afferent in weakly electric fish. These receptors encode random amplitude modulations of an external electric field (stimulus) which, in this case is white noise with a cut-off frequency of ≈ 10 Hz and a standard deviation equal to 0.24 of the mean stimulus amplitude. The neuron fires 314 spk/s (bottom spike train) and the estimated stimulus is shown on top. The coding fraction equals 0.83 in this example. **B.** Signal-to-noise ratio computed as in Eq. (23.4). Adapted from Gabbiani and Metzner (1999).

Second, we assume that for $\tau \neq 0$,

$$E[(Y(t) - m_Y)(Y(t+\tau) - m_Y) \,|\, X] = E[(Y(t) - m_Y) \,|\, X]E[(Y(t+\tau) - m_Y) \,|\, X].$$

In other words, the correlation between single spikes is entirely determined by the stimulus since they are uncorrelated given the stimulus. After averaging over the stimulus, we obtain for $\tau \neq 0$

$$R_{YY}(\tau) = (k \star \tilde{k}) \star R_{XX}(\tau),$$

and hence

$$R_{YY}(\tau) = \lambda\delta(\tau) + (k \star \tilde{k}) \star R_{XX}(\tau).$$

Therefore the optimal filter is given by

$$\hat{h}(\omega) = \frac{\hat{k}^*(\omega)S_{XX}(\omega)}{\lambda + |\hat{k}(\omega)|^2 S_{XX}(\omega)}. \qquad (23.5)$$

This formula is formally identical to that obtained from the mean instantaneous firing rate (Exercise 2).

23.3 SUMMARY AND SOURCES

The reverse-correlation technique is a natural extension of the stochastic estimation techniques covered in Chapter 22, since it is based on spike trains rather than instantaneous firing rates. It was originally developed for auditory system neurons in the early seventies, see the review of Eggermont et al. (1983). Since then, it has been rapidly extended to other sensory systems and is now part of the standard toolbox to characterize the receptive field properties of neurons. The framework of stimulus reconstruction from spike trains of neuronal populations was proposed by Gielen et al. (1988). Since then, it has been applied to many sensory systems. The stimulus reconstruction method described in §23.2 is known as a Wiener–Kolmogorov filter in the engineering literature and was introduced in Bialek et al. (1991). It allows one to assess how accurately the spike train of a single neuron conveys the dynamics of a time-varying stimulus based on changes in its instantaneous firing rate. The analytical result, Eq. (23.5), is derived in Gabbiani and Koch (1996) and Gabbiani (1996). For further results, see also Gabbiani and Koch (1998). The example stimulus reconstruction illustrated in Figure 23.4 has an exceptionally high signal-to-noise ratio, the highest ever reported in any sensory system to the best of our knowledge. For more typical values in the electrosensory system of weakly electric fish, see Wessel et al. (1996).

23.4 EXERCISES

1. Replicate the results illustrated in Figure 23.1.
   (i) Generate a white noise stimulus with a sampling step of 1 ms (yielding a cut-off frequency of 500 Hz) as in Exercise 22.5.
   (ii) Convolve this white noise stimulus with the same LGN filter as in Exercise 22.5, but with a peak at 20 spk/s.
   (iii) Add a mean rate of 100 spk/s and clip the resulting firing rate below zero to obtain a positive rate.
   (iv) Use this rate to drive an inhomogeneous Poisson process (time step $dt = 1$ ms) and the resulting spike train to estimate the optimal reconstruction filter (using `tfestimate` and `ifft`, as in Exercise 22.5).
   (v) Repeat the same procedure, but use Exercise 18.12 to generate a white noise with a cut-off frequency of 50 Hz sampled at $dt = 1$ ms.

2. Given a random, zero mean stimulus $X(t)$, assume that the changes in the instantaneous firing rate $Y(t)$ of a neuron are given by $Y(t) = k \star X(t) + N(t)$, where the noise term $N(t)$ is zero mean and independent of X. Show that the optimal reconstruction filter is

$$\hat{h}(\omega) = \frac{\hat{k}^*(\omega)S_{XX}(\omega)}{S_{NN}(\omega) + |\hat{k}(\omega)|^2 S_{XX}(\omega)}. \qquad (23.6)$$

3. Replicate the results illustrated in Figure 23.3.
   (i) Generate a white noise stimulus with a cut-off frequency of 10 Hz sampled at $dt = 0.5$ ms and consisting of 524,288 sample points (see Exercise 18.12).
   (ii) Low-pass filter the white noise using an exponential filter, $\exp(-t/\tau)$, with $\tau = 20$ ms.
   (iii) Scale the resulting waveform so that on average its positive and negative portions yield a mean firing rate of 50 spk/s.
   (iv) Use the resulting positive and negative portions to drive two inhomogeneous Poisson processes.

(v) Combine the resulting spike trains, $X_{comb}(t) = \sum_i \delta(t - t_{i\,pos}) - \sum_j \delta(t - t_{j\,neg})$, where $t_{i\,pos}$ and $t_{j\,neg}$ are the spike times of the two inhomogeneous Poisson processes encoding the positive and negative part of the stimulus, respectively. Use $X_{comb}(t)$ to estimate the optimal reconstruction filter using `tfestimate` with a window of 8192 points and an overlap of 1/2 the window length.

(vi) Set to zero the filter components that are above/below $\pm$ the cut-off frequency of the white noise, since they are irrelevant to the reconstruction.

(vii) Recover the optimal estimation filter in the time domain using `ifft`.

(viii) After "unwrapping" the filter (§7.2), use `fftfilt` to estimate the stimulus.

(ix) Finally, use `pwelch`, with an 8192 point window and 1/2 overlap, to estimate the power spectrum of the stimulus and of the reconstruction noise. Derive the signal-to-noise ratio and plot it as in Figure 23.3B.

(x) Repeat for various firing rates to replicate Figure 23.3C.

(xi) Replace the exponentially distributed random threshold of the inhomogeneous Poisson process by a gamma distributed random threshold (see Exercise 16.16) to arrive at Figure 23.3D.

Signal Detection Theory

OUTLINE

24.1 Testing Hypotheses   343   24.5 Fisher Linear Discriminant*   351

24.2 Ideal Decision Rules   346   24.6 Summary and Sources   354

24.3 ROC Curves*   348   24.7 Exercises   354

24.4 Multidimensional Gaussian Signals*   348

Signal detection theory, as its name implies, is the mathematical theory used to optimally detect signals embedded in noise. If the noise is a random variable with a known probability distribution, then it is possible to exploit this knowledge to determine an optimal method of detecting the signal. More generally, we may think of signal detection in noise as the testing of a hypothesis with two alternatives: is the signal present or absent in the noisy background? Under this formulation the theory is broadly applicable to neuroscience to quantify the information conveyed by neurons or ensemble of neurons about sensory stimuli. In §§24.1–24.3 we introduce the basic concepts and results of signal detection theory. In §§24.4 and 24.5 we generalize them to multidimensional signals, a step that allows us to analyze the coding of information in populations of neurons and in the time-varying firing rate or membrane potential of single neurons.

24.1 TESTING HYPOTHESES

We consider information encoded in spike trains under two noise models: Poisson and Gaussian.

Poisson noise model. Assume that a neuron responds with a mean number of spikes m_1 in a given time interval following a stimulus and a mean number m_0 if no stimulus is present. The neuron could, e.g., be a retinal ganglion cell and the stimulus a brief light flash, as considered in the next chapter. On a given trial when the stimulus is present, the number of spikes will typically be variable and may follow a Poisson distribution, as assumed here. If we denote the stimulus by s_1, we may then write down the probability of observing k spikes given the stimulus:

$$P(k \,|\, s_1) = \frac{m_1^k}{k!} e^{-m_1}, \quad k = 0, 1 \ldots$$

Similarly, if no stimulus is present we call this condition s_0 and,

$$P(k \,|\, s_0) = \frac{m_0^k}{k!} e^{-m_0}, \quad k = 0, 1 \ldots$$

(see Figure 24.1A). The questions that we are interested in addressing are the following: given that we observe k spikes in a given trial, should we guess that the stimulus was present or absent and how should we decide between the two alternatives? Given a decision rule, how accurate will our decision be?

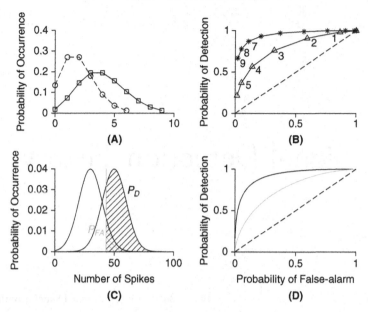

FIGURE 24.1   Signal detection using Poisson and Gaussian noise models. **A**. Distribution of the number of spikes for $m_0 = 2$ (circles) and $m_1 = 4$ (squares). **B**. Corresponding probabilities of detection as a function of the probability of false-alarm (triangles). The number next to each symbol indicates the corresponding threshold in the number of spikes. As the threshold increases, the false-alarm rate decreases but so does the detection rate. The asterisks correspond to the case $m_0 = 4$ and $m_1 = 10$. **C**. When the number of spikes is large a Gaussian approximation may be appropriate. In this case $n_0 = 30$, $n_1 = 50$, and $\sigma_n = 10$. The vertical red line illustrates a possible threshold value and the corresponding probability of detection (P_D, hatched black) and false-alarm (P_{FA} hatched red). **D**. Probability of detection as a function of the probability of false-alarm corresponding to C (black trace). The red trace corresponds to the case $d = 1$. (poiss1.m)

For a fixed number of observed spikes, k, the probabilities $P(k|s_0)$ and $P(k|s_1)$ can be thought of as the likelihood of observing k under conditions s_0 and s_1, respectively. Thus, a natural quantity to consider is the *likelihood ratio*,

$$l_r(k) = \frac{P(k|s_1)}{P(k|s_0)} = (m_1/m_0)^k e^{-(m_1 - m_0)}.$$

The ratio $l_r(k)$ will be large when k is much more likely to originate from s_1 than from s_0 and vice-versa. Thus, a plausible decision rule is to opt for s_1 when $l_r(k)$ exceeds a threshold η, i.e.,

$$l_r(k) \geq \eta \Rightarrow s_1,$$
$$l_r(k) < \eta \Rightarrow s_0.$$

We will now see that the choice of a particular value for the threshold η entails a trade-off between two types of error that may arise in this detection task. But first, we note that one may consider the threshold $\log \eta$ on the log-likelihood ratio $l = \log l_r$ since the logarithm is monotone increasing. Because $l = k(\log m_1 - \log m_0) - (m_1 - m_0)$ this decision rule is equivalent to imposing a threshold on the number of spikes,

$$k \geq k_{th} \Rightarrow s_1$$
$$k < k_{th} \Rightarrow s_0$$

with

$$k_{th} = \frac{\log(\eta) + m_1 - m_0}{\log m_1 - \log m_0}.$$

This decision rule will result in two possible types of error:

1. Calling the stimulus present when it was not, i.e., a *false-alarm*.
2. Calling the stimulus absent when it was present, i.e., a *miss*.

We denote the probability of false-alarm by P_{FA} and the miss probability by P_M. Of course, the probability of miss is equal to $1 - P_D$, where P_D is the probability of correct detection of the stimulus. The probabilities of correct detection and false-alarm are given by

$$P_D = \sum_{k \geq k_{th}} \frac{m_1^k}{k!} e^{-m_1}, \quad \text{and} \quad P_{FA} = \sum_{k \geq k_{th}} \frac{m_0^k}{k!} e^{-m_0}. \tag{24.1}$$

Thus, fixing a threshold $k_{th} = k_0$ gives a probability of false-alarm P_{FA0} and a corresponding probability of correct detection P_{D0} as determined by Eq. (24.1). If $k_{th} = k_1 = k_0 + 1$ then $P_{FA1} < P_{FA0}$ and $P_{D1} < P_{D0}$. Therefore, as we increase the threshold, we decrease our probability of false-alarm at the expense of decreasing our probability of correct detection. A plot of the probability of detection (P_D) as a function of the probability of false-alarm (P_{FA}) is called a *receiver-operating characteristic* (ROC) curve, an arcane term that originated in the initial application of signal detection theory to radar signals during World War II. The ROC curve fully characterizes the performance of the decision rule based on a threshold number of spikes (Figure 24.1B).

Randomized decision rules. What if we would like to obtain a probability of correct detection between P_{D1} and P_{D0}, say $(P_{D1} + P_{D0})/2$? This can be achieved by the following strategy: if $k \geq k_0 + 1$ choose s_1 and if $k < k_0$ choose s_0. If $k = k_0$ choose s_0 with probability $1/2$ and s_1 with probability $1/2$. This corresponds to using the decision rule determined by k_0 and the one determined by $k_0 + 1$ with probability $1/2$ and yields a probability of correct detection that is the average of those two decision rules, i.e., $(P_{D1} + P_{D0})/2$. Such a decision rule is called a *randomized decision rule*. Although this may seem rather artificial at this point, we will see in §24.2 how this example helps one understand a fundamental result of optimal decision rules called the Neyman–Pearson lemma. Two ROC curves for such a decision rule are plotted in Figure 24.1B.

Gaussian noise model. We now consider the situation where the observed random variable is continuous. This could, e.g., be the peak membrane potential of a neuron following the stimulus. Alternatively, in a spiking neuron this situation will occur if the distribution of spikes can be approximated by a Gaussian density. We thus assume

$$p(n|s_0) = \frac{1}{\sqrt{2\pi}\sigma_n} e^{-(n-n_0)^2/2\sigma_n^2} \quad \text{and} \quad p(n|s_1) = \frac{1}{\sqrt{2\pi}\sigma_n} e^{-(n-n_1)^2/2\sigma_n^2}. \tag{24.2}$$

In this case the log-likelihood ratio l is given by:

$$l = \frac{n_1 - n_0}{\sigma_n^2} \left(n - \frac{n_1 + n_0}{2} \right) \tag{24.3}$$

(Exercise 2). Just as in the Poisson case, imposing a threshold on the likelihood ratio is equivalent to imposing a threshold on the number of spikes n. Moreover, since l is a linear transform of n, it will be a Gaussian random variable when n is Gaussian. This is of course the case under assumptions s_0 and s_1 and after defining $d^2 = (n_1 - n_0)^2/\sigma_n^2$ it follows that

$$p(l|s_0) \sim \mathcal{N}(-d^2/2, d^2) \quad \text{and} \quad p(l|s_1) \sim \mathcal{N}(d^2/2, d^2) \tag{24.4}$$

(Exercise 3). From this result we can compute the probability of false-alarm and detection given the threshold ξ imposed on l. The probability of false-alarm and correct detection are given by

$$P_{FA} = \int_\xi^\infty p(l|s_0) \, dl \quad \text{and} \quad P_D = \int_\xi^\infty p(l|s_1) \, dl$$

and a change in integration variables shows that

$$P_{FA} = 1 - \Phi(\xi_0) \quad \text{and} \quad P_D = 1 - \Phi(\xi_0 - d) \tag{24.5}$$

with $\xi_0 = (\xi + d^2/2)/d$ and

$$\Phi(x) = \frac{1}{\sqrt{2\pi}} \int\limits_{-\infty}^{x} \exp(-y^2/2)\,\mathrm{d}y.$$

This last expression is the cumulative probability function of the unit Gaussian random variable, see Exercise 4. The minimum error is achieved for $\xi = 0$ and the corresponding probability of correct response, P_C, is given by

$$P_C = 1 - \Phi(-d/2). \tag{24.6}$$

Note also that d^2 plays the role of a "signal-to-noise ratio" since it measures the squared distance between the means of the likelihood distributions normalized by their variance (Eq. (24.4)). This example is illustrated in Figure 24.1C and D.

24.2 IDEAL DECISION RULES

We are now ready to define more precisely the decision rules introduced above and to state the basic result asserting that optimal (ideal) decisions are always based on the likelihood ratio. Let X be the set of values that can be taken by the observed variable under s_0 and s_1, irrespective of whether stimulus 0 or 1 is presented. In the first example above, $X = \mathbb{N}$ (positive integers) and in the second example, $X = \mathbb{R}$ (real numbers). A *decision rule* (or equivalently a *test*) is a map $\phi : X \to \{0,1\}$ assigning to each possible observation $x \in X$ either stimulus s_0 or stimulus s_1.

There are many ways of defining ideal or optimal decision rules depending on the optimality criterion chosen. We focus on the *Neyman–Pearson* and *minimum error* criteria. A Neyman–Pearson ideal observer is one that maximizes the probability of detection P_D for a fixed value, say α, of the probability of false-alarm, P_{FA}. Such a decision rule is called the most *powerful* test of size α. The achieved probability of correct detection, β, is called the power of the test. A minimum error ideal observer is one that minimizes the probability of error ε or equivalently maximizes the probability of correct decisions, P_C. If the stimulus is presented in one half of the trials, then $\varepsilon = (P_{FA} + 1 - P_D)/2$. Clearly, the minimum error ideal observer will be most powerful of size α, where α is equal to the probability of false-alarm corresponding to the minimum error. Thus, characterizing the ideal, Neyman–Pearson observer also yields a characterization of the ideal, minimum error observer. The fundamental result is the following:

Neyman–Pearson lemma. Let P_0 and P_1 be two probability distributions with densities p_0 and p_1 corresponding to two conditions s_0 and s_1. A test of the form

$$\phi(x) = \begin{cases} 1 & \text{if} \quad p_1(x) > kp_0(x), \\ \gamma & \text{if} \quad p_1(x) = kp_0(x), \\ 0 & \text{if} \quad p_1(x) < kp_0(x), \end{cases}$$

for some threshold $k \geq 0$ and a number $0 \leq \gamma \leq 1$ is the most powerful test of size $\alpha > 0$. When $\phi(x) = 0$ choose s_0 and when $\phi(x) = 1$ choose s_1. If $\phi(x) = \gamma$ flip a "γ-coin" and choose s_1 with probability γ (the probability that the coin turns up heads). The test defined above is essentially unique (up to changes on a subset of values $x \in X$ with zero probability of occurrence).

The test may also be formulated in terms of the likelihood ratio, i.e.,

$$\phi(x) = \begin{cases} 1 & \text{if} \quad l_r(x) > k, \\ \gamma & \text{if} \quad l_r(x) = k, \\ 0 & \text{if} \quad l_r(x) < k. \end{cases}$$

Proof.* First we note that if α is the size of the test ϕ, and β its power, then

$$\alpha = P_{FA} = E[\phi(x)\,|\,s_0], \quad \text{and} \quad \beta = P_D = E[\phi(x)\,|\,s_1].$$

Next, define

$$D_> = \{x : p_1(x) - kp_0(x) > 0\}, \quad D_< = \{x : p_1(x) - kp_0(x) < 0\}.$$

Consider a test $\phi^\sharp(x)$, $0 \le \phi^\sharp(x) \le 1$, with a smaller size than ϕ:

$$\alpha^\sharp = E[\phi^\sharp(x) \,|\, s_0] \le E[\phi(x) \,|\, s_0] = \alpha. \tag{24.7}$$

Then the following inequality holds:

$$\int_X (\phi(x) - \phi^\sharp(x))(p_1(x) - kp_0(x)) \, dx \ge 0. \tag{24.8}$$

This follows by writing the integral in Eq. (24.8) as a sum of two integrals over the domains $D_>$ and $D_<$. On $D_>$, we have $(1 - \phi^\sharp(x)) \ge 0$ and $(p_1(x) - kp_0(x)) > 0$ so that their product in Eq. (24.8) is positive. Similarly, on $D_<$ we have $(0 - \phi^\sharp(x)) \le 0$ and $(p_1(x) - kp_0(x)) < 0$, thus establishing the inequality. By carrying out the multiplication on the left hand side of Eq. (24.8) we obtain $(\beta - \beta^\sharp) + k(\alpha^\sharp - \alpha) \ge 0$ and combining this with Eq. (24.7)

$$\beta - \beta^\sharp \ge k(\alpha - \alpha^\sharp) \ge 0.$$

This shows that the power of $\phi^\sharp$ cannot be larger than that of ϕ. To choose the threshold, write the size α as follows:

$$\alpha = E[\phi(x) \,|\, s_0] = 1 - P(p_1(x) \le kp_0(x) \,|\, s_0) + \gamma P(p_1(x) = kp_0(x)).$$

If there exists a k_0 such that

$$P(p_1(x) \le kp_0(x) \,|\, s_0) = 1 - \alpha \tag{24.9}$$

then we select it as the threshold and set $\gamma = 0$. Otherwise, select k_0 such that

$$P(p_1(x) < k_0 p_0(x) \,|\, s_0) < 1 - \alpha \le P(p_1(x) \le k_0 p_0(x) \,|\, s_0).$$

Then use k_0 to solve for γ from the following equation:

$$\gamma P(p_1(x) = k_0 p_0(x) \,|\, s_0) = P(p_1(x) \le k_0 p_0(x) \,|\, s_0) - (1 - \alpha).$$

$\square$

In most cases, the probability that $l_r(x) = k$ is effectively zero, which implies $\gamma = 0$. In the Gaussian noise model of the previous paragraph for example, both probability densities are Gaussians and thus probabilities are only nonzero over intervals of finite length. In such cases, Eq. (24.9) tells us that the threshold k is determined by

$$\alpha = P(l_r > k \,|\, s_0) = \int_k^\infty q(l_r \,|\, s_0) \, dl_r, \tag{24.10}$$

where $q(l_r | s_0)$ is the probability distribution of the likelihood ratio when s_0 is in effect. The probability of correct detection is similarly given by

$$P_D = \int_k^\infty q(l_r \,|\, s_1) \, dl_r. \tag{24.11}$$

In the case of the Poisson noise model, the probability of false-alarm α may lie between two values α_0 and α_1 determined by discrete thresholds k_0 and k_1. When this occurs, one sets $k = k_1$ and a randomized test is needed.

Minimum error test. Assume that s_0 and s_1 are presented with equal probability $(1/2)$. In the Gaussian model of the previous section, the minimum error test is a likelihood ratio test with threshold $k = 1$ (Exercise 4). In the next section, we will show that this holds independent of the Gaussian assumption. The minimum error test can also be determined directly from the ROC curve by computing $(P_{FA} + 1 - P_D)/2$ as a function of P_{FA} and selecting the minimum value.

24.3 ROC CURVES*

ROC curves have some important properties. First note that the diagonal $P_D = P_{FA}$ corresponds to chance performance while perfect performance essentially means $P_D = 1$ independent of P_{FA}. In addition, ROC curves are concave and their slope determines the threshold value of the corresponding optimal test.

Concavity of ROC curves. The fact that ROC curves are concave follows by an argument similar to that used in the first example of §24.1. If we have two points (tests) (P_{FA1}, P_{D1}) and (P_{FA2}, P_{D2}) on a ROC curve, the randomized tests built as linear combinations of these two tests yields a straight line connecting the two points. The most powerful tests of the Neyman–Pearson lemma have to be at least as performant as the randomized tests, i.e., they have to lie above the straight line connecting (P_{FA1}, P_{D1}) and (P_{FA2}, P_{D2}). By definition, this means that an ROC curve is concave.

Slope of ROC curves. The slope of an ROC curve is the threshold value of the corresponding Neyman–Pearson test. This means that

$$\left. \frac{dP_D}{dP_{FA}} \right|_\alpha = k, \qquad (24.12)$$

where k is determined by Eq. (24.10). Since the likelihood ratio is greater than or equal to zero, k is as well, and Eq. (24.12) implies that the ROC curve cannot decrease.

Proof. To derive Eq. (24.12) first note that

$$E[l_r^n(x) \, | \, s_1] = \int p_1(x) \frac{p_1^n(x)}{p_0^n(x)} \, dx = \int p_0(x) \frac{p_1^{n+1}(x)}{p_0^{n+1}(x)} \, dx = E[l_r^{n+1}(x) \, | \, s_0].$$

This result may also be written as

$$\int l_r^n q(l_r | s_1) \, dl_r = \int l_r^{n+1} q(l_r | s_0) \, dl_r, \quad \text{for } n = 0, 1, \ldots$$

and implies that

$$l_r q(l_r | s_0) = q(l_r | s_1). \qquad (24.13)$$

We can now compute

$$\frac{dP_D}{dP_{FA}} = \frac{dP_D}{dk} \frac{dk}{dP_{FA}} = \frac{q(k | s_1)}{q(k | s_0)} = k.$$

$\square$

Eq. (24.13) can be used to show from Eqs. (24.10) and (24.11) that the minimum error always occurs for $k = 1$ (Exercise 5).

24.4 MULTIDIMENSIONAL GAUSSIAN SIGNALS*

We now generalize the one-dimensional Gaussian model of §24.1 to the multidimensional case. This will allow us to treat two examples: (i) signal detection using neuronal populations and (ii) signal detection using time-varying neuronal responses.

Assume a population of k neurons whose spikes number $\mathbf{v}_X = (X_1, \ldots, X_k)^T$ follow a multidimensional Gaussian distribution under assumptions s_0 and s_1, with the same covariance matrix $\mathbf{C}$:

$$p(\mathbf{x}|s_0) = \frac{1}{(2\pi)^{k/2}} \frac{1}{|\det \mathbf{C}|^{1/2}} \exp(-(\mathbf{x} - \mathbf{n}_0)^T \mathbf{C}^{-1}(\mathbf{x} - \mathbf{n}_0)/2),$$

$$p(\mathbf{x}|s_1) = \frac{1}{(2\pi)^{k/2}} \frac{1}{|\det \mathbf{C}|^{1/2}} \exp(-(\mathbf{x} - \mathbf{n}_1)^T \mathbf{C}^{-1}(\mathbf{x} - \mathbf{n}_1)/2).$$

The log-likelihood ratio is given by

$$l(\mathbf{x}) = (\mathbf{n}_1 - \mathbf{n}_0)^T \mathbf{C}^{-1}(\mathbf{x} - \mathbf{x}_0), \quad \mathbf{x}_0 = \frac{1}{2}(\mathbf{n}_0 + \mathbf{n}_1) \tag{24.14}$$

(Exercise 6). Therefore $l(\mathbf{x}) = \mathbf{w}^T(\mathbf{x} - \mathbf{x}_0)$ with $\mathbf{w} = \mathbf{C}^{-1}(\mathbf{n}_1 - \mathbf{n}_0)$. Thus the maximum likelihood decision rule assigns an observed set of firing rates to s_0 or s_1 depending on whether its scalar product with $\mathbf{w}$ is greater or smaller than a fixed threshold η. Geometrically, this corresponds to assigning firing rate vectors on either side of a line perpendicular to $\mathbf{w}$ to the alternatives s_0 and s_1, respectively. This is illustrated in Figure 24.2 for the threshold value $\eta = 0$ which corresponds to the minimum error test.

Note that since $l(\mathbf{x})$ is a linear function of $\mathbf{x}$, it is a Gaussian random variable whenever $\mathbf{x}$ is Gaussian. Under s_1, $\mathbf{x} \sim \mathcal{N}(\mathbf{n}_1, \mathbf{C})$ and

$$l_1 = E[l \,|\, s_1] = \frac{1}{2} \mathbf{w}^T(\mathbf{n}_1 - \mathbf{n}_0) \tag{24.15}$$

(Exercise 7). Similarly,

$$E[(l - l_1)^2 \,|\, s_1] = (\mathbf{n}_1 - \mathbf{n}_0)^T \mathbf{C}^{-1}(\mathbf{n}_1 - \mathbf{n}_0) \tag{24.16}$$

(Exercise 8). If we define $d^2 = (\mathbf{n}_1 - \mathbf{n}_0)^T \mathbf{C}^{-1}(\mathbf{n}_1 - \mathbf{n}_0)$ then $l_1 = d^2/2$ and $l \sim \mathcal{N}(d^2/2, d^2)$ under s_1 (Exercise 9). The corresponding equations for s_0 show that $l \sim \mathcal{N}(-d^2/2, d^2)$ under s_0. Therefore d^2 is again the "signal-to-noise ratio" for this signal detection task, just as in the one-dimensional case.

We first consider the example of a population of k uncorrelated neurons that respond to s_0 and s_1 with mean firing rates $\mathbf{n}_0$ and $\mathbf{n}_1$, respectively. If the noise has uniform variance, σ_n^2, we have $\mathbf{C} = \sigma_n^2 \mathbf{I}$. Therefore $\mathbf{C}^{-1} = \mathbf{I}/\sigma_n^2$, $\mathbf{w} = (\mathbf{n}_1 - \mathbf{n}_0)/\sigma_n^2$, and $d^2 = \|\mathbf{n}_1 - \mathbf{n}_0\|^2/\sigma_n^2$. For each neuron i let $v_i = n_{1i} - n_{0i}$ be the mean difference in firing rate between conditions s_0 and s_1 ($\mathbf{v} = \mathbf{n}_1 - \mathbf{n}_0$). The average firing rate difference and its variance across the population are given by

$$\mu_v = \frac{1}{k} \sum_{i=1}^k v_i, \quad \sigma_v^2 = \frac{1}{k} \sum_{i=1}^k (v_i - \mu_v)^2. \tag{24.17}$$

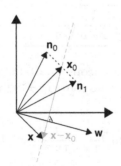

FIGURE 24.2 The dashed red line that lies perpendicular to the vector $\mathbf{w}$ and intersects with $\mathbf{x}_0$ corresponds to the set of vectors $\mathbf{x}$ such that $l(\mathbf{x}) = 0$. Other values of the log-likelihood threshold η correspond geometrically to lines parallel to the red line.

The signal-to-noise ratio for a single neuron is given by $d_{si}^2 = v_i^2/\sigma_n^2$ and its average across the population is

$$E[d_s^2] = \frac{1}{k}\sum_{i=1}^{k} d_{si}^2 = \frac{1}{\sigma_n^2}(\mu_v^2 + \sigma_v^2). \tag{24.18}$$

We may now rewrite the signal-to-noise ratio for the population in terms of the mean signal-to-noise ratio for single neurons:

$$d^2 = kE[d_s^2].$$

Therefore, the signal-to-noise ratio rises linearly with the number of neurons. If the neurons are uniformly correlated, the covariance matrix is given by

$$\mathbf{C} = (C_{ij}), \quad C_{ij} = \sigma_n^2(\delta_{ij} + c(1-\delta_{ij})), \quad i,j = 1,\ldots,k,$$

where δ_{ij} is the Kronecker delta and c is the correlation coefficient between any two neurons of the population. The inverse of $\mathbf{C}$ is

$$\mathbf{C}^{-1} = (C_{ij}^{-1}), \quad C_{ij}^{-1} = \frac{1}{\sigma_n^2}(a\delta_{ij} + b(1-\delta_{ij})), \tag{24.19}$$

with

$$a = \frac{-(1+(k-2)c)}{(k-1)c^2 - (k-2)c - 1}, \quad b = \frac{c}{(k-1)c^2 - (k-2)c - 1} \tag{24.20}$$

(Exercise 10). We may now compute the signal-to-noise ratio

$$d^2 = \mathbf{v}^T\mathbf{C}^{-1}\mathbf{v} = \frac{1}{\sigma_n^2}\left(a\sum_{i=1}^{k} v_i^2 + b\sum_{i=1}^{k} v_i \sum_{j=1,j\neq i}^{k} v_j\right). \tag{24.21}$$

After some algebra we obtain

$$d^2 = \frac{\mu_v^2}{\sigma_n^2}\left(\frac{k}{kc-c+1} + \frac{k}{1-c}\frac{\sigma_v^2}{\mu_v^2}\right) \tag{24.22}$$

(Exercise 11) and by using Eqs. (24.17) and (24.18) above we can rewrite this expression in terms of the mean single neuron signal-to-noise ratio $E[d_s^2]$ and the squared coefficient of variation of the firing rate difference across the population, $\rho = \sigma_v^2/\mu_v^2$,

$$\boxed{d^2 = E[d_s^2]\frac{k}{1+\rho}\left(\frac{1}{kc-c+1} + \frac{\rho}{1-c}\right)} \tag{24.23}$$

(Exercise 12). If the population response is homogeneous ($\rho = 0$) then d^2 saturates for large k, $d^2 \to E[d_s^2]/c$ ($k \to \infty$). In contrast, if there is variability in the population response ($\rho \neq 0$) the signal-to-noise ratio still grows linearly with the number of neurons:

$$d^2 \to kE[d_s^2]\frac{\rho}{1+\rho}\frac{1}{1-c} \quad \text{as} \quad k \to \infty,$$

albeit more slowly than for independent neurons. Thus we are led to the important conclusion that inhomogeneities in the population response improve coding in this case (Figure 24.3).

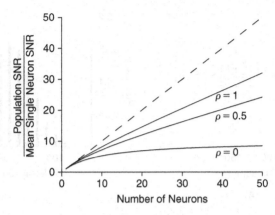

FIGURE 24.3 Plot of the signal-to-noise ratio of a population (d^2) normalized by the average single neuron signal-to-noise ratio ($E[d_s^2]$) as a function of the number of neurons in the population. The dashed line is the case where $c = 0$. The other curves are for $c = 0.1$ and three values of ρ (0, 0.5, and 1, respectively). The case $\rho = 0$ corresponds to a uniform population. (sdpop.m)

The multidimensional Gaussian result, Eq. (24.14), also allows us to consider the detection of signals based on a time-varying firing rate rather than its mean over a fixed interval of length T. For concreteness, we assume a fixed sampling interval $\Delta t = 10$ ms and describe the time-varying firing rate $x(t)$ by its samples $(x(\Delta t), \ldots, x(n\Delta t))$ over $[0, T]$. In condition s_1, a stimulus presented at time zero elicits a response in a neuron that consists on average of a time-varying increase in firing rate above baseline, followed by a smaller and longer lasting decrease. The average response, $f(t)$, under s_1 is illustrated by the red line in Figure 24.4A, while the baseline firing rate (f_0) in condition s_0 is illustrated by the dashed black line. We also assume that the firing rate samples $x(i\Delta t)$, $i = 1, \ldots, n$ are independent and Gaussian distributed, with a standard deviation of 5 spk/s. Thus, the covariance matrix between firing rate samples along the trial is diagonal. Since the average firing rate over the entire interval ($T = 250$ ms) is nearly the same under both conditions, using the total number of spikes from a single trial to detect the stimulus leads to a poor performance (Figure 24.4D, dashed line): the minimum error amounts to 0.49, only 1% better than chance, which lies at 0.50. A better strategy is to use the mean firing rate or the number of spikes over the first 50 ms of the trial, since the firing rate difference between the two conditions is highest there. As illustrated in Figure 24.4B and D, this leads to a better performance (error: 0.25). According to Eq. (24.14), optimal detection is obtained by correlating the time-varying firing rate sample relative to baseline, $x(t) - f_0$, with the vector $f(t) - f_0$. This is often called a *matched filter*, a concept already encountered in §14.3 and Exercise 14.7. As illustrated by the red line in Figure 24.4C and D, this leads to the best performance (error: 0.17).

24.5 FISHER LINEAR DISCRIMINANT*

If the Gaussian distributions characterizing the observed data under the two stimulus conditions s_0 and s_1 have different covariances, i.e.,

$$p(\mathbf{x}|s_0) \sim \mathcal{N}(\mathbf{n}_0, \mathbf{C}_0), \quad p(\mathbf{x}|s_1) \sim \mathcal{N}(\mathbf{n}_1, \mathbf{C}_1)$$

then the log-likelihood ratio has a quadratic dependence on $\mathbf{x}$, leading to a complicated optimal decision rule that cannot be expressed in closed form. An alternative is to project $\mathbf{x}$ onto a vector $\mathbf{w}$ so that its assignment to s_0 or s_1 is based on the condition

$$\tilde{l}(\mathbf{x}) = \mathbf{w}^T \mathbf{x} \gtrless \xi,$$

just as in Eq. (24.14). The function $\tilde{l}(\mathbf{x})$ is called a linear discriminant function. Of course the decision rule is not optimal in the sense of §24.2 and its performance will depend on the choice of an appropriate vector $\mathbf{w}$. To motivate the selection of $\mathbf{w}$, first note that $\tilde{l}(\mathbf{x})$ is Gaussian under s_0 and s_1, i.e., $p(\tilde{l}|s_0) \sim \mathcal{N}(\mu_0, \sigma_0^2)$ and $p(\tilde{l}|s_1) \sim \mathcal{N}(\mu_1, \sigma_1^2)$, with

$$\mu_i = \mathbf{w}^T \mathbf{n}_i \quad \text{and} \quad \sigma_i^2 = \mathbf{w}^T \mathbf{C}_i \mathbf{w}, \quad i = 0, 1.$$

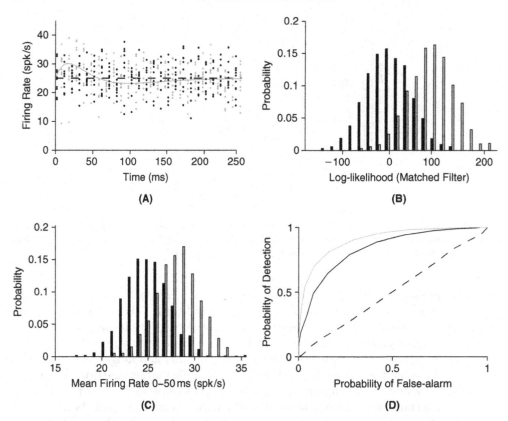

FIGURE 24.4   **A.** Simulated mean firing rate of a neuron in response to a brief stimulus at time zero (red line) and in response to no stimulus (black dashed line). The corresponding dots were obtained by assuming that in a single trial the firing rate follows a Gaussian distribution centered around its mean with a standard deviation of 5 spk/s. At each sampling point $i\Delta t$, ten different samples are depicted for s_0 and s_1 and have been slightly shifted in time for better visibility. **B.** Distribution of the mean firing rate averaged over the first 50 ms after stimulus presentation in the absence (blue) and presence of the stimulus (red). **C.** Distribution of the log-likelihood ratio obtained by projecting each trial onto the matched filter associated with the neuron's response. **D.** ROC curves computed for the mean firing rate on the first 50 ms of the trial (black) and using the matched filter (red). The dashed line is the ROC curve computed with the mean firing rate over the 250 ms of the response and is close to chance level. (`matched.m`)

We can therefore look for a vector $\mathbf{w}$ that maximizes the squared distance between μ_0 and μ_1. However, an increase in $(\mu_1 - \mu_0)^2$ is only meaningful if the scatter of the distributions is not increased in the process. For example, multiplying $\mathbf{w}$ by $\lambda > 0$ will increase the squared difference between μ_0 and μ_1, but since σ_0 and σ_1 are increased proportionally, this does not improve classification. Thus, only the direction of $\mathbf{w}$ matters. A natural measure of scatter is the average of the variances of the projected distributions, $(\sigma_0^2 + \sigma_1^2)/2$, and we therefore maximize

$$f(\mathbf{w}) = \frac{(\mu_1 - \mu_0)^2}{(\sigma_0^2 + \sigma_1^2)/2} = \frac{\mathbf{w}^T (\mathbf{n}_1 - \mathbf{n}_0)(\mathbf{n}_1 - \mathbf{n}_0)^T \mathbf{w}}{\mathbf{w}^T (\frac{1}{2}\mathbf{C}_1 + \frac{1}{2}\mathbf{C}_0)\mathbf{w}}.$$

Note that $f(\lambda \mathbf{w}) = f(\mathbf{w})$ and therefore f depends only on the direction of $\mathbf{w}$, as expected. Note also that when $\sigma_1 = \sigma_2$ the first equality shows that $f(\mathbf{w})$ is equal to the signal-to-noise ratio d^2 of §24.1. The vector $\mathbf{w}$ that maximizes this quotient can be obtained as in Exercise 14.7. Alternatively, if we define $\mathbf{S}_n = (\mathbf{n}_1 - \mathbf{n}_0)(\mathbf{n}_1 - \mathbf{n}_0)^T$ and $\mathbf{S}_C = (\mathbf{C}_1 + \mathbf{C}_0)/2$ then $f(\mathbf{w}) = (\mathbf{w}^T \mathbf{S}_n \mathbf{w})/(\mathbf{w}^T \mathbf{S}_C \mathbf{w})$ and the vector $\mathbf{w}$ that maximizes f must satisfy the following equation:

$$\mathbf{S}_n \mathbf{w} = \lambda \mathbf{S}_C \mathbf{w} \quad \text{or, equivalently} \quad \mathbf{S}_C^{-1} \mathbf{S}_n \mathbf{w} = \lambda \mathbf{w} \quad \text{where} \quad \lambda = f(\mathbf{w}) \qquad (24.24)$$

(Exercise 13). Note that the matrix $\mathbf{S}_n$ is simply a projection onto the vector $\mathbf{n} = \mathbf{n}_1 - \mathbf{n}_0$ since $\mathbf{S}_n \mathbf{w} = (\mathbf{n}^T \mathbf{w})\mathbf{n}$. Therefore, a solution to Eq. (24.24) is given by $\mathbf{w} = \mathbf{S}_C^{-1}(\mathbf{n}_1 - \mathbf{n}_0)$. If $\mathbf{C}_0 = \mathbf{C}_1$ this reduces to the solution of Eq. (24.14). An example is illustrated in Figure 24.5 below.

We illustrate the use of a Fisher linear discriminant in Figure 24.6. Panel A shows the spike train of a pyramidal cell in the electrosensory lateral line lobe (ELL) of weakly electric fish in response to a random electric field amplitude

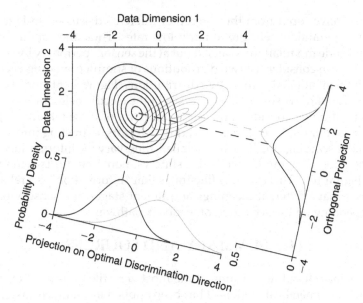

FIGURE 24.5   Contour plots of iso-probability for two Gaussian distributions as well as the projected distributions along the optimal discrimination direction (determined by solving Eq. (24.24)) and the direction orthogonal to it. (fisher_fig.m)

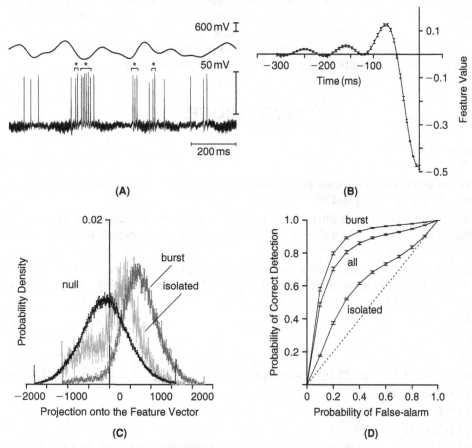

FIGURE 24.6   **A.** Random electric field amplitude modulation (top) and simultaneous recording of an I-type pyramidal cell in the ELL of weakly electric fish. This neuron fires isolated spikes and short spike bursts in response to downstrokes in the amplitude modulation (indicated by *'s). **B.** Fisher linear discriminant (feature) allowing to distinguish stimuli preceding spikes and no-spikes after simultaneous binning of the stimulus and spike train (10 ms bins). **C.** Distribution of the stimuli projected on the feature vector split in three categories depending on whether no-spike, an isolated spike or a burst occurred in the associated bin. These distributions correspond to distributions projected on the optimal discrimination direction of Figure 24.5. **D.** Corresponding ROC curves for an ideal observer based on the distributions in C. Adapted from Gabbiani et al. (1996).

modulation. These neurons receive input from the P-receptor afferents discussed in Figure 23.4. In contrast to the P-receptor afferents, however, pyramidal cells fire at fairly low rates. Thus, they are unable to encode the detailed time course of a random amplitude modulation as carried out at the sensory periphery by the afferents. By discretizing the time axis in 10 ms bins, we can consider the two distributions of stimuli preceding each bin that contains a spike or not. A Fisher linear discriminant applied to these two distributions (Figure 24.6B and D) reveals that the pyramidal cells encode well the occurrence of downstrokes or upstrokes in the electric field amplitude modulation, depending on the particular pyramidal cell under consideration. The occurrence of these features is particularly well encoded by short bursts of spikes. Thus, pyramidal cells act as feature detectors, extracting information that is behaviorally relevant to the animal while discarding much of the detailed time-varying information originally sampled at the periphery. The mode of operation of pyramidal cells (bursting vs. nonbursting) is actually controlled by feedback pathways, as illustrated in Figure 10.6. This example illustrates that "information" is a relative concept in the context of the nervous system. It may have different meanings at different stages of a sensory pathway and may even be dynamically modulated depending on the activation of feedback pathways.

24.6 SUMMARY AND SOURCES

Signal detection theory, as introduced here, is one of the most versatile tools used by neuroscientists to analyze experimental data and formulate theoretical models. It has been applied in countless cases, from the analysis of ionic currents to that of cognitive systems. In this chapter, we have seen how it can be used to analyze single neuron spike counts, the time-varying firing rate of a neuron in response to a stimulus, and population activity. We will encounter further applications of signal detection theory in the next chapter. Most of the material covered in this chapter can be found in many textbooks on statistical signal processing. We recommend Scharf (1991) and Duda et al. (2000) for the material covered in §24.5. The derivation leading to Eq. (24.23) follows Sompolinsky et al. (2001). The variable ρ in Eq. (24.23) corresponds to $\kappa/(1-\kappa)$ in Sompolinsky et al. (2001). See Borghuis et al. (2009) for an application of the matched filter illustrated in Figure 24.4. In deriving Eq. (24.13) we have assumed that both distributions $q(l_r|s_0)$ and $q(l_r|s_1)$ are determined by their moments, the so-called *moment problem*. For further information, see, e.g., Billingsley (1995, §30).

24.7 EXERCISES

1. Reproduce Figure 24.1.
2. Prove Eq. (24.3).
3. Show that the mean and variance of l under the assumption that n is Gaussian with mean n_0 (resp. n_1) and variance σ_n^2 are given by $-d^2/2$ (resp. $d^2/2$) and d^2.
4. Compute P_{FA} and P_D under the Gaussian model, Eq. (24.5). Use these results to show that the minimum error occurs for a log-likelihood ratio $\xi = 0$ or equivalently a likelihood ratio $k = 1$. Compute the correct response probability, P_C, when the error is minimum.
5. Prove that $\varepsilon(k) = (P_{FA}(k) + 1 - P_D(k))/2$ has a minimum at $k = 1$ under the assumption that $q(l_r|s_0) \neq 0$ for $l_r \neq 0$. In this equation, $P_{FA}(k)$ and $P_D(k)$ are defined through Eqs. (24.10) and (24.11), respectively. Hint: Differentiate with respect to k and use Eq. (24.13).
6. †Prove Eq. (24.14).
7. †Prove Eq. (24.15).
8. Prove Eq. (24.16).
9. †In the context of Eqs. (24.15) and (24.16), show that $l_1 = d^2/2$ and $l_0 = -d^2/2$ under s_1 and s_0, respectively.
10. Prove Eqs. (24.19) and (24.20).
11. Derive Eq. (24.22) from Eq. (24.21).
12. Derive Eq. (24.23) from Eq. (24.22).
13. Prove Eq. (24.24). Hint: Argue that the matrix $\mathbf{S}_C$ is positive definite, given that $\mathbf{C}_0$ and $\mathbf{C}_1$ are, and use its Cholesky decomposition, $\mathbf{S}_C = \mathbf{U}^T\mathbf{U}$ to rewrite

$$f(\mathbf{w}) = \frac{\mathbf{x}^T(\mathbf{U}^{-1})^T\mathbf{S}_n\mathbf{U}^{-1}\mathbf{x}}{\mathbf{x}^T\mathbf{x}}$$

where $\mathbf{x} = \mathbf{U}\mathbf{w}$. Now use the result derived in Exercise 18.15.

Relating Neuronal Responses and Psychophysics

OUTLINE

25.1 Single Photon Detection   355   25.4 Summary and Sources   363

25.2 Signal Detection Theory and Psychophysics   359   25.5 Exercises   364

25.3 Motion Detection   361

Studying how sensory perception and behavior arise from the encoding and processing of information by nerve cells and neuronal networks is one of the most fascinating and challenging aspects of neuroscience. The sensory stimuli to which animal species respond and the behaviors that they elicit are so diverse that a multitude of approaches and techniques have been devoted to this goal. We will focus on a very restricted set of sensory perception tasks involving the detection of signals embedded in noise. These tasks have been studied at the level of individual human subjects, a field called *psychophysics*. Many of the methods used in psychophysics are closely related to those originally developed in signal detection theory. We will see how these methods can also be applied to study perception in animals and to analyze neuronal signals, thus opening a way to relate perception and behavior to neuronal processing.

25.1 SINGLE PHOTON DETECTION

A series of experiments first reported in 1942 investigated the threshold of human subjects for detecting brief, weak light flashes. The experimental conditions were carefully optimized to maximize the sensitivity of human subjects. Prior to the task, the subjects were kept in the dark for at least 30 mins to ensure full dark-adaptation of their visual system. The flashes were delivered at a horizontal distance 20 degrees away from the fovea in a region where the density of rod photoreceptors is high. The area covered by the stimulus (10 mins of arc) was also optimized to yield the highest sensitivity. Stimuli were presented for 1 ms and the wavelength of the light stimulus was 510 μm (green, Figure 19.1), a value at which the eye is known to be most sensitive for dim vision (Figure 19.2A). In the experiments, the energy of the light flash or equivalently the mean number of photons delivered at the cornea was varied and the frequency at which the observers detected the flashes was recorded.

The results of the experiments are illustrated in Figure 25.1. Typically, the number of photons at the cornea needed to detect 60% of the flashes ranged between an average of 54 and 148 light quanta. Based on the data available at the time, the authors estimated that 4% of the light would be reflected by the cornea, 50% of the remaining photons would be absorbed by the ocular media before reaching the retina, and 80% of the light would pass through the retina without being absorbed by photoreceptors. Thus, only about 9.6% of the photons available at the cornea could be responsible for light detection in these experiments. This corresponds to an average of 5–14 light quanta. This number is surprisingly small and suggests that absorption of two photons by the same photoreceptor is highly improbable. In particular, if the area covered by the light stimulus contains, say, 500 photoreceptors then the likelihood of 2 out

Mathematics for Neuroscientists. DOI: 10.1016/B978-0-12-374882-9.00025-3

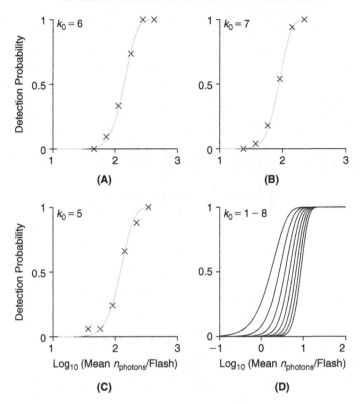

FIGURE 25.1   **A–C.** Experimental data from three subjects and corresponding fits using Eq. (25.1). **D.** Cumulative Poisson distribution for $k_0 = 1 - 8$. (hsp.m)

of 7 quanta being absorbed by the same photoreceptor is $(7 \cdot 6/2)/500 \approx 0.04$. Thus, one predicts that rods should be sensitive to *single photons* and that the simultaneous absorption of a small number of them leads to conscious sensation.

Because the average number of absorbed photons is so small, one expects considerable fluctuations in the number of photons absorbed from trial to trial. Thus, it is conceivable that a large fraction of the subject's response variability is caused by fluctuations in the absorbed photon number. If we assume that photon absorptions are independent random events of constant probability, we expect their distribution to follow a Poisson distribution, just as the number of photons emitted by the light source and observed at the cornea. Let a be the average number of absorbed photons for a given average flash intensity. The authors assumed that $a = \alpha n$, where n is the average number of photons measured at the cornea and α is an attenuation factor related to the optical properties of the eye and retina. Let $P(k)$ denote the probability of k photons being absorbed, then

$$P(k) = \frac{a^k}{k!} e^{-a}.$$

If a human observer sees the experimental light flash only when a fixed threshold number of photons k_0 is absorbed, we expect a probability of seeing the stimulus given by

$$P_D(a) = \sum_{k \geq k_0} \frac{a^k}{k!} e^{-a}. \tag{25.1}$$

The curves P_D are plotted as a function of $\log_{10}(a)$ for various values of k_0 in Figure 25.1D. The average number of absorbed photons (a) for a given average number of corneal photons (n) is of course unknown. If the probability of seeing P_D is plotted as a function of $\log_{10}(n)$, the curve becomes identical in shape to that determined by P_D as a function of $\log_{10}(a)$ except for a shift along the horizontal axis, since $\log_{10}(a) = \log_{10}(n) + \log_{10}(\alpha)$. Fitting the appropriate value of k_0 to the experimental data then becomes very easy: it simply amounts to matching the curve's shape to that of the cumulative Poisson distributions of Eq. (25.1). Thus, the two parameters of the model, k_0 and α, are determined by the slope of the frequency of seeing the curve and its shift along the abscissa, respectively. The fits obtained in Figure 25.1A and C for the probability of seeing as a function of the average number of corneal photons matches well this expectation for values of k_0 between 5 and 7.

The dark light hypothesis. The experiment discussed above suggests that most of the variability in the observers' responses is due to noise in the physical stimulus rather than biological noise. As pointed out a decade later, the experimental design and its interpretation have, however, several shortcomings:

1. If rods are indeed sensitive to single photons, why would observers not be as well, given that biological noise is assumed to be nonexistent?

2. The experiment described above is by itself somewhat ambiguous: an observer could always lower its threshold and thus give the appearance of "seeing" better.

A solution to these two problems is obtained by interpreting the results differently and by proposing a modified model of photon absorption. Although rods may be sensitive to single photons, it could be that several rods must be activated simultaneously when a weak flash is detected to overcome biological noise. One plausible source of noise is the random spontaneous decay of the rod photopigments (rhodopsin) in the absence of light. This decay would give the illusion of photon arrival and thus the registration of a single photon would in turn be unreliable to signal the presence of weak light flashes. Other sources of noise might result from central nervous system processing and can be lumped together with spontaneous rhodopsin decay for modeling purposes.

Let us assume that in the absence of light the mean number of absorbed photons (dark light) is x and follows a Poisson distribution. When presented with "blank" trials where no flash occurs, an observer is expected to report a light flash (even if none occurred) in a fraction of the trials because of this noise. If we call P_{FA} the probability of such "false-alarms," it is given by

$$P_{FA}(x) = \sum_{k \geq k_0} \frac{x^k}{k!} e^{-x}. \tag{25.2}$$

It depends both on the amount of noise (x) and the detection threshold (k_0) of the observer. In the presence of a light flash, the mean number of absorbed photons will be due both to absorption related to the light flash, αn, and to the noise, x. If both processes follow independent Poisson distributions, their sum is also Poisson with mean $a = \alpha n + x$ (Exercise 11.22). Thus,

$$P_D(a) = \sum_{k \geq k_0} \frac{(\alpha n + x)^k}{k!} e^{-(\alpha n + x)}. \tag{25.3}$$

The model has three parameters (instead of two in the formulation of the previous section): the threshold level, k_0, the fraction of absorbed photons, α, and the "dark light level" x. Formally, Eqs. (25.2) and (25.3) are identical to (24.1). Fitting the model to the data now becomes more complex because the parameters cannot be simply interpreted geometrically. The additional parameter can be fit to the data by using the false-alarm rate obtained from presenting "blank" trials. As illustrated in Figure 25.2A, the model offers good fits to the data collected in the experiments

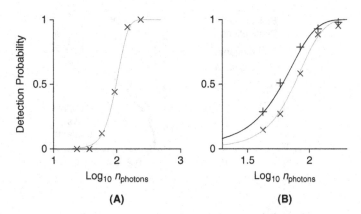

FIGURE 25.2 **A.** Example fit of the data taken from the same experiments as in Figure 25.1 with the dark noise model (the parameters are as follows: $\alpha = 0.13$, $x = 8.9$, $k_0 = 21$). **B.** Fit of the dark noise model for one subject asked to be very conservative in detecting the flashes (crosses and red curve, probability of false-alarms equal to zero) and less conservative (pluses and black curve, probability of false-alarms equal to 0.1). The parameters are as follows: $\alpha = 0.13$, $x = 9.8$, $k_0 = 19, 17$. (darknoise.m)

described above. Typically, the fraction of absorbed photons α is predicted to be higher in the presence of noise $x \neq 0$; this is consistent with later estimates of the probability of photon absorption (predicted to be higher, $\approx 20\%$ than at the time of the original experiment). Furthermore, by encouraging subjects to report less probable stimuli, the threshold is observed to decrease in parallel with an increase in the probability of false-alarms (Figure 25.2B). This is in agreement with point 2 above and emphasizes the needs to monitor thresholds with independent data.

Detection of light in dark-adapted retinal ganglion cells. How does the performance of neurons in detecting weak light flashes compare with the observer's performance? Since retinal ganglion cells are the first spiking neurons that convey information to the central nervous system, it is natural to investigate their responses to such weak light flashes. The experiments were performed in the cat using ON-center retinal ganglion cells and a representative experimental result is illustrated in Figure 25.3. The stimulus consisted either of a weak light flash (five photons on average) of 10 ms duration or of a "blank" trial. The spiking response of the retinal ganglion cell was recorded during a time window of 200 ms starting at flash onset. In the absence of light, the cell was spontaneously active with an average of 4.14 spikes whereas in the presence of light the mean spike count was increased to 6.62. Does the distribution of spike counts match the model described above? If this were the case, one would expect the spike counts to be Poisson distributed both for the spontaneous and evoked response with a difference in means equal to the mean number of absorbed photons, $\Delta m = q_a = \alpha n$ and a difference in variance $\Delta \sigma^2 = q_a$ so that the Fano factor would be $\Delta \sigma^2 / \Delta m = 1$. However, the experimentally measured difference in variance is usually larger than that expected from a Poisson distribution. Let us assume that for each absorbed photon an average of λ spikes are produced. Then $\Delta m = \lambda q_a$ and $\Delta \sigma^2 = \lambda^2 q_a$ so that $\Delta \sigma^2 / \Delta m = \lambda$. The variance in the evoked spike count distributions is consistent with the assumption that between 2 and 3 spikes are fired in response to each absorbed photon (i.e., $2 \leq \lambda \leq 3$). Thus, the response of retinal ganglion cells is consistent with a process of *amplification* of the absorbed photons at low light levels.

The performance of retinal ganglion cells at detecting light can be assessed by choosing a fixed threshold spike count λ_{thres} and computing the corresponding probability of detecting the light flash in the above experiment. According to §§24.1 and 24.2 this procedure is optimal in the case of Poisson spike trains. In a trial that consists with equal probability

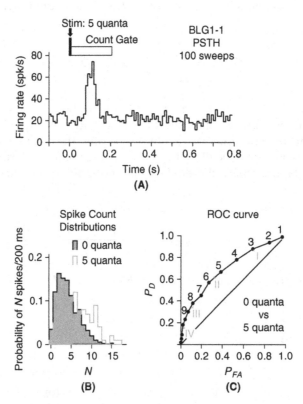

FIGURE 25.3 Responses of a single retinal ganglion cell to 5 quanta (average) of light. **A.** Poststimulus time histogram, 10 ms bin width, 100 repetitions. **B.** Spike count distributions in the presence (red outline) and absence (gray area) of the stimulus. **C.** ROC curve, i.e., probability of λ_{thres} or more spikes in the presence of "dark light" only, P_{FA}, vs. probability of λ_{thres} or more spikes in the presence of the flash plus "dark light", P_D. Arabic numerals and black dots indicate different threshold values λ_{thres}. Roman numerals and crosses in red indicate values for an ideal detector assuming $\alpha = 0.18$, $x = 6.5$, and $k_0 = 14$, respectively. Adapted from Barlow et al. (1971).

of a light flash or a "blank," the observer will report that a light flash occurred if λ_{thres} or more spikes are counted. Otherwise the observer reports that no flash occurred ("blank" trial). As pointed out above, the probability of detection, $P_D = P(\lambda \geq \lambda_{thres}|\text{flash})$ will of course depend on the selected threshold: decreasing λ_{thres} leads to higher probabilities of detection. This is, however, offset by an increase in the probability of false-alarms, $P_{FA} = P(\lambda \geq \lambda_{thres}|\text{blank})$, i.e., the probability of reporting a flash in a "blank" trial. A plot of P_D as a function of P_{FA} (i.e., an ROC curve) is illustrated in Figure 25.3C for the retinal ganglion cell of Figure 25.3A. Each labeled dot $(1,2,3,\dots)$ represents the performance for a spike count threshold $\lambda_{tresh} = 1,2,3,\dots$. Plotting P_D as a function of P_{FA} (instead of using directly the threshold λ_{thres}) is a better representation of the data because this fully characterizes the performance of the observer and is independent of the particular way in which the classification decision was made. This allows one to compare performance with that of an observer based on the model in Eqs. (25.2) and (25.3): the Roman numerals correspond to the (P_{FA}, P_D) values obtained from the model with parameters $\alpha = 0.18$, $x = 6.5$ at detection thresholds of 1, 2, and 3 absorbed quantas, respectively. Because this model accurately describes the psychophysical performance of human observers, it suggests that the performance of single retinal ganglion cells is comparable to that of humans. This conclusion is based on the assumption that cats would report light flash occurrences in a similar manner to humans or *vice-versa*, that human retinal ganglion cells respond like cat retinal ganglion cells to light flashes.

Single photon sensitivity in rods. Do rods really respond to single light quanta? The answer to this question had been known to be affirmative for invertebrate photoreceptors since the mid 1960s. The same answer was obtained for rods at the end of the 1970s when a technique was developed for recording responses of single rods isolated from the retina of salamanders to weak flashes of light. The results unambiguously demonstrated responses to single photons, thus verifying the claim, about 40 years after the original experiment of Figure 25.1, that dark-adapted rod photoreceptors are highly sensitive detection devices.

25.2 SIGNAL DETECTION THEORY AND PSYCHOPHYSICS

Psychophysics is the subfield of psychology devoted to the study of physical stimuli and their interaction with sensory systems. Psychophysical tasks have been extensively used to draw conclusions on how information is processed by the visual and other sensory systems. These tasks often resemble the one described in the previous section and use weak visual stimuli or stimuli embedded in noise. The subject's performance can then be analyzed using the signal detection theory methods introduced in the previous chapter. In this section, we present some of the additional formal framework used to describe and analyze psychophysical experiments. We start with a description of task design.

Yes-no rating experiments. Experiments like those described in §25.1 are called *yes-no rating experiments*. In these experiments, either one of two stimuli (s_0 and s_1) is randomly presented with equal probability. An observer is to report after each stimulus presentation which one of s_0 or s_1 was presented. The time course of the task is illustrated in Figure 25.4A. In a typical situation s_0 is "noise" and s_1 corresponds to a signal presented simultaneously with the noise ("signal plus noise"). In §25.1 the noise condition would correspond to the "blank" stimulus and the "signal plus noise" condition to the flash stimulus. The responses are denoted $r = 0$ or 1 depending on whether "noise" or "signal plus noise" is chosen by the observer.

Two-alternative forced-choice experiments. A two-alternative forced-choice (2-AFC) experiment is one in which the subject is required to respond only after *two* successive stimulus presentations, as illustrated in Figure 25.4B. Both s_0 and s_1 are presented exactly once with equal probability in the two presentation intervals. After the second interval, the subject is asked to report in which interval s_1 ("signal plus noise") was presented. In the flash detection experiments described above, this corresponds to presenting the "blank" stimulus in one interval and the flash in the other interval and subsequently asking the subject to report in which of the two intervals the flash appeared. In this case, responses $r = 0$ or 1 indicate the first or second interval, respectively.

Correct detection and false-alarm probabilities. In a yes-no rating experiment, the *probability of correct detection*, P_D, is the probability of reporting the signal when it was indeed present, i.e., $P_D = P(r = 1|s_1)$ and the probability of false-alarm is the probability of incorrectly reporting the signal when it was absent, i.e., $P_{FA} = P(r = 1|s_0)$. The total error rate of the observer is given by averaging both types of errors by their probability of occurrence,

$$\varepsilon = \frac{1}{2}P_{FA} + \frac{1}{2}(1 - P_D).$$

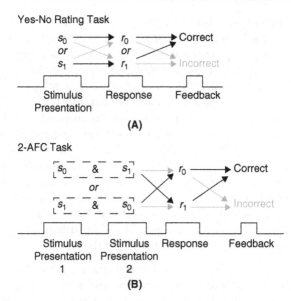

FIGURE 25.4 **A.** Schematic representation of the yes-no experiment. **B.** Schematic of the 2-AFC experiment. Black arrows trace the correct trials and red arrows incorrect ones. In some (but not all) psychophysical experiments, a feedback may be given following the subject's response, as depicted schematically for both tasks.

The corresponding probability of correct response is $P_C = 1 - \varepsilon$. In a 2-AFC experiment, the probability, P_C, of correct response is defined similarly (i.e., probability of $r = 0$ when s_1 was presented in the first interval and $r = 1$ when s_1 was presented in the second interval).

Psychometric functions. When the strength of the signal is continuously varied over a range of values in a yes-no rating task, a plot of the detection probability as a function of signal strength is called a *psychometric function* (e.g., Figures 25.1 and 25.2). The term psychometric function is also applied to the probability of correct response in a 2-AFC task as a function of signal strength and sometimes to the same quantity in a yes-no rating task. It is usual to define from a psychometric function a *detection threshold* to be able to compare the responses of subjects across different conditions. Typically, detection thresholds are defined as 50% correct performance for yes-no rating experiments and 75% correct performance for 2-AFC experiments. These definitions are somewhat arbitrary and some authors define detection thresholds using different values (such as 68% correct performance for 2-AFCs).

ROC curves. For a yes-no rating experiment, the ROC curve is a plot of P_D as a function of P_{FA} for a fixed signal strength. In psychophysical experiments, ROC curves are often plotted for a signal strength equal to the psychophysical threshold. As explained above, such ROC curves fully characterize the performance of the observer for a fixed set of physical stimulus conditions.

Statistical distribution of responses. If we have access to some physiological variable such as the number of spikes fired by a neuron in response to "noise" and "signal plus noise" the question then arises as to how that information can be used to "optimally" decide which of the two stimuli was presented. This question has been addressed in the previous chapter for the yes-no rating experiments. We address it here for the 2-AFC experiment.

Minimum error in a 2-AFC experiment. If the observer's response is not biased towards one of the two presentation intervals, the minimum error test in a 2-AFC experiment is to compare the likelihood ratio based on the outcome of the two presentations (x_1, x_2) and select response $r = 1$ for the presentation interval with the highest likelihood ratio:

$$l_r(x_1) > l_r(x_2) \Rightarrow r = 0, \quad l_r(x_1) < l_r(x_2) \Rightarrow r = 1 \tag{25.4}$$

This result can be immediately derived by computing the Neyman–Pearson test corresponding to a threshold $k = 1$, assuming that the presentations are independent (Exercise 3). Note that no threshold is needed, in contrast to the yes-no rating experiments considered previously. This can be understood intuitively from the fact that one presentation interval effectively serves as the threshold for the other one.

Area under an ROC curve. The area under an ROC curve for a yes-no rating task equals the expected ideal observer performance in the corresponding 2-AFC task, i.e.,

$$P_C = \int_0^1 P_D(P_{FA}) \, dP_{FA} \tag{25.5}$$

(Exercise 4). The area under an ROC curve in a yes-no experiment is thus often used as a measure of discrimination performance, since it is independent of the chosen threshold and since it predicts performance in the corresponding 2-AFC task, under the assumption that the observer treats both intervals identically.

2-AFC Gaussian model. The correct response probability for the Gaussian noise model is given by

$$\boxed{P_C = 1 - \Phi(-d/\sqrt{2})} \tag{25.6}$$

(Exercise 5). Comparing this equation with the equivalent one for the yes-no rating task, Eq. (24.6), shows that the parameter d_{YN} characterizing correct detection in the yes-no rating task is related to the equivalent parameter d_{2AFC} by $d_{2AFC} = \sqrt{2} d_{YN}$.

25.3 MOTION DETECTION

We now discuss electrophysiological and psychophysical experiments aimed at understanding the relation between the activity of single neurons and perception in the context of a motion detection task. These experiments are similar in spirit to the ones described in §25.1. An important difference is that both electrophysiological recordings and behavior were performed simultaneously in trained awake behaving monkeys, thus allowing a direct comparison of the single neuron responses with behavior.

Experimental configuration. Monkeys were trained to perform a two alternative discrimination task in which dots moved within a circular window on a video screen (Figure 25.5). A fraction of the dots were updated from frame to frame in such a way as to move coherently in a specified direction while the remaining dots were updated randomly.

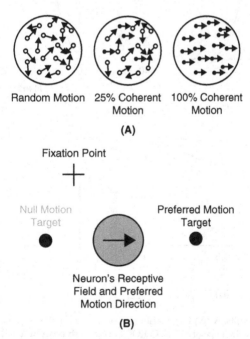

Random Motion   25% Coherent Motion   100% Coherent Motion

(A)

Fixation Point

Null Motion Target   Preferred Motion Target

Neuron's Receptive Field and Preferred Motion Direction

(B)

FIGURE 25.5 Schematic representation of the MT motion detection experiments. **A.** Three motion coherence levels. **B.** The gray disc illustrates the receptive field of the neuron, where the stimuli shown in A are presented. The fixation point maintained by the animal during the trial is indicated by a cross, and the two LEDs to which the animal makes an eye movement following the stimulus presentation, by the two black dots.

After the stimulus presentation started, the animal could report his guess of the dots' direction of motion by making an eye movement towards one of two lights. If the response was correct, the animal was rewarded. By changing the level of coherent motion, the difficulty of the task could be varied from easy (100% coherence) to difficult (close to 0% coherence, i.e., random motion of the dots in any possible direction). Note that the structure of the task is equivalent to that of a yes-no rating task (Figure 25.4A) and should not be confused with the 2-AFC task described in the previous section.

The activity of neurons in the middle temporal area (MT) was recorded simultaneously during the task. MT neurons receive inputs from V1 and most of them ($\approx$ 90%) are directionally selective. Their responses are thought to be well described by variants of the motion-energy model described in §21.4. The receptive fields of MT neurons are typically considerably larger than those of V1 neurons, suggesting a convergence of information from V1 cells with different receptive fields. During the recordings, the direction of preferred motion of the recorded cell was first determined and the stimulus was displayed in a circular region optimally covering the cell's receptive field. The direction of dot motion was matched to the preferred or antipreferred direction of the cell, to maximize the likelihood that the recorded cell contributed to the motion detection task.

Comparison of neuronal and behavioral performance. Figure 25.6A and B illustrates typical distributions for the number of spikes generated by MT neurons during motion in the preferred and null direction at two coherence levels. On average, the firing rate (in spk/s) in response to the stimulus was equal to

$$f_{preferred} = 0.265c + 23.32 \quad \text{and} \quad f_{null} = 0.072c + 23.32, \tag{25.7}$$

where "preferred" and "null" denote the neuron's optimal motion direction and its opposite, respectively. The number, c, is the coherence level of the stimulus, ranging from 0 to 100 (in percent). The typical time used by monkeys to make their decision amounted to $T \approx 500$ ms. This allows us, together with Eq. (25.7), to compute the mean number of spikes in a single trial: $m_{preferred} = f_{preferred}T$ and $m_{null} = f_{null}T$. These numbers were variable and well fit by a Gaussian distribution, a situation similar to that of the second example in §24.1. However, the variance of the distribution scaled

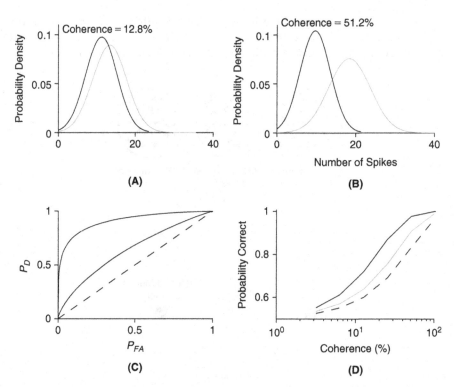

FIGURE 25.6 Summary of experimental results. **A.** Typical distribution of spike number for preferred (red) and null (black) motion directions at a coherence of 12.8%. **B.** Same as A, but for a coherence of 51.2%. **C.** ROC curves derived from A and B. **D.** Typical probability of correct detection as a function of coherence for the animal (solid black line). The dashed black line is the probability of correct detection of an ideal observer based on the distribution of spikes obtained in a single trial from a single MT neuron. The red line is the probability of detection based on two, identical neurons, with opposite preferred directions (area under the ROC curves in C). (mt_perf.m)

linearly with the mean number of spikes (see Figure 15.4):

$$\sigma^2_{preferred} = 1.5 m_{preferred} \quad \text{and} \quad \sigma^2_{null} = 1.5 m_{null}.$$

Therefore the variance was different for the null and preferred distributions, in contrast to Eq. (24.2). As the coherence of dot motion increased, the two distributions of spikes became better separated, thus conveying more information about the presence of preferred *vs.* null motion stimuli. A representative example of the animal's performance in detecting motion direction as a function of coherence is illustrated in Figure 25.6D (solid black line). This curve corresponds to

$$p_c = 1 - 0.5 \exp((c/\alpha)^\beta),$$

with $\alpha = 20$ and $\beta = 1.2$.

To compare the neuron's performance with the observer's performance, we compute the ideal, minimum error observer based on distributions such as those of Figure 25.6A and B. Because the variance of the two distributions differ, the simple results of the previous chapter do not hold. However, the ideal observer for a fixed false-alarm rate can nonetheless be computed numerically, based on the Neyman–Pearson lemma (Exercise 6). The corresponding ROC curves are illustrated in Figure 25.6C for the two coherence levels of Figure 25.6A and B. From such ROC curves, we then derive the minimum error ideal observer, based on a single neuron. The corresponding correct probability is plotted as a function of coherence in Figure 25.6D (dashed black line). Comparing with the monkey's performance (solid black line), we see that a single neuron performs considerably less well than the animal, in contrast to the result suggested by Figure 25.3. What would the ideal performance be, if we had access not only to the number of spikes of the recorded neuron, but also to that of a perfectly mirror-symmetric one, tuned to the opposite motion direction? This assumption is equivalent to recording the response of the same neuron to *two* stimulus presentations, one in the neuron's preferred and one in the neuron's null direction, respectively. Hence, the two mirror-symmetric neurons yield the same information as in a 2-AFC task (Figure 25.4B) and thus, optimal performance is equal to the area under the ROC curve characterizing the single neuron's performance. The performance of the mirror-symmetric pair of neurons is illustrated by the solid red line in Figure 25.6D. Not surprisingly, it is better than that of a single neuron, but still worse than that of the animal. Thus, the animal's performance can only be explained by pooling information across multiple neurons. Here, the results of §24.4 are relevant: if the pool of neurons used to make the decision are correlated and have identical mean responses to the preferred and null stimuli, then discrimination performance will saturate as the size of the pool increases (see Figure 24.3, $\rho = 0$). If, however, the neuron's properties are inhomogeneous, performance will increase with pool size (Figure 24.3, $\rho \neq 0$).

Brain lesion studies. The visual cortex consists of a large number of areas besides V1 and MT and neurons sensitive to motion stimuli are found in many of these areas (Figure 20.1). Thus, it is entirely possible that the correlation between average neuronal performance and behavior described above is not due to a causal relation. An alternative possibility is that behavior is determined in another brain area and that MT neurons merely reflect the outcome of computations carried out in that area. This can be ruled by making a brain lesion restricted to area MT and measuring the behavioral performance of the animal before and after the lesion. The threshold for 82% correct performance in the motion coherence task before and immediately after the lesion to MT typically increases by about a factor 10. The effect is specific: if the motion stimulus is presented in the opposite half of the visual field motion information will be represented in the MT area located on the opposite side of the brain. Since that area was not lesioned, one would expect unchanged performance if the effect of the lesion were specific to the lesioned area. This is indeed the case. Thus area MT is necessary to perform the psychophysical motion task. Over the course of several weeks following the lesion, the ability of the monkey to carry out the task recovers to levels comparable to those achieved before the lesion. Thus other areas of the brain are indeed able to take over the role of MT in motion detection.

25.4 SUMMARY AND SOURCES

This chapter has highlighted the main issues in relating neuronal activity to perception and behavior: how many neurons are involved in carrying out a specific task, what is the algorithm used by nervous tissue to extract the necessary information and convert it into motor commands, and what is the impact of neuronal response variability? The answers clearly depend on the level at which each system is analyzed (e.g., closer to the sensory periphery or to the motor output). In very special cases, single neurons often called *command neurons* may determine a specific behavior by themselves, see, e.g., Korn and Faber (2005). In most cases, however, networks or populations of neurons are thought to determine perception and behavior. We will present some of the theoretical tools used to analyze population activity in Chapters 26 and 27 and an example of how population activity is related to behavior in §26.6. Heiligenberg (1991) reviews a particularly well worked out case. The exact mechanisms linking neuronal activity to perception and behavior are still the focus of intense debate across species and sensory modalities. In most studied higher vertebrate cases, the relation between the activity of single sensory neurons and perceptual decisions has proven elusive. See Nienborg and Cumming (2009) for a perspective in the context of monkey visual cortex and Houweling and Brecht (2008) in the barrel cortex of rats.

Our discussion of single photon detection follows closely the original papers of Hecht et al. (1942) and Barlow (1956). In particular, Figure 25.1 is directly adapted from table V of Hecht et al. (1942), see also their Figures 6 and 7. Figure 25.2 corresponds to Figures 1 and 2 of Barlow (1956). In rods, single photon detection was reported by Baylor et al. (1979). This article also references the earlier invertebrate literature. At intermediate light levels, both rod and cone pathways contribute to light detection. See Borghuis et al. (2009) for a discussion of how retinal neurons from photoreceptors to ganglion cells are involved in this process. A classical reference on signal detection theory and psychophysics is Green and Swets (1966). See also, e.g., Wickens (2001). Section 25.3 is based mainly on Cohen and Newsome (2009), which also provides references to much of the earlier literature. See Maunsell and VanEssen (1983) for a characterization of MT neuron tuning properties. The lesion experiments described at the end of §25.3 were reported in Newsome and Paré (1988). Exercise 7 is derived from Saleh and Teich (1985).

25.5 EXERCISES

1. Reproduce Figure 25.1. For A, use the following data set:

$$\{(46.9\ 0.0)\ (73.1\ 9.4)\ (113.8\ 33.3)\ (177.4\ 73.5)\ (276.1\ 100.0)\ (421.7\ 100.0)\}.$$

   Each pair represents the mean number of photons per flash and their probability of detection. For B use,

$$\{(24.1\ 0.0)\ (37.6\ 4.0)\ (58.6\ 18.0)\ (91.0\ 54.0)\ (141.9\ 94.0)\ (221.3\ 100.0)\}$$

   and for C,

$$\{(37.6\ 6.0)\ (58.6\ 6.0)\ (91.0\ 24.0)\ (141.9\ 66.0)\ (221.3\ 88.0)\ (342.8\ 100.0)\}.$$

2. Reproduce Figure 25.2. For A, use the following data set:

$$\{(23.5\ 0.0)\ (37.1\ 0.0)\ (58.5\ 12.0)\ (92.9\ 44.0)\ (148.6\ 94.0)\ (239.3\ 100.0)\}.$$

   As in Exercise 1, each pair represents the mean number of photons per flash and their probability of detection. For B use

$$\{(1.63\ 0.15)\ (1.76\ 0.27)\ (1.93\ 0.58)\ (2.07\ 0.88)\ (2.23\ 0.95)\}$$

   and

$$\{(1.63\ 0.29)\ (1.76\ 0.51)\ (1.93\ 0.79)\ (2.07\ 0.93)\ (2.23\ 0.98)\}$$

   where the first column is the base 10 logarithm of the number of photons.

3. Show that the minimum error test for the 2-AFC task consists in comparing the likelihood ratios obtained from the responses in the two intervals, as in Eq. (25.4). Hint: Consider the vector $\mathbf{x} = (x_1, x_2)^T$ where x_1 is the value of X in the first presentation interval and x_2 the value of X in the second presentation interval. Compute the associated likelihood ratio of x and then apply the Neyman–Pearson lemma.

4. Prove Eq. (25.5). Hint: Show first that

$$P_C = \int\limits_0^\infty q(k\,|\,s_0) \int\limits_k^\infty q(l_r\,|\,s_1)\,\mathrm{d}l_r \mathrm{d}k. \tag{25.8}$$

Then carry out the change of variables $P_{FA} \to k$ in Eq. (25.5) by using Eqs. (24.10) and (24.11) to show that it is equal to the right hand side of Eq. (25.8).

5. Show that P_C in the 2-AFC Gaussian model is given by Eq. (25.6). Hint: Argue that the decision variable is $l_s - l_n$ where l_s is the log-likelihood ratio in the case of stimulus and l_n in the case of noise. Compute the distribution of $l_s - l_n$ in the Gaussian case.

6. Compute the ideal observer for the case of two Gaussian distributions with unequal variance considered in §25.3. Hint: Consider the transformed variable $Y = (X - m_{null})/\sigma_{null}$ and show that selection of the optimal threshold for $\log p(y|s)/p(y|n)$ leads to a quadratic equation for y with two solutions, $y_{\pm}$. This allows us to write

$$P_D = P(Y > y_+ | s) + P(Y < y_- | s) \quad \text{and} \quad P_{FA} = P(Y > y_+ | n) + P(Y < y_0 | n).$$

These two equations can be solved numerically, given the distribution of Y under the two hypotheses.

7. [†]A model describing the discharge of retinal ganglion cells in response to weak light flashes assumes that photons are absorbed according to a Poisson process and filtered through an exponential low-pass filter,

$$f(t) = Ce^{-t/\tau} \mathbb{1}(t)$$

with a time constant $\tau = 30$ ms. The resulting continuous waveform is then used to drive an inhomogeneous Poisson process that represents the ganglion cell spike train. The constant C is chosen such that

$$\int_0^\infty f(t)\, dt = 2.$$

This implies that, on average, two spikes are generated per absorbed photon.

   (i) Generate a 500 ms long Poisson train (each event represents the absorption of one photon) with a mean value of 10 absorbed photons per second. Filter this sequence with $f(t)$ and plot five samples of the resulting continuous waveform.

   (ii) Use this waveform to drive an inhomogeneous Poisson process. Plot a sample spike train for each of the corresponding waveforms in (i). Compute and plot from 1000 such sample spike trains (obtained from 1000 different waveforms) the corresponding distribution of spike number over the 500 ms period.

   (iii) Compute the mean spike number and the Fano factor of the spike count distribution. How does the distribution compare to a Poisson distribution with the same mean number of spikes?

   (iv) Assume that spontaneous activity is described by the same model but with a mean number of absorbed photons equal to 6 per second. Compute and plot the corresponding spike count distribution. Plot the ROC curve based on a spike count threshold. Compute the minimum error of an observer based on a spike threshold.

Hint: Use a time step of 0.1 ms for (i) and (ii). For (iii), use bins centered at integer values from 0 to 30 to compute the ROC curve.

Population Codes*

OUTLINE

26.1 Cartesian Coordinate Systems   367   26.5 Estimation Error and the Cramer–Rao Bound* 374

26.2 Overcomplete Representations   369   26.6 Population Coding in the Superior Colliculus 375

26.3 Frames   370   26.7 Summary and Sources   376

26.4 Maximum Likelihood   372   26.8 Exercises   378

In many instances, sensory and motor information is encoded by mean firing rates across a population of neurons. Although this is by no means the only way sensory information is encoded in neural populations and networks, it is the best understood. In this chapter, we introduce the tools used to describe the encoding of information across neural populations. We start with a simple example: the encoding of wind direction in sensory neurons of the cricket cercal system (§26.1). From there, we work our way towards a general theory applicable to large neuron populations in the presence of neuronal noise (§§26.2–26.5). Finally, in §26.6 we describe experimental results demonstrating population coding in the superior colliculus, one of the best understood examples in monkeys.

26.1 CARTESIAN COORDINATE SYSTEMS

Two simple and well-studied examples of population codes are found in the central nervous system of crickets and leeches. In crickets, wind stimuli are encoded in the mean firing rate of four interneurons that receive information gathered by receptors located on two specialized sensory organs called the *cerci* (Figure 26.1). Together, these four interneurons form a Cartesian coordinate system representing information about wind stimuli. We number these four neurons with indices $1, 2, -1$, and -2, respectively. If 0 degrees represents the animal's front, each neuron responds best to the wind direction θ_i, $i = 1, 2, -1,$ and -2, that is equal to 45, 135, -135, and -45 degrees, respectively. The neurons are broadly tuned with substantial responses over a range of wind directions spanning approximately 90 degrees (Figure 26.2A). In addition, their responses vary linearly with the logarithm of wind velocity over a ten-fold range (Figure 26.2B). These neurons can also be characterized by the corresponding unit vectors $\boldsymbol{\phi}_i$, $i = 1, 2, -1, -2$ that lie orthogonal to each other in the two-dimensional wind plane (inset of Figure 26.2B). Let $\mathbf{e}_1$, $\mathbf{e}_2$ be an orthonormal basis of the vector space used to describe wind direction and speed. Each wind vector $\mathbf{v}$ is characterized by its direction, θ_v, and length, $\|\mathbf{v}\|$, which we take to be equal to the logarithm of the wind speed. For a given wind stimulus vector $\mathbf{v} = v_1 \mathbf{e}_1 + v_2 \mathbf{e}_2$, each neuron responds with a mean firing rate

$$f_i = C \lfloor \mathbf{v}^T \boldsymbol{\phi}_i \rfloor_+ = C \|\mathbf{v}\| \cos(\theta_v - \theta_i) \mathbb{1}(\mathbf{v}^T \boldsymbol{\phi}_i). \tag{26.1}$$

The constant C converts the logarithm of wind speed to firing rate, within its linear range. In the following, we will normalize wind speed such that C is equal to 1 to simplify the notation. Equivalently, the length of $\mathbf{v}$ determines the

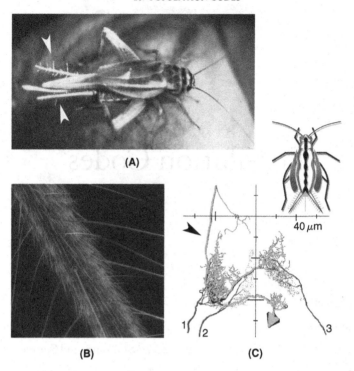

FIGURE 26.1   The cricket cercal system. **A**. The two cerci can be seen extending from the rear of the abdomen (white arrowheads). They resemble antennas and are covered with fine hairs. **B**. Scanning electron micrograph of a cercus showing more closely the hairs. **C**. Reconstruction of three primary sensory afferents conveying signals from the cerci (1–3) and a primary sensory interneuron (approximate outline in red, black arrowhead). The top inset shows a section through the cricket nervous system, that consists of a chain of ganglia connected together by nerve bundles. The terminal ganglion (red arrow) is where sensory neurons and interneurons processing wind information are located. Adapted from Jacobs et al. (2008).

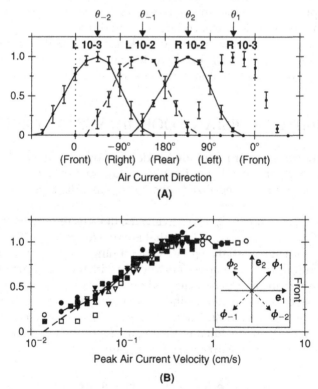

FIGURE 26.2   **A**. Wind direction tuning curves for four identified interneurons of the cricket cercal system (left, L, and right, R, 10-2 and 10-3 neurons). **B**. Wind speed tuning curve for the same neurons. The inset on the right shows the definition of the vectors e_1, e_2 (basis vectors for wind direction and intensity) and the four preferred direction vectors (ϕ_1, ϕ_{-1}, ϕ_2, ϕ_{-2}) corresponding to the neurons' tuning curves depicted in **A**. Adapted from Miller et al. (1991).

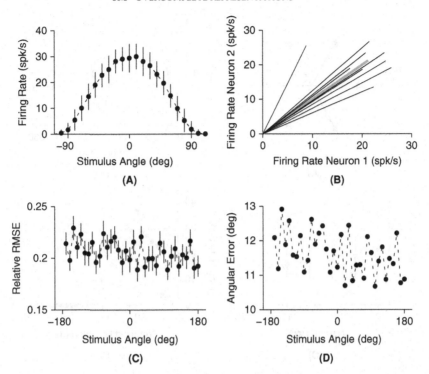

FIGURE 26.3 **A.** Tuning curve as function of stimulus angle for a neuron obeying Eq. (26.1). The angle value of 0 degree corresponds to the neuron's preferred orientation. The mean and standard deviations are obtained over 100 trials. The mean peak firing rate elicited by the stimulus at the neuron's preferred orientation is 30 spk/s and the standard deviation is 5 spk/s. **B.** Vector representation of the stimulus (in red) and of 10 firing rate vectors corresponding to the responses of two neurons with orthogonal preferred orientations. **C.** Root mean square error (RMSE) in estimating the stimulus as a function of its orientation. The stimulus elicits a mean response of 30 spk/s when aligned with a neuron's preferred orientation (standard deviation 5 spk/s). The RMSE is normalized by the average peak response elicited by the stimulus (30 spk/s). **D.** Equivalent mean angular error. (`tuning_rec.m`)

corresponding peak firing rate of a neuron best tuned to its direction. A similar encoding scheme is found in leeches, where four sensory neurons encode the location and strength of touch stimuli around the body wall of the animal.

Since neurons 1 and -1 are tuned to opposite wind directions, they never fire together to a directional wind stimulus and the same holds true for neurons 2 and -2. We can therefore represent their activity by the single variable $g_1 = f_1 - f_{-1}$ and $g_2 = f_2 - f_{-2}$, with the understanding that $g_1 = f_1$ when $g_1 > 0$ and $g_1 = -f_{-1}$ when $g_1 < 0$. Hence, the neural activity vector (g_1, g_2) allows one to reconstruct wind direction, $\mathbf{v} = g_1 \boldsymbol{\phi}_1 + g_2 \boldsymbol{\phi}_2$ with $g_i = \mathbf{v}^T \boldsymbol{\phi}_i$, $i = 1, 2$. In other words, $\boldsymbol{\phi}_1$ and $\boldsymbol{\phi}_2$ or equivalently the pairs of neurons ± 1 and ± 2 build an orthonormal basis representation of wind stimuli. The example of two such pairs of neurons with peak firing rates of 30 spk/s and zero mean Gaussian noise with standard deviation $\sigma = 5$ spk/s added to g_i, $i = 1, 2$, is illustrated in Figure 26.3.

26.2 OVERCOMPLETE REPRESENTATIONS

What happens if we have more than two pairs of neurons representing a two-dimensional stimulus? Such a situation is encountered, e.g., in the motor cortex of monkeys where neurons encode the direction of arm movements when one of their arms is restricted to move in a two-dimensional plane. Each neuron has a preferred direction and is tuned broadly to movement direction, with a tuning curve that approximates a cosine, as in Eq. (26.1). Typically, many neurons encode the arm movement, with preferred directions distributed roughly evenly in the two-dimensional plane.

To illustrate this case, we start by considering a set of m neuron pairs with neurons $1, \dots, m$ having preferred directions $\boldsymbol{\phi}_1, \dots, \boldsymbol{\phi}_m$ equally spaced in the plane, as illustrated in Figure 26.4 for $m = 3$. As above, the preferred direction of the second neuron of each pair is given by $\boldsymbol{\phi}_{-i} = -\boldsymbol{\phi}_i$. For example, in the case $m = 3$, we have $\boldsymbol{\phi}_1 = \mathbf{e}_1$, $\boldsymbol{\phi}_2 = -(1/2)\mathbf{e}_1 + (\sqrt{3}/2)\mathbf{e}_2$, and $\boldsymbol{\phi}_3 = -(1/2)\mathbf{e}_1 - (\sqrt{3}/2)\mathbf{e}_2$. For a given stimulus $\mathbf{v}$, the activity associated with each neuron pair is given by $g_i = \mathbf{v}^T \boldsymbol{\phi}_i$, $i = 1, \dots, m$. Therefore each stimulus is uniquely associated with an activity vector $(g_1, \dots, g_m)^T$. Clearly, many different activity vectors could represent the same two-dimensional stimulus vector $\mathbf{v}$

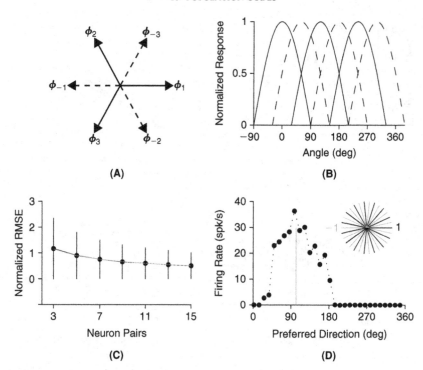

FIGURE 26.4 **A.** Preferred direction tuning of three neuron pairs encoding two-dimensional stimuli. **B.** Corresponding normalized cosine tuning curves as a function of stimulus angle. **C.** RMSE for reconstruction of the stimulus from the neurons' firing rates, normalized by the firing rate standard deviation for each neuron pair ($\sigma = 5$ spk/s) as a function of the number of neuron pairs. The plot shows mean and standard deviation over 1000 simulated stimuli, with uniformly distributed angles and with lengths uniformly distributed between 0 and 3 times the neurons' peak firing rate (30 spk/s). The red line is the theoretical value obtained from Eq. (26.3). **D.** Example firing rates in the case of a stimulus with angular direction indicated by the red line for 15 neuron pairs (30 neurons total). The stimulus would evoke an average response of 30 spk/s when aligned with the preferred direction of one of the neurons. The inset on the right shows the preferred directions for each neuron pair. (over_rep.m)

since $\phi_1, \ldots, \phi_m$ are not linearly independent. Thus the representation is redundant. The formula for reconstructing $\mathbf{v}$ from $(g_1, \ldots, g_m)^T$ is

$$\mathbf{v} = \frac{d}{m} \sum_{i=1}^{m} g_i \phi_i \tag{26.2}$$

with $d = 2$, as may be easily verified by direct computation in the case $m = 3$ (Exercise 1).

Redundancy is useful to minimize the effects of noise on the reconstruction from the neurons' firing rates. This can be simply illustrated by assuming that the firing rate coefficients g_i, corresponding to the activity of the neuron pairs $\phi_{\pm i}$ with $i = 1, \ldots, m$, are affected by Gaussian noise having zero mean and variance σ^2, independent of each other. The reconstruction formula is then contaminated by the noise term $\mathbf{w} = (d/m) \sum_{i=1}^{m} w_i \phi_i$, where the w_i are independent Gaussian random variables with zero mean and variance σ^2. A simple calculation shows that

$$E(\|\mathbf{w}\|^2) = (d^2/m)\sigma^2 \tag{26.3}$$

(Exercise 2). Therefore, increasing the number m of neurons encoding stimulus direction reduces the noise in its reconstruction from their firing rates.

26.3 FRAMES

We now consider the general case of m vectors ϕ_i, $i = 1, \ldots, m$, not necessarily of the same length, corresponding to neurons that may have different peak firing rates. For a given stimulus vector $\mathbf{v}$ the firing rate of the corresponding

m neuron pairs determines a matrix $\mathbf{U} \in \mathbb{R}^{m \times 2}$ with $g_i = (\mathbf{U}\mathbf{v})_i = \mathbf{v}^T \boldsymbol{\phi}_i$. In matrix notation $\mathbf{v} = v_1 \mathbf{e}_1 + v_2 \mathbf{e}_2$ and

$$\mathbf{U}\mathbf{v} = \begin{pmatrix} u_{11} & u_{12} \\ u_{21} & u_{22} \\ \vdots & \vdots \\ u_{m1} & u_{m2} \end{pmatrix} \begin{pmatrix} v_1 \\ v_2 \end{pmatrix} \tag{26.4}$$

with $u_{i1} = \mathbf{e}_1^T \boldsymbol{\phi}_i$ and $u_{i2} = \mathbf{e}_2^T \boldsymbol{\phi}_i$. For example, if $\boldsymbol{\phi}_1 = \mathbf{e}_1$, $\boldsymbol{\phi}_2 = -\mathbf{e}_1 + \mathbf{e}_2$ and $\boldsymbol{\phi}_3 = -(1/2)\mathbf{e}_1 - \mathbf{e}_2$, then

$$\mathbf{U}\mathbf{v} = \begin{pmatrix} 1 & 0 \\ -1 & 1 \\ -1/2 & -1 \end{pmatrix} \begin{pmatrix} v_1 \\ v_2 \end{pmatrix}. \tag{26.5}$$

Reconstructing $\mathbf{v}$ from the neuronal activity vector $\mathbf{U}\mathbf{v}$ amounts to finding a matrix $\mathbf{V} \in \mathbb{R}^{2 \times m}$ such that $\mathbf{V}\mathbf{U}\mathbf{v} = \mathbf{v}$. In other words, $\mathbf{V}$ is an inverse of $\mathbf{U}$ for the vectors in $\mathbb{R}^m$ that belong to its range. To construct $\mathbf{V}$ we first note that $\mathbf{U}^T\mathbf{U}$ is symmetric and positive semidefinite. If we denote its two eigenvalues by $0 \le \lambda_2 \le \lambda_1$ we may invoke Exercise 6.8 to conclude that

$$\lambda_2 \mathbf{v}^T \mathbf{v} \le \mathbf{v}^T \mathbf{U}^T \mathbf{U} \mathbf{v} \le \lambda_1 \mathbf{v}^T \mathbf{v}. \tag{26.6}$$

If $\lambda_2 > 0$ then $\mathbf{U}^T\mathbf{U}$ is invertible and the reciprocated form of Eq. (26.6) holds. That is,

$$\frac{1}{\lambda_1} \|\mathbf{v}\|^2 \le \mathbf{v}^T (\mathbf{U}^T\mathbf{U})^{-1} \mathbf{v} \le \frac{1}{\lambda_2} \|\mathbf{v}\|^2.$$

As $(\mathbf{U}\mathbf{v})_i = \mathbf{v}^T \boldsymbol{\phi}_i$, we may express Eq. (26.6) in terms of the preferred directions, $\{\boldsymbol{\phi}_i\}$, as

$$\lambda_2 \|\mathbf{v}\|^2 \le \sum_{i=1}^{m} (\mathbf{v}^T \boldsymbol{\phi}_i)^2 \le \lambda_1 \|\mathbf{v}\|^2. \tag{26.7}$$

The two inequalities in Eq. (26.7) define a **frame** $\{\boldsymbol{\phi}_i\}_{i=1}^m$. We can now show that $\mathbf{V} = (\mathbf{U}^T\mathbf{U})^{-1}\mathbf{U}^T$ since for $\mathbf{v} \in \mathbb{R}^2$, $\mathbf{V}\mathbf{U}\mathbf{v} = (\mathbf{U}^T\mathbf{U})^{-1}\mathbf{U}^T\mathbf{U}\mathbf{v} = \mathbf{v}$. For $\mathbf{U}$ given by Eq. (26.5), this yields

$$\mathbf{V} = \frac{4}{17} \begin{pmatrix} 2 & -3/2 & -3/2 \\ 1/2 & 7/4 & -10/4 \end{pmatrix}$$

and it is easy to show directly that $\mathbf{V}\mathbf{U}\mathbf{v} = \mathbf{v}$ in this case.

Pseudoinverse. If $\mathbf{R}\boldsymbol{\Sigma}\mathbf{S}^T = \mathbf{U}$ is the singular value decomposition of $\mathbf{U}$ (Chapter 14), then $\mathbf{U}^T\mathbf{U} = \mathbf{S}\boldsymbol{\Sigma}^2\mathbf{S}^T$ and $(\mathbf{U}^T\mathbf{U})^{-1} = \mathbf{S}(\boldsymbol{\Sigma}^+)^2\mathbf{S}^T$ so that

$$\mathbf{V} = (\mathbf{U}^T\mathbf{U})^{-1}\mathbf{U}^T = \mathbf{S}(\boldsymbol{\Sigma}^+)^2\mathbf{S}^T\mathbf{S}\boldsymbol{\Sigma}\mathbf{R}^T = \mathbf{S}\boldsymbol{\Sigma}^+\mathbf{R}^T = \mathbf{U}^+$$

which is the pseudoinverse of $\mathbf{U}$. Therefore, for any $\mathbf{g} \in \mathbb{R}^m$, $\mathbf{v}_0 = \mathbf{V}\mathbf{g} = \mathbf{U}^+\mathbf{g}$ is a solution that minimizes $\|\mathbf{U}\mathbf{v} - \mathbf{g}\|^2$ (Exercise 14.4).

Dual frame. If we define the dual frame vectors through $\tilde{\boldsymbol{\phi}}_i = (\mathbf{U}^T\mathbf{U})^{-1}\boldsymbol{\phi}_i$, then the following equation holds for any $\mathbf{v} \in \mathbb{R}^2$

$$\mathbf{v} = \sum_{i=1}^{m} (\mathbf{v}^T \boldsymbol{\phi}_i) \tilde{\boldsymbol{\phi}}_i. \tag{26.8}$$

Thus, the dual frame allows one to reconstruct $\mathbf{v}$ from its coefficients. To see how Eq. (26.8) arises, let $\mathbf{f}_i, i = 1, \ldots, m$ be the standard basis of $\mathbb{R}^m$. Since $(\mathbf{U}^T\mathbf{f}_i)^T\mathbf{v} = \mathbf{f}_i^T\mathbf{U}\mathbf{v} = (\mathbf{U}\mathbf{v})_i = \mathbf{v}^T\boldsymbol{\phi}_i$ it follows that $\mathbf{U}^T\mathbf{f}_i = \boldsymbol{\phi}_i$. Consequently,

$$\mathbf{U}^T\mathbf{g} = \sum_{i=1}^{m} g_i\boldsymbol{\phi}_i$$

and therefore

$$\mathbf{V}\mathbf{g} = (\mathbf{U}^T\mathbf{U})^{-1}\sum_{i=1}^{m} g_i\boldsymbol{\phi}_i = \sum_{i=1}^{m} g_i\tilde{\boldsymbol{\phi}}_i.$$

If $\mathbf{g} = \mathbf{U}\mathbf{v}$ we obtain immediately Eq. (26.8). A frame is *tight* if its frame bounds λ_2 and λ_1 coincide. In this case, $\mathbf{U}^T\mathbf{U} = \lambda_1\mathbf{I}$, $(\mathbf{U}^T\mathbf{U})^{-1} = \mathbf{I}/\lambda_1$, and so each $\tilde{\boldsymbol{\phi}}_i = \boldsymbol{\phi}_i/\lambda_1$.

26.4 MAXIMUM LIKELIHOOD

For a given stimulus vector $\mathbf{v}$, assume that the neurons' firing rates are given by $\mathbf{g} = \mathbf{U}\mathbf{v} + \mathbf{n}$ with the noise $\mathbf{n} \sim \mathcal{N}(0, \sigma^2\mathbf{I})$. This means that $E[n_i] = 0$ and $E[n_in_j] = \sigma^2\delta_{ij}$. Therefore the noise for each pair of neurons, $\boldsymbol{\phi}_{\pm i}$, is independent of that of other neuron pairs, $\boldsymbol{\phi}_{\pm j}$, for $i, j = 1, \ldots, m$. The conditional probability density of observing $\mathbf{g}$ given $\mathbf{v}$ is therefore given by

$$\begin{aligned} p(\mathbf{g}|\mathbf{v}) &= \prod_{i=1}^{m}(2\pi)^{-1/2}\sigma^{-1}e^{-(g_i-(\mathbf{U}\mathbf{v})_i)^2/2\sigma^2} \\ &= (2\pi)^{-m/2}\sigma^{-m}\exp(-\|\mathbf{g}-\mathbf{U}\mathbf{v}\|^2/(2\sigma^2)). \end{aligned} \tag{26.9}$$

According to the maximum likelihood principle, we select the estimator $\check{\mathbf{v}}$ that maximizes $p(\mathbf{g}|\mathbf{v})$ for a given observed firing rate $\mathbf{g}$. In other words,

$$p(\mathbf{g}|\check{\mathbf{v}}) = \max_{\mathbf{v}} p(\mathbf{g}|\mathbf{v}). \tag{26.10}$$

As the logarithm is a monotone increasing function, maximizing $p(\mathbf{g}|\mathbf{v})$ is identical to maximizing the log-likelihood, $L(\mathbf{v}, \mathbf{g}) = \log p(\mathbf{g}|\mathbf{v})$. In the present case,

$$\log p(\mathbf{g}|\mathbf{v}) = \frac{-m}{2}\log 2\pi - m\log\sigma - \frac{1}{2\sigma^2}\|\mathbf{g}-\mathbf{U}\mathbf{v}\|^2.$$

Therefore maximizing the log-likelihood is equivalent to minimizing $\|\mathbf{g}-\mathbf{U}\mathbf{v}\|^2$. If the neurons' firing rates are still Gaussian, but are correlated with each other, the noise will be distributed as $\mathbf{n} \sim \mathcal{N}(0, \mathbf{C})$. The covariance matrix of the noise, $\mathbf{C}$, is assumed to be invertible. The conditional probability density is given by

$$p(\mathbf{g}|\mathbf{v}) = (2\pi)^{-m/2}|\det\mathbf{C}|^{-1/2}\exp(-(\mathbf{g}-\mathbf{U}\mathbf{v})^T\mathbf{C}^{-1}(\mathbf{g}-\mathbf{U}\mathbf{v})/2) \tag{26.11}$$

thus, maximizing the log-likelihood is equivalent to minimizing

$$(\mathbf{g}-\mathbf{U}\mathbf{v})^T\mathbf{C}^{-1}(\mathbf{g}-\mathbf{U}\mathbf{v}). \tag{26.12}$$

Since $\mathbf{C}$ is symmetric it is diagonalizable and $\boldsymbol{\Sigma} = \mathbf{W}\mathbf{C}\mathbf{W}^T$ has positive diagonal elements. Therefore $\mathbf{C}^{-1} = \mathbf{W}^T\boldsymbol{\Sigma}^{-1/2}\boldsymbol{\Sigma}^{-1/2}\mathbf{W}$ which means that minimizing Eq. (26.12) is equivalent to minimizing $\|\boldsymbol{\Sigma}^{-1/2}\mathbf{W}(\mathbf{g}-\mathbf{U}\mathbf{v})\|^2$. With $\mathbf{f} = \boldsymbol{\Sigma}^{-1/2}\mathbf{W}\mathbf{g}$ and $\mathbf{V} = \boldsymbol{\Sigma}^{-1/2}\mathbf{W}\mathbf{U}$ we obtain the solution by computing the pseudoinverse of $\mathbf{f}$, as in the previous section:

$$\begin{aligned} (\mathbf{V}^T\mathbf{V})^{-1}\mathbf{V}^T\mathbf{f} &= (\mathbf{U}^T\mathbf{W}^T\boldsymbol{\Sigma}^{-1/2}\boldsymbol{\Sigma}^{-1/2}\mathbf{W}\mathbf{U})^{-1}\mathbf{U}^T\mathbf{W}^T\boldsymbol{\Sigma}^{-1/2}\boldsymbol{\Sigma}^{-1/2}\mathbf{W}\mathbf{g} \\ &= (\mathbf{U}^T\mathbf{C}^{-1}\mathbf{U})^{-1}\mathbf{U}^T\mathbf{C}^{-1}\mathbf{g}. \end{aligned} \tag{26.13}$$

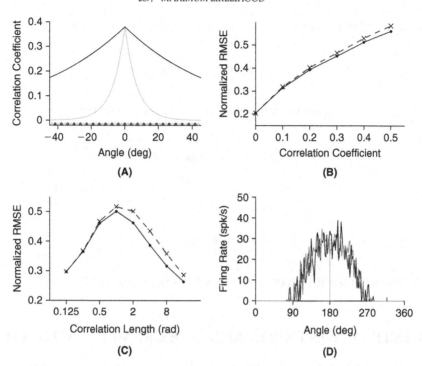

FIGURE 26.5 **A.** Exponentially decaying correlation between neuron pairs whose preferred directions are indicated by the circles at bottom (95 pairs). The red trace corresponds to $c = 0.38$ and $\rho = 0.125$ radians in Eq. (26.14). The black trace depicts $\rho = 1$ rad (≈ 57 degrees). **B.** Normalized RMSE in estimating randomly distributed stimuli as a function of the correlation coefficient c for $\rho = 1$. The dots indicate the optimal solution, Eq. (26.13), and the crosses the optimal solution for uncorrelated neurons ($\mathbf{C} = \mathbf{I}$). **C.** Normalized RMSE for $c = 0.38$ as a function of ρ (symbols have the same meaning as in **B**). **D.** Sample firing rate distribution for a stimulus directed at 180 degrees that elicits a maximal average firing rate of 30 spk/s (red line) as a function of the neurons' preferred directions. The black line depicts uncorrelated neurons and the gray line exponentially decaying correlations with $c = 0.38$, $\rho = 1$ rad. (`pop_corr.m`)

This last result allows us to investigate the effect of correlations on the encoding of a two-dimensional stimulus vector. We assume that the correlation matrix among m neuron pairs is given by $\mathbf{C} = (C_{ij})_{i,j=1,\ldots,m}$, with

$$C_{ij} = \sigma^2(\delta_{ij} + C(\boldsymbol{\phi}_i - \boldsymbol{\phi}_j)(1 - \delta_{ij})) \quad \text{and} \quad C(\boldsymbol{\phi}) = c\exp(-|\boldsymbol{\phi}|/\rho). \tag{26.14}$$

The firing rate variance of each neuron is equal to $C_{ii} = \sigma^2$ and the correlation between neurons i and j decays exponentially with the angular difference, $|\boldsymbol{\phi}_i - \boldsymbol{\phi}_j|$, in their preferred directions. The results are illustrated in Figure 26.5. As the correlation coefficient c increases, the RMSE increases as well (Figure 26.5B). The RMSE in the reconstructions is lower with the optimal algorithm (dots) than with the suboptimal algorithm of Eq. (26.2) (crosses) when $c \neq 0$, as expected. Figure 26.5C shows that increasing the spatial extent of the correlations among neurons initially increases the RMSE up to $\rho = 1$ but somewhat counterintuitively, beyond that point the reconstructions improve rapidly with ρ.

Maximum likelihood is not the only way of selecting an estimator for a given variable, such as stimulus direction and strength, from noisy observations. We introduce two popular alternatives.

Maximum a posteriori estimator. If $p(\mathbf{v})$ is nonuniform, then $p(\mathbf{g}|\mathbf{v})p(\mathbf{v}) = p(\mathbf{g}, \mathbf{v})$. Integration over $\mathbf{v}$ yields $p(\mathbf{g})$ and we may define $p(\mathbf{v}|\mathbf{g})$ through

$$p(\mathbf{v}|\mathbf{g}) = \frac{p(\mathbf{g}, \mathbf{v})}{p(\mathbf{g})} \quad \text{for} \quad p(\mathbf{g}) \neq 0.$$

The function $p(\mathbf{v}|\mathbf{g})$ is the posterior probability of $\mathbf{v}$ given $\mathbf{g}$. The maximum a posteriori estimator is the vector, $\mathbf{v}_{MAP}$, that maximizes this posterior probability. Since

$$\log p(\mathbf{v}|\mathbf{g}) = \log p(\mathbf{g}|\mathbf{v}) + \log p(\mathbf{v}) - \log p(\mathbf{g})$$

and the last term is independent of $\mathbf{v}$, this is equivalent to maximizing $\log p(\mathbf{g}|\mathbf{v}) + \log p(\mathbf{v})$.

Conditional mean. We may also minimize the mean square error of the estimator $\check{\mathbf{v}}(\mathbf{g})$,

$$\int \|\mathbf{v} - \check{\mathbf{v}}\|^2 p(\mathbf{v}\,|\,\mathbf{g})\,d\mathbf{v}.$$

By taking the derivative $\partial/\partial \check{v}_i$ with respect to each of the components of $\check{\mathbf{v}}$ we obtain

$$-2\int (v_i - \check{v}_i)p(\mathbf{v}|\mathbf{g})\,d\mathbf{v} = 0$$

and this yields

$$\check{\mathbf{v}} = \int \mathbf{v}p(\mathbf{v}\,|\,\mathbf{g})\,d\mathbf{v}.$$

This is precisely the conditional mean of $\mathbf{v}$ given $\mathbf{g}$, also denoted $E[\mathbf{v}\,|\,\mathbf{g}]$, see §22.1.

26.5 ESTIMATION ERROR AND THE CRAMER–RAO BOUND*

Given an estimator of $\mathbf{v}$ like that derived in Eq. (26.13) of the previous section for correlated neuron pairs, $\check{\mathbf{v}} = \mathbf{F}\mathbf{g}$, $\mathbf{F} = (\mathbf{U}^T\mathbf{C}^{-1}\mathbf{U})^{-1}\mathbf{U}^T\mathbf{C}^{-1}$, the question arises of how well it performs compared to other possible estimators. In Figure 26.5 we have, e.g., compared its performance to that of Eq. (26.2). We now address the same question from a more general point of view. First we observe that for different random values of $\mathbf{g}$, $\check{\mathbf{v}}$ is a random variable. We can therefore define the covariance error matrix as

$$\mathbf{C}_e = E[(\check{\mathbf{v}} - \mathbf{v})(\check{\mathbf{v}} - \mathbf{v})^T] = \begin{pmatrix} E[(\check{v}_1 - v_1)^2] & E[(\check{v}_1 - v_1)(\check{v}_2 - v_2)] \\ E[(\check{v}_1 - v_1)(\check{v}_2 - v_2)] & E[(\check{v}_2 - v_2)^2] \end{pmatrix},$$

where the expectation is taken over $\mathbf{g}$. The covariance error matrix can be written as follows:

$$\mathbf{C}_e = E[(\check{\mathbf{v}} - E[\check{\mathbf{v}}])(\check{\mathbf{v}} - E[\check{\mathbf{v}}])^T] + (E[\check{\mathbf{v}}] - \mathbf{v})(E[\check{\mathbf{v}}] - \mathbf{v})^T \tag{26.15}$$

(Exercise 3). The first term describes the covariance of the estimator and the second one its bias (§18.2). The estimator is unbiased if $E[\check{\mathbf{v}}] = \mathbf{v}$, in which case the second term in Eq. (26.15) vanishes. In the case of $\check{\mathbf{v}} = \mathbf{F}\mathbf{g}$, with $\mathbf{g} = \mathbf{U}\mathbf{v} + \mathbf{n}$ and $E[\mathbf{n}] = 0$ as in the previous paragraph, it follows immediately that $E[\check{\mathbf{v}}] = \mathbf{v}$ (Exercise 4).

Fisher information matrix. Assume that $p(\mathbf{g}|\mathbf{v}) = f_\mathbf{v}(\mathbf{g})$ is a differentiable function of $\mathbf{v}$. Then at the optimal (maximum likelihood) value of $\mathbf{v}$, Eq. (26.10), the gradient, with respect to $\mathbf{v}$, of $f_\mathbf{v}(\mathbf{g})$ vanishes. Equivalently,

$$\nabla_\mathbf{v} \log f_\mathbf{v}(\mathbf{g}) = \begin{pmatrix} \frac{\partial}{\partial v_1} \log f_\mathbf{v}(\mathbf{g}) \\ \frac{\partial}{\partial v_2} \log f_\mathbf{v}(\mathbf{g}) \end{pmatrix} = 0.$$

The function $\mathbf{s}(\mathbf{v}, \mathbf{g}) \equiv \nabla_\mathbf{v} \log f_\mathbf{v}(\mathbf{g})$ is called the *score function*. By taking its expectation with respect to $\mathbf{g}$ given $\mathbf{v}$ and exchanging this operation with the derivative, we can show that the score function has zero mean: $E[\mathbf{s}(\mathbf{v}, \mathbf{g})] = 0$ (Exercise 5). The covariance matrix of the score function,

$$\mathbf{J} = E[\mathbf{s}(\mathbf{v}, \mathbf{g})\mathbf{s}(\mathbf{v}, \mathbf{g})^T]$$

is called the Fisher information matrix. Note that $\mathbf{J}$ is symmetric and that its eigenvalues are nonnegative, since it is the covariance of a random vector. For an unbiased estimator, $E[\check{\mathbf{v}}] = \mathbf{v}$, the Fisher information matrix has the following property:

$$E[\mathbf{s}(\mathbf{v},\mathbf{g})(\check{\mathbf{v}} - \mathbf{v})^T] = \mathbf{I} \tag{26.16}$$

(Exercise 6).

Cramer–Rao bound. If $\mathbf{J} \in \mathbb{R}^{n \times n}$ is positive definite then $\mathbf{J}^{-1}$ exists and Eq. (26.16) allows us to establish the following bound on the covariance error matrix of an unbiased estimator ($E[\check{\mathbf{v}}] = \mathbf{v}$):

$$\boxed{\mathbf{x}^T \mathbf{C}_e \mathbf{x} \ge \mathbf{x}^T \mathbf{J}^{-1} \mathbf{x} \qquad \text{for all } \mathbf{x} \in \mathbb{R}^n,} \tag{26.17}$$

(Exercise 7).

To illustrate the significance of this result, let us start by assuming that we want to estimate a one-dimensional quantity, e.g., the direction, θ, of the vector $\mathbf{v}$ with respect to the first coordinate axis rather than $\mathbf{v}$ itself, as in the following §27.6. In this case, the Fisher information matrix is actually a scalar. Let $f_\theta(\mathbf{g}) = p(\mathbf{g}|\theta)$ and $J = E[(\mathrm{d}\,f_\theta(\mathbf{g})/\mathrm{d}\theta)^2]$ then the Cramer–Rao bound states that $E[(\check{\theta} - \theta)^2] \ge J^{-1}$ for any unbiased estimator $\check{\theta}$ of θ. Similarly, in the multidimensional case the diagonal elements, J_{ii}^{-1}, of $\mathbf{J}^{-1}$ provide lower bounds on the variance of any estimator for the components of $\mathbf{v} = (v_1\ v_2)^T$:

$$E[(\check{v}_i - v_i)^2] \ge J_{ii}^{-1}, \quad \text{for} \quad i = 1, 2.$$

The Fisher information matrix is thus a useful quantity to study population coding since it gives an absolute lower bound on the error that *any* estimator based on experimental data may achieve, provided a model of the probability distribution $p(\mathbf{g}|\mathbf{v})$ exists.

In the case of a Gaussian noise vector, $\mathbf{g} = \mathbf{U}\mathbf{v} + \mathbf{n}$, $\mathbf{n} \sim \mathcal{N}(0, \mathbf{C})$, $f_{\mathbf{v}}(\mathbf{g})$ is given by Eq. (26.11) so that

$$\mathbf{s}(\mathbf{v},\mathbf{g}) = \nabla_{\mathbf{v}} \log f_{\mathbf{v}}(\mathbf{g}) = -\frac{1}{2} \nabla_{\mathbf{v}} \mathrm{tr}(\mathbf{C}^{-1}(\mathbf{g} - \mathbf{U}\mathbf{v})(\mathbf{g} - \mathbf{U}\mathbf{v})^T) = \mathbf{U}^T \mathbf{C}^{-1}(\mathbf{g} - \mathbf{U}\mathbf{v}), \tag{26.18}$$

(Exercise 8). In this equation, tr is the trace of the matrix, i.e., the sum of its diagonal elements (Exercise 5.6). Consequently, the Fisher information matrix is given by

$$\mathbf{J} = E[\mathbf{U}^T \mathbf{C}^{-1}(\mathbf{g} - \mathbf{U}\mathbf{v})(\mathbf{g} - \mathbf{U}\mathbf{v})^T \mathbf{C}^{-1}\mathbf{U}] = \mathbf{U}^T \mathbf{C}^{-1}\mathbf{U}.$$

On the other hand, since $\check{\mathbf{v}} = \mathbf{F}\mathbf{g} = \mathbf{F}\mathbf{U}\mathbf{v} + \mathbf{F}\mathbf{n} = \mathbf{v} + \mathbf{F}\mathbf{n}$ we have

$$\mathbf{C}_e = E[(\check{\mathbf{v}} - \mathbf{v})(\check{\mathbf{v}} - \mathbf{v})^T] = (\mathbf{U}^T \mathbf{C}^{-1}\mathbf{U})^{-1} = \mathbf{J}^{-1} \tag{26.19}$$

(Exercise 9). Therefore the maximum likelihood estimator is efficient, since it saturates the Cramer–Rao bound.

26.6 POPULATION CODING IN THE SUPERIOR COLLICULUS

The superior colliculus is a small bilaterally symmetric nucleus located at the top of the midbrain of mammals (Figure 26.6A). It is involved in the generation of rapid eye movements called *saccades* that are used several times per second to shift the gaze to different parts of the visual field. Neurons in the superior colliculus fire a high frequency burst of action potentials just before each saccade (Figure 26.6B). Each neuron fires maximally before a specific eye movement, but will typically fire to a broad range of eye movements (Figure 26.6C). The superior colliculus is organized into a two-dimensional map of eye movements, with amplitudes coded along one axis and angles with respect to the horizontal along the other (Figure 26.6D). The direction of eye movement is thought to be determined by the vector average of the neurons' activity weighted by their preferred eye movement as in Eq. (26.2).

Because of the orderly two-dimensional mapping of eye movement amplitude and angle with respect to the horizontal in the superior colliculus, this population coding hypothesis can be tested by chemically inactivating a specific location in the map. This makes the prediction that some eye movements will overshoot or undershoot their

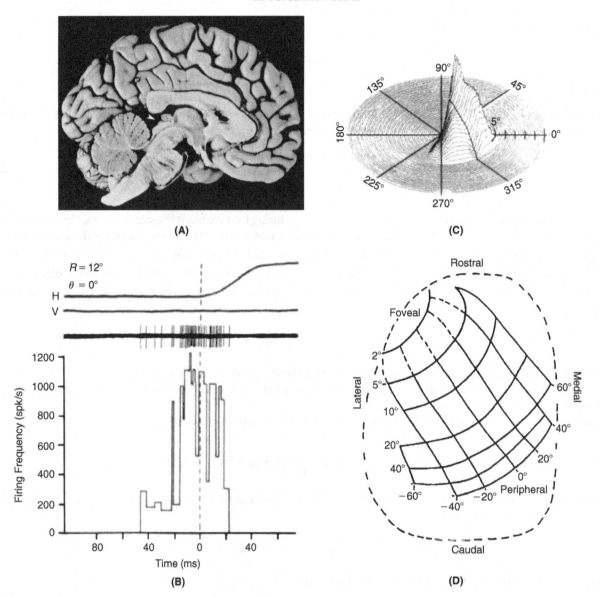

FIGURE 26.6   **A.** Vertical section of the human brain through the midline. The superior colliculus is indicated by the white arrowhead.
B. Trajectory of an eye-movement (top horizontal, H, and vertical, V, traces) in the horizontal plane as well as action potential firing of a superior
colliculus neuron (raw discharge trace shown in the middle) and histogram of firing rates (bottom). **C.** Relative peak firing frequency of the neuron
as a function of the amplitude and direction of the eye movement. **D.** Two-dimensional map of saccadic eye movements in the superior colliculus.
The amplitude is roughly mapped from front to back (rostral to caudal) and the direction relative to the horizontal from medial to lateral. Adapted
from Sparks and Nelson (1987).

intended targets, depending on their position relative to the inactivated spot (Figure 26.7A). Such predictions can be
verified experimentally (Figure 26.7B).

26.7 SUMMARY AND SOURCES

This chapter has presented the basic mathematical tools used to investigate neural population codes. The main
idea is to estimate a stimulus given the firing rate of a population of neurons encoding its strength and direction.
We started by considering neurons that form a Cartesian coordinate system for wind stimuli in the cricket cercal
system. In this case, stimulus reconstruction amounts to a simple addition of weighted orthonormal basis vectors
as in Cartesian geometry. Next we looked at oversampled representations, where many more neurons sample the
stimulus than the minimal number required for an orthonormal decomposition. The general case was treated in

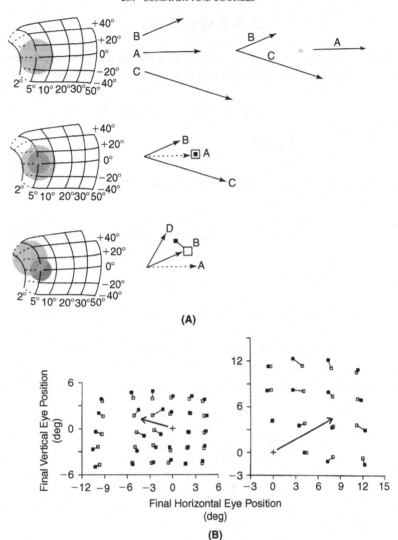

(A)

(B)

FIGURE 26.7   **A.** Predictions of the population vector hypothesis. If spot A in the map is inactivated, the eye movements to the corresponding location in space will not be affected (middle row) because summating the activity of the surrounding neurons yields the same population vector (top row). In contrast an eye movement towards position B will lead to an overshoot towards D, since neurons flanking B are inactivated (bottom row). **B.** Experimental validation in two examples. The arrow indicates the eye movement corresponding to the inactivated region (approx. 6 degrees horizontal on the left panel). Note that movements beyond that amplitude result in an overshoot (−9 degrees) and smaller eye movements result in an undershoot compared to those elicited when inactivation is absent (white squares). Eye movements to the opposite side are unaffected, because they are encoded by the superior colliculus on the opposite side of the brain. Adapted from Lee et al. (1988).

§26.3 where sensory neurons have heterogeneous properties, which from the mathematical point of view correspond to frames. For simplicity, our treatment always considered pairs of neurons that have equal and opposite response properties. Although this assumption considerably simplifies the mathematical exposition, it does not affect the concepts presented here. Finally, we introduced the maximum likelihood method to estimate the stimulus in the presence of neural noise and the general bounds on the resulting estimation error that can be derived using the Fisher information matrix. The last section on the superior colliculus illustrates how these concepts make specific predictions that can be tested experimentally, at least qualitatively.

We recommend the following two reviews on population codes: Sanger (2003) and Zhang and Sejnowski (2001). The first one includes a discussion and references on population coding in motor cortex. The second one reviews theoretical papers and summarizes additional theoretical results. For population coding in the leech, see Lewis and Kristan (1998). A recent review that places the results of §26.6 in a more general context is Sparks (2002). For additional results on frames, see Daubechies (1992, Chapter 3) or Mallat (2008, Chapter 5). We recommend Scharf (1991) for additional reading on the material of §§26.4 and 26.5.

26.8 EXERCISES

1. Derive Eq. (26.2) by direct computation in the case $m = 3$. To generalize the result to arbitrary positive values of m, first note that $\boldsymbol{\phi}_j = (\Re(z_{j-1})\ \Im(z_{j-1}))^T$ with $z_j = \exp(2\pi i j/m)$, $j = 1, \ldots, m$. Start by showing that

$$
\mathbf{U}^T \mathbf{U} = \begin{pmatrix} \sum_{j=0}^{m-1} \cos^2 \frac{2\pi j}{m} & \sum_{j=0}^{m-1} \cos \frac{2\pi j}{m} \sin \frac{2\pi j}{m} \\ \sum_{j=0}^{m-1} \cos \frac{2\pi j}{m} \sin \frac{2\pi j}{m} & \sum_{j=0}^{m-1} \sin^2 \frac{2\pi j}{m} \end{pmatrix}
$$

where $\mathbf{U}$ is the frame operator defined in Eq. (26.4). Next, show that

$$
\sum_{j=0}^{m-1} z_j^2 = 0
$$

and derive the identities

$$
\cos 2\alpha = \cos^2 \alpha - \sin^2 \alpha, \quad \cos^2 \alpha = \frac{1 + \cos 2\alpha}{2}
$$

$$
\sin 2\alpha = 2 \sin \alpha \cos \alpha, \quad \sin^2 \alpha = \frac{1 + \cos 2\alpha}{2}.
$$

Hint: Use Euler's formula for the complex exponential, $\exp i\alpha = \cos \alpha + i \sin \alpha$. Use these two results to conclude that

$$
\sum_{j=0}^{m-1} \cos^2 \frac{2\pi j}{m} = \sum_{j=0}^{m-1} \sin^2 \frac{2\pi j}{m} = \frac{m}{2}
$$

$$
\sum_{j=0}^{m-1} \cos \frac{2\pi j}{m} \sin \frac{2\pi j}{m} = 0.
$$

Finally, apply Eq. (26.8).

2. †Derive Eq. (26.3).

3. Prove Eq. (26.15). Hint: Replace $\check{\mathbf{v}} - \mathbf{v}$ by $(\check{\mathbf{v}} - E[\check{\mathbf{v}}]) + (E[\check{\mathbf{v}}] - \mathbf{v})$ in the original definition of $\mathbf{C}_e$.

4. Show that if $\check{\mathbf{v}} = \mathbf{Fg}$ with $\mathbf{g} = \mathbf{Uv} + \mathbf{n}$ and $E[\mathbf{n}] = 0$ then $E[\check{\mathbf{v}}] = \mathbf{v}$.

5. Show that the score function satisfies $E[\mathbf{s}(\mathbf{v}, \mathbf{g})] = 0$. Hint: Start from the definition of the expectation

$$
E[\mathbf{s}(\mathbf{v}, \mathbf{g})] = \int \mathbf{s}(\mathbf{v}, \mathbf{g}) p(\mathbf{g}|\mathbf{v}) \, d\mathbf{g}.
$$

Plug in the definition of $\mathbf{s}$, compute the derivative and exchange it with the integral.

6. Prove Eq. (26.16). Hint: Since the estimator is unbiased,

$$
0 = E[(\check{\mathbf{v}} - \mathbf{v})^T] = \int f_{\mathbf{v}}(\mathbf{g})(\check{\mathbf{v}} - \mathbf{v})^T \, d\mathbf{g}.
$$

Now take the gradient, $\nabla_{\mathbf{v}}$, exchange with the integral sign and compute it using the product rule for derivatives. Use also the following equality: $\nabla_{\mathbf{v}} \log(f_{\mathbf{v}}(\mathbf{g})) = (\nabla_{\mathbf{v}} f_{\mathbf{v}}(\mathbf{g})) / f_{\mathbf{v}}(\mathbf{g})$.

7. Prove Eq. (26.17) by proceeding as follows. First show that the vector

$$
\mathbf{q} = \begin{pmatrix} \check{\mathbf{v}} - \mathbf{v} \\ \mathbf{s}(\mathbf{v}, \mathbf{g}) \end{pmatrix}
$$

has zero mean and covariance matrix

$$Q = \begin{pmatrix} C & I \\ I & J \end{pmatrix}.$$

Then show that $A^T Q A$ is diagonal, where

$$A = \begin{pmatrix} I & 0 \\ -J^{-1} & I \end{pmatrix}.$$

Use now the fact that $Q \geq 0$ (since it is a covariance matrix) and $J > 0$ to conclude that $C - J^{-1} \geq 0$.

8. Prove Eq. (26.18) as follows. First show that

$$\nabla_v \log(f_v(g)) = -\frac{1}{2} \nabla_v \left((g - Uv)^T C^{-1} (g - Uv) \right).$$

Then show that for two vectors a, b

$$a^T b = \mathrm{tr}\, ba^T. \tag{26.20}$$

Use this result to rewrite

$$\nabla_v \log(f_v(g)) = -\frac{1}{2} \nabla_v \mathrm{tr}\, C^{-1}(g - Uv)(g - Uv)^T.$$

Now show that

$$-\frac{1}{2} \frac{\partial}{\partial v_i} \mathrm{tr}\, C^{-1}(g - Uv)(g - Uv)^T = (Uf_i)^T C^{-1}(g - Uv),$$

where $f_i \in \mathbb{R}^m$ is the vector of zeros save a 1 in position i. Hint: Use again Eq. (26.20). This last result will allow you to complete the proof.

9. †Prove Eq. (26.19).

Neuronal Networks

OUTLINE

27.1 Hopfield Networks 382

27.2 Leaky Integrate-and-Fire Networks 383

27.3 Leaky Integrate-and-Fire Networks with Plastic Synapses 389

27.4 Hodgkin–Huxley Based Networks 392

27.5 Hodgkin–Huxley Based Networks with Plastic Synapses 397

27.6 Rate Based Networks 397

27.7 Brain Maps and Self-Organizing Maps 401

27.8 Summary and Sources 403

27.9 Exercises 404

The human brain is comprised of over 100 billion neurons, each of which receives on average 10,000 "inputs" from neighboring neurons. To tackle such complexity we naturally restrict ourselves to well-defined subnetworks of the brain. Even then, however, we are far from constructing (for lack of data as well as computational resources) detailed models that capture network architecture, cell morphology, cell biophysics, and synaptic plasticity. Most existing strategies fall into one of four large subfields; Hopfield networks, conductance based networks, rate based networks, and self-organized maps. The rate at which these areas are growing would quickly obsolete any attempt at a systematic survey. For the reader who wishes to gain hands-on experience we therefore present a guided tour, via representative examples, of the methods of each subfield.

In Hopfield networks, §27.1, each cell, at a given instant, can take on but two values, e.g., ±1. Furthermore, time evolves in discrete steps. The activity of N cells is therefore abstracted to discrete time dynamics on the vertices of the N-dimensional cube. One marches from one instant to the next by applying a threshold to a weighted sum of inputs at each cell. This permits experimentation, and often analytical treatment, with relatively large networks, but suffers in translation to biology.

The modeling of conductance based networks retains continuous time, membrane conductances, and potential, but typically sacrifices ionic machinery and/or cell morphology. The simplest approach adopts the leaky integrate-and-fire (LIF) cell model of Chapter 10 and so sacrifices both, but in a way that makes it relatively straightforward to reincorporate ion channels and/or dendrites. In §27.2 we carefully formulate and illustrate the full set of conductance and voltage equations for networks of excitatory and inhibitory LIF cells. We augment this system, in §27.3, with a learning rule that updates the synaptic weights between cells in a fashion that is spike time-dependent.

We generalize this approach, with a focus on synchrony and rhythmogenesis, to multicompartment cells with Hodgkin–Huxley type ion channels and calcium-dependent learning rules in §§27.4 and 27.5. During rhythmic network activity, a cell's firing rate typically agrees with the average firing rate of the network. In §27.6 we formulate and analyze a simple model for evolving a network's average firing rate in response to average synaptic input.

In the final section we transcend spikes and rates and consider learning rules associated with self-organized maps for evolving the weights between parametrized activity patterns. Although this ignores the bulk of the biophysics developed in the previous chapters, it nonetheless reproduces a number of the brain maps that appear during early learning, or development, of the nervous system. We concentrate here on the maps of orientation and direction preference in visual cortex.

27.1 HOPFIELD NETWORKS

The state of a Hopfield network with N cells is specified by $\mathbf{s} \in \mathbb{R}^N$ where each $s_i \in \{-1,1\}$. These two values could represent, e.g., high and low activity states of the corresponding neurons. We advance, from time j to time $j+1$, for $j = 1, 2, \ldots$, by thresholding a linear combination of state elements. In particular, state $\mathbf{s}^j$ is advanced to

$$\mathbf{s}^{j+1} = \mathrm{Hop}(\mathbf{W}\mathbf{s}^j) \quad \text{where} \quad \mathrm{Hop}(x) \equiv \begin{cases} 1 & \text{if } x > 0 \\ -1 & \text{if } x \le 0 \end{cases} \tag{27.1}$$

is applied to each component of $\mathbf{W}\mathbf{s}^j$ in the Hopfield net. Here $\mathbf{W} \in \mathbb{R}^{N \times N}$ is the synaptic weight matrix. This net can be trained to remember an input pattern $\mathbf{p} \in \{-1,1\}^N$ by setting the weights to $\mathbf{W} = \mathbf{p}\mathbf{p}^T$. In this case, proceeding from an arbitrary state $\mathbf{s}$, we find

$$\mathbf{W}\mathbf{s} = \mathbf{p}\mathbf{p}^T\mathbf{s} = \mathbf{p}(\mathbf{p}^T\mathbf{s}) = (\mathbf{p}^T\mathbf{s})\mathbf{p}$$

and so

$$\mathrm{Hop}(\mathbf{W}\mathbf{s}) = \begin{cases} \mathbf{p} & \text{if } \mathbf{p}^T\mathbf{s} > 0 \\ -\mathbf{e} & \text{if } \mathbf{p}^T\mathbf{s} = 0, \\ -\mathbf{p} & \text{if } \mathbf{p}^T\mathbf{s} < 0. \end{cases} \quad \text{where} \quad \mathbf{e} \equiv \texttt{ones(N,1)}.$$

In particular, both $\mathbf{p}$ and $-\mathbf{p}$ are *fixed points* of the associated Hopfield net in the sense that

$$\mathrm{Hop}(\mathbf{W}\mathbf{p}) = \mathbf{p} \quad \text{and} \quad \mathrm{Hop}(\mathbf{W}(-\mathbf{p})) = -\mathbf{p}.$$

Furthermore, these are the only fixed points unless $\mathbf{p}$ is balanced in the sense that $\mathbf{p}^T\mathbf{e} = 0$, in which case, $-\mathbf{e}$ is the only other fixed point. These fixed points are *attractors* in the sense that the Hopfield trajectory, Eq. (27.1), will terminate (rapidly) in one of these fixed points regardless of the initial state.

All of this generalizes nicely to multiple training patterns. In fact, if $\mathbf{p}_1$ and $\mathbf{p}_2$ are two such patterns, we set $\mathbf{P} = (\mathbf{p}_1 \ \mathbf{p}_2)$ and $\mathbf{W} = \mathbf{P}\mathbf{P}^T$. Arguing as above, we find

$$\mathbf{W}\mathbf{s} = \mathbf{P}\mathbf{P}^T\mathbf{s} = (\mathbf{s}^T\mathbf{p}_1)\mathbf{p}_1 + (\mathbf{s}^T\mathbf{p}_2)\mathbf{p}_2.$$

Evaluating Hop of this is now a much more interesting affair. If $\mathbf{p}_1$ and $\mathbf{p}_2$ are orthogonal, i.e., $\mathbf{p}_1^T\mathbf{p}_2 = 0$, then it is not hard to see that both $\pm\mathbf{p}_1$ and $\pm\mathbf{p}_2$ will be fixed points. In the nonorthogonal case the input patterns may combine to form phantom fixed points. As a simple example we consider the binary visual stimuli of Figure 27.1.

We reshape each input pattern of Figure 27.1 into a long vector and lay these into the columns of $\mathbf{P} = (\mathbf{p}_1 \ \mathbf{p}_2)$ and assemble the weight matrix $\mathbf{W} = \mathbf{P}\mathbf{P}^T$ as above. We then present the network with noisy copies of "I" and "O," as in Figure 27.2, and record the next state.

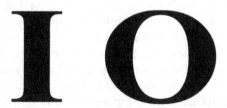

FIGURE 27.1   Binary visual patterns to be learned by a Hopfield network. Each of these letters is comprised of a 67-by-71 rectangular field of pixels, where black $= 1$ and white $= -1$. (`hop.m`)

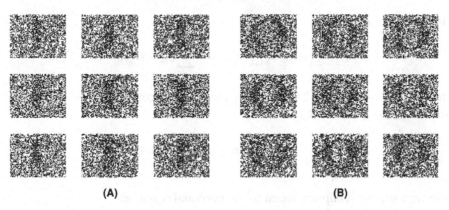

FIGURE 27.2 **A.** Nine noisy copies of "I" that the Hopfield network successfully identified. In other words, iterated application of Hop converged towards the left pattern in Figure 27.1. **B.** Nine noisy copies of "O" that the Hopfield network successfully identified. (hop.m)

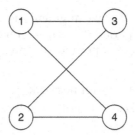

FIGURE 27.3 A four-cell network with bidirectional synapses between nodes 1 and 3, 1 and 4, 2 and 3, and 2 and 4.

We should note that fixed points are not the only possible attractors. Indeed, it is quite possible that the network may "oscillate" by periodically bouncing between several states. As a concrete example we consider the network of Figure 27.3. If we assume reciprocal unit weights along each of the edges in Figure 27.3 then we arrive at the symmetric weight matrix

$$\mathbf{W} = \begin{pmatrix} 0 & 0 & 1 & 1 \\ 0 & 0 & 1 & 1 \\ 1 & 1 & 0 & 0 \\ 1 & 1 & 0 & 0 \end{pmatrix}.$$

If initially we excite cells 1 and 2 then $\mathbf{s}^1 = (1\ 1\ -1\ -1)$. It then follows that $\mathbf{s}^2 = -\mathbf{s}^1$ and $\mathbf{s}_3 = -\mathbf{s}_2 = \mathbf{s}_1$ and we say that the network has an attractor of period 2. We shall see in Exercise 2 that this example captures the general result, in the sense that no undirected Hopfield net may have an attractor with period greater than 2.

27.2 LEAKY INTEGRATE-AND-FIRE NETWORKS

We now move from one discrete, on/off, variable to three continuous variables per cell: voltage as well as synaptic excitatory and inhibitory conductances. We begin with the simple two-cell network of Figure 27.4.

The circuit in Figure 27.4 is comprised of two cells driven by two excitatory conductances. We denote the membrane potentials by V_1 and V_2 and conductances by $g_{E,1}$ and $g_{E,2}$. The circuit is driven by an excitatory input train that spikes at $T_{inp} \equiv \{T_{inp}^n : n = 1, 2, \ldots\}$. Each such spike increments $g_{E,1}$, the excitatory conductance at cell 1, by a fixed amount, w^{inp}/τ_E. Between such spikes we assume that $g_{E,1}$ returns to zero at the fixed rate τ_E. In other words, we suppose that

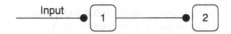

FIGURE 27.4 The smallest network, consisting of two cells driven by two excitatory conductances.

$g_{E,1}$ is governed by the differential equation

$$\tau_E g'_{E,1}(t) = -g_{E,1}(t) + w^{inp} \sum_n \delta(t - T^n_{inp}). \tag{27.2}$$

Similarly, the excitatory conductance at cell 2 is driven by the spikes of cell 1, at times $T_1 \equiv \{T^n_1 : n = 1, 2, \ldots\}$ and with weight w_{21}. It follows that $g_{E,2}$ is governed by

$$\tau_E g'_{E,2}(t) = -g_{E,2}(t) + w_{21} \sum_n \delta(t - T^n_1). \tag{27.3}$$

These conductances in turn supply synaptic current to the potential equations

$$C_m V'_i(t) = g_L(V_L - V_i(t)) + g_{E,i}(t)(V^{syn}_E - V_i(t)), \quad \text{while } V_i(t) < V_{thr} \tag{27.4}$$

and cell i is not refractory. When $V_i(t)$ exceeds V_{thr} we augment the spike time sequence, T_i, and we reset $V_i(t)$ to a fixed reset potential, V_{res}, for a set refractory period, t_{ref}. These spike times couple the conductance and potential equations. We decouple this system by choosing a time step, dt, and specifying an order of operation. In particular, we adopt the marching scheme:

1. check for an input spike at the **current** time, t, and for network spikes from the **previous** time, $t - dt$,
2. update conductances based on the input spikes and network spikes recorded in (1),
3. update potentials, record spikes, and return to (1).

In our graphical representation of the potential, e.g., Figure 27.5, the presence of a spike can be inferred from the hard reset to V_{res}. Accordingly, if cell 1 receives an input spike in the interval $(j dt, [j+1)dt)$ then the trapezoid rule on (27.2), applied to $g^j_{E,1} \approx g_{E,1}((j-1)dt)$, requires

$$\tau_E(g^{j+1}_{E,1} - g^j_{E,1}) = -(g^{j+1}_{E,1} + g^j_{E,1})dt/2 + w^{inp}$$

which may be rearranged to read

$$g^{j+1}_{E,1} = a_E g^j_{E,1} + b_E w^{inp}$$

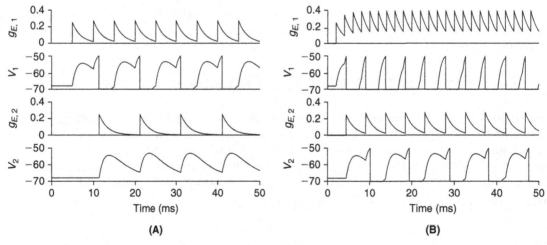

FIGURE 27.5 Response of the two-cell net to a low frequency periodic input with period, $P = 5$ ms, and a high frequency, $P = 2$ ms, stimulus. Voltage is in mV and conductance in mS/cm^2. The stimuli and cell are parametrized in Eqs. (27.6) and (27.7). In each case we see that cell 1 fires following every second input spike. In the low frequency case the resultant spike rate of cell 1 is not sufficient to bring cell 2 to threshold. (twocell.m)

where

$$a_E = \frac{2\tau_E - dt}{2\tau_E + dt} \quad \text{and} \quad b_E = \frac{2}{2\tau_E + dt}.$$

Similarly, if cell 1 was found to spike in the previous interval, i.e., in $[(j-1)dt, jdt)$, then we update the conductance via

$$g_{E,2}^{j+1} = a_E g_{E,2}^{j} + b_E w_{21}.$$

If cell 1 did not fire in that interval then simply $g_{E,2}^{j+1} = a_E g_{E,2}^{j}$. Regarding the potentials, when cell i is nonrefractory, i.e., when

$$(j+1)dt - \acute{T}_i > t_{ref} \tag{27.5}$$

where $\acute{T}_i$ is the last time that cell i spiked, the trapezoid rule in Eq. (27.4) requires

$$V_i^{j+1} = \frac{(2C_m/dt - (g_L + g_{E,i}^j))V_i^j + 2g_L V_L + (g_{E,i}^{j+1} + g_{E,i}^j)V_E^{syn}}{2C_m/dt + g_L + g_{E,i}^{j+1}}.$$

If Eq. (27.5) is not satisfied we enforce $V_i^{j+1} = V_{res}$. We have coded this update procedure in `twocell.m` and illustrate our findings, see Figure 27.5, for periodic input trains that spike at

$$T_{inp}^n = nP, \quad n = 1, 2, \ldots \tag{27.6}$$

where P is the period (in ms). Throughout we shall use

$$\tau_E = 2 \text{ ms}, \ V_E^{syn} = 0 \text{ mV}, \ g_L = 0.3 \text{ mS/cm}^2, \ V_L = -68 \text{ mV}, \ C_m = 1 \ \mu\text{F/cm}^2,$$
$$w^{inp} = 0.5 \text{ mS ms/cm}^2, \ w_{21} = 0.5 \text{ mS ms/cm}^2, \ t_{ref} = 3 \text{ ms}, \ V_{thr} = -50, \ V_{res} = -70 \text{ mV}. \tag{27.7}$$

As most cells receive input from more than one neighbor we move on to the three-cell net of Figure 27.6. We retain periodic input and add to the parameter set above $w_{32} = w_{31} = 0.5$. We have coded the subsequent model in `threecell.m`. This code is a considerable refinement of the two-cell version. In particular, we have laid the weights in a weight matrix, **W**, and we have "vectorized" the computations of both g_E and V. We illustrate its use in Figure 27.7.

We next suppose, see Figure 27.8, that cell 3 inhibits cell 1. This new conductance is governed by

$$g_{I,1}^{j+1} = a_I g_{I,1}^j + b_I w_{inh} s_3^j$$

where $s_3^j \equiv \mathbb{1}(V_3^j - V_{th})$ is one if cell 3 spiked at time j, and is zero otherwise (recall the definition of the Heaviside function, $\mathbb{1}$, Eq. (1.6)). In addition, as in the excitatory case,

$$a_I = \frac{2\tau_I - dt}{2\tau_I + dt} \quad \text{and} \quad b_I = \frac{2}{2\tau_I + dt}.$$

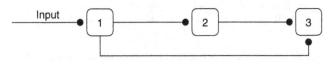

FIGURE 27.6　A three-cell network.

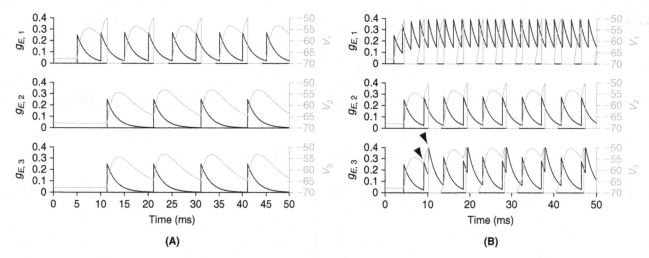

FIGURE 27.7 Response of the three-cell net to low frequency, $P = 5$ ms (**A**), and high frequency, $P = 2$ ms (**B**), periodic stimulus. Observe in the lower right panel that the third conductance receives a double kick (arrowheads) as cell 2 fires just after each second spike of cell 1. (threecell.m)

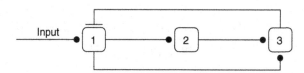

FIGURE 27.8 A three-cell network with feedback inhibition.

The potential at cell 1 now follows

$$V_1^{j+1} = \frac{\left(2C_m/dt - \left(g_L + g_{E,1}^j + g_{I,1}^j\right)\right)V_1^j + 2g_L V_L + \left(g_{E,1}^{j+1} + g_{E,1}^j\right)V_E^{syn} + \left(g_{I,1}^{j+1} + g_{I,1}^j\right)V_I^{syn}}{2C_m/dt + g_L + g_{E,1}^{j+1} + g_{I,1}^{j+1}}.$$

We set

$$\tau_I = 2 \text{ ms}, \quad V_I^{syn} = -70 \text{ mV}, \quad \text{and} \quad w_{inh} = 3 \text{ mS ms/cm}^2,$$

and arrive at the trajectories of Figure 27.9.

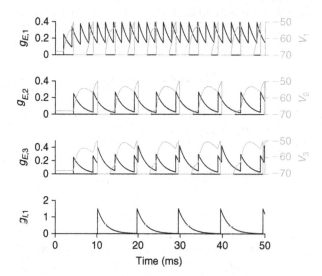

FIGURE 27.9 Response of the network in Figure 27.8 to high frequency, $P = 2$ ms, periodic stimulus. We note that cell 3 now staggers the firing of cell 1. (threecellI.m)

In the simulation of large networks, one computes, but does not typically report, the conductances and potentials at each time step. Rather one reports the times at which each cell spikes. We have trimmed `threecell.m` and `threecellI.m` down to `threecellrast.m` and `threecellIrast.m` and illustrated their use in Figure 27.10.

Proceeding to larger networks, we suppose that $\mathbf{W} \in \mathbb{R}^{n \times n}$ denotes the matrix of weights between n excitatory cells and $\mathbf{W}_{inp} \in \mathbb{R}^{n \times n}$ denotes the weight of input spikes upon excitatory cells, then, arguing as above, the network equations take the form

$$g_E^{j+1} = a_E g_E^j + b_E \left(\mathbf{W} s^j + \mathbf{W}_{inp} s_{inp}^{j+1} \right)$$

$$v^{j+1} = \frac{(2C_m/dt - (g_L + g_E^j)) v^j + 2g_L V_L + (g_E^{j+1} + g_E^j) V_E^{syn}}{2C_m/dt + g_L + g_E^{j+1}}$$

(27.8)

$$s^{j+1} = \mathbb{1}(V^{j+1} - V_{thr})$$

where all operations in the voltage update are elementwise. Here s^j and s_{inp}^j are vectors with binary, i.e., $\{0,1\}$, elements. We set $s_{inp,i}^j = 1$ if cell i receives an input spike at time jdt. Similarly, via the Heaviside function $\mathbb{1}$, we set $s_i^j = 1$ if cell i spiked (exceeded threshold) at time jdt. We have coded this in `Enet.m` with the help of MATLAB's `sprand` function, which generates sparse matrices from the uniform distribution on $[0,1]$ with a prescribed fraction of nonzeros.

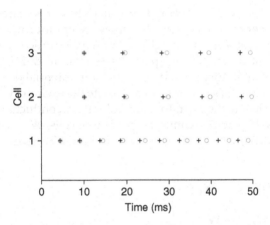

FIGURE 27.10 Raster plots of spike times of the three-cell net without (black plus) and with (red circle) inhibition, subject to the same high frequency, $P = 2$ ms, periodic stimulus. (`threecellrast.m` and `threecellIrast.m`)

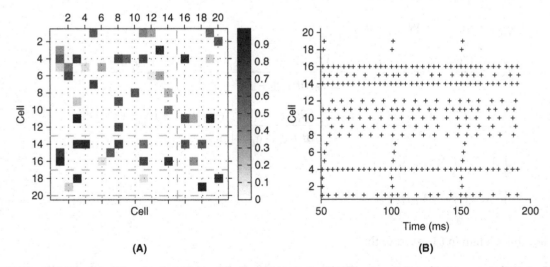

(A)

(B)

FIGURE 27.11 Weight matrix (**A**) and spikes (**B**) in a 20-cell excitatory net with 15% connectivity subject to a periodic train, $P = 50$ ms, with $W_{inp} = 1$, delivered to the first 20% of the cells. The red dashed lines in **A** indicate the three rows and single column with vanishing weights. (`Enet.m`)

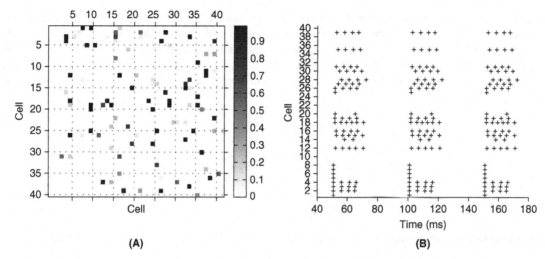

FIGURE 27.12 Weight matrix (**A**) and spikes (**B**) in a 40-cell excitatory net with 7% connectivity subject to a periodic train, $P = 50$ ms, with $W_{inp} = 1$, delivered to the first 20% of the cells. (Enet.m)

Regarding the weight matrix of Figure 27.11A, note that cell 15 has *no* squares in its column and hence has no impact on the behavior of the net. Every row has a nonzero entry, except for rows 13, 17, and 20. So in fact every cell except those three receives input from at least one neighbor. We have stripped the diagonal clean and hence no cell excites itself. These nets are capable of generating rich patterns, see Figure 27.12B.

We now introduce a population of inhibitory cells. We denote their potentials by V_I and those of the excitatory cells by V_E. Now each cell has two conductances; g_{EE} and g_{IE} will denote the excitatory and inhibitory conductances on an excitatory cell while g_{EI} and g_{II} will denote the excitatory and inhibitory conductances on an inhibitory cell. Coupling occurs through the weight matrices; $\mathbf{W}_{EE}$ which connects E cells to E cells, $\mathbf{W}_{EI}$ which connects E cells to I cells, $\mathbf{W}_{IE}$ which connects I cells to E cells, and $\mathbf{W}_{II}$ which connects I cells to I cells. The subsequent network equations are

$$g_{EE}^{j+1} = a_E\, g_{EE}^j + b_E\left(\mathbf{W}_{EE} s_E^j + \mathbf{W}_{EE}^{inp} s_{inp,E}^{j+1}\right)$$

$$g_{EI}^{j+1} = a_E\, g_{EI}^j + b_E\left(\mathbf{W}_{EI} s_E^j + \mathbf{W}_{EI}^{inp} s_{inp,E}^{j+1}\right)$$

$$g_{II}^{j+1} = a_I\, g_{II}^j + b_I\left(\mathbf{W}_{II} s_I^j + \mathbf{W}_{II}^{inp} s_{inp,I}^{j+1}\right)$$

$$g_{IE}^{j+1} = a_I\, g_{IE}^j + b_I\left(\mathbf{W}_{IE} s_I^j + \mathbf{W}_{IE}^{inp} s_{inp,I}^{j+1}\right)$$

$$V_E^{j+1} = \frac{\left(2C_m/dt - \left(g_L + g_{EE}^j + g_{IE}^j\right)\right)V_E^j + 2g_L V_L + \left(g_{EE}^{j+1} + g_{EE}^j\right)V_E^{syn} + \left(g_{IE}^{j+1} + g_{IE}^j\right)V_I^{syn}}{2C_m/dt + g_L + g_{EE}^{j+1} + g_{IE}^{j+1}}$$

$$V_I^{j+1} = \frac{\left(2C_m/dt - \left(g_L + g_{II}^j + g_{EI}^j\right)\right)V_I^j + 2g_L V_L + \left(g_{II}^{j+1} + g_{II}^j\right)V_I^{syn} + \left(g_{EI}^{j+1} + g_{EI}^j\right)V_E^{syn}}{2C_m/dt + g_L + g_{II}^{j+1} + g_{EI}^{j+1}}$$

$$s_E^{j+1} = \mathbb{1}\left(V_E^{j+1} - V_{thr}\right)$$

$$s_I^{j+1} = \mathbb{1}\left(V_I^{j+1} - V_{thr}\right).$$

We have coded this system in EInet.m with

$$\tau_I = 1\,\text{ms} \quad \text{and} \quad V_I^{syn} = -70\,\text{mV}$$

and illustrate its findings in Figure 27.13.

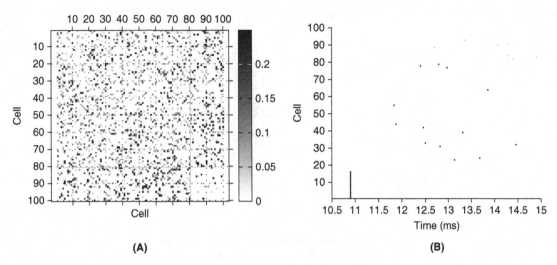

FIGURE 27.13 Weight matrices (**A**) and spikes (**B**) in an EI net with 80 E cells and 20 I cells. **A.** W_{EE}, W_{EI}, and W_{IE} each have 25% connectivity while W_{II} has 5%. Red lines differentiate the respective weight matrices. **B.** The spikes (black for excitatory and red for inhibitory cells) associated with simultaneous input delivered to the excitatory conductances of the first 16 E cells, causing them to fire synchronously 10.9 ms after the beginning of the simulation. (EInet.m)

27.3 LEAKY INTEGRATE-AND-FIRE NETWORKS WITH PLASTIC SYNAPSES

Spikes not only increment transient synaptic conductances, but also impact the associated elements of the synaptic weights. In §§12.6, 12.7, and 13.4 we discussed a number of biophysical mechanisms that are suspected to underlie such synaptic plasticity. In this section we will implement and analyze a Hebbian rule that goes by the name *spike time-dependent plasticity*, or STDP, which has been characterized in several experimental preparations. More precisely, if $W_{i,j}$ is the weight of cell j upon cell i then STDP dictates that we increment $W_{i,j}$ when cell j spikes before cell i and that we decrement $W_{i,j}$ when cell i spikes before cell j. The size of the weight change is a function of the time between spikes and the current weights. Let us begin with the simple four-cell net of Figure 27.14.

We excite cell 1 every 40 ms. This activity propagates quickly to fire cells 2 and 4 and eventually cell 3. As 1 fires 4 we expect this weight, $W_{4,1}$, to increase, and as 3 does not fire 4 we expect $W_{4,3}$ to decrease. To do this, when a cell fires we potentiate the weights from presynaptic cells that have recently fired and depress the weights to postsynaptic cells that have recently fired. We quantify "recent" by adopting a scheme that is in line with observations that the degree of both potentiation and depression decays exponentially with the interval between the presynaptic and postsynaptic spikes, see Figure 27.15.

As a concrete example, we denote by T_1 and T_3 the most recent times at which cells 1 and 3 fired, respectively. If cell 2 is the next to fire, at time T_2, we update the associated conductances via

$$W_{2,1}(T_2^+) = W_{2,1}(T_2^-) + A_P \exp((T_1 - T_2)/\tau_P)$$
$$W_{3,2}(T_2^+) = W_{3,2}(T_2^-) - A_D \exp((T_3 - T_2)/\tau_D). \tag{27.9}$$

When called repeatedly these increments may lead to runaway weight loss and gain. There are a number of remedies, e.g., Oja's Rule of Eq. (14.14), for this. The simplest is to set to zero any weights that become negative and to set to W_{max} all weights that exceed this specified maximum. A smoother way of enforcing these bounds is to replace Eq. (27.9) with

$$W_{2,1}(T_2^+) = W_{2,1}(T_2^-) + A_P \exp((T_1 - T_2)/\tau_P)(W_{max} - W_{2,1}(T_2^-))$$
$$W_{3,2}(T_2^+) = W_{3,2}(T_2^-) - A_D \exp((T_3 - T_2)/\tau_D)W_{3,2}(T_2^-). \tag{27.10}$$

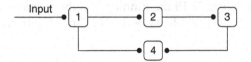

FIGURE 27.14 A four-cell net.

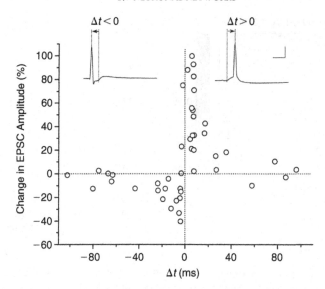

FIGURE 27.15 Spike time-dependent plasticity in cultures of dissociated rat hippocampal neurons. The change in the (peak) amplitude of the Excitatory Postsynaptic Current (EPSC), at subthreshold glutamatergic synapses 20–30 minutes after repetitive correlated spiking, is plotted as a function of Δt, the time interval (see inset) between the onset of the EPSC and the peak of the postsynaptic action potential. Correlated spiking was produced by stimulating the presynaptic cell with 60 suprathreshold pulses at 1 Hz and stimulating the postsynaptic cell at a set time within each cycle. The scale bars in the inset denote 10 ms and 50 mV. These data suggest potentiation of the form $A_P \exp(-\Delta t/\tau_P)$ when pre precedes post, i.e., when $\Delta t > 0$, and depression of the form $A_D \exp(\Delta t/\tau_D)$ when post precedes pre, i.e., when $\Delta t < 0$. From Bi and Poo (1998).

Another advantage of this procedure is that now the maximum adjustments, A_P and A_D, are dimensionless. Regarding the implementation of these general rules, if our marching scheme determines that cell k fires in the interval $[j\mathrm{d}t, (j+1)\mathrm{d}t)$ we potentiate its presynaptic weights and depress its postsynaptic weights via

$$W_{k,k_{pre}}^{j+1} = W_{k,k_{pre}}^{j} + A_P \exp\left((T_{k_{pre}} - (j+1)\mathrm{d}t)/\tau_P\right)\left(W_{max} - W_{k,k_{pre}}^{j}\right)$$

$$W_{k_{post},k}^{j+1} = W_{k_{post},k}^{j} - A_D \exp\left((T_{k_{post}} - (j+1)\mathrm{d}t)/\tau_D\right)W_{k_{post},k}^{j}.$$

We have coded these rules for the four-cell net, with

$$A_P = A_D = 0.3 \quad \text{and} \quad \tau_P = \tau_D = 10 \text{ ms} \tag{27.11}$$

and initial weights

$$W_{2,1} = W_{3,2} = W_{4,1} = 0.75 \quad \text{and} \quad W_{4,3} = 0.7 \text{ mS ms/cm}^2, \tag{27.12}$$

and illustrate our findings in Figure 27.16. We next apply this learning rule on E-to-E connections of the large net studied in Figure 27.13A. We suppose

$$\tau_E = 2, \ \tau_I = 1, \ \tau_P = 5, \ \tau_D = 5 \text{ ms}, \ A_P = 0.1, \ A_D = 0.3, \ W_{EE,max} = 0.2 \text{ mS ms/cm}^2,$$

and as above drive the first 20% of the E cells with the same synchronous input delivered to their excitatory conductances and repeated with a period of 100 ms. We permit STDP to act on the E-to-E connections and arrive at the new weights in Figure 27.17. Since the gray-scale weight plots of Figures 27.13 and 27.17 are not the best means of tracking weight shifts over time, we report in Figure 27.18 the running weight distribution. To the question, "What has the network learned?" we answer that it has learned to associate the "input pattern," comprised of simultaneous firing of cells

$$\text{in} \equiv \{1:16\},$$

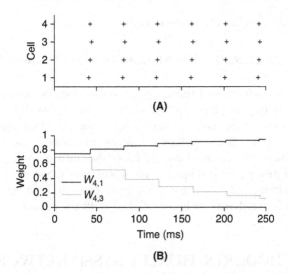

FIGURE 27.16 Spike (**A**) and weight (**B**) evolution via STDP in the four-cell net parametrized by Eqs. (27.11) and (27.12). We see indeed that the direct connection, $W_{4,1}$, is strengthened (up to $W_{max} = 1$) while the indirect connection, $W_{4,3}$, is diminished. (`fourcell.m`)

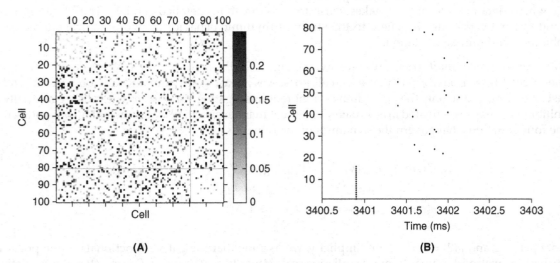

FIGURE 27.17 Weights (**A**) and spikes (**B**) after 5 seconds of STDP learning with $dt = 0.02$ ms. **A**. On comparing to the initial weights in Figure 27.13A we notice a striking depression in the weights between input cells (for they are firing independently of their network neighbors) and a striking potentiation of the input to output connections (columns 1:16 and selected rows between 20 and 80). **B**. The resulting spike pattern associated with input at $t = 3.4$ seconds. (`EInetH.m`)

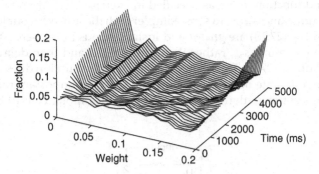

FIGURE 27.18 Running histogram of E-to-E synaptic weights for the network of Figure 27.13. As in the four-cell example, we see that most weights shift to the two extremes over time. (`EInetH.m`)

with the output pattern of Figure 27.17B, i.e., the firing of cells

$$\text{out} \equiv \{22:24, 26, 31:33, 39, 41, 42, 44, 48, 49, 51, 55, 64, 66, 77:79\}$$

within the next few milliseconds. In order to test the strength of this association we measure the learned network's ability to complete incomplete input. In particular, we systematically drop input spikes and count the average number of dropped output spikes. We implement this test in `EInetComp.m` and find that dropping one input spike produces no loss in output fidelity. Dropping two input spikes produces an average loss of 4% of the output spikes and dropping three input spikes produces an average loss of 34% of the output spikes. Each average is computed over $16!/(d!(16-d)!)$ random trials of d dropped input spikes. We see no loss when $d=1$ and substantial loss when $d=3$. At the intermediate stage we note that $d=2$ produces 12.5% input error and yet our output is only off by 4%. In that sense, STDP has endowed the random network of Figure 27.13A with the power of "pattern completion."

27.4 HODGKIN–HUXLEY BASED NETWORKS

The leaky integrate-and-fire setting provides a close to minimal model of the salient properties of a network. In instances where there remain large gaps in our understanding of network architecture, cell morphology and electrophysiology, this approach allows one to probe hypotheses concerning the behavior of large ensembles of cells. In settings where data are available it makes sense to consider more detailed models. The literature is vast and growing and so we restrict ourselves here to the study of rhythmic behavior in two canonical situations, namely, mutual inhibition and mutual excitation.

Oscillations via reciprocal inhibition. We consider, see Figure 27.19, a pair of driven Morris Lecar cells that inhibit one another. Recall from Exercise 5.11 that each cell possesses a leak, potassium and calcium current and that the latter is fast activating and so only the potassium current requires a gating variable, n. The cells are mutually coupled through inhibitory synapses activated in a voltage-dependent manner specified by the instantaneous gating functional $s_\infty(V)$. The four equations that govern the dynamics of the two cells are

$$
\begin{aligned}
C_m V_i'(t) &+ \overline{g}_{Ca} m_\infty(V_i)(V_i - V_{Ca}) + \overline{g}_K n_i(V_i - V_K) + g_{Cl}(V_i - V_L) \\
&+ w_i s_\infty(V_{p(i)})(V_i - V_{syn}) = I_{stim} \\
n_i'(t) &= (n_\infty(V_i) - n_i)/\tau_n(V_i) \quad i = 1, 2.
\end{aligned}
\tag{27.13}
$$

Furthermore $p(1) = 2$ and $p(2) = 1$, and, for simplicity, we assume that the gating functionals of the potassium and calcium currents as well as the synaptic one are all identical sigmoids, $n_\infty(V) = s_\infty(V) = m_\infty(V)$. The synaptic weights and reversal potential are

$$w_1 = w_2 = 30 \ \mu S/cm^2 \quad \text{and} \quad V_{syn} = -80 \ mV, \tag{27.14}$$

and the remaining constants and functionals are as specified in Exercise 5.11. Although this model exhibits complex action potentials, its synaptic conductances are in a sense simpler than those used in our leaky integrate-and-fire model. More precisely, the synapses in Eq. (27.13) are *graded* and instantaneous in the sense that the presynaptic potential $V_{p(i)}$ is merely passed through a sigmoid, s_∞, rather than thresholded and then delayed via integration through a conductance equation, like that of Eq. (27.2). Thus, graded synaptic transmission does not require presynaptic action potentials. It is ubiquitous in invertebrate nervous systems and plays an important role in vertebrates as well, e.g., at the synapses made by photoreceptors with their target neurons, the bipolar cells of the retina.

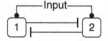

FIGURE 27.19 Using reciprocal graded inhibition to build an oscillator.

We approximate Eq. (27.13) via the hybrid Euler scheme

$$n_i^j = \frac{\tau_n\left(V_i^{j-1}\right)n_i^{j-1} + n_\infty\left(V_i^{j-1}\right)dt}{dt + \tau_n\left(V_i^{j-1}\right)}$$

(27.15)

$$V_i^j = \frac{(C_m/dt)V_i^{j-1} + \overline{g}_{Ca}m_\infty\left(V_i^{j-1}\right)V_{Ca} + \overline{g}_K n_i^j V_K + g_{Cl}V_L + w_i s_\infty\left(V_{p(i)}^{j-1}\right)V_{syn} + I_{stim}^j}{(C_m/dt) + \overline{g}_{Ca}m_\infty\left(V_i^{j-1}\right) + \overline{g}_K n_i^j + g_{Cl} + w_i s_\infty\left(V_{p(i)}^{j-1}\right)}$$

and illustrate first, see Figure 27.20, that each cell, in isolation, oscillates when driven by current in a particular interval. That interval corresponds to the values of I_{stim} for which the gating nullcline, $n = m_\infty(V)$ (black dashed "sigmoid" in Figure 27.20B) intersects the voltage nullcline,

$$n = f(V) \equiv \frac{I_{stim} - \overline{g}_{Ca}m_\infty(V)(V - V_{Ca}) - g_{Cl}(V - V_{Cl})}{\overline{g}_K(V - V_K)}$$

(27.16)

(black dotted "cubic" in Figure 27.20) on the increasing branch of f. In analyzing network behavior it will be useful to consider the inhibited nullcline

$$n = F(V) \equiv \frac{I_{stim} - \overline{g}_{Ca}m_\infty(V)(V - V_{Ca}) - g_{Cl}(V - V_{Cl}) - w(V - V_{syn})}{\overline{g}_K(V - V_K)}.$$

(27.17)

Figure 27.21 depicts the membrane potential trajectories of two coupled Morris Lecar cells under low current stimulation. In the subsequent three Figures 27.22–27.24, we illustrate that slight changes in I_{stim} are sufficient to switch the network between four quite distinct regimes. Each of these oscillatory patterns are highly dependent on the coupling weights, w_1 and w_2 specified in Eq. (27.14). In §27.5 we will investigate means for the self-tuning of these weights.

The Pinksy–Rinzel CA3 network. We construct a network comprised of N two-compartment E cells of Eq. (10.8). We denote the network adjacency matrix by **A**. It is a binary, $\{0,1\}$, matrix for which $A_{ij} = 1$ if cell j is presynaptic to cell i. For the small circuit of Figure 27.25, e.g.,

$$\mathbf{A} = \begin{pmatrix} 0 & 0 \\ 1 & 0 \end{pmatrix}.$$

We suppose that each dendritic compartment has both AMPA and NMDA receptors. The vector representing total synaptic current is then

$$\mathbf{I}_{syn} = \mathbf{I}_{AMPA} + \mathbf{I}_{NMDA}$$

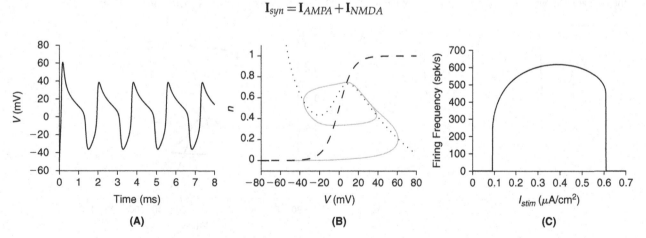

(A) (B) (C)

FIGURE 27.20 **A, B.** The response of a single Morris Lecar cell to constant current injection, $I_{stim} = 0.55 \ \mu A/cm^2$. The voltage trace is plotted in A and the full phase trajectory (solid red) in B. Also in B we have plotted the gating nullcline, $n = m_\infty(V)$ (black dashed "sigmoid"), and the voltage nullcline, Eq. (27.16) (black dotted "cubic"). The cell responds in an oscillatory fashion to those I_{stim} for which the nullclines intersect on the increasing branch of f. We quantify this in panel **C**. (ml1pp.m and ml1.m)

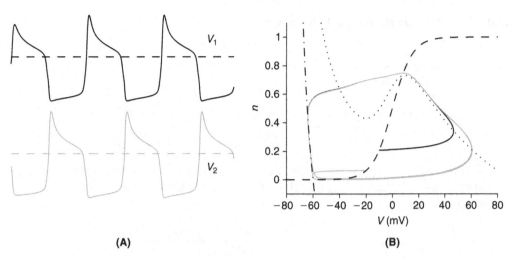

(A)   **(B)**

FIGURE 27.21   The voltages responses (**A**), and phase plane (**B**) of the coupled system with $I_{stim} = 0.55 \ \mu A/cm^2$ delivered to each cell. The time and voltage scales in **A** are the same as in Figure 27.20A. The two solid traces in **B** are the respective trajectories of cell 1 and cell 2. The dashed and dotted curves are the two nullclines of Figure 27.20B, while the dash-dot curve is the inhibited nullcline of Eq. (27.17). We note that cell 1 fires first. Its voltage then declines gradually until the phase trajectory nears the maximum of f, at which point the voltage declines rapidly, hence releasing cell 2 from inhibition. Skinner et al. (1994) refer to this mechanism as "intrinsic release." (m12.m)

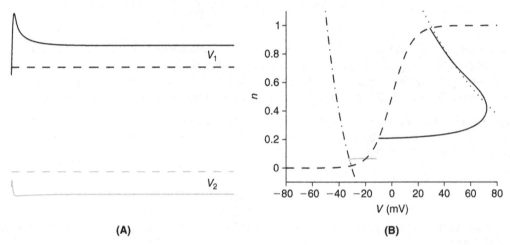

(A)   **(B)**

FIGURE 27.22   As we increase I_{stim} we enter a regime of bistability with one cell resting at a high state and the other resting at a low state. Here, the voltages responses (**A**), and phase plane (**B**) of the coupled system are depicted for $I_{stim} = 1.55 \ \mu A/cm^2$. (m12.m)

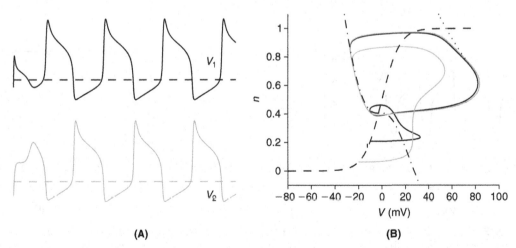

(A)   **(B)**

FIGURE 27.23   Voltages responses (**A**), and phase plane (**B**) of the coupled system with additional current, here $I_{stim} = 2.55 \ \mu A/cm^2$. We see that network oscillation resumes and, as the inhibited cell slowly depolarizes, the phase trajectory nears a minimum of the inhibited nullcline, F, and escapes its inhibition. Skinner et al. (1994) refer to this mechanism as "intrinsic escape." (m12.m)

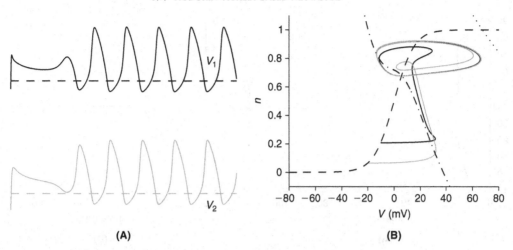

(A)   **(B)**

FIGURE 27.24 Voltages responses (**A**), and phase plane (**B**) of the coupled system as we inject still more current, here $I_{stim} = 3.05\,\mu\text{A}/\text{cm}^2$. We find that the lower branch of the inhibited nullcline, F, crosses the synaptic threshold, $V_{th} = 0$. Hence, as the voltage of the inhibited cell increases past V_{th} it forces the trajectory of the free cell to follow the inhibited nullcline, and so permit the former to escape from inhibition. Skinner et al. (1994) refer to this mechanism as "synaptic escape." (m12.m)

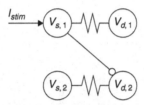

FIGURE 27.25 A pair of two-compartment cells, with current injection into the somatic compartment of cell 1 and an excitatory synaptic connection to the dendritic compartment of cell 2 from the somatic compartment of cell 1. Compare with Figure 10.10A.

where the AMPA current into the ith cell is

$$I_{AMPA,i}(t) = \bar{g}_{AMPA} x_i(t)(V_{d,i}(t) - V_{syn}), \quad \mathbf{x}' = \mathbf{A}\mathbb{1}(\mathbf{V}_s(t) - V_{\theta,x}) - \mathbf{x}/\tau_x, \quad V_{\theta,x} = 20\text{ mV}, \quad \tau_x = 2\text{ ms} \tag{27.18}$$

and the associated NMDA current is

$$I_{NMDA,i}(t) = \bar{g}_{NMDA} y_i(t) M(V_{d,i}(t))(V_{d,i}(t) - V_{syn}), \quad \mathbf{y}' = \mathbf{A}\mathbb{1}(\mathbf{V}_s(t) - V_{\theta,y}) - \mathbf{y}/\tau_y, \quad V_{\theta,y} = 10\text{ mV}, \quad \tau_y = 150\text{ ms.} \tag{27.19}$$

The function M encodes the voltage-dependent magnesium block via

$$M(V) = \frac{1}{1 + 0.28\exp(-0.062(V - 60))},$$

a simple variant of Eq. (9.20). The parameters that govern the time course of the AMPA and NMDA conductances, Eqs. (27.18) and (27.19), are chosen to mimic a rapid rise and rapid fall in the former as opposed to a slow rise and slow fall in the latter. We suppose that each y_i in Eq. (27.19) saturates, i.e., may not exceed, 125. In addition we set

$$\bar{g}_{AMPA} = 0.0045, \quad \bar{g}_{NMDA} = 0.014\text{ mS}/\text{cm}^2, \quad \text{and} \quad V_{syn} = 60\text{ mV}, \tag{27.20}$$

and, as in §10.3, we deliver a tonic current of $-0.5\,\mu\text{A}/\text{cm}^2$ to each soma. Into the first soma we inject an additional short current pulse and illustrate the response in Figure 27.26. We now consider large random networks of such cells.

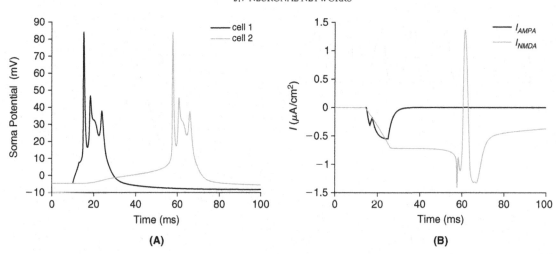

FIGURE 27.26 Response of the two-cell net of Figure 27.25 to transient current injection, $10\,\mathbb{1}_{(10,13)}(t)\ \mu\text{A/cm}^2$, into the soma of cell 1. The single cell parameters are as specified in Exercise 10.8 and the synaptic parameters in Eq. (27.20). The time step $dt = 0.01$ ms. **A.** The two soma potentials. **B.** The AMPA and NMDA currents in the dendritic compartment of cell 2. The AMPA current is confined, in time, to the burst in cell 1 while the NMDA current, also activated by this burst, is then further amplified by the subsequent burst in cell 2. Compare with Figure 9.11. (hyEprnetdemo.m)

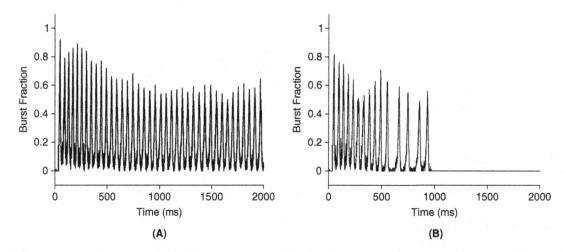

FIGURE 27.27 Response of a random 100-cell, 20% dense, network of Pinsky–Rinzel cells to transient current injection, $30\,\mathbb{1}_{(10,13)}(t)\ \mu\text{A/cm}^2$, into the soma of cell 1. The single cell parameters are as specified in Exercise 10.8 and the synaptic parameters as in Eq. (27.20), except $\overline{g}_{NMDA} = 0.007$ in (**A**) and $\overline{g}_{NMDA} = 0.005\ \text{mS/cm}^2$ in (**B**). (hyEprnet.m)

Application to epileptic rhythmic activity. Rhythmic activity across populations of neurons is thought to play an important role in the processing of sensory information (see Figure 10.6) as well as in diseases such as epilepsy. During epileptic seizures for instance, neurons of the hippocampus tend to fire rhythmic bursts of action potentials synchronized across a large neural population. Rhythmic activity is also well documented in the olfactory system of vertebrates and invertebrates for instance. We now investigate, in Figures 27.27 and 27.28, the roles played by the AMPA and NMDA conductances in rhythmogenesis in large random networks. In each case we suppose that there are $N = 100$ cells and that each cell receives input from approximately 20 of its neighbors. Rather than tracking individual spikes we instead record the fraction of bursting cells, i.e., the fraction of cells with soma potential in excess of 20 mV. We see that both the network frequency and its ability to sustain rhythms is highly dependent on the NMDA conductance. We next exhibit the impact of blocking AMPA receptors after rhythmogenesis. We note that the rhythms of Figures 27.27 and 27.28 emerge from the cell and synapse models and the number, but not the pattern, of E-to-E connections. Rhythms are, of course, also initiated and modulated by inhibition. In Exercise 7 we investigate the role of inhibition on burst duration and composition.

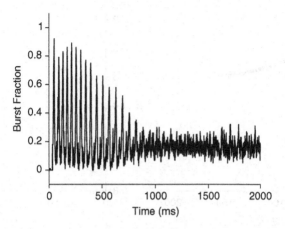

FIGURE 27.28 The setting of Figure 27.27A with $\overline{g}_{AMPA}$ set to zero for $t > 400$ ms. (hyEprnet.m)

27.5 HODGKIN–HUXLEY BASED NETWORKS WITH PLASTIC SYNAPSES

We return to the two-cell inhibitory network of Eq. (27.13) and investigate a learning rule that leads to rhythmic behavior. We append to Eq. (27.13) equations that govern the evolution of synaptic weights, w_i, in terms of the concentration of intracellular calcium, $c_i(t)$, in cell i. As Faraday's constant permits us to tie coulombs to moles and as calcium enters through membrane currents in amperes per unit area, we choose to represent concentration in units of $\mu C/cm^2$. We pose the simplest possible dynamics,

$$\tau_w w_i'(t) = \frac{c_i(t) - C}{C} w_i(t)$$

$$c_i'(t) = -\overline{g}_{Ca} m_\infty(V_i)(V_i - V_{Ca}) - c_i(t)/\tau_{Ca}.$$

(27.21)

The first equation serves to steer w_i to that configuration in which its calcium concentration hits the target value, C. The latter equation dictates that calcium enter through calcium channels and that it decays at rate τ_{Ca}. We adopt the parameters

$$\tau_w = 35\,s, \quad C = 9000\,\mu C/cm^2, \quad \text{and} \quad \tau_{Ca} = 10\,s,$$

(27.22)

and functionals

$$m_\infty(V) = (1 + \tanh((V + 10)/20))/2, \quad \tau_n(V) = 125/\cosh(V/30),$$

$$n_\infty(V) = (1 + \tanh((V + 10)/5))/2, \quad s_\infty(V) = 1/(1 + \exp(-(V + 58)/10)),$$

(27.23)

and demonstrate in Figure 27.29 that each uncoupled cell is tonically depolarized to approximately 5.6 mV. We now couple two such cells, as in Eq. (27.13), and permit the weights to evolve according to Eq. (27.21). The results of

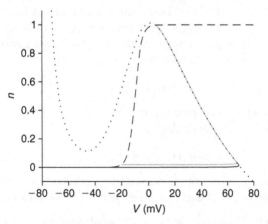

FIGURE 27.29 The phase plane and individual trajectories (solid) associated with uncoupled ($w_1 = w_2 = 0$) Morris Lecar cells, commencing from $V_1(0) = -80$ mV (black) and $V_2(0) = -20$ mV (red), that each obey Eqs. (27.13), (27.22), and (27.23). The dashed and dotted curves are the respective n and V nullclines. Compare with Figure 27.22B. (soto.m)

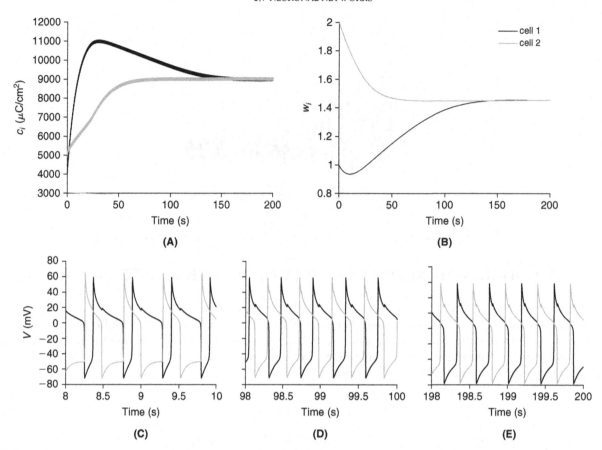

FIGURE 27.30 Convergence of cell calcium levels (**A**), and synaptic weights (**B**), in accordance with the learning rule, Eq. (27.21). Evolution of the oscillator is traced in panels (**C**) early, (**D**) middle, and (**E**) late. Initial values were, $\mathbf{V} = (-80\ -40)$ mV, $\mathbf{n} = n_\infty(\mathbf{V})$, $\mathbf{c} = (4000\ 5000)\ \mu C/cm^2$, and $\mathbf{w} = (1\ 2)$ mS/cm^2. The time step $dt = 1$ ms. (soto.m)

one such simulation are presented in Figure 27.30. Commencing from distinct calcium levels, i.e., $c_1(0) \neq c_2(0)$ as well as distinct weights, $w_1 \neq w_2$, this figure reveals the convergence of $c_1(t)$ and $c_2(t)$ onto their target level and the convergence of $w_1(t)$ and $w_2(t)$ to a common value and subsequent antiphase oscillation in the membrane potentials.

27.6 RATE BASED NETWORKS

As pointed out earlier, the instantaneous firing rate captures a substantial fraction of the information conveyed either by single neurons (Chapters 20 and 25) or neuronal populations (Chapter 26). Thus, network models are often formulated in terms of instantaneous firing rates. Here $f(t)$ will denote the average firing rate, at time t, of a population of cells, in response to its average synaptic input, $u(t)$. The spike generating machinery of the individual cells is collapsed into a single threshold. In particular, we will assume that

$$f(t) = \sigma(u(t)) \tag{27.24}$$

for some sigmoidal function σ. The mean synaptic input is then assumed to evolve in a manner reminiscent of the conductance equations (27.2) and (27.3). In particular

$$\tau u'(t) = -u(t) + w(t)f(t), \tag{27.25}$$

where $w(t)$ is the average synaptic weight at time t. We will now consider a specific example that will yield insight into the firing rate dynamics of a network of head direction cells in the rat's brain.

Head direction cells. Animals moving in a complex environment need to keep track of their head direction if they are to navigate successfully towards a desired target location, such as a source of food. In the rat brain, cells whose firing rates are strongly correlated with a fixed head direction during locomotion have been discovered in numerous regions of the brain, see Figure 27.31 for two examples. For a preferred direction θ_0 it is common to fit the rate curves of Figure 27.31 to functions of the form

$$f(\theta - \theta_0) = A + B\exp(K\cos(\theta - \theta_0)). \tag{27.26}$$

Here A and $B\exp(K)$ specify the respective background and peak rates, and K determines the width of the distribution. We proceed with the concrete choice in Figure 27.32A. For the threshold function we use

$$\sigma(u) \equiv a(\log(1 + \exp(b(u+c))))^{\beta} \tag{27.27}$$

with parameter values as specified in Figure 27.32B.

To consider the interaction of head direction (HD) cells, we denote, respectively, by $u(\theta, t)$ and $f(\theta, t)$ the average synaptic input and firing rate over all HD cells with preferred direction θ. We continue to assume that f is determined by u via the static threshold $f(\theta, t) = \sigma(u(\theta, t))$ and now assume that HD cells with distinct preferred directions, say θ_1 and θ_2, influence one another through synaptic weights that depend solely on the difference, $\theta_1 - \theta_2$. In particular, we suppose that u obeys

$$\tau u_t(\theta, t) = -u(\theta, t) + w(\theta, t) \star \sigma(u(\theta, t)), \tag{27.28}$$

where $w \star \sigma$ denotes the angular convolution

$$w(\theta, t) \star \sigma(u(\theta, t)) \equiv \frac{1}{2\pi} \int_0^{2\pi} w(\theta - \phi, t)\sigma(u(\phi, t)) \, d\phi. \tag{27.29}$$

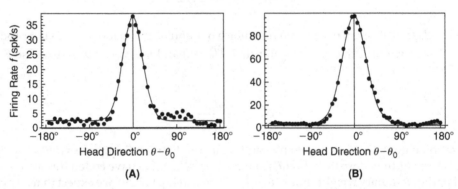

FIGURE 27.31 Firing rates of a head direction cell from (A) the anterior thalamus, and (B) the postsubiculum. Here, θ is the head direction of the rat moving in the environment, while θ_0 is the cell's preferred direction. Adapted from Zhang (1996).

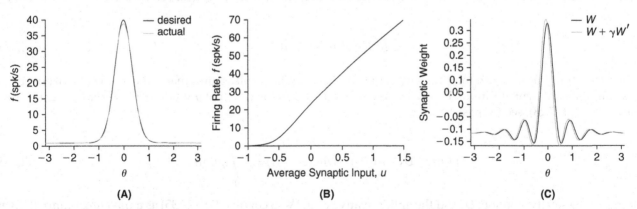

FIGURE 27.32 A. The graph (black) of Eq. (27.26) when $A = 1$ spk/s, $K = 8$, $B\exp(K) = 39$ spk/s, and $\theta_0 = 0$. The red curve is the result of regularized deconvolution, $\sigma(W \star f)$, where W is the (black) weight function in C and f is the desired tuning curve. B. The sigmoid threshold function, Eq. (27.27), with parameters $a = 6.34$, $b = 10$, $c = 0.5$, and $\beta = 0.8$. C. The stationary weight function, W, (black) computed from Eq. (27.33) with $\lambda = 10^{-3}max|\hat{f}_n|^2$. The dynamic weight function, $w = W + \gamma W'$, (red) computed from Eq. (27.34) with $\gamma = 0.063$ rad. (hdnet.m)

We now discuss how to choose the synaptic weight function, w, in order to reproduce two fundamental behaviors of the observed HD network:

HD1. When the rat is stationary the HD population behavior simply mirrors the single HD cell behavior. More precisely, when stationary, cells of preferred direction θ spike at rates described by Figure 27.32A, where θ_0 is the current head direction with respect to a fixed reference frame. We will assume $\theta_0 = 0$ in the following, corresponding to the head aligned with the body.

HD2. In a controlled environment, the rotation of a single salient visual cue associated with the animal's reference frame leads to a near equal rotation of the preferred direction of every HD cell. Equivalently, as the rat rotates its head, the spike rate of the population shifts in a rigid fashion.

Regarding HD1, in the stationary case we presume in response to an initial disturbance $\sigma(u_0(\theta))$, that $u(\theta, t)$ converges over time to $U(\theta)$. If the weight function, $w(\theta, t)$, likewise converges to some $W(\theta)$, then Eq. (27.28) yields

$$U(\theta) = W(\theta) \star \sigma(U(\theta)). \tag{27.30}$$

As we expect the limiting firing rate to coincide with the known f, we recognize that Eq. (27.30) is

$$U(\theta) = W(\theta) \star f(\theta), \tag{27.31}$$

where f and $U(\theta) = \sigma^{-1}(f(\theta))$ are both known and so W, the limiting weight distribution, may be determined via deconvolution. From the Convolution Theorem, Eq. (7.11), we recognize that their Fourier coefficients obey

$$\hat{U}_n = \hat{W}_n \hat{f}_n, \quad n = 0, \pm 1, \pm 2, \ldots \tag{27.32}$$

and so, formally, $\hat{W}_n = \hat{U}_n / \hat{f}_n$. Unfortunately, given our choice of f and σ, this quotient does not produce a suitable W. More precisely, as $|n| \to \infty$ we find that $\hat{f}_n \to 0$ faster than $\hat{U}_n \to 0$ and so $\hat{W}_n \to \infty$. In Exercise 8 we will derive a "regularized" solution

$$\hat{W}_n = \frac{\hat{U}_n \hat{f}_n^*}{\lambda + |\hat{f}_n|^2}, \tag{27.33}$$

where the regularization parameter, λ, is chosen by hand, to insure that the firing rate $\sigma(u(\theta, t))$ indeed converges to $f(\theta)$ when the initial state $u(\theta, 0)$ is close to $\sigma^{-1}(f(\theta))$ and $w(\theta, t) = W(\theta)$. We have coded this in hdnet.m and illustrate it in Figure 27.32B. For the stationary weight choice, $w(\theta, t) = W(\theta)$, in Eq. (27.29), we expect that any initial disturbance will settle into a translate of f. We illustrate this in Figure 27.33A with a noisy combination of two competing head directions.

We now take up HD2 and argue that the dynamic shift in firing rate may be achieved by a dynamic weight of the form

$$w(\theta, t) = W(\theta) + \gamma(t)W'(\theta) \tag{27.34}$$

where $\gamma(t)/\tau$ (rad/ms) is the angular velocity of the rat's head, and we will assume that τ, the time constant governing the dynamics of the synaptic input, Eq. (27.28), is equal to 10 ms. In the case that $u(\theta, 0) = U(\theta)$ we may write the exact solution to Eq. (27.28), see Exercise 9,

$$u(\theta, t) = U(\theta + \Gamma(t)) \quad \text{where} \quad \Gamma(t) = \frac{1}{\tau} \int_0^t \gamma(s) \, ds \tag{27.35}$$

in terms of the steady solution, U, and the antiderivative of γ. We recognize Eq. (27.35) as a traveling bump. If given general initial conditions, we discretize knowns and unknowns,

$$u_j(\theta) \approx u(\theta, (j-1)dt) \quad \text{and} \quad w_j(\theta) = w(\theta, (j-1)dt)$$

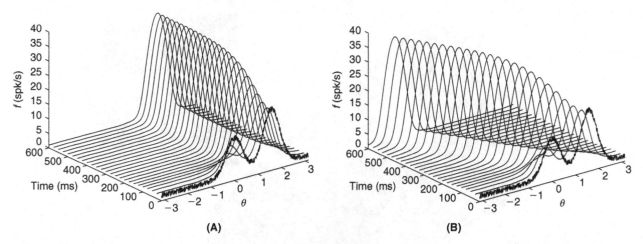

FIGURE 27.33 The evolution of the population firing rate, $f = \sigma(u)$, where u is the solution to Eq. (27.28), obtained via Eq. (27.36) with $dt = 1$ ms, of the synaptic input equation, Eq. (27.28), with initial data corresponding to a noisy sum of two shifted copies of the desired f in Figure 27.32A. **A.** The stationary case, $w = W$. By symmetry every translate, $f(\theta + \theta_0)$, of $f(\theta)$, is a steady solution of Eq. (27.28) when the rat is stationary. The resulting peak firing rate direction, θ_0, is the direction in which the initial population firing rate was strongest. **B.** The dynamic case, $w = W + \gamma W'$ with $\gamma = 0.063$ rad and $\tau = 10$ ms. We observe that the population response shifts, with the rat's head, at approximately 2π rad/s. (hdnet.m)

and solve Eq. (27.28) via the hybrid Euler rule

$$(\tau/dt)(u_{j+1}(\theta) - u_j(\theta)) = -u_{j+1}(\theta) + w_{j+1}(\theta) \star \sigma(u_j(\theta))$$

or

$$u_{j+1}(\theta) = \frac{\tau u_j(\theta) + dt w_{j+1}(\theta) \star \sigma(u_j(\theta))}{\tau + dt}. \tag{27.36}$$

We plot in Figure 27.33B the spike rate of the population of head direction cells during a head rotation at speed $\gamma(t)/\tau \approx 2\pi$ rad/s (achieved by setting $\gamma = 0.063$ rad since the time constant $\tau = 10$ ms). We have plotted the associated shifted weight function, $W + \gamma W'$, in Figure 27.32C.

27.7 BRAIN MAPS AND SELF-ORGANIZING MAPS

A fascinating feature of visual cortex is that it is organized in an orderly manner with nearby neurons sharing many common features that vary relatively smoothly as one travels along the cortical surface. This leads to the concept of *topographic maps* that underlies the organization of both sensory and motor areas of the brain. Thus, in visual cortex nearby neurons will usually have nearby receptive fields in visual space, but the topographic organization is more refined than that. Usually, nearby neurons will also share the same orientation preference, the same direction of motion preference, as well as preference for the same eye. Thus, multiple features are jointly represented in topographic maps. Figure 27.34A illustrates the map of orientation preference in the primary visual cortex of the tree shrew. In most regions of the map, orientation preference varies smoothly (Figure 27.34B, left), except for singular points close to which all possible orientation preferences are found (Figure 27.34B, right). These points are called *pinwheels*. A central question of developmental neurobiology is how such maps arise. Two broadly defined mechanisms are thought to be at play. The first one is based on molecular guidance cues, which are thought, e.g., to help growing axons find the appropriate subregion where they should be making synapses with target neurons. The second mechanism is visual experience which is thought to trigger learning, allowing maps to be refined over time.

Here, we examine a high level approach to the problem of development of maps of orientation and direction preference in visual cortex using a learning rule based on visual experience. To begin we suppose that a retinal square, $[0, L] \times [0, L]$, is mapped (fairly regularly) onto a square grid of N^2 cortical cells. In particular, we suppose that the center of the receptive field of cortical cell C_{ij} lies at

$$x_{ij} = iL/N + \mathcal{U}(0, \sigma_r), \quad y_{ij} = jL/N + \mathcal{U}(0, \sigma_r), \quad i = 1, 2, \ldots, N, \quad j = 1, 2, \ldots, N \tag{27.37}$$

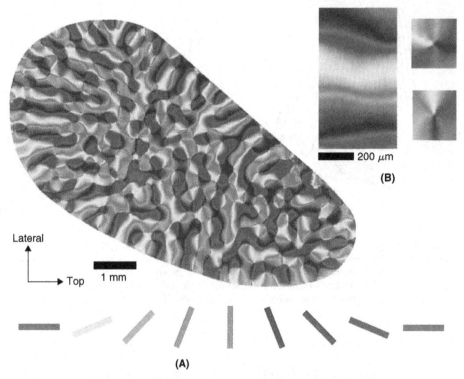

(B)

(A)

FIGURE 27.34   **A.** Map of orientation preference in the primary visual cortex of the tree shrew obtained by intrinsic imaging. The local orientation preference is coded in gray scale according to the key shown below. **B.** Three enlarged portions of the orientation preference map of **A** illustrate linear zones (left) and pinwheel arrangements (right). Adapted from Bosking et al. (1997).

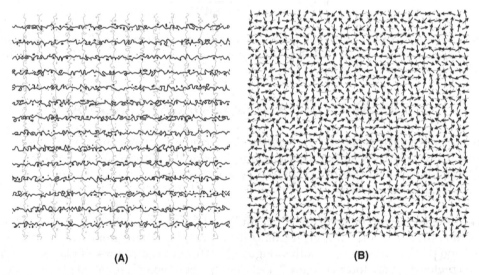

(A)   **(B)**

FIGURE 27.35   Initial cortical map. **A.** Lines of constant x (red, $x = 1, 2, \ldots, 14$) and constant y (black, $y = 1, 2, \ldots, 14$) determined by Eq. (27.37) with $L = 15$, $N = 128$, and $\sigma_r = 0.5$. **B.** Random preferred orientations (red) and directions (black arrows) of the first 32-by-32 block of cortical cells. (codpm.m)

where $\mathcal{U}(0, \sigma_r)$ is the uniform distribution with mean 0 and width σ_r. This leads to a retinotopic map like the one of Figure 27.35A. We next denote the preferred orientation of cell C_{ij} by $(a_{ij} \; b_{ij})$ and its preferred direction by $(c_{ij} \; d_{ij})$ and commence from the random distribution of preferred orientations and directions depicted in Figure 27.35B. The receptive field of cell C_{ij} is thus parametrized by

$$\mathbf{w}_{ij} \equiv (x_{ij} \; y_{ij} \; a_{ij} \; b_{ij} \; c_{ij} \; d_{ij})$$

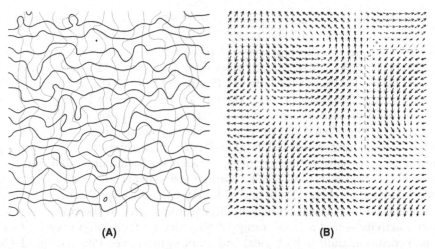

(A)   **(B)**

FIGURE 27.36   Final cortical map achieved after 7×10^5 stimulus presentations. **A.** Lines of constant x (red, $x = 1, 2, \ldots, 14$) and constant y (black, $y = 1, 2, \ldots, 14$). **B.** Preferred orientations (red) and directions (black arrows) of the first 32-by-32 block of cortical cells. Line lengths reflect vector magnitudes. A pinwheel is indicated by the gray asterisk and a linear fracture by the dashed gray line. (codpm.m)

and we investigate a simple learning rule that adapts $\mathbf{w}$ to stimuli. Given a visual stimulus, $\mathbf{v} = (x\ y\ a\ b\ c\ d)$, centered at $(x\ y)$, with orientation $(a\ b)$ and direction $(c\ d)$, we find the cell, C_{IJ}, with the closest receptive field, $\mathbf{w}_{IJ}$, by solving

$$\|\mathbf{v} - \mathbf{w}_{IJ}\| = \min_{ij} \|\mathbf{v} - \mathbf{w}_{ij}\|. \tag{27.38}$$

We then bring the receptive fields of those cells close to C_{IJ} into alignment with the stimulus $\mathbf{v}$ via the update rule

$$\mathbf{w}_{ij} = \mathbf{w}_{ij} + \varepsilon e^{-((i-I)^2 + (j-J)^2)/(2\sigma^2)}(\mathbf{v} - \mathbf{w}_{ij}). \tag{27.39}$$

This two-step process, Eqs. (27.38) and (27.39), when applied to a large and varied set of stimuli, has the power to organize the highly disordered map of Figure 27.35 in a fashion that agrees with experimental findings. The result is known as a self-organized map, and the process itself is often interpreted in broad physiological terms as a competitive mechanism that detects, via Eq. (27.38), the cortical region that responds maximally to a given stimulus followed by enhancement, Eq. (27.39), of the neighboring active synapses. Its application to the problem at hand, with

$$\varepsilon = 0.02 \quad \text{and} \quad \sigma = 2.5$$

results in the map of Figure 27.36. We note that Figure 27.36B concurs with several key experimental findings. In addition to orientation being orthogonal to direction, we observe (i) in regions of small orientation magnitude the orientation varies by 180° around a "singularity," or pinwheel, and (ii) regions of small direction magnitude are separated by "linear fractures" that run either vertically or horizontally.

27.8 SUMMARY AND SOURCES

As recently as ten years ago, simultaneous recordings from large populations of neurons were still fairly rare. Thus, most models of network activity are either higher level abstractions (e.g., Hopfield networks), or have been inferred indirectly through repeated single neuron recordings and anatomical data. Nowadays, technical advances such as multielectrode arrays and optical imaging techniques have rendered population recordings fairly common, opening the way for a more refined understanding of neuronal networks. Yet, these new techniques also have substantial limitations. For instance the synaptic connections between simultaneously recorded neurons are usually unknown, and although many cells are recorded simultaneously, this is often at the expense of a detailed characterization of individual ones. For a glimpse at this rapidly growing experimental literature, we recommend Zochowski et al. (2000), McLean et al. (2007), Perez-Orive et al. (2002), Ohki et al. (2006), and Airan et al. (2007).

Hopfield networks go back to Hopfield (1982). See Amit (1992) for a thorough treatment. Exercise 2 is drawn from Goles-Chacc et al. (1985). STDP was first observed by Levy and Steward (1983). In weakly electric fish, its role is particularly well understood. See, e.g., Bell et al. (1997). Song et al. (2000) is an excellent theoretical counterpart to the experimental work of Bi and Poo (1998). We demonstrate in Exercise 5 that STDP in an LIF model may produce the backward shift in hippocampal place fields observed by Mehta et al. (1997). Our work on Hodgkin–Huxley based networks is based on Skinner et al. (1994), Soto-Treviño et al. (2001), and Pinsky and Rinzel (1994). We consider the extension of the latter by Booth and Bose (2001) in Exercise 7. The important question of the degree to which the dynamics of Hodgkin–Huxley based networks may be approximated by those of Hopfield-like networks is addressed by Terman et al. (2008). Our exposition of rate based networks, including Exercises 8–10, is drawn from Zhang (1996). For a review of head direction cells, see Taube (2007). Shriki et al. (2003) establish conditions under which Hodgkin–Huxley based networks may be approximated by rate based networks. The section on self-organizing maps is based on Swindale and Bauer (1998). Self-organizing maps are due to Kohonen, see Kohonen (2001) for a comprehensive overview. For further neuronal application of self-organizing maps see Ritter et al. (1992). Traub and Miles (1991) discuss synchronization mechanisms in the hippocampus. For synchronization mechanisms based on electrical synapses in the cortex, see Mancilla et al. (2007). Synchronized oscillatory activity across a broad range of olfactory systems is reviewed by Gelperin (2006). For a broader perspective on synchronization in biological and other systems, see Pikovsky et al. (2003). For an experimental approach to the role of network architecture in synchronization see Bonifazi et al. (2009). For the theory, in a neurobiological context, behind such scale-free networks we recommend Freeman and Kozma (2009).

27.9 EXERCISES

1. Argue that, for a given weight matrix, $\mathbf{W}$, we may sharpen the Hopfield threshold function by showing that there exists a $\mathbf{b} \in \mathbb{R}^N$ such that if

$$\text{Hop}_i^{\sharp}(x) \equiv \begin{cases} 1 & \text{if } x > b_i \\ -1 & \text{if } x < b_i, \end{cases} \tag{27.40}$$

then in fact $\text{Hop}(\mathbf{Ws}) = \text{Hop}^{\sharp}(\mathbf{Ws})$ for all $\mathbf{s} \in \{-1, 1\}^N$.

2. †In a Hopfield net with undirected edges, we observe that $\mathbf{W} = \mathbf{W}^T$. Use this symmetry, the $\mathbf{b}$ vector of the previous exercise and the "energy" functional

$$E(j) \equiv -(\mathbf{s}^{j-1})^T \mathbf{Ws}^j + \mathbf{b}^T(\mathbf{s}^j + \mathbf{s}^{j-1}) \quad \text{where} \quad \mathbf{s}^j = \text{Hop}^{\sharp}(\mathbf{Ws}^{j-1}),$$

to argue that the energy difference $\Delta E \equiv E(j+1) - E(j)$ is simply

$$\Delta E = -(\mathbf{s}^{j+1} - \mathbf{s}^{j-1})^T(\mathbf{Ws}^j - \mathbf{b}).$$

Use this to show that if $\mathbf{s}^{j+1} \neq \mathbf{s}^{j-1}$ then $\Delta E < 0$ and so conclude that no attractor of an undirected Hopfield net can have period greater than 2.

3. †In the case of periodic input, Eq. (27.6), for the two-cell network we may solve Eq. (27.2) for $g_{E,1}$ by hand. In particular, please show that

$$g_{E,1}(t) = \frac{w_{inp}}{\tau_E} \exp((P-t)/\tau_E) \frac{1 - \exp(P\lfloor t/P \rfloor / \tau_E)}{1 - \exp(P/\tau_E)} \tag{27.41}$$

where $\lfloor x \rfloor$ denotes the largest integer less than x. First show that $g_{E,1}(P^+) = w_{inp}/\tau_E$, then $g_{E,1}(t) = \exp((P-t)/\tau_E)w_{inp}/\tau_E$ for $P \leq t < 2P$, then $g_{E,1}(2P^+) = (1 + \exp(-P/\tau_E))w_{inp}/\tau_E$ and so

$$g_{E,1}(t) = \exp((P-t)/\tau_E)(1 + \exp(P/\tau_E))w_{inp}/\tau_E, \quad 2P \leq t < 3P.$$

Continuing in this fashion you will find a (summable) finite geometric series.

4. Experiment with `threecell.m` to further delay the spiking of cell 3. In particular, retain $P = 2$ but set $W_{3,1} = W_{3,2} = w$ and find the smallest w (to two decimal places) such that cell 3 fires once for every two spikes of cell 2.

5. [†]The rat hippocampus is known to contain cells that fire when the rat is near a particular place within a given environment. For this exercise we will suppose that the rat is running clockwise, at a fixed velocity, along a circular track. As the rat traverses the track the associated "place cell" receives input. We consider a ring, Figure 27.37, of 120 leaky integrate-and-fire cells with reciprocal excitatory connections among immediate neighbors and excitatory input into each cell. We suppose that the rat spends 100 ms in each place field and that the associated cell receives a kick, $w_{inp} = 10$, every 20 ms. The cell parameters are

$$\tau_m = 20, \quad \tau_{gE} = 5, \quad t_{ref} = 5, \quad V_{rest} = -70, \quad V_{thr} = -54, \quad V_{reset} = -60,$$

where times are in ms and voltages in mV.

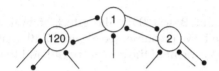

FIGURE 27.37   A segment of a ring of 120 "place cells."

We set the plasticity parameters

$$w_{max} = 5, \quad w_{init} = 0.5, \quad \tau_+ = 20, \quad \tau_- = 20, \quad A_+ = 8, \quad A_- = 8.4,$$

and note that as the rat travels clockwise and excites cell j then the connection to cell $j+1$ will **increase** for when the rat enters the place field of cell $j+1$ its presynaptic cell will have just fired. Conversely, as cell j fires independently of cell $j+1$ we expect to see a **decrease** in the associated weight. The effect of this weight change is a slight backward shift in all of the place fields.

Please illustrate this by coding the small ring and tracking the spikes in cell 2 and the weights between cells 1 and 2, as in Figure 27.38, as the simulated rat completes 20 laps of the ring with a time step of $dt = 1$ ms. With 120 place cells, each receives external input over a 3 degree window.

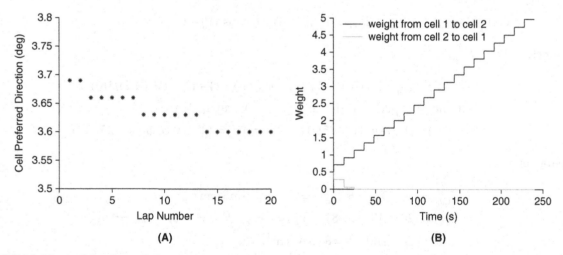

FIGURE 27.38   **A.** The angle at which cell 2 fires as a function of lap number. **B.** The forward and backward weights as a function of time. (`bkwshift.m`)

6. Show that the calcium target, C, determines the oscillator frequency by adapting `soto.m` and producing Figure 27.39.

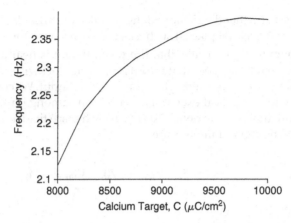

FIGURE 27.39 The calcium target, C, in Eq. (27.21) determines the oscillator frequency. (sotofreq.m)

7. [†]We investigate, following Booth and Bose (2001), the effect of inhibition on the burst shape of the two-compartment Pinksy–Rinzel CA3 cell. We presume, see Figure 27.40, that the inhibitory cell is isopotential and that it is driven by the somatic compartment of the excitatory cell and that it in turn inhibits that cell's dendritic compartment.

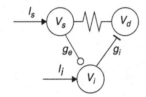

FIGURE 27.40 The simple EI net of Booth and Bose (2001).

We suppose that the inhibitory cell follows Morris Lecar dynamics and that the full network is described by

$$C_m V_s' = -g_L(V_s - V_L) - I_{Na}(V_s) - I_{K,DR}(V_s) + \frac{g_c(V_d - V_s) + I_s}{p}$$

$$C_m V_d' = -g_L(V_d - V_L) - I_{Ca}(V_d) - I_{K,AHP}(V_d) - I_{K,C}(V_d) + \frac{g_c(V_s - V_d)}{1-p} - g_i s_i(V_d - V_{inh})$$

$$C_m V_i' = -g_{L,i}(V_i - V_{L,i}) - I_{Ca,i}(V_i) - I_{K,i}(V_i) + I_i - g_e s_e(V_i - V_{exc}),$$

with functionals

$$I_{Ca,i}(V) = \bar{g}_{Ca,i} m_\infty(V)(V - V_{Ca,i}), \quad m_\infty(V) = (1 + \tanh((V + 1.2)/18))/2$$
$$I_{K,i}(V,w) = \bar{g}_{K,i} w(V - V_K), \quad w' = (w_\infty(V_i) - w)/\tau_w(V_i)$$
$$w_\infty(V) = (1 + \tanh((V + 25)/11))/2, \quad \tau_w(V) = (25/4)/\cosh((V + 25)/22),$$

and parameters

$$\bar{g}_{Ca,i} = 4.4, \quad \bar{g}_{K,i} = 8, \quad g_{L,i} = 2, \quad g_e = 5\,\text{mS/cm}^2$$
$$V_{Ca,i} = 120, \quad V_{K,i} = -84, \quad V_{L,i} = -60, \quad V_{inh} = -80, \quad V_{exc} = 0\,\text{mV}$$
$$I_s = 0.3, \quad \text{and} \quad I_i = 88\,\mu\text{A/cm}^2,$$

and synaptic kinetics

$$s_e' = 2\mathbb{1}(V_s + 10)(1 - s_e) - \mathbb{1}(-10 - V_s)s_e$$
$$s_i' = 2\mathbb{1}(V_i + 10)(1 - s_i) - \mathbb{1}(-10 - V_i)s_i,$$

and initial conditions, $V_d(0) = V_s(0) = 0$ mV, $V_i(0) = -35$ mV, $w(0) = w_\infty(-35)$, and $q(0) = 0.1$. Code this system and investigate (by reproducing Figure 27.41) the impact of the inhibitory weight, w_i, on the burst frequency and shape in the somatic compartment, V_s, of the excitatory cell.

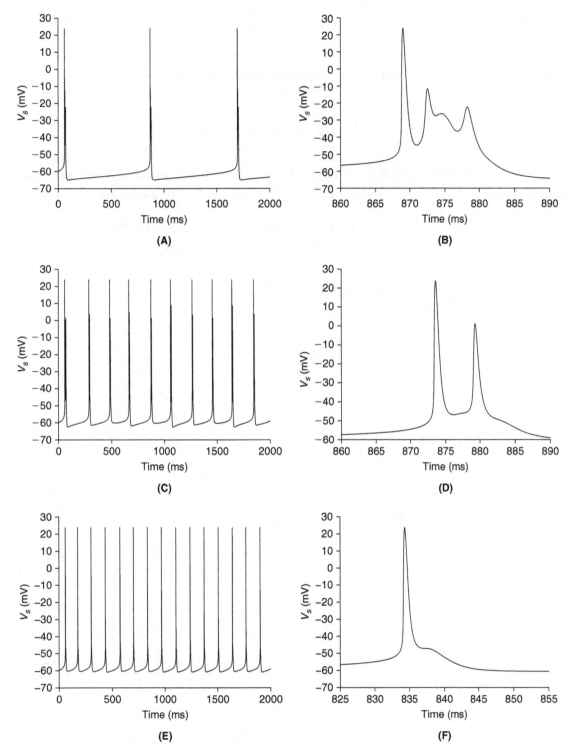

FIGURE 27.41 The effect of inhibition on frequency and burst shape. (A) $g_i = 0$. (B) Zoom on (A). (C) $g_i = 0.0315$ mS/cm^2. (D) Zoom on (C). (E) $g_i = 0.034$ mS/cm^2. (F) Zoom on (E). (hyprEInet.m)

8. [†]Recall that the naive solution, $\hat{W}_n = \hat{U}_n / \hat{f}_n$, to the deconvolution problem Eq. (27.31), led to infinite growth in the high frequencies of W. One means of controlling this growth is to introduce a regularization, or penalization,

parameter into an associated minimization problem. In particular, rather than attempting to minimize the average squared distance of $W(\theta) \star f(\theta)$ from $U(\theta)$, we minimize

$$E(W) = \int_0^{2\pi} (W(\theta) \star f(\theta) - U(\theta))^2 \, d\theta + \lambda \int_0^{2\pi} W(\theta)^2 \, d\theta \qquad (27.42)$$

for some $\lambda > 0$. We see that λ mediates a trade-off between fidelity and size. Use Parseval's identity, Eq. (7.10), to arrive at

$$E(W) = \sum_{n=-\infty}^{\infty} |\hat{W}_n \hat{f}_n - \hat{U}_n|^2 + \lambda |\hat{W}_n|^2. \qquad (27.43)$$

Do not be dismayed by these infinities, for this is simply a sum of *independent* squares, and as such we can minimize them one at a time. In particular, argue that the choice of $\hat{W}_n$ that minimizes $|\hat{W}_n \hat{f}_n - \hat{U}_n|^2 + \lambda |\hat{W}_n|^2$ is the one featured in Eq (27.33).

9. Confirm that Eq. (27.35) is indeed a solution to Eq. (27.28) when w is of the form Eq. (27.34). Hint: Use Exercise 7.4.

10. †Given the even tuning function, $f(\theta) = f(-\theta)$, of Figure 27.32(A), argue that

   (i) $\hat{f}_n = \hat{f}_{-n}$.

   (ii) As $U(\theta) = \sigma^{-1}(f(\theta))$ then U is also even and so $\hat{U}_n = \hat{U}_{-n}$.

   (iii) Eq. (27.33) now implies that W is even.

   (iv) As W is even W' must be odd, i.e., $W'(-\theta) = -W'(\theta)$.

Solutions to Selected Exercises

OUTLINE

28.1 Chapter 2	409	28.14 Chapter 15	433
28.2 Chapter 3	411	28.15 Chapter 16	436
28.3 Chapter 4	413	28.16 Chapter 17	442
28.4 Chapter 5	414	28.17 Chapter 18	445
28.5 Chapter 6	416	28.18 Chapter 19	452
28.6 Chapter 7	419	28.19 Chapter 20	453
28.7 Chapter 8	421	28.20 Chapter 21	453
28.8 Chapter 9	422	28.21 Chapter 22	455
28.9 Chapter 10	422	28.22 Chapter 23	458
28.10 Chapter 11	423	28.23 Chapter 24	459
28.11 Chapter 12	428	28.24 Chapter 25	464
28.12 Chapter 13	430	28.25 Chapter 26	466
28.13 Chapter 14	431	28.26 Chapter 27	470

28.1 CHAPTER 2

Exercise 1. Setting $V'(t) = 0$ in Eq. (2.12) yields $I_{stim} - Ag_{Cl}(V_{max} - V_{Cl})$ and so

$$V_{max} = V_{Cl} + \frac{I_{stim}}{Ag_{Cl}} = -68 \text{ mV} + \frac{10 \text{ pA}}{4\pi 10^{-6} \text{ cm}^2 \cdot 0.3 \text{ mS/cm}^2} \approx -65.35 \text{ mV}.$$

Exercise 2. Without loss we set $t_1 = 0$ and study $g_{syn}(t) = g_{max}(t/\tau_\alpha)\exp(1 - t/\tau_\alpha)$. We note that

$$g'_{syn}(t) = (g_{max}/\tau_\alpha)\exp(1 - t/\tau_\alpha)(1 - t/\tau_\alpha)$$

vanishes only at $t = \tau_\alpha$. As g_{syn} is positive and decays at both ends its only critical point must be a maximum. Next,

$$\int_0^\infty g_{max}(t/\tau_\alpha) \exp(1 - t/\tau_\alpha)\, dt = -g_{max}(\tau_\alpha + t) \exp(1 - t/\tau_\alpha)\Big|_{t=0}^\infty = g_{max}\tau_\alpha \exp(1).$$

Exercise 3. For constant g_{syn} Eq. (2.15) reads

$$C_m V'(t) + (g_{Cl} + g_{syn})V(t) = g_{Cl}V_{Cl} + g_{syn}V_{syn}$$

and so we arrive at Eq. (2.22) with

$$\tau_{eff} = \frac{C_m}{g_{Cl} + g_{syn}} \quad \text{and} \quad V_{ss} = \frac{g_{Cl}V_{Cl} + g_{syn}V_{syn}}{g_{Cl} + g_{syn}}.$$

Note that the membrane time constant is decreased relative to its original value of C_m/g_{Cl} since the membrane is more leaky as a result of the opening of the synaptic channels. On setting $V_{syn} = 0$ and $c_e = g_{syn}/g_{Cl}$ in V_{ss} we arrive at

$$V_{ss} = \frac{V_{Cl}}{1 + c_e}.$$

This is graphed in Figure 2.8 by `sse.m`.

Exercise 4. We rearrange Eq. (2.23) to Eq. (2.24) with

$$\tau_{eff,2} = \frac{\tau}{1 + c_1 + c_2} \quad \text{and} \quad V_{ss} = \frac{V_{Cl} + c_1 V_{syn1} + c_2 V_{syn2}}{1 + c_1 + c_2}. \tag{28.1}$$

Exercise 5. Setting $V_{syn1} = V_{syn2} = 0$ and $c_1 = c_2 = c_e$ in Eq. (28.1) gives Eq. (2.25). Figure 2.9 is generated by `ss2e.m`.

Exercise 7.

(i) Use Kirchhoff's Current Law and follow the arrows on Figure 2.11A.

(ii) With regard to Eq. (2.29), the derivatives vanish for constant conductances, and, with $v_p \equiv V_p - V_{Cl}$, we arrive at the pair of algebraic equations,

$$(g_p + g_i)v_p = g_c(V_d - V_{Cl} - v_p)$$
$$g_d(V_d - V_{Cl}) + g_e(V_d - V_e) = g_c(v_p + V_{Cl} - V_d).$$

We rearrange the former to

$$(g_p + g_i + g_c)v_p = g_c(V_d - V_{Cl}) \tag{28.2}$$

and solve the latter for

$$V_d = \frac{g_d V_{Cl} + g_e V_e + g_c(v_p + V_{Cl})}{g_d + g_e + g_c}.$$

On its substitution into Eq. (28.2) we find

$$(g_p + g_i + g_c)v_p = g_c \frac{g_d V_{Cl} + g_e V_e + g_c(v_p + V_{Cl}) - V_{Cl}(g_d + g_e + g_c)}{g_d + g_e + g_c}$$
$$= g_c \frac{g_e(V_e - V_{Cl}) + g_c v_p}{g_d + g_e + g_c}$$

and, upon clearing the fraction, find

$$((g_p+g_i+g_c)(g_d+g_e+g_c)-g_c^2)v_p=g_cg_ev_e,$$

from which the desired form, Eq. (2.30), immediately follows.

(iii) Substitute into Eq. (2.30) and divide top and bottom by g_d^2. For graph code see `Comp2syn.m`.

(iv) Apply l'Hôpital's rule to Eq. (2.30) to arrive at (2.32).

Exercise 9. We define $R \equiv \mathcal{O}/(\mathcal{O}+\mathcal{C})$ and note that $R'=\mathcal{O}'/(\mathcal{O}+\mathcal{C})$ because $\mathcal{O}+\mathcal{C}$ is constant. Hence, dividing Eq. (2.20) by $\mathcal{O}+\mathcal{C}$ brings

$$R'(t)=k_+T(t)\frac{\mathcal{C}(t)}{\mathcal{O}+\mathcal{C}}-k_-\frac{\mathcal{O}(t)}{\mathcal{O}+\mathcal{C}}=k_+T(t)(1-R(t))-k_-R(t),$$

on account of

$$\frac{\mathcal{C}}{\mathcal{O}+\mathcal{C}}=1-\frac{\mathcal{O}}{\mathcal{O}+\mathcal{C}}.$$

28.2 CHAPTER 3

Exercise 1. Substituting $I_{stim}=te^{-t}$ into Eq. (3.2) yields

$$V(T)=V_{Cl}+\frac{1}{AC_m}e^{-T/\tau}\int_0^T te^{ct}\,dt$$

where $c=1/\tau-1$. On integrating by parts we find

$$V(T)=V_{Cl}+\frac{e^{-T/\tau}+e^{-T}(cT-1)}{AC_mc^2}.$$

Exercise 3.

$$\mathcal{L}(c)(s)=\int_0^\infty e^{-st}c\,dt=-c\int_0^\infty (\exp(-st)/s)'\,dt$$

$$=-(c/s)\lim_{t\to\infty}(\exp(-st)-1)=c/s,$$

$$\mathcal{L}(e^{-ct})(s)=\int_0^\infty \exp(-(s+c)t)dt=-\int_0^\infty (\exp(-(s+c)t)/(s+c))'\,dt$$

$$=-1/(s+c)\lim_{t\to\infty}(\exp(-(s+c)t)-1)=1/(s+c),$$

$$\mathcal{L}(\sin(ct))(s)=\int_0^\infty \sin(ct)\exp(-st)dt=\frac{-\exp(-st)}{c^2+s^2}(s\sin(ct)+c\cos(st))\Big|_{t=0}^{t=\infty}$$

$$=\frac{c}{s^2+c^2}.$$

Exercise 4. Applying Eq. (3.16) with $V(t)=t$, and since $V'(t)=1$, $V(0)=0$ we obtain

$$\mathcal{L}(1)(s)=s\mathcal{L}(t)(s) \quad \text{or} \quad \mathcal{L}(t)(s)=\frac{1}{s^2},$$

using $\mathcal{L}(1)(s)=1/s$ (Eq. (3.14)). Similarly, with $V(t)=t^2$, $V'(t)=2t$, $V(0)=0$, we obtain

$$2\mathcal{L}(t)(s)=s\mathcal{L}(t^2)(s) \quad \text{or} \quad \mathcal{L}(t^2)(s)=\frac{2}{s^3}.$$

Exercise 6.

(i) If $g(t)=f(t-a)$ then, with $y=t-a$,

$$\mathcal{L}(g)(s)=\int_0^\infty f(t-a)\exp(-st)\,dt=\int_0^\infty f(y)\exp(-s(y+a))\,dy=e^{-as}\mathcal{L}(f)(s).$$

(ii) If $g(t)=f(t/a)$ then, with $y=t/a$,

$$\mathcal{L}(g)(s)=\int_0^\infty f(t/a)\exp(-st)\,dt=\int_0^\infty f(y)\exp(-say))a\,dy=a\mathcal{L}(f)(as).$$

Exercise 7. For $n=1$,

$$\mathcal{L}(p_1)(s)=\int_0^\infty \varrho e^{-\varrho x}e^{-sx}\,dx=\varrho\int_0^\infty \frac{-1}{\varrho+s}\frac{d}{dx}e^{-(\varrho+s)x}\,dx=\frac{-\varrho}{s+\varrho}e^{-(\varrho+s)x}\Big|_0^\infty=\frac{\varrho}{\varrho+s}.$$

For $n>1$,

$$\mathcal{L}(p_n)(s)=\int_0^\infty \varrho\frac{(\varrho x)^{n-1}}{(n-1)!}e^{-\varrho x}e^{-sx}\,dx.$$

Integration by parts, $\int_a^b u\,dv=uv|_a^b-\int_a^b v\,du$ with

$$u=\frac{(\varrho x)^{n-1}}{(n-1)!} \quad \text{and} \quad dv=e^{-(\varrho+s)x}\,dx$$

so that

$$\frac{du}{dx}=(n-1)\frac{(\varrho x)^{n-2}}{(n-1)!}\varrho=\varrho\frac{(\varrho x)^{n-2}}{(n-2)!}$$

and

$$\frac{dv}{dx}=e^{-(\varrho+s)x}=\frac{-\varrho}{\varrho+s}\frac{d}{dx}e^{-(\varrho+s)x} \quad \text{so that} \quad v=\frac{-1}{\varrho+s}e^{-(\varrho+s)x}$$

yields

$$\mathcal{L}(p_n)(s) = uv\big|_0^\infty - \int_0^\infty v\,du$$

$$= \varrho\,\frac{(\varrho x)^{n-1}}{(n-1)!}\left(\frac{-1}{\varrho+s}\right)\bigg|_0^\infty - \varrho\int_0^\infty \varrho\,\frac{(\varrho x)^{n-2}}{(n-2)!}\left(\frac{-1}{\varrho+s}\right)e^{-(\varrho+s)x}\,dx$$

$$= \frac{\varrho}{\varrho+s}\int_0^\infty \varrho\,\frac{(\varrho x)^{n-2}}{(n-2)!}e^{-\varrho x}e^{-sx}\,dx$$

$$= \frac{\varrho}{\varrho+s}\mathcal{L}(p_{n-1})(s).$$

Exercise 9. The marching scheme that arises from backward Euler is

$$V_j = (V_{j-1} + dt\,f_j)/(1 + dt/\tau) = V_{j-1}/(1+dt/\tau) + dt\,f_j/(1+dt/\tau).$$

Commencing from $V_1 = b$, we get

$$V_j = b/(1+dt/\tau)^{j-1} + \sum_{i=1}^{j-1} dt\,f_i/(1+dt/\tau)^i.$$

This remains finite so long as f_i is bounded and $(1+dt/\tau) > 1$. As the latter is true for every $dt \geq 0$ we conclude that backward Euler is absolutely stable.

If we examine the trapezoid rule, we see that

$$V_j = \left(\frac{2-dt/\tau}{2+dt/\tau}\right)^{j-1} b + \sum_{i=1}^{j-1}\left(\frac{dt}{2+dt/\tau}\right)^{i-1}(f_{i-1}+f_i).$$

This remains finite so long as f_i is bounded and $2 - dt/\tau < 2 + dt/\tau$. As the latter is true for every $dt \geq 0$ we conclude that the trapezoid scheme is absolutely stable.

Exercise 10. be_vs_trap.m.

Exercise 11. curvssyn.m.

28.3 CHAPTER 4

Exercise 1. See clamp.m.

Exercise 2. See stErefracdrive.m.

Exercise 3. See stEfreq.m.

Exercise 4. See molifreq.m.

Exercise 5. See stEKstimdrive.m.

Exercise 6. See stE2d.m.

Exercise 7.

(i) If $m(t) = m_\infty(V(t))$ and $h(t) = 0.7 - n^2(t)$ then the Hodgkin–Huxley system takes the form

$$C_m V'(t) = -\bar{g}_{Na} m_\infty^3(V)(0.7 - n^2)(V - V_{Na}) - \bar{g}_K n^4(V - V_K) - g_{Cl}(V - V_{Cl}) + I_{stim}/A$$
$$n'(t) = \alpha_n(V)(1 - n) - \beta_n(V)n.$$

We write the right hand side of the V equation as a biquadratic $a(V)n^4 + b(V)n^2 + c(V) + I_{stim}/A$ by defining

$$a(V) \equiv -\bar{g}_K(V - V_K), \quad b(V) \equiv \bar{g}_{Na} m_\infty^3(V)(V - V_{Na}),$$
$$c(V) \equiv -0.7\bar{g}_{Na} m_\infty^3(V)(V - V_{Na}) - g_{Cl}(V - V_{Cl}).$$

Two applications of the quadratic formula takes one from Eq. (4.32) to Eq. (4.33).

(ii) If t is such that $(V(t), n(t))$ lies on the n nullcline the tangent vector to the solution trajectory is $(V'(t), n'(t)) = (V'(t), 0)$ hence the crossing is horizontal. Similarly if $(V(t), n(t))$ lies on the V nullcline then the tangent vector to the solution trajectory is $(V'(t), n'(t)) = (0, n'(t))$ and the crossing is vertical.

(iii) From (ii), if t is such that $(V(t), n(t))$ lies on both nullclines then $(V'(t), n'(t)) = (0, 0)$ and the system is at rest. To be on the n nullcline requires $n = n_\infty(V)$. On substituting this into Eq. (4.32) we arrive at Eq. (4.34).

For graphs use `fhpp.m`.

28.4 CHAPTER 5

Exercise 1. See `getVrJacfull.m`.

Exercise 2.

(i) Multiply $\mathbf{E}_1$ by this putative $\mathbf{E}_1^{-1}$ and arrive at $\mathbf{I}$.

(ii) In a similar fashion, as

$$\mathbf{E}_2 = \begin{pmatrix} 1 & 0 & 0 & 0 \\ 0 & 1 & 0 & 0 \\ 0 & 0 & 1 & 0 \\ 0 & b & 0 & 1 \end{pmatrix} \quad \text{and} \quad \mathbf{E}_3 = \begin{pmatrix} 1 & 0 & 0 & 0 \\ 0 & 1 & 0 & 0 \\ 0 & 0 & 1 & 0 \\ 0 & 0 & c & 1 \end{pmatrix}$$

we find

$$\mathbf{E}_2^{-1} = \begin{pmatrix} 1 & 0 & 0 & 0 \\ 0 & 1 & 0 & 0 \\ 0 & 0 & 1 & 0 \\ 0 & -b & 0 & 1 \end{pmatrix} \quad \text{and} \quad \mathbf{E}_3^{-1} = \begin{pmatrix} 1 & 0 & 0 & 0 \\ 0 & 1 & 0 & 0 \\ 0 & 0 & 1 & 0 \\ 0 & 0 & -c & 1 \end{pmatrix}.$$

(iii) Given $\mathbf{U} = \mathbf{E}_3 \mathbf{E}_2 \mathbf{E}_1 \mathbf{A}$ we multiply each side by $\mathbf{E}_3^{-1}$ and find $\mathbf{E}_3^{-1}\mathbf{U} = \mathbf{E}_2 \mathbf{E}_1 \mathbf{A}$. Next, multiply through by $\mathbf{E}_2^{-1}$, and finally by $\mathbf{E}_1^{-1}$.

(iv) If $\mathbf{C} = \mathbf{AB}$ where $\mathbf{A}$ and $\mathbf{B}$ are lower triangular then

$$C_{ii} = \sum_{j=1}^{n} A_{ij} B_{ji} = A_{ii} B_{ii}$$

because $A_{ij} = 0$ for $j > i$ and $B_{ij} = 0$ for $j < i$. If $A_{ii} = B_{ii} = 1$ then of course $C_{ii} = 1$.

(v) It follows from (iv) that $\mathbf{L} \equiv \mathbf{E}_1^{-1}\mathbf{E}_2^{-1}\mathbf{E}_3^{-1}$ is lower triangular and has only ones on its diagonal. It follows from (iii) that $\mathbf{A} = \mathbf{LU}$.

(vi) From $\mathbf{U} = \mathbf{E}_2 \mathbf{P}_2 \mathbf{E}_1 \mathbf{P}_1 \mathbf{A}$ and $\mathbf{F}_1 \equiv \mathbf{P}_2 \mathbf{E}_1 \mathbf{P}_2$ we use $\mathbf{P}_2^2 = \mathbf{I}$ to write

$$\mathbf{U} = \mathbf{E}_2 \mathbf{P}_2 \mathbf{E}_1 \mathbf{P}_2 \mathbf{P}_2 \mathbf{P}_1 \mathbf{A} = \mathbf{E}_2 \mathbf{F}_1 \mathbf{P}_2 \mathbf{P}_1 \mathbf{A}$$

and so $\mathbf{A} = \mathbf{PLU}$ where $\mathbf{L} = \mathbf{F}_1^{-1}\mathbf{E}_2^{-1}$. To see that $\mathbf{F}_1$ is lower triangular note that as $\mathbf{E}_1$ is diagonal save for column 1, $\mathbf{P}_2\mathbf{E}_1$ exchanges row 2 for row j the only violation of triangularity is the rise of the one at (j,j) to $(2,j)$ (coupled with the fall of the one at $(2,2)$ to $(j,2)$). Now the action of $\mathbf{P}_2$ from the right serves to exchange the associated columns of $\mathbf{P}_2\mathbf{E}_1$. This will serve to shift (left) the offending one in slot $(2,j)$ to safe haven on the diagonal at $(2,2)$ while shifting (right) the benign one at $(j,2)$ back to the diagonal at (j,j).

Exercise 6. The eigenvalues are roots of the quadratic given by Eq. (5.15), $(-2-z)(-2-z)-1$. These are $z_1 = -3$ and $z_2 = -1$. The associated eigenvectors, $\mathbf{w}_j$, obey $(\mathbf{B} - z_j\mathbf{I})\mathbf{w}_j = 0$, i.e.,

$$\begin{pmatrix} 1 & 1 \\ 1 & 1 \end{pmatrix}\begin{pmatrix} w_{11} \\ w_{12} \end{pmatrix} = \begin{pmatrix} 0 \\ 0 \end{pmatrix} \quad \text{and so} \quad \mathbf{w}_1 = \begin{pmatrix} 1 \\ -1 \end{pmatrix},$$

and

$$\begin{pmatrix} -1 & 1 \\ 1 & -1 \end{pmatrix}\begin{pmatrix} w_{21} \\ w_{22} \end{pmatrix} = \begin{pmatrix} 0 \\ 0 \end{pmatrix} \quad \text{and so} \quad \mathbf{w}_2 = \begin{pmatrix} 1 \\ 1 \end{pmatrix}.$$

Figure 5.8 was achieved by `distort.m`.

The ellipse in Figure 5.8A has a major axis of length $|z_1| = 3$ and a minor axis of length $|z_2| = 1$. The area of an ellipse is π times the product of the lengths of its minor and major axes, and so is 3π in our case.

We divide the parallelogram in Figure 5.8B into 2 equal isosceles triangles. The base of each triangle is the diagonal of the square. The length of this diagonal is $\sqrt{2}$. The height of each triangle may be computed directly as $3/\sqrt{2}$. It follows that the area of the parallelogram is 3.

In the 2-by-2 case the eigenvalues are roots of the quadratic equation, Eq. (5.15),

$$(z - z_1)(z - z_2) = z^2 - (B_{11} + B_{22})z + B_{11}B_{22} - B_{12}B_{21} = 0.$$

It follows immediately from this that $z_1 z_2 = B_{11}B_{22} - B_{12}B_{21}$ and $z_1 + z_2 = B_{11} + B_{22}$.

Exercise 9. We use the symbolic toolbox

```
>> syms tm th tn z1 z2 z3 z4 I
>> W = [1/(1+z1*tm) 1/(1+z2*tm) 1/(1+z3*tm) 1/(1+z4*tm)
        1/(1+z1*th) 1/(1+z2*th) 1/(1+z3*th) 1/(1+z4*th)
        1/(1+z1*tn) 1/(1+z2*tn) 1/(1+z3*tn) 1/(1+z4*tn)
        1           1           1           1];
>> f = [0; 0; 0; I];
>> c = simple(W\f)
```

Exercise 10. See `fhpp3.m`.

Exercise 11. The rest potential, V_r, is a root of

$$\bar{g}_{Ca}m_\infty(V)(V - V_{Ca}) + \bar{g}_K w_\infty(V)(V - V_K) + g_{Cl}(V - V_L)$$

while the quasi-active system is governed by

$$\mathbf{B} = \begin{pmatrix} -1/\tau_w(V_r) & w'_\infty(V_r)/\tau_w(V_r) \\ -(V_r - V_K)/\tau_K & -(m'_\infty(V_r)(V_r - V_{Ca}) + m_\infty(V_r))/\tau_{Ca} - w_\infty(V_r)/\tau_K - 1/\tau_L \end{pmatrix}.$$

Using the stated parameters, we find, see `mlsym.m`, $V_r = -51.84$,

$$\mathbf{B} = \begin{pmatrix} -0.7 & 0.001 \\ -1453 & -21.5 \end{pmatrix}$$

and eigenvalues $z_1 = -0.8$ and $z_2 = -21.4$. As both have negative real part we find the rest state stable.

Exercise 13.

(i) Thanks to the Laplace derivative identity Eq. (3.16) the Laplace transform of the m equation in Eq. (5.2) reveals

$$s\mathcal{L}\tilde{m} = (\overline{m}'_\infty \mathcal{L}\tilde{V} - \mathcal{L}\tilde{m})/\overline{\tau}_m$$

which yields Eq. (5.53) once rearranged.

(ii) In a similar fashion, the Laplace transform of the potential equation reveals

$$C_{ms}\mathcal{L}\tilde{V} = -\overline{g}_{Na}\{\overline{m}^3\overline{h}\mathcal{L}\tilde{V} + (3\overline{m}^2\overline{h}\mathcal{L}\tilde{m} + \overline{m}^3\mathcal{L}\tilde{h})v_{Na}\} - \overline{g}_K\{\overline{n}^4\mathcal{L}\tilde{V} + 4\overline{n}^3 v_K \mathcal{L}\tilde{n}\} - g_{Cl}\mathcal{L}\tilde{V} + \mathcal{L}\tilde{I}/A.$$

On substituting for $\mathcal{L}\tilde{m}$, $\mathcal{L}\tilde{h}$, and $\mathcal{L}\tilde{m}$ from (i) we may solve for $\mathcal{L}\tilde{V}$ as a multiple of $\mathcal{L}\tilde{I}$. On dividing this into $\mathcal{L}\tilde{I}$ we achieve the stated G_{in}.

(iii) The derivatives in Eq. (5.54) follow from the fact that

$$\frac{d^j}{ds^j}\frac{1}{1+s\tau}\bigg|_{s=0} = (-\tau)^j.$$

The derivatives in Eq. (5.55) follow from

$$M_j(f) = (-1)^j \frac{d^j}{ds^j}(\mathcal{L}f)(s)\bigg|_{s=0}.$$

(iv) See Cox and Griffith (2001).

28.5 CHAPTER 6

Exercise 1. Given the $\mathbf{S}$ of Eq. (6.9) and $\mathbf{u} \in \mathbb{R}^N$ we find

$$
\begin{aligned}
dx^2\mathbf{u}^T\mathbf{S}\mathbf{u} &= \sum_{i=1}^N \mathbf{u}_i \sum_{j=1}^N \mathbf{S}_{ij}\mathbf{u}_j \\
&= \mathbf{u}_1(\mathbf{u}_2 - \mathbf{u}_1) + \sum_{i=2}^{N-1}\mathbf{u}_i(\mathbf{u}_{i-1} - 2\mathbf{u}_i + \mathbf{u}_{i+1}) + \mathbf{u}_N(\mathbf{u}_{N-1} - \mathbf{u}_N) \\
&= \mathbf{u}_1(\mathbf{u}_2 - \mathbf{u}_1) + \mathbf{u}_1\mathbf{u}_2 - \mathbf{u}_2^2 - \sum_{i=2}^{N-2}(\mathbf{u}_i - \mathbf{u}_{i+1})^2 - \mathbf{u}_{N-1}^2 + \mathbf{u}_{N-1}\mathbf{u}_N + \mathbf{u}_N(\mathbf{u}_{N-1} - \mathbf{u}_N) \\
&= -\sum_{i=1}^{N-1}(\mathbf{u}_i - \mathbf{u}_{i+1})^2.
\end{aligned}
$$

Exercise 2.

(i) $(z\mathbf{u})^* = z^*\mathbf{u}^* = (A\mathbf{u})^* = A\mathbf{u}^*$.

(ii) $\mathbf{u}^H A\mathbf{u} = z\|\mathbf{u}\|^2$ and $\mathbf{u}^T A\mathbf{u}^* = z^*\|\mathbf{u}\|^2$. As $\mathbf{u}^H A\mathbf{u}$ is scalar it must coincide with its transpose. As such, recalling Eq. (1.3),

$$\mathbf{u}^H A\mathbf{u} = (\mathbf{u}^H A\mathbf{u})^T = \mathbf{u}^T A^T (\mathbf{u}^H)^T = \mathbf{u}^T A\mathbf{u}^*.$$

It follows that $z\|\mathbf{u}\|^2 = z^*\|\mathbf{u}\|^2$, and, as $\|\mathbf{u}\| > 0$ that $z = z^*$.

Exercise 6. From $\mathbf{q}_m^T\mathbf{q}_n = \delta_{mn}$ and $\mathbf{Q} = (\mathbf{q}_0 \ \mathbf{q}_1 \cdots \mathbf{q}_{N-1})$ follows

$$
\mathbf{Q}^T\mathbf{Q} = \begin{pmatrix} \mathbf{q}_0^T\mathbf{q}_0 & \cdots & \mathbf{q}_{N-1}^T\mathbf{q}_0 \\ \vdots & \ddots & \vdots \\ \mathbf{q}_0^T\mathbf{q}_{N-1} & \cdots & \mathbf{q}_{N-1}^T\mathbf{q}_{N-1} \end{pmatrix} = \mathbf{I}
$$

from which we can conclude that $\mathbf{Q}^T = \mathbf{Q}^{-1}$.

Exercise 7.

(i) From Exercise 5.2 we know $\mathbf{A} = \mathbf{LT}$ where $\mathbf{L}$ is lower triangular with ones on its diagonal and $\mathbf{T}$ is upper triangular. If $\mathbf{D}$ is the diagonal of $\mathbf{T}$ and $\mathbf{U}$ is derived by dividing each row i of $\mathbf{T}$ by T_{ii} then $\mathbf{T} = \mathbf{DU}$ and so $\mathbf{A} = \mathbf{LDU}$.

(ii) If $\mathbf{A} = \mathbf{A}^T$ then $\mathbf{LDU} = (\mathbf{LDU})^T = \mathbf{U}^T \mathbf{DL}^T$. On multiplying this by $\mathbf{L}^{-1}$ on the left and $\mathbf{L}^{-T}$ on the right we find $\mathbf{L}^{-1} \mathbf{U}^T \mathbf{D} = \mathbf{DUL}^{-T}$.

(iii) On following the Gauss–Jordan method of Exercise 5.3 we conclude that the inverse of a lower triangular matrix is lower triangular. From Exercise 5.2 we learned that products of lower triangular matrices are lower triangular. Hence, $\mathbf{L}^{-1} \mathbf{U}^T \mathbf{D}$ is lower triangular. By the same reasoning, $\mathbf{DUL}^{-T}$ is upper triangular. As these two coincide they must each be diagonal. By Exercise 5.2 $\mathbf{L}^{-1} \mathbf{U}^T$ is lower triangular with ones on its diagonal, hence the diagonal of $\mathbf{L}^{-1} \mathbf{U}^T \mathbf{D}$ is the diagonal of $\mathbf{D}$. As both are diagonal it follows that $\mathbf{L}^{-1} \mathbf{U}^T \mathbf{D} = \mathbf{D}$. Multiplying this by $\mathbf{D}^{-1}$ reveals $\mathbf{U} = \mathbf{L}^T$ and $\mathbf{A} = \mathbf{LDL}^T$.

(iv) If $\mathbf{A}$ is positive definite then, for each $\mathbf{x} \in \mathbb{R}^n$,

$$0 < \mathbf{x}^T \mathbf{A}\mathbf{x} = \mathbf{x}^T \mathbf{LDL}^T \mathbf{x} = (\mathbf{L}^T \mathbf{x})^T \mathbf{D}(\mathbf{L}^T \mathbf{x}) = \sum_{j=1}^{n} D_{jj} (\mathbf{L}^T \mathbf{x})_j^2$$

and so each $D_{jj} > 0$. It follows that $\mathbf{D} = \mathbf{D}^{1/2} \mathbf{D}^{1/2}$ and $\mathbf{A} = (\mathbf{LD}^{1/2})(\mathbf{LD}^{1/2})^T$.

Exercise 9. The key identities, Eqs. (6.65), (6.68), and (6.71) follow from setting $x = 0$ in Eq. (6.45) and integrating in time precisely as in Eqs. (3.9) and (3.11).

Exercise 11.

(i) $v_\infty(x) = c \exp(\alpha x)$ into Eq. (6.32) brings $\lambda^2 \alpha^2 c \exp(\alpha x) = c \exp(\alpha x)$ and so $\alpha = \pm 1/\lambda$ and $v_\infty(x) = c_1 \exp(x/\lambda) + c_2 \exp(-x/\lambda)$.

(ii) The boundary conditions, Eq. (6.33), impose

$$v'_\infty(0) = (c_1 - c_2)/\lambda = -R_a I_0/(\pi a^2),$$
$$v'_\infty(\ell) = c_1 \exp(\ell/\lambda)/\lambda - c_2 \exp(-\ell/\lambda)/\lambda = 0,$$

and so $c_2 = c_1 \exp(2\ell/\lambda)$ and $c_1(1 - \exp(2\ell/\lambda)) = -R_a \lambda I_0/(\pi a^2)$.

(iii) It follows that

$$v_\infty(x) = \frac{R_a \lambda I_0}{\pi a^2 (\exp(2\ell/\lambda) - 1)} \{\exp(x/\lambda) + \exp((2\ell - x)/\lambda)\}$$

$$= \frac{R_a \lambda I_0 \exp(\ell/\lambda)}{\pi a^2 (\exp(2\ell/\lambda) - 1)} \{\exp((x - \ell)/\lambda) + \exp((\ell - x)/\lambda)\}$$

$$= \frac{R_a \lambda I_0}{\pi a^2} \frac{\cosh((x - \ell)/\lambda)}{\sinh(\ell/\lambda)}$$

as desired.

Exercise 13. The first inequality in Eq. (6.73) uses only the fact that exp is nonnegative. The second inequality follows from direct integration and the fact that $\zeta_n = -(1 + (\lambda n \pi/\ell)^2)/\tau$. Eq. (6.66) demonstrates that such M_n are explicitly summable.

Exercise 14. We proceed, as above, from Eqs. (6.41) and (6.44). In this case, Eq. (6.43) reads (with $r \equiv 1/(2\pi a g_{Cl})$),

$$\tau p'_n(t) = \tau \int_0^\ell q_n(x) \frac{\partial v}{\partial t}(x, t) dx = \int_0^\ell q_n(x) \left(\lambda^2 \frac{\partial^2 v}{\partial x^2}(x, t) - v(x, t) + rI(x, t) \right) dx$$

$$= \lambda^2 \int_0^\ell q_n(x) \frac{\partial^2 v}{\partial x^2}(x, t) dx - p_n(t) + rI_n(t)$$

$$= (\lambda^2 \vartheta_n - 1) p_n(t) + rI_n(t),$$

where $I_n(t)$ is as in Eq. (6.77) and we have used the fact that the cable is sealed at both ends. This establishes Eq. (6.76). On solving this for p_n and substituting it into Eq. (6.41) we arrive at Eq. (6.78). Now, if $I(x,t) = -q_1(x)(e^{-t} - e^{-2t})/500$ then $I_n(t) = -\delta_{1,n}(e^{-t} - e^{-2t})/500$ and so

$$v(x,t) = \frac{q_1(x)}{C_m 2a\pi} \int_0^t I_1(s) \exp((t-s)\zeta_1) ds.$$

Evaluation of the integral yields Eq. (6.80). For the graph see `pfibexact.m`.

Exercise 15.

(i) For $x < x_s$ we integrate Eq. (6.52) in time and find

$$0 = \tau \int_0^\infty \frac{\partial v}{\partial t}(x,t) dt + \int_0^\infty v(x,t) dt - \lambda^2 \int_0^\infty \frac{\partial^2 v}{\partial x^2}(x,t) dt$$
$$= v(x,\infty) - v(x,0) + M_L(x) - \lambda^2 M_L''(x).$$

As $v(x,0)$ begins and returns to rest we find $v(x,\infty) = v(x,0) = 0$ and so M_L obeys $M_L(x) = \lambda^2 M_L''(x)$. By the same reasoning M_R obeys the same equation.

(ii) The left seal imposes $M_L'(0) = 0$ and so $M_L(x) = c_L \cosh(\lambda x)$ for some c_L. As $M_L(0) = c_L$ it follows that $c_L = M_0(v(0,\cdot))$. By the same reasoning, $M_R(x) = M_0(v(\ell,\cdot)) \cosh((\ell - x)/\lambda)$.

(iii) As $x \mapsto v(x,t)$ is continuous at $x = x_s$ so too must be its zero order moment, i.e., $M_L(x_s) = M_R(x_s)$. Given the forms achieved in (ii) we find

$$M_0(v(0,\cdot)) \cosh(x_s/\lambda) = M_0(v(\ell,\cdot)) \cosh((\ell - x_s)/\lambda),$$

or

$$\frac{\cosh((\ell - x_s)/\lambda)}{\cosh(x_s/\lambda)} = \frac{M_0(v(0,\cdot))}{M_0(v(\ell,\cdot))}.$$

The right hand side is constant while the left side, call it $\sigma(x_s)$, has the slope

$$-\frac{\sinh(\ell/\lambda)}{\lambda \cosh^2(x_s/\lambda)}.$$

As this is strictly negative it follows that Eq. (6.81) uniquely determines x_s.

Exercise 16. From the fact that $\mathbf{F}\mathbf{q}_n = \gamma_n \mathbf{q}_n$ we discern $(\mathbf{F}\mathbf{q}_0 \cdots \mathbf{F}\mathbf{q}_{N-1}) = (\gamma_0 \mathbf{q}_0 \cdots \gamma_{N-1}\mathbf{q}_{N-1})$ and recognize that this may be expressed $\mathbf{F}\mathbf{Q} = \mathbf{Q}\boldsymbol{\Gamma}$. On multiplying each side by $\mathbf{Q}^T$ we arrive at $\mathbf{F} = \mathbf{Q}\boldsymbol{\Gamma}\mathbf{Q}^T$. Next

$$\mathbf{F}^2 = \mathbf{F}\mathbf{F} = \mathbf{Q}\boldsymbol{\Gamma}\mathbf{Q}^T\mathbf{Q}\boldsymbol{\Gamma}\mathbf{Q}^T = \mathbf{Q}\boldsymbol{\Gamma}\mathbf{I}\boldsymbol{\Gamma}\mathbf{Q}^T = \mathbf{Q}\boldsymbol{\Gamma}^2\mathbf{Q}^T.$$

Multiplying by subsequent powers of $\mathbf{F}$ shifts those powers onto $\boldsymbol{\Gamma}$. It follows that $\mathbf{F}^j$ remains bounded so long as the largest eigenvalue of $\mathbf{F}$ has magnitude less than one. Recalling the ordering of the θ_n, stability requires that $(dt/\tau)(\lambda^2\theta_{N-1} - 1) > -2$. That is

$$dt < \frac{2\tau}{1 + 4(N/\ell)^2 \sin^2((N-1)\pi/(2N))}.$$

For large N the right hand side becomes prohibitively small.

28.6 CHAPTER 7

Exercise 1.

$$1 + 2\sum_{n=1}^{N}\cos(2\pi nx) = 1 + \sum_{n=1}^{N}(\exp(i2\pi nx) + \exp(-i2\pi nx)) = \sum_{n=-N}^{N}\exp(i2\pi nx)$$

$$= e^{-2\pi iNx}\sum_{n=0}^{2N}\exp(i2\pi nx) = e^{-2\pi iNx}\frac{1 - \exp(i2\pi(2N+1)x)}{1 - \exp(i2\pi x)}$$

$$= e^{-2\pi i(N+1/2)x}\frac{1 - \exp(i2\pi 2Nx)}{\exp(-i\pi x) - \exp(i\pi x)} = \frac{\sin((N+1/2)2\pi x)}{\sin(\pi x)}.$$

Exercise 3. We proceed exactly as in Eq. (7.9)

$$\int_{-1/2}^{1/2} f(x)g(y-x)\,dx = \int_{-1/2}^{1/2} f(x)\sum_{n=-\infty}^{\infty}\hat{g}_ne^{2\pi in(y-x)}\,dx = \sum_{n=-\infty}^{\infty}\hat{g}_ne^{2\pi iny}\int_{-1/2}^{1/2} f(x)e^{-2\pi inx}\,dx$$

$$= \sum_{n=-\infty}^{\infty}\hat{f}_n\hat{g}_ne^{2\pi iny}.$$

Exercise 4. On differentiating Eq. (7.3) we find

$$f'(x) = \sum_{n=-\infty}^{\infty} 2\pi in\hat{f}_ne^{2\pi inx}$$

and so, $\widehat{(f')}_n$, the nth Fourier coefficient of f', is $2\pi in\hat{f}_n$. Hence,

$$f' \star g = \sum_{n=-\infty}^{\infty} 2\pi in\hat{f}_n\hat{g}_ne^{2\pi iny} = \frac{d}{dy}\sum_{n=-\infty}^{\infty}\hat{f}_n\hat{g}_ne^{2\pi iny} = (f \star g)'.$$

Exercise 6. The eigenvectors are simply the four columns of the Fourier matrix, Eq. (7.15), with $N=4$ and $w = \exp(2\pi i/N) = i$. The eigenvalues lie in the discrete Fourier transform of the first column of $\mathbf{B}$,

$$\begin{pmatrix} 1 & 1 & 1 & 1 \\ 1 & -i & -1 & i \\ 1 & -1 & 1 & -1 \\ 1 & i & -1 & i \end{pmatrix}\begin{pmatrix} 1 \\ 0 \\ 1 \\ 0 \end{pmatrix} = \begin{pmatrix} 2 \\ 0 \\ 2 \\ 0 \end{pmatrix}.$$

Now take the real part of the eigen-equation $\mathbf{B}\mathbf{x}_j = \lambda_j\mathbf{x}_j$,

$$\Re(\mathbf{B}\mathbf{x}_j) = \Re(\lambda_j\mathbf{x}_j) \Rightarrow \mathbf{B}(\Re\mathbf{x}_j) = \lambda_j(\Re\mathbf{x}_j)$$

as $\mathbf{B}$ and λ_j are real. It follows that the real parts of each of the vectors in Eq. (7.38), i.e.,

$$\begin{pmatrix} 1 \\ 1 \\ 1 \\ 1 \end{pmatrix} \quad \begin{pmatrix} 1 \\ 0 \\ -1 \\ 0 \end{pmatrix} \quad \begin{pmatrix} 1 \\ -1 \\ 1 \\ -1 \end{pmatrix} \quad \begin{pmatrix} 1 \\ 0 \\ -1 \\ 0 \end{pmatrix} \tag{28.3}$$

comprise an orthogonal basis of eigenvectors of $\mathbf{B}$.

Exercise 8. The Fourier transform of the derivative of u is, via integration by parts,

$$\widehat{u'}(\omega) = \int\limits_{-\infty}^{\infty} e^{-2\pi i\omega t} u'(t)\,dt = u(t)e^{-2\pi i\omega t}\Big|_{t=-\infty}^{\infty} + 2\pi i\omega \int\limits_{-\infty}^{\infty} e^{-2\pi i\omega t} u(t)\,dt = 2\pi i\omega\hat{u}(\omega),$$

so long as u vanishes at $\pm\infty$.

Exercise 10. Both assertions follow from the commutativity and associativity of the multiplication operation, namely

$$\widehat{u \star v} = \hat{u}\hat{v} = \hat{v}\hat{u} = \widehat{v \star u}$$

and

$$u \star (\widehat{v \star w}) = \hat{u}(\widehat{v \star w}) = \hat{u}(\hat{v}\hat{w}) = (\hat{u}\hat{v})\hat{w} = (\widehat{u \star v})\hat{w} = (\widehat{u \star v}) \star w.$$

Exercise 11. We use the fact that $\cos x = \frac{1}{2}(e^{ix} + e^{-ix})$ with Eq. (7.27),

$$\int\limits_{-\infty}^{\infty} \cos(2\pi a t)e^{-2\pi i\omega t}\,dt = \int\limits_{-\infty}^{\infty} \frac{1}{2}(e^{2\pi iat} + e^{-2\pi iat})e^{-2\pi i\omega t}\,dt$$

$$= \frac{1}{2}\int\limits_{-\infty}^{\infty} e^{-2\pi i(\omega - a)t}\,dt + \frac{1}{2}\int\limits_{-\infty}^{\infty} e^{-2\pi i(\omega + a)t}\,dt$$

$$= \frac{1}{2}(\delta(\omega - a) + \delta(\omega + a)).$$

Since $\sin x = (e^{ix} - e^{-ix})/(2i)$, we conclude that its Fourier transform is

$$\frac{1}{2i}(\delta(\omega - a) - \delta(\omega + a)).$$

Exercise 13. If $v(x)$ is real, then $v(x)^* = v(x)$. We use this fact and $(e^{ix})^* = e^{-ix}$ to show that,

$$\hat{v}(-\omega)^* = \left(\int\limits_{-\infty}^{\infty} v(t)e^{-2\pi i(-\omega)t}\,dt\right)^* = \int\limits_{-\infty}^{\infty} v(t)^* (e^{2\pi i\omega t})^*\,dt = \int\limits_{-\infty}^{\infty} v(t)e^{-2\pi i\omega t}\,dt = \hat{v}(\omega).$$

Exercise 20. The linearity of the Dirac distribution follows immediately from its definition. The second assertion follows from the change of variables $t \to s = t - \tau$ in the following integral

$$\int\limits_{-\infty}^{\infty} \delta(t - \tau)f(t)\,dt = \int\limits_{-\infty}^{\infty} \delta(s)f(s + \tau)\,ds = f(\tau).$$

The linearity of D_g follows immediately from the linearity of the integral.

Exercise 21.

$$D_g'(f) = D_g(-f') = -\int\limits_{-\infty}^{\infty} g(t)f'(t)\,dt = \int\limits_{-\infty}^{\infty} g'(t)f(t)\,dt = D_{g'}(f).$$

The first equality is the definition of the derivative, and the second one the definition of D_g. The third equality is obtained by integration by parts and using the fact that $f(t)$ is equal to zero outside a bounded interval. The last equality is again the definition of D_g. The equation $\mathbb{1}'(f) = \delta(f)$ follows from

$$\mathbb{1}'(f) = -\mathbb{1}(f') = \int_0^\infty f'(x)\,dx = -(f(\infty) - f(0)) = f(0),$$

since $f(\infty) = 0$. Furthermore, $f(0) = \delta(f)$.

28.7 CHAPTER 8

Exercise 1. We find

$$(\mathbf{DH})_{ij} = \sum_{k=1}^N D_{ik} H_{kj} = D_{ii} H_{ij} \quad \text{and} \quad (\mathbf{DH})_{ji} = \sum_{k=1}^N D_{jk} H_{ki} = D_{jj} H_{ji}.$$

We must now show that $D_{ii}H_{ij} = D_{jj}H_{ji}$. We follow the block structure of $\mathbf{D}$ and $\mathbf{H}$ and do this in pieces.

If $1 \le i, j \le N_1$ then $D_{ii} = D_{jj} = a_1$ and $H_{ij} = H_{ji}$. The same argument holds in the other safe diagonal blocks, $N_1 + 1 \le i, j \le N_1 + N_2 - 1$, and $N_1 + N_2 + 1 \le i, j \le N_1 + N_2 + N_3$, where $\mathbf{D}$ is constant and $\mathbf{H}$ symmetric.

In the far-off diagonal place, $i = N_1 + N_2 + 1$ and $j = N_1$ we find $D_{ii} = a_3$, $D_{jj} = a_1$, $H_{ij} = a_1\lambda_1^2/a_3$, and $H_{ji} = \lambda_1^2$, and so $D_{ii}H_{ij} = D_{jj}H_{ji}$.

Similarly, at the off-diagonal asymmetry, $i = N_1 + N_2 + 1$ and $j = N_1 + N_2$, we find $D_{ii} = a_3$, $D_{jj} = a_2$, $H_{ij} = a_2\lambda_2^2/a_3$, and $H_{ji} = \lambda_2^2$ and so $D_{ii}H_{ij} = D_{jj}H_{ji}$.

Finally, at the somatic asymmetry, $i = N$ and $j = N-1$, $D_{ii} = a_3/\rho$, $D_{jj} = a_3$, $H_{ij} = \rho\lambda_3^2$, and $H_{ji} = \lambda_3^2$ and indeed $D_{ii}H_{ij} = D_{jj}H_{ji}$.

Next, given $\mathbf{DH} = (\mathbf{DH})^T = \mathbf{H}^T\mathbf{D}$ we multiply on the right by $\mathbf{D}^{-1}$ and find $\mathbf{DHD}^{-1} = \mathbf{H}^T$. We now place this $\mathbf{H}^T$ in

$$\mathbf{A}^T = (\mathbf{D}^{1/2}\mathbf{HD}^{-1/2})^T = (\mathbf{D}^{-1/2})^T\mathbf{H}^T(\mathbf{D}^{1/2})^T = (\mathbf{D}^{-1/2})^T\mathbf{DHD}^{-1}\mathbf{D}^{1/2} = \mathbf{D}^{1/2}\mathbf{HD}^{-1/2} = \mathbf{A},$$

as desired.

Exercise 5. f is periodic and unbounded and so crosses the line, g, at infinitely many points. For large n, the crossings approach the asymptotes of $\tan(zL)$. These occur at the zeros of $\cos(zL)$, i.e., $z_n = (n+1/2)\pi/L$.

Exercise 6. We use Eq. (8.21) and integration by parts

$$\vartheta_n \int_0^L q_n(X)q_m(X)\,dX = \int_0^L q_n''(X)q_m(X)\,dX$$

$$= q_n'(X)q_m(X)\big|_0^L - \int_0^L q_n'(X)q_m'(X)\,dX$$

$$= -\vartheta_n q_n(X)q_m(X)/h - \int_0^L q_n'(X)q_m'(X)\,dX$$

$$= -\vartheta_n q_n(L)q_m(L)/h - q_n(X)q_m'(X)\big|_0^L + \int_0^L q_n(X)q_m''(X)\,dX$$

$$= -\vartheta_n q_n(L)q_m(L)/h + \vartheta_m q_n(L)q_m(L)/h + \vartheta_m \int_0^L q_n(X)q_m(X)\,dX$$

$$= q_m(L)q_n(L)(\vartheta_m - \vartheta_n)/h + \vartheta_m \int_0^L q_n(X)q_m(X)\,dX.$$

Simple rearrangement brings Eq. (8.24).

Exercise 8. In this case Eq. (8.20) takes the form

$$\frac{\partial U}{\partial T}(X,T)+U(X,T)=\frac{\partial^2 U}{\partial X^2}(X,T)+\mathbb{1}_{(0,L_1)}(X)I_{stim}(X,T),$$

$$\frac{\partial U}{\partial X}(0,T)=0,$$

$$\frac{\partial U}{\partial T}(L,T)+U(L,T)+h\frac{\partial U}{\partial X}(L,T)=0,$$

$$U(X,0)=0,$$

where the stimulus is removed from the soma condition and inserted into the partial differential equation with the help of the characteristic function of the daughter.

Exercise 9. See `trapforkd.m`.

Exercise 11. The symbolic toolbox reveals the four eigenvectors via

```
>> syms b1 b2 b3
>> c = sqrt(b1^2+b2^2+b3^2);
>> A = [0 0 0 b1; 0 0 0 b2; 0 0 0 b3; b1 b2 b3 0]/c;
>> I = eye(4);
>> null(A)
>> null(A-I)
>> null(A+I)
```

The splitting $\vartheta=-n^2\pi^2$ or $\cos(\sqrt{-\vartheta})=z_j$ corresponds precisely with our splitting $\sin(\sqrt{-\vartheta})=0$ or $\cos(\sqrt{-\vartheta})=0$, with $L=1$ and $z_j=0$.

28.8 CHAPTER 9

Exercise 1. See `stEcabsdriver.m` and `stEcabgNadriver.m`.

Exercise 3. See `myelins.m`.

Exercise 5. See `demyelin.m`.

Exercise 6. See `drfsenoper.m`.

28.9 CHAPTER 10

Exercise 1. See `lif_rand_inp.m`.

Exercise 2. See `lif_rand_inp.m`.

Exercise 3. See `lif_rand_inp.m`.

Exercise 4. See `lif_rand_inp.m`.

Exercise 5. See `thresh_fatigue.m`.

Exercise 6. See `wang_ss.m`.

Exercise 7. See `wang_mod.m`.

Exercise 8. See `pr_sodca_spike.m`, `pr_modes.m`, and `pr_complex.m`.

28.10 CHAPTER 11

Exercise 1. The probability p_k represents the probability of k successes among n synaptic release trials. The probability that sites $1, \ldots, k$ are successful and sites $k+1, \ldots, n$ fail is $p^k q^{n-k}$. Because we are not interested in which particular synaptic release site is successful, this probability has to be multiplied by the number of different ways to obtain exactly k successes among n different sites. This number is

$$\frac{n!}{k!(n-k)!}.$$

To see why this is so, we decide on a fixed strategy: draw from $1, \ldots, n$ at random and assign the first k draws to releases and the last $n-k$ draws to failures. There are $n!$ ways of doing such draws, but of course any permutations in each of the success and failure sets leads to the same assignment of failures and successes. Since there are respectively $k!$ and $(n-k)!$ such permutations we need to divide by the product of these factors.

Exercise 2. Let X and Y be two random variables that take values $x_1, \ldots, x_n$ and $y_1, \ldots, y_m$ and denote by $P(x_i, y_j)$ their joint probability distributions. Then

$$\sum_{i=1}^{n} P(x_i, y_j) = P(y_j) \quad \text{and} \quad \sum_{j=1}^{m} P(x_i, y_j) = P(x_i)$$

so that

$$E[X+Y] = \sum_{i=1}^{n} \sum_{j=1}^{m} (x_i + y_j) P(x_i, y_j)$$

$$= \sum_{i=1}^{n} x_i \sum_{j=1}^{m} P(x_i, y_j) + \sum_{j=1}^{m} y_j \sum_{i=1}^{n} P(x_i, y_j)$$

$$= \sum_{i=1}^{n} x_i P(x_i) + \sum_{j=1}^{m} y_j P(y_j) = E[X] + E[Y].$$

The same argument generalizes to several variables and shows that taking expectations is a linear operation.

The random variables X and Y are independent if and only if the probability $P(X = x_i, Y = y_j)$ factors to $P(X = x_i) \cdot P(Y = Y_j) = p_i q_j$. We can then compute

$$E[(X+Y-m_X-m_Y)^2] = E[(X-m_X)^2 + (Y-m_Y)^2 + (X-m_X)(Y-m_Y)]$$

$$= E[(X-m_X)^2] + E[(Y-m_Y)^2] + E[(X-m_X)(Y-m_Y)]$$

$$= \sigma_X^2 + \sigma_Y^2 + E[(X-m_X)(Y-m_Y)].$$

The next step is to show that $E[(X-m_X)(Y-m_Y)] = 0$:

$$E[(X-m_X)(Y-m_Y)] = E[XY - Xm_Y - m_X Y + m_X m_Y]$$

$$= E[XY] - m_X m_Y - m_X m_Y + m_X m_Y$$

$$= E[XY] - m_X m_Y.$$

But

$$E[XY] = \sum_{i=1}^{n} \sum_{j=1}^{m} x_i y_j p_i q_j = \left(\sum_{i=1}^{n} x_i p_i \right) \left(\sum_{j=1}^{m} y_j q_j \right) = m_X m_Y.$$

Exercise 3. We set $\lambda = n \cdot p$ and assume n large, $p \to 0$ for λ fixed. We start by an approximation of p_0 in this limit:

$$p_0 = (1-p)^n = \left(1 - \frac{\lambda}{n}\right)^n.$$

Taking the logarithm on both sides yields:

$$\log(p_0) = n \log\left(1 - \frac{\lambda}{n}\right).$$

For x small, $\log(1-x) \cong -x - \frac{1}{2}x^2 - \cdots$ and plugging this approximation in the previous equation, we see that the leading term is $-\lambda$ and therefore,

$$p_0 \cong e^{-\lambda}$$

(up to terms of order $1/n$). We can also compute

$$\frac{p_k}{p_{k-1}} = \frac{n-k+1}{k} \cdot \frac{p}{q} = \frac{\lambda - (k-1)p}{k(1-p)} \cong \frac{\lambda}{k},$$

for p small. This last equation allows us to compute p_1 from p_0, p_2 from p_1, etc. We obtain

$$p_1 = \lambda e^{-\lambda}, \quad p_2 = \frac{\lambda^2}{2} e^{-\lambda}, \ldots \quad p_k = \frac{\lambda^k}{k!} e^{-\lambda}, \ldots$$

Exercise 4. We compute

$$m_S = \sum_{k=0}^{\infty} k \frac{\lambda^k e^{-\lambda}}{k!} = e^{-\lambda}\left(\lambda + \frac{\lambda^2}{1!} + \frac{\lambda^3}{2!} + \cdots\right) = e^{-\lambda}\lambda\left(1 + \frac{\lambda}{1!} + \frac{\lambda^2}{2!} + \cdots\right) = \lambda,$$

since the infinite sum in the inner parenthesis is the power expansion of the exponential, e^λ.

We now compute $e^\lambda E[S^2]$, to cancel out the factor $e^{-\lambda}$ that arises just as in the previous computation:

$$
\begin{aligned}
e^\lambda E[S^2] &= \sum_{k=0}^{\infty} \frac{k^2 \lambda^k}{k!} = \lambda + 2\frac{\lambda^2}{1!} + 3\frac{\lambda^3}{2!} + \cdots \\
&= \lambda + \frac{\lambda^2}{1!} + \frac{\lambda^3}{2!} + \cdots + \frac{\lambda^2}{1!} + 2\frac{\lambda^3}{2!} + 3\frac{\lambda^4}{3!} + \cdots \\
&= \lambda\left(1 + \frac{\lambda}{1!} + \frac{\lambda^2}{2!} + \cdots\right) + \lambda^2\left(1 + \frac{\lambda}{1!} + \frac{\lambda^2}{2!} + \cdots\right) \\
&= \lambda e^\lambda + \lambda^2 e^\lambda = e^\lambda(\lambda + \lambda^2).
\end{aligned}
$$

Therefore, $E[S^2] = \lambda + \lambda^2$.

Exercise 5. Proof of the identity, Eq. (11.28), follows exactly as for Exercise 1. Next according to the discrete convolution formula, Eq. (11.12),

$$P(Z=k) = \sum_{n=0}^{k} e^{-\lambda} \frac{\lambda^n}{n!} e^{-\mu} \frac{\mu^n}{n!} = e^{-(\lambda+\mu)} \sum_{n=0}^{k} \frac{\lambda^n}{n!} \frac{\mu^{n-k}}{(n-k)!} = \frac{(\lambda+\mu)^k}{k!}$$

which completes the proof.

Exercise 6.

(i) The mean of the standard normal distribution,

$$p(x) = \frac{1}{\sqrt{2\pi}} e^{-x^2/2},$$

is clearly equal to zero since $p(x)$ is symmetric around zero. The variance is obtained by integrating by part, $\int_a^b v \, du = uv|_a^b - \int_a^b u \, dv$ with $u = e^{-x^2/2}$ and $v = -x$, so that

$$\frac{1}{\sqrt{2\pi}} \int_{-\infty}^{+\infty} x^2 e^{-x^2/2} \, dx = \frac{1}{\sqrt{2\pi}} \left(-xe^{-x^2/2}|_{-\infty}^{+\infty} + \int_{-\infty}^{+\infty} e^{-x^2/2} \, dx \right)$$

$$= \frac{1}{\sqrt{2\pi}} (0 + \sqrt{2\pi}) = 1.$$

The last integral has been computed in Exercise 7.15.

(ii) According to §11.8, if X has density $p(x) = \sqrt{2\pi}^{-1} \exp(-x^2/2)$ and $y = g(x) = ax + b$ then $Y = g(X)$ has density $p(y) = p(g^{-1}(y))/|g'(g^{-1}(y))|$. Since $g'(x) = a$ and $g^{-1}(y) = (y-b)/a$ we obtain

$$p(y) = \frac{1}{\sqrt{2\pi}a} e^{(y-b)^2/2a^2}$$

and thus $Y \sim \mathcal{N}(b, a^2)$. The converse argument follows at once.

(iii) By definition, the expectation $E[\cdot]$ is linear. Thus $E[Y] = E[aX + b] = aE[X] + b$. Furthermore, $E[(Y - m_Y)^2] = E[(aX - am_X)^2] = E[a^2(X - m_X)^2] = a^2 E[(X - m_X)^2]$.

Exercise 8. If $X \sim \mathcal{N}(\mu, \sigma^2)$, then

$$p_X(x) = \frac{1}{\sqrt{2\pi}\sigma} e^{-(x-\mu)^2/2\sigma^2} = \frac{1}{\sqrt{2\pi}\sigma} u((x-\mu)/\sigma),$$

where $u(t) = \exp(-t^2/2)$. Using Exercises 7.12 and 7.15,

$$\hat{p}_X(\omega) = \frac{1}{\sqrt{2\pi}\sigma} \widehat{u((x-\mu)/\sigma)}(\omega) = \frac{1}{\sqrt{2\pi}} \widehat{u(x-\mu)}(\sigma\omega) = \frac{1}{\sqrt{2\pi}} e^{-2\pi i\mu\omega} \hat{u}(\sigma\omega) = e^{-2\pi i\mu\omega} e^{-(2\pi\omega\sigma)^2/2}.$$

Since

$$\hat{p}_Z(\omega) = \hat{p}_X(\omega)\hat{p}_Y(\omega) = e^{-2\pi i\omega(m_1+m_2)} e^{-(2\pi\omega)^2(\sigma_1^2+\sigma_2^2)/2}$$

we conclude that $Z \sim \mathcal{N}(m_1 + m_2, \sigma_1^2 + \sigma_2^2)$.

Exercise 11. After replacing x_1 by $x_1 - m_1$ and x_2 by $x_2 - m_2$, it is sufficient to consider the case where x_1 and x_2 have zero mean. The density $p(x_1, x_2)$ is obtained from Eq. (11.18) by inverting $\mathbf{C}$. According to Eq. (5.39),

$$\mathbf{C}^{-1} = \frac{1}{1-\rho^2} \begin{pmatrix} \sigma_1^{-2} & -\rho\sigma_1\sigma_2 \\ -\rho\sigma_1\sigma_2 & \sigma_2^{-2} \end{pmatrix}.$$

Plugging this result in Eq. (11.18), we obtain

$$p(x_1, x_2) = \frac{1}{2\pi\sigma_1\sigma_2\sqrt{1-\rho^2}} \exp\left(-\frac{1}{2(1-\rho^2)} \left(\frac{x_1^2}{\sigma_1^2} - \frac{2\rho}{\sigma_1\sigma_2} x_1 x_2 + \frac{x_2^2}{\sigma_2^2} \right) \right).$$

Since

$$p(x_1) = \frac{1}{\sqrt{2\pi}\sigma_1} \exp(-x_1^2/2\sigma_1)$$

it follows that

$$p(x_2|x_1) = \frac{1}{\sqrt{2\pi}\sigma_2\sqrt{1-\rho^2}} \exp\left(\frac{-1}{2(1-\rho^2)}\left(\frac{x_1^2}{\sigma_1^2} - \frac{x_2^2}{\sigma_2^2} - \frac{2\rho x_1 x_2}{\sigma_1\sigma_2}\right) + \frac{x_1^2}{2\sigma_1^2}\right)$$

$$= \frac{1}{\sqrt{2\pi}\sigma_2\sqrt{1-\rho^2}} \exp\left(\frac{-1}{2\sigma_2^2(1-\rho^2)}\left(x_2 - \frac{\rho\sigma_2 x}{\sigma_1}\right)^2\right).$$

Exercise 12. If $Z = X_1 + X_2$ and $p(x_1, x_2)$ is the joint density of $(X_1, X_2)^T$, then the density $q(z)$ of Z is given by

$$q(z) = \int_{-\infty}^{\infty} p(x, z - x)\mathrm{d}x.$$

Since $Z = (X_1 - m_1) + (X_2 - m_2) + (m_1 + m_2)$, it is sufficient to consider the case of zero mean Gaussian variables with correlation matrix

$$\mathbf{C} = \begin{pmatrix} \sigma_1^2 & \sigma_1\sigma_2\rho \\ \sigma_1\sigma_2\rho & \sigma_2^2 \end{pmatrix}.$$

The density $p(x_1, x_2)$ was obtained in the previous exercise:

$$p(x_1, x_2) = \frac{1}{2\pi\sigma_1\sigma_2\sqrt{1-\rho^2}} \exp\left(-\frac{1}{2(1-\rho^2)}\left(\frac{x_1^2}{\sigma_1^2} - \frac{2\rho}{\sigma_1\sigma_2}x_1 x_2 + \frac{x_2^2}{\sigma_2^2}\right)\right)$$

which implies

$$q(z) = \frac{1}{2\pi\sigma_1\sigma_2\sqrt{1-\rho^2}} \int_{-\infty}^{\infty} \exp\left(-\frac{1}{2(1-\rho^2)}\left(\frac{x^2}{\sigma_1^2} - \frac{2\rho}{\sigma_1\sigma_2}x(z-x) + \frac{(z-x)^2}{\sigma_2^2}\right)\right)\mathrm{d}x.$$

To "complete the square," we rewrite

$$\frac{x^2}{\sigma_1^2} - \frac{2\rho}{\sigma_1\sigma_2}x(z-x) + \frac{(z-x)^2}{\sigma_2^2} = \frac{\sigma_1^2 + 2\rho\sigma_1\sigma_2 + \sigma_2^2}{\sigma_1^2 + \sigma_2^2}\left(x - \frac{\rho\sigma_1\sigma_2 + \sigma_1^2}{\sigma_1^2 + 2\rho\sigma_1\sigma_2 + \sigma_2^2}z\right)^2 + \frac{1-\rho^2}{\sigma_1^2 + 2\rho\sigma_1\sigma_2 + \sigma_2^2}z^2.$$

This leads to

$$q(z) = \frac{1}{2\pi\sigma_1\sigma_2\sqrt{1-\rho^2}} \exp\left(-\frac{1}{2}\frac{z^2}{\sigma_1^2 + 2\rho\sigma_1\sigma_2 + \sigma_2^2}\right) I_2 \qquad (28.4)$$

where

$$I_2 = \int_{-\infty}^{\infty} \exp\left(-\frac{1}{2}\frac{\sigma_1^2 + 2\sigma_1\sigma_2 + \sigma_2^2}{(1-\rho^2)\sigma_1^2\sigma_2^2}\left(x - \frac{\rho\sigma_1\sigma_2 + \sigma_1^2}{\sigma_1^2 + 2\rho\sigma_1\sigma_2 + \sigma_2^2}z\right)^2\right)\mathrm{d}x.$$

After a shift in the integration variable to recenter the Gaussian at zero, we recognize that this integral is of the form (see Exercise 7.15),

$$\int_{-\infty}^{\infty} \exp\left(-\frac{1}{2}\frac{x^2}{\alpha^2}\right)\mathrm{d}x = \sqrt{2\pi}\alpha, \quad \text{with} \quad \alpha^2 = \frac{(1-\rho^2)\sigma_1^2\sigma_2^2}{\sigma_1^2 + 2\rho\sigma_1\sigma_2 + \sigma_2^2}$$

and so

$$I_2 = \sqrt{2\pi}\,\frac{\sqrt{1-\rho^2}\sigma_1\sigma_2}{\sqrt{\sigma_1^2+\rho\sigma_1\sigma_2+\sigma_2^2}}.$$

Plugging this result in Eq. (28.4),

$$q(z) = \frac{1}{\sqrt{2\pi}}\frac{1}{\sqrt{\sigma_1^2+2\rho\sigma_1\sigma_2+\sigma_2^2}}\exp\!\left(-\frac{1}{2}\frac{z^2}{\sigma_1^2+2\rho\sigma_1\sigma_2+\sigma_2^2}\right).$$

Thus Z is Gaussian with variance $\sigma_Z^2 = \sigma_1^2 + 2\rho\sigma_1\sigma_2 + \sigma_2^2$.

Exercise 13.

$$\sum_{n=0}^{\infty}\int_0^T\!\int_{t_1}^T\cdots\int_{t_{n-1}}^T p_{(0,T]}(s_1,\ldots,s_n)\,\mathrm{d}s_1\cdots\mathrm{d}s_n = \sum_{n=0}^{\infty}\int_0^T\!\int_{t_1}^T\cdots\int_{t_{n-1}}^T e^{-\varrho T}\varrho^n\,\mathrm{d}s_1\cdots\mathrm{d}s_n$$

$$= e^{-\varrho T}\sum_{n=0}^{\infty}\varrho^n\int_0^T\!\int_{t_1}^T\cdots\int_{t_{n-1}}^T \mathrm{d}s_1\cdots\mathrm{d}s_n.$$

The multiple integral is $1/n!$ times the integral over the hypercube $[0;T]^n$ since we need to carry out all possible permutations of the lower boundary indices to fully cover it,

$$\int_0^T\!\int_{t_1}^T\cdots\int_{t_{n-1}}^T \mathrm{d}s_1\cdots\mathrm{d}s_n = \frac{1}{n!}\int_0^T\!\int_0^T\cdots\int_0^T \mathrm{d}s_1\cdots\mathrm{d}s_n = \frac{1}{n!}T^n.$$

The infinite sum is therefore equal to

$$\sum_{n=0}^{\infty}\frac{1}{n!}\varrho^n T^n = e^{\varrho T},$$

completing the proof.

Exercise 14. With

$$\mathbf{A} = \begin{pmatrix} a & b \\ c & d \end{pmatrix},$$

$\mathbf{A}^T\mathbf{A} = \mathbf{I}$ implies

$$a^2+b^2 = 1, \quad c^2+d^2 = 1, \quad \text{and} \quad ac+bd = 0.$$

We set $a=\cos\theta$, $b=\sin\theta$, $c=\sin\phi$, $d=\cos\phi$, for $\theta,\phi\in[0;2\pi)$ to satisfy the first two equations. The last equation leads to

$$\frac{\sin\theta}{\cos\theta} = -\frac{\sin\phi}{\cos\phi} \tag{28.5}$$

provided $\cos\theta$, $\cos\phi \neq 0$. If $\cos\theta=0$ then $\sin\theta=1$ and $\cos\phi=0$ so that $\sin\phi=1$. Therefore $\mathbf{A}=\mathbf{R}(\pi/2)$, the same argument holds for $\cos\phi=0$. The solutions to Eq. (28.5) are $\phi=\pi-\theta$ and $2\pi-\theta$ (mod 2π). In the first case,

$c = \sin \pi - \theta = \sin \theta$ and $d = \cos \pi - \theta = -\cos \theta$. The corresponding matrix has, however, $\det \mathbf{A} = -1$, while in the second case $\sin 2\pi - \theta = -\sin \theta$ and $\cos 2\pi - \theta = \cos \theta$, which leads to $\det \mathbf{A} = 1$.

Exercise 15. By definition, $C_{ij} = E[(X_i - m_i)(X_j - m_j)]$, $i, j = 1, \ldots, n$ and

$$\mathbf{y}^T \mathbf{C} \mathbf{y} = \sum_{i=1}^{n} \sum_{j=1}^{n} y_i E[(X_i - m_i)(X_j - m_j)] y_j = E\left[\left(\sum_{i=1}^{n} (X_i - m_i) y_i \right)^2 \right] \geq 0.$$

The remainder of the proof proceeds as in Exercises 6.2 and 3.

Exercise 16. ρ is the off-diagonal element of the covariance matrix of the centered and normalized variables Z_1 and Z_2, Eq. (11.23). Since the covariance matrix is symmetric and positive semidefinite, we have $\det \mathbf{C}_Z = 1 - \rho^2 \geq 0$, which implies $-1 \leq \rho \leq 1$. When $\rho = \pm 1$ it is easy to see that $E[(Z_1 \mp Z_2)^2] = 0$ which implies $Z_1 = \pm Z_2$ or equivalently

$$\frac{X_1 - m_1}{\sigma_1} = \pm \frac{X_2 - m_2}{\sigma_2}$$

which implies that

$$X_2 = \pm \sigma_2 \frac{X_1 - m_1}{\sigma_1} + m_2.$$

Exercise 20. The result follows from

$$\mathcal{L}(q)(s) = \int_0^\infty e^{-sx} q(x) \, dx = E[e^{-sY}] = E[e^{-sX_1} e^{-sX_2}]$$

$$= E[e^{-sX_1}] E[e^{-sX_2}] = \mathcal{L}(p_1)(s) \mathcal{L}(p_2)(s),$$

where the fourth equality results from the independence of X_1 and X_2. Clearly the generalization is

$$\mathcal{L}(q)(s) = \mathcal{L}(p_1)(s) \cdots \mathcal{L}(p_n)(s).$$

Exercise 21. See `plot_pp.m`.

Exercise 22. The result follows immediately from Exercise 5 by verifying the two properties defining the Poisson process. (i) The probability of two events occurring at the same time is zero for N_1 and N_2 and is therefore also zero for $N_3 = N_1 + N_2$. (ii) Since $N_3(a,b) = N_1(a,b) + N_2(a,b)$, it will be Poisson with rate $\varrho_1 + \varrho_2$, according to Exercise 5. Finally, $N_3(a,b)$ and $N_3(c,d)$ are independent when $(a,b] \cap (c,d] = \emptyset$ since this property is true for each of N_1 and N_2, and since N_1 and N_2 are independent.

28.11 CHAPTER 12

Exercise 1. See `boyd_martin2.m`.

Exercise 2. See `mt_mod6.m`.

Exercise 3. According to Eq. (12.12), between two action potentials the resources relax exponentially towards their steady-state value of 1 from the initial condition r_{init}:

$$r(t) = r_{init} e^{-\Delta t / \tau_{rec}} + (1 - e^{\Delta t / \tau_{rec}}).$$

Immediately after the nth action potential, the resources are reset according to $r_n^+ = (1-u_0)r_n$. Therefore, if r_n denotes the resources at the time of the nth action potential,

$$r_{n+1} = (1-u_0)r_n e^{-\Delta t/\tau_{rec}} + (1-e^{\Delta t/\tau_{rec}}).$$

At steady state, $r_{n+1} = r_n = r_{ss}$ which leads to

$$r_{ss} = (1-u)r_{ss}e^{-\Delta t/\tau_{rec}} + (1-e^{-\Delta t/\tau_{rec}})$$

or

$$r_{ss} = \frac{1-re^{-\Delta t/\tau_{rec}}}{1-(1-u_0)e^{-\Delta t/\tau_{rec}}} \quad \text{and} \quad q_{ss} = q_{max}u_0 r_{ss}. \tag{28.6}$$

Similarly, Eq. (12.13) implies

$$v_{n+1} = \left(v_n + q_n \frac{R_{in}}{\tau_m}\right) e^{-\Delta t/\tau_m}$$

and at steady state

$$v_{ss} = v_{ss}e^{-\Delta t/\tau_m} + q_{ss}\frac{R_{in}}{\tau_m}e^{-\Delta t/\tau_m}.$$

Rearranging,

$$v_{ss} = q_{ss}\frac{R_{in}}{\tau_m}\frac{1}{1-e^{-\Delta t/\tau_m}}$$

and during two pulses,

$$v(t) = q_{ss}\frac{R_{in}}{\tau_m}\frac{1}{1-e^{-\Delta t/\tau_m}}e^{-t/\tau_m}.$$

The average over the interpulse interval is

$$\bar{v} = \frac{1}{\Delta t}\int_0^{\Delta t} v(t)\,dt$$

$$= \frac{q_{ss}R_{in}}{\tau_m \Delta t}\frac{1}{1-\exp(-\Delta t/\tau_m)}\int_0^{\Delta t} e^{-t/\tau_m}\,dt$$

$$= \frac{q_{ss}R_{in}}{\tau_m \Delta t}\frac{1}{1-\exp(-\Delta t/\tau_m)}(-\tau_m)\,e^{-t/\tau_m}\Big|_0^{\Delta t} = \frac{q_{ss}R_{in}}{\Delta t}.$$

If $\Delta t \ll \tau_{rec}$ and τ_m then

$$e^{-\Delta t/\tau_{rec}} \approx 1 - \frac{\Delta t}{\tau_{rec}} \quad \text{and} \quad 1-e^{-\Delta t/\tau_{rec}} \approx \frac{\Delta t}{\tau_{rec}}$$

so that

$$q_{ss} \approx \frac{q_{max}u_0\Delta t/\tau_{rec}}{1-(1-u_0)(1-\Delta t/\tau_{rec})} \approx \frac{q_{max}u_0\Delta t/\tau_{rec}}{u_0\left(1+\Delta t/\tau_{rec}\left(\frac{1+u_0}{u_0}\right)\right)}.$$

Since

$$\frac{1}{1-x} = 1 + x + x^2 + \cdots$$

we obtain

$$q_{ss} = \frac{q_{max}u_0}{u_0}\frac{\Delta t}{\tau_{rec}}\left(1 - \frac{\Delta t}{\tau_{rec}}\frac{1+u_0}{u_0} + \cdots\right) \approx \frac{q_{max}\Delta t}{\tau_{rec}}.$$

For $v_{peak,ss}$ we have

$$v_{peak,ss} = q_{ss}\frac{R_{in}}{\tau_m}\frac{1}{1-e^{\Delta t/\tau_m}} \approx \frac{q_{max}\Delta t}{\tau_{rec}}\frac{R_{in}}{\tau_m}\frac{1}{\Delta t/\tau_m} \approx \frac{q_{max}R_{in}}{\tau_{rec}}.$$

For $v_{av,ss}$ we have

$$v_{av,ss} = q_{ss}\frac{R_{in}}{\Delta t} \approx q_{max}\frac{\Delta t}{\tau_{rec}}\frac{R_{in}}{\Delta t} = q_{max}\frac{R_{in}}{\tau_{rec}}.$$

Exercise 4. See `mt_mod12.m`.

Exercise 5. According to the facilitation model, if an action potential occurs at time t, $r(t)$ is updated to $r(t^+) = r - u \cdot r$ and $u(t^+) = u + u_0(1-u)$. For a regular train,

$$r_1 = r(t_1) = 1, \ u_1 = u_{ss}, \ r_1^+ = r(t_1^+) = (1-u_1)r_1, \ u_1^+ = u_1 + u_0(1-u_1), \ q_1 = q_{max}u_1r_1.$$

Thereafter, both $r(t)$ and $u(t)$ relax exponentially to their steady state so that

$$r_2 = (1-u_1)r_1e^{-\Delta t/\tau_{rec}} + (1-e^{-\Delta t/\tau_{rec}}),$$
$$u_2 = (u_1 + u_0(1-u_1))e^{-\Delta t/\tau_{facil}} + u_0(1-e^{-\Delta t/\tau_{facil}})$$
$$= u_1e^{-\Delta t/\tau_{facil}} + u_0(1 - u_1e^{-\Delta t/\tau_{facil}}).$$

Similarly,

$$r_{n+1} = (1-u_n)r_ne^{-\Delta t/\tau_{rec}} + (1-e^{-\Delta t/\tau_{rec}}),$$
$$u_{n+1} = u_ne^{-\Delta t/\tau_{facil}} + u_0(1 - u_ne^{-\Delta t/\tau_{facil}}).$$

At steady state, $r_{ss} = r_n = r_{n+1}$ and $u_{ss} = u_n = u_{n+1}$ so that

$$u_{ss} = u_{ss}e^{-\Delta t/\tau_{facil}} + u_0(1 - u_{ss}e^{-\Delta t/\tau_{facil}}) = \frac{u_0}{1 - (1-u_0)e^{-\Delta t/\tau_{facil}}},$$
$$r_{ss} = (1-u_{ss})r_{ss}e^{-\Delta t/\tau_{rec}} + (1-e^{-\Delta t/\tau_{rec}}) = \frac{1 - e^{-\Delta t/\tau_{rec}}}{1 - (1-u_{ss})e^{-\Delta t/\tau_{rec}}}.$$

28.12 CHAPTER 13

Exercise 1. See `hyEcabCa3traindrive.m`.

Exercise 3. See `haircell1.m` and `haircell2.m`.

Exercise 4. The system Eq. (13.61) is a direct translation of Figure 13.10. The exponents on c correspond to the requisite number of binding sites. If the a and b pathways are fast then C_1 and O_1 are in relative equilibrium, as are O_1 and O_2. More precisely, we set $C_1' = O_2' = 0$ in Eq. (13.61) and arrive at Eq. (13.62) where

$$K_a = k_a^-/k_a^+ \quad \text{and} \quad K_b = k_b^-/k_b^+.$$

Equations (13.63) and (13.64) now follow by direct substitution. Regarding w',

$$\begin{aligned} w' &= -C_2' = k_c^- C_2 - k_c^+ O_1 \\ &= k_c^-(1-w) - k_c^+(c/K_a)^4 C_1 = k_c^-(1-w) - k_c^+(c/K_a)^4(w-O) \\ &= k_c^-(1-w) - \frac{k_c^+ w}{1 + (K_a/c)^4 + (c/K_b)^3} \\ &= k_c^- - w\frac{k_c^-(1 + (K_a/c)^4 + (c/K_b)^3) + k_c^+}{1 + (K_a/c)^4 + (c/K_b)^3} \end{aligned}$$

and so, with $K_c = k_c^-/k_c^+$,

$$\frac{1}{k_c^-}\frac{1 + (K_a/c)^4 + (c/K_b)^3}{1 + (K_a/c)^4 + (c/K_b)^3 + 1/K_c}w' = \frac{1 + (K_a/c)^4 + (c/K_b)^3}{1 + (K_a/c)^4 + (c/K_b)^3 + 1/K_c} - w,$$

in agreement with Eqs. (13.19) and (13.20).

Exercise 7. See `camk2.m`.

Exercise 8.

(i) The scheme Eq. (13.68) dictates that b obey $b' = k_1 cB - k_2 b$ and so at rest, where $b' = 0$, we find $b = cB/K_d$. Clearly, if $c = K_d$ then $b = B$ and we see that half of the available buffer is indeed bound.

(ii) We substitute Eq. (13.70) into Eq. (13.69) and find $F_1 = (S_{f_1} + S_{b_1}c/K_d)B$ and $F_2 = (S_{f_2} + S_{b_2}c/K_d)B$ and so their ratio is

$$R = \frac{F_1}{F_2} = \frac{S_{f_1} + S_{b_1}c/K_d}{S_{f_2} + S_{b_2}c/K_d}. \tag{28.7}$$

Solving this for c produces Eq. (13.71).

(iii) For small c in Eq. (28.7) we find $R \approx S_{f_1}/S_{f_2} \equiv R_{min}$ while for large c, $R \approx S_{b_1}/S_{b_2} \equiv R_{max}$. Substituting these ratios back into Eq. (28.7) yields the desired Eq. (13.72).

28.13 CHAPTER 14

Exercise 1. As the nonzero eigenvalues of $\mathbf{AA}^T$ and $\mathbf{A}^T\mathbf{A}$ must coincide it follows that

$$\mathbf{\Sigma} = \begin{pmatrix} \sqrt{2} & 0 & 0 & 0 \\ 0 & \sqrt{2} & 0 & 0 \end{pmatrix}.$$

We now use Eq. (14.3) to find that $\mathbf{x}_1$ and $\mathbf{x}_2$ must obey

$$\mathbf{Ax}_1 = \sqrt{2}\,(1\,0)^T, \quad \mathbf{Ax}_2 = \sqrt{2}\,(0\,1)^T, \quad \text{and} \quad \mathbf{x}_i^T\mathbf{x}_j = \delta_{ij}.$$

It follows that

$$\mathbf{x}_1 = (1\,0\,1\,0)^T/\sqrt{2} \quad \text{and} \quad \mathbf{x}_2 = (0\,1\,0\,1)^T/\sqrt{2}.$$

Next, we need an orthonormal pair of solutions to $\mathbf{A}\mathbf{x} = 0$. The simplest seems to be

$$\mathbf{x}_3 = (1\ 0\ -1\ 0)^T/\sqrt{2} \quad \text{and} \quad \mathbf{x}_4 = (0\ 1\ 0\ -1)^T/\sqrt{2}.$$

Finally, as $\mathbf{Y} = \mathbf{I}$,

$$\mathbf{Y}\mathbf{\Sigma}\mathbf{X}^T = \mathbf{\Sigma}\mathbf{X}^T = \frac{1}{\sqrt{2}}\begin{pmatrix} \sqrt{2} & 0 & 0 & 0 \\ 0 & \sqrt{2} & 0 & 0 \end{pmatrix}\begin{pmatrix} 1 & 0 & 1 & 0 \\ 0 & 1 & 0 & 1 \\ 1 & 0 & -1 & 0 \\ 0 & 1 & 0 & -1 \end{pmatrix} = \begin{pmatrix} 1 & 0 & 1 & 0 \\ 0 & 1 & 0 & 1 \end{pmatrix} = \mathbf{A}$$

as desired.

Exercise 2.

$$
\begin{aligned}
(\mathbf{A}^T\mathbf{A})\mathbf{A}^+\mathbf{b} &= \mathbf{X}\mathbf{\Lambda}_n\mathbf{X}^T\mathbf{X}\mathbf{\Sigma}^+\mathbf{Y}^T\mathbf{b} && \text{by (14.4)} \\
&= \mathbf{X}\mathbf{\Lambda}_n\mathbf{\Sigma}^+\mathbf{Y}^T\mathbf{b} && \text{because } \mathbf{X}^T\mathbf{X} = \mathbf{I} \\
&= \mathbf{X}\mathbf{\Sigma}^T\mathbf{\Sigma}\mathbf{\Sigma}^+\mathbf{Y}^T\mathbf{b} && \text{by (14.6)} \\
&= \mathbf{X}\mathbf{\Sigma}^T\mathbf{Y}^T\mathbf{b} && \text{because } \mathbf{\Sigma}^T\mathbf{\Sigma}\mathbf{\Sigma}^+ = \mathbf{\Sigma}^T \\
&= \mathbf{A}^T\mathbf{b} && \text{by (14.7).}
\end{aligned}
$$

Exercise 5. Given $v_j = \mathbf{w}_j^T\mathbf{x}_j$ we define

$$
\begin{aligned}
F(\gamma_j) &\equiv \frac{1}{\|\mathbf{w}_j + \gamma_j v_j \mathbf{x}_j\|} \\
&= \{(\mathbf{w}_j + \gamma_j v_j \mathbf{x}_j)^T(\mathbf{w}_j + \gamma_j v_j \mathbf{x}_j)\}^{-1/2} \\
&= \{\|\mathbf{w}_j\|^2 + 2\gamma_j v_j^2 + (\gamma_j v_j)^2\|\mathbf{x}_j\|^2\}^{-1/2},
\end{aligned}
$$

and develop F in the MacLaurin series $F(\gamma_j) = F(0) + \gamma_j F'(0) + O(\gamma_j^2)$. The $F(0)$ term is immediate. We compute

$$F'(\gamma_j) = (-1/2) = \{\|\mathbf{w}_j\|^2 + 2\gamma_j v_j^2 + (\gamma_j v_j)^2\|\mathbf{x}_j\|^2\}^{-1/2}(2v_j^2 + 2\gamma_j v_j^2\|\mathbf{x}_j\|^2)$$

and so $F'(0) = -v_j^2/\|\mathbf{w}_j\|$. If we now use this in Eq. (14.14), with $\|\mathbf{w}_j\| = 1$, we find

$$
\begin{aligned}
\mathbf{w}_{j+1} &= \frac{\mathbf{w}_j + \gamma_j v_j \mathbf{x}_j}{\|\mathbf{w}_j + \gamma_j v_j \mathbf{x}_j\|} = (\mathbf{w}_j + \gamma_j v_j \mathbf{x}_j)\big(1 - \gamma_j v_j^2 + O(\gamma_j^2)\big) \\
&= \mathbf{w}_j + \gamma_j(\mathbf{x}_j\mathbf{x}_j^T - \mathbf{w}_j^T\mathbf{x}_j\mathbf{x}_j^T\mathbf{w}_j\mathbf{I})\mathbf{w}_j + O(\gamma_j^2)
\end{aligned}
$$

where we have used $v_j = \mathbf{w}_j^T\mathbf{x}_j$.

Exercise 8. We differentiate Eq. (5.30) and find

$$
\begin{aligned}
\frac{\mathrm{d}}{\mathrm{d}t}\exp(t\mathbf{B}) &= \frac{\mathrm{d}}{\mathrm{d}t}(\mathbf{I} + t\mathbf{B} + (t\mathbf{B})^2/2 + (t\mathbf{B})^3/3! + \cdots) \\
&= \mathbf{B} + t\mathbf{B}^2 + t^2\mathbf{B}^3/2 + \cdots = \mathbf{B}(\mathbf{I} + t\mathbf{B} + (t\mathbf{B})^2/2 + (t\mathbf{B})^3/3! + \cdots) \\
&= \mathbf{B}\exp(t\mathbf{B}) = \exp(t\mathbf{B})\mathbf{B}.
\end{aligned}
$$

As the identical result holds for $\mathbf{B}^T$ we may differentiate Eq. (14.26) and find

$$\mathbf{E}'(t) = \mathbf{B}\exp(t\mathbf{B})\mathbf{C}\mathbf{C}^T\exp(t\mathbf{B}^T) + \exp(t\mathbf{B})\mathbf{C}\mathbf{C}^T\exp(t\mathbf{B}^T)\mathbf{B}^T$$

as claimed. The equation for $\mathbf{F}'(t)$ is obtained in exactly the same fashion.

Exercise 9. The zeros in column 1 of Eq. (14.40) derive from the simple fact that

$$\mathbf{B}\mathbf{y}_1 = \lambda\mathbf{y}_1 = (\mathbf{y}_1\,\mathbf{y}_2\,\cdots\,\mathbf{y}_N)(\lambda\,0\,\cdots\,0)^T = \mathbf{Y}\begin{pmatrix}\lambda\\0\end{pmatrix}.$$

To show that $\mathbf{X}$ is unitary we use the fact that $\mathbf{Y}$ and $\mathbf{Z}$ are unitary.

$$\mathbf{X}^H\mathbf{X} = \begin{pmatrix}1 & 0\\0 & \mathbf{Z}^H\end{pmatrix}\mathbf{Y}^H\mathbf{Y}\begin{pmatrix}1 & 0\\0 & \mathbf{Z}\end{pmatrix} = \begin{pmatrix}1 & 0\\0 & \mathbf{Z}^H\end{pmatrix}\begin{pmatrix}1 & 0\\0 & \mathbf{Z}\end{pmatrix} = \begin{pmatrix}1 & 0\\0 & \mathbf{Z}^H\mathbf{Z}\end{pmatrix} = \mathbf{I}.$$

To show that $\mathbf{X}^H\mathbf{B}\mathbf{X}$ is upper triangular we note that $\mathbf{W} = \mathbf{Z}^H\mathbf{V}\mathbf{Z}$ is upper triangular.

$$\begin{aligned}
\mathbf{X}^H\mathbf{B}\mathbf{X} &= \begin{pmatrix}1 & 0\\0 & \mathbf{Z}^H\end{pmatrix}\mathbf{Y}^H\mathbf{B}\mathbf{Y}\begin{pmatrix}1 & 0\\0 & \mathbf{Z}\end{pmatrix}\\
&= \begin{pmatrix}1 & 0\\0 & \mathbf{Z}^H\end{pmatrix}\mathbf{Y}^H\mathbf{Y}\begin{pmatrix}\lambda & \mathbf{v}\\0 & \mathbf{V}\end{pmatrix}\begin{pmatrix}1 & 0\\0 & \mathbf{Z}\end{pmatrix}\\
&= \begin{pmatrix}1 & 0\\0 & \mathbf{Z}^H\end{pmatrix}\begin{pmatrix}\lambda & \mathbf{v}\\0 & \mathbf{V}\end{pmatrix}\begin{pmatrix}1 & 0\\0 & \mathbf{Z}\end{pmatrix}\\
&= \begin{pmatrix}\lambda & \mathbf{v}\mathbf{Z}\\0 & \mathbf{Z}^H\mathbf{V}\mathbf{Z}\end{pmatrix} = \begin{pmatrix}\lambda & \mathbf{v}\mathbf{Z}\\0 & \mathbf{W}\end{pmatrix}.
\end{aligned}$$

Exercise 13. See `stEQcabBT2.m`.

28.14 CHAPTER 15

Exercise 4. See `neg_corr.m`.

Exercise 5. Since for a Poisson process $f(x) = \varrho\exp(-\varrho x)$, integration yields $F(x) = 1 - \exp(-\varrho x)$ and $f_1(x) = (1 - F(x))/m_{\Delta t} = \varrho\exp(-\varrho x)$ which is identical to $f(x)$. The cumulative distribution function of a gamma process was computed in Eq. (15.1). This yields

$$1 - F(x) = \sum_{r=0}^{n-1} e^{-\varrho x}\frac{(\varrho x)^r}{r!}.$$

Plugging in this equation $n = 2$, $m_{\Delta t} = n/\varrho$ and using the formula $f_1(x) = (1 - F(x))/m_{\Delta t}$, we obtain

$$f_1(x) = \frac{\varrho}{2}(\varrho x + 1)e^{-\varrho x}.$$

The numerical implementation is in `gamma_frect.m`.

Exercise 6. Since $f_1(x) = (1 - F(x))/m_{\Delta t}$

$$\mathcal{L}(f_1)(s) = \mathcal{L}\left(\frac{1 - F(x)}{m_{\Delta t}}\right) = \mathcal{L}\left(\frac{1}{m_{\Delta t}}\right) - \frac{1}{m_{\Delta t}}\mathcal{L}(F)(s) = \frac{1}{m_{\Delta t}s} - \frac{1}{m_{\Delta t}}\mathcal{L}(F)(s).$$

But $F(0) = 0$ and $F'(x) = f(x)$, so that $\mathcal{L}(F)(s) = (1/s)\mathcal{L}(f)(s)$ and plugging this result in the previous equation yields

$$\mathcal{L}(f_1)(s) = \frac{1 - \mathcal{L}(F)}{m_{\Delta t}}.$$

Exercise 8. Since

$$P(N(0,t) < l) = P(S_l > t) = 1 - K_l(t), \quad \text{and} \quad K_0(t) = 1$$

we have

$$
\begin{aligned}
P(N(0,t)=l) &= P(N(0,t)<l+1) - P(N(0,t)<l) \\
&= 1 - K_{l+1}(t) - (1 - K_l(t)) = K_l(t) - K_{l+1}(t).
\end{aligned}
$$

Consequently,

$$
\begin{aligned}
E[N(0,t)] &= \sum_{l=1}^{\infty} l(K_l(t) - K_{l+1}(t)) = \sum_{l=1}^{\infty} lK_l(t) - \sum_{l=1}^{\infty} lK_{l+1}(t) \\
&= \sum_{l=1}^{\infty} lK_l(t) - \sum_{l=2}^{\infty} (l-1)K_l(t) = \sum_{l=1}^{\infty} K_l(t).
\end{aligned}
$$

Exercise 9. We use the fact that the Laplace transform of $K_l(t)$ is given by

$$
\mathcal{L}(K_l)(s) = \frac{1}{s}\mathcal{L}(k_l)(s) - K_l(0) = \frac{1}{s}\mathcal{L}(k_l)(s)
$$

(see Eq. (3.16)). Furthermore, $\mathcal{L}(k_l)(s) = \mathcal{L}(p_n)(s)^l$ by a straightforward generalization of Exercise 11.20. Plugging these results in Eq. (15.7) we obtain

$$
\mathcal{L}(m_{N(0,t)})(s) = \sum_{l=1}^{\infty} \mathcal{L}(K_l)(s) = \frac{1}{s}\sum_{l=1}^{\infty} \mathcal{L}(k_l)(s) = \frac{1}{s}\sum_{l=1}^{\infty} \mathcal{L}(p_n)(s)^l = \frac{1}{s}\frac{\mathcal{L}(p_n)(s)}{1-\mathcal{L}(p_n)(s)}.
$$

The last equality follows from the identity $\sum_{l=1}^{\infty} x^l = x/(1-x)$ for $|x|<1$.

Exercise 10. For $n=2$, $p_n(x) = \varrho^2 x \exp(-\varrho x)$ and $\mathcal{L}(p_n)(s) = \varrho^2/(\varrho+s)^2$. Therefore,

$$
\begin{aligned}
\mathcal{L}(m_{N(0,t)})(s) &= \frac{1}{s}\frac{\varrho^2}{(\varrho+s)^2}\frac{1}{1-\varrho^2/(\varrho+s)^2} = \frac{1}{s}\frac{\varrho^2}{(\varrho+s)^2-\varrho^2} \\
&= \frac{1}{s}\frac{\varrho^2}{(\varrho+s-\varrho)(\varrho+s+\varrho)} = \frac{\varrho^2}{s^2(\sigma+2\varrho)}.
\end{aligned}
$$

The partial fraction expansion

$$
\begin{aligned}
\frac{\varrho^2}{s^2(s+2\varrho)} &= \frac{A}{s^2}+\frac{B}{s}+\frac{C}{s+2\varrho} \\
&= \frac{A(s+2\varrho)+Bs(s+2\varrho)+Cs^2}{s^2(s+2\varrho)} \\
&= \frac{(C+B)s^2+(A+2\varrho B)s+2\varrho A}{s^2(s+\varrho)}
\end{aligned}
$$

leads to: $2\varrho A = \varrho^2$ or $A = \varrho/2$, $A+2\varrho B = 0$ or $B = -A/2\varrho = -1/4$, and $C = -B-1/4$. Summing up,

$$
\mathcal{L}(m_{N(0,t)})(s) = \frac{\varrho}{2}\frac{1}{s^2} - \frac{1}{4s} + \frac{1}{4}\frac{1}{s+2\varrho}
$$

which implies

$$
m_{N(0,t)} = \frac{\varrho}{2}t - \frac{1}{4} + \frac{1}{4}e^{-2\varrho t}.
$$

Exercise 11. Since

$$\sigma^2_{N(0,t)} = E[N(0,t)^2] - E[N(0,t)]^2 \quad \text{and} \quad \xi(t) = E[N(0,t)^2] + E[N(0,t)]$$

the result is immediate.

Exercise 12. By definition of $\xi(t)$,

$$\xi(t) = \sum_{l=0}^{\infty} l(l+1)P(N(0,t)=l) = \sum_{l=0}^{\infty} l(l+1)(K_l(t) - K_{l+1}(t)).$$

Taking the Laplace transform yields

$$\mathcal{L}(\xi)(s) = \sum_{l=0}^{\infty} l(l+1)\frac{1}{s}(\mathcal{L}(k_l)(s) - \mathcal{L}(k_{l+1}(s))$$

$$= \frac{2}{s}\sum_{l=1}^{\infty} l\mathcal{L}(k_l)(s) = \frac{2}{s}\sum_{l=1}^{\infty} l\mathcal{L}(p_n)(s)^l = \frac{2}{s}\frac{\mathcal{L}(p_n)}{(1-\mathcal{L}(p_n))^2}.$$

Exercise 14. For a stationary renewal process with interspike interval distribution density $f(x)$, the distribution of the first interval W_1 is given by $f_1(x) = 1 - F(x)/m_{\Delta t}$ (the forward recurrence time, Exercise 5). Consequently, the lth interval S_l is the sum $W_1 + X_2 + \cdots + X_l$ of $l-1$ identically distributed random variables and W_1. According to Exercises 6 and 11.20, the Laplace transform of the corresponding density is

$$\mathcal{L}(k_l)(s) = \frac{1 - \mathcal{L}(f)(s)}{m_{\Delta t}}\mathcal{L}(f)(s)^{l-1}.$$

In Exercise 9 we showed that

$$\mathcal{L}(m_{N(0,t)})(s) = \frac{1}{s}\sum_{l=1}^{\infty}\mathcal{L}(k_l)(s) = \frac{1 - \mathcal{L}(f)(s)}{m_{\Delta t}s^2}\sum_{l=1}^{\infty}\mathcal{L}(f)(s)^{l-1} = \frac{1}{m_{\Delta t}s^2},$$

where we used the identity $\sum_{l=0}^{\infty} x^l = 1/(1-x)$ for $|x| < 1$. Taking the inverse Laplace transform immediately yields $m_{N(0,t)} = t/m_{\Delta t}$.

Exercise 15. Using the results derived in Exercises 12 and 14, we have

$$\mathcal{L}(\xi)(s) = \frac{2}{s}\sum_{l=1}^{\infty} l\mathcal{L}(k_l)(s) = \frac{2}{s}\sum_{l=1}^{\infty} l\mathcal{L}(p_n)(s)^{l-1}\frac{1 - \mathcal{L}(p_n)(s)}{m_{\Delta t}s}$$

$$= \frac{2}{m_{\Delta t}s^2}(1 - \mathcal{L}(p_n)(s))\mathcal{L}(p_n)(s)^{-1}\sum_{l=1}^{\infty} l\mathcal{L}(p_n)(s)^l = \frac{2}{m_{\Delta t}s^2}\frac{1}{1 - \mathcal{L}(p_n)(s)}.$$

Exercise 16. Since $\mathcal{L}(p_2) = \varrho^2/(\varrho+s)^2$, we have

$$\mathcal{L}(\xi)(s) = \frac{2}{m_{\Delta t}s^2}\frac{(\varrho+s)^2}{(\varrho+s)^2 - \varrho^2} = \frac{2}{m_{\Delta t}s^2}\frac{(\varrho+s)^2}{s(s+2\varrho)} = \frac{2}{m_{\Delta t}s^3}\frac{(\varrho+s)^2}{(s+2\varrho)}.$$

We carry out the partial fraction expansion

$$\frac{1}{s^3}\frac{(s+\varrho)^2}{(s+2\varrho)} = \frac{A}{s^3} + \frac{B}{s^2} + \frac{C}{s} + \frac{D}{s+2\varrho}$$

with the numerator on the left hand side being given by $(s+\varrho)^2 = s^2 + 2\varrho s + \varrho^2$ and that on the right hand side by

$$A(s+2\varrho) + Bs(s+2\varrho) + Cs^2(s+2\varrho) + Ds^3 = s^3(C+D) + s^2(B+2\varrho C) + s(A+2\varrho B) + 2\varrho A.$$

This yields the following equations:

1. $C+D=0 \Rightarrow C=-D$.
2. $2\varrho A = \varrho^2 \Rightarrow A = \varrho/2$.
3. $A+2\varrho B = 2\varrho \Rightarrow 2\varrho B + 2\varrho - \varrho/2$, or $B=3/4$.
4. $B+2\varrho C = 1 \Rightarrow 3/4 + 2\varrho C = 1$ or $C = 1/(8\varrho)$.
5. $D = -C = -1/(8\varrho)$.

Summing up,

$$\mathcal{L}(\xi)(s) = \frac{\varrho^2}{2s^3} + \frac{3\varrho}{4s^2} + \frac{1}{8s} - \frac{1}{8(s+2\varrho)},$$

which can be immediately inverted

$$\xi(t) = \frac{\varrho^2 t^2}{4} + \frac{3\varrho t}{4} + \frac{1}{8} - \frac{1}{8}e^{-2\varrho t}.$$

Combining this result with $m_{N(0,t)} = t/m_{\Delta t}$ we arrive at Eq. (15.10).

Exercise 17. For the numerics, see `gamma_char.m`. Practically, the two graphs coincide. Thus it is very difficult to distinguish an ordinary gamma two process from a stationary one based on the first two moments of spike counts.

28.15 CHAPTER 16

Exercise 1. By definition,

$$C_X(\tau) = E[(X(t) - m_V)(X(t+\tau) - m_V)]$$
$$C_X(-\tau) = E[(X(t) - m_V)(X(t-\tau) - m_V)].$$

By stationarity and interchange of the order of the multiplication terms,

$$E[(X(t) - m_X)(X(t+\tau) - m_X)] = E[(X(t-\tau) - m_X)(X(t) - m_X)]$$
$$= E[(X(t) - m_X)(X(t-\tau) - m_X)].$$

Combining these two sets of equations, we obtain the desired result.

Exercise 2. See `rand_fig2.m` for the associated numerics.

Exercise 3. According to Eq. (16.4),

$$p(w_1, w_2) = \frac{1}{2\pi} \frac{1}{\sqrt{t_1(t_2 - t_1)}} e^{-\frac{1}{2}\left(\frac{w_1^2}{t_1} + \left(\frac{(w_2 - w_1)^2}{t_2 - t_1}\right)\right)}.$$

By definition

$$E[W(t_1)W(t_2)] = \int\!\!\!\int_{-\infty}^{\infty} p(w_1, w_2)w_1 w_2 dw_1 dw_2$$

$$= \frac{1}{\sqrt{2\pi t_1}} \int_{-\infty}^{\infty} w_1 e^{-\frac{w_1^2}{2t_1}} \left(\frac{1}{\sqrt{2\pi(t_2 - t_1)}} \int_{-\infty}^{\infty} w_2 e^{\frac{(w_2 - w_1)^2}{2(t_2 - t_1)}} dw_2\right) dw_1.$$

The integral in parentheses is equal to the mean of the integrated Gaussian distribution, w_1. This results in

$$E[W(t_1)W(t_2)] = \frac{1}{\sqrt{2\pi t_1}} \int_{-\infty}^{\infty} w_1^2 e^{-\frac{w_1^2}{2t_1}} \, dw_1 = t_1.$$

Exercise 4. We first show $E[M_P(t)] = \varrho$. Since $M_P(t) = 0$ when $n = 0$,

$$E[M_P(t)] = \sum_{n=1}^{\infty} \int_0^T \int_{t_1}^T \cdots \int_{t_{n-1}}^T p_{(0,T]}(t_1,\ldots,t_n) M_P(t) \, dt_1 \ldots dt_n.$$

Using the argument presented in Exercise 11.13 we may replace the lower integration boundaries by 0 if we divide each term by $1/n!$ since the integrand is totally symmetric in $(t_1,\ldots t_n)$. This leads to

$$E[M_P(t)] = \sum_{n=1}^{\infty} \frac{1}{n!} \int_0^T \int_0^T \cdots \int_0^T p_{(0,T]}(t_1,\ldots,t_n) M_P(t) \, dt_1 \ldots dt_n$$

$$= \sum_{n=1}^{\infty} \frac{1}{n!} \int_0^T \cdots \int_0^T \varrho^n e^{-\varrho T} \sum_{i=1}^n \delta(t - t_i) dt_1 \ldots dt_n$$

$$= \sum_{n=1}^{\infty} \frac{1}{n!} \varrho^n e^{-\varrho T} n \int_0^T \delta(t - t_1) \, dt_1 \cdot T^{n-1}$$

$$= \sum_{n=1}^{\infty} \frac{1}{(n-1)!} \varrho^n e^{-\varrho T} T^{n-1} = \varrho \left(\sum_{n=1}^{\infty} \frac{1}{(n-1)!} \varrho^{n-1} T^{n-1} \right) e^{-\varrho T} = \varrho.$$

Similarly,

$$E[M_P(t_a)M_P(t_b)] = \sum_{n=1}^{\infty} \frac{1}{n!} \int_0^T \cdots \int_0^T p_{(0,T]}(t_1,\ldots,t_n) M_P(t_a) M_P(t_b) dt_1 \cdots dt_n$$

$$= \varrho e^{-\varrho T} \int_0^T \delta(t_a - t_1)\delta(t_b - t_1) \, dt_1 + \sum_{n=2}^{\infty} \frac{1}{n!} \varrho^n e^{-\varrho T} \int_0^T \cdots \int_0^T \sum_{i,j=1}^n \delta(t_a - t_i)\delta(t_b - t_j) \, dt_1 \cdots dt_n$$

$$= \varrho e^{-\varrho T} \delta(t_b - t_a) + \sum_{n=2}^{\infty} \frac{1}{n!} \varrho^n e^{-\varrho T} \left(\sum_{i \neq j} \int_0^T \cdots \int_0^T \delta(t_a - t_i)\delta(t_b - t_j) dt_1 \cdots dt_n \right.$$

$$\left. + \sum_{i=1}^n \int_0^T \cdots \int_0^T \delta(t_a - t_i)\delta(t_b - t_i) \, dt_1 \cdots dt_n \right).$$

Since

$$\sum_{i=1}^n \int_0^T \cdots \int_0^T \delta(t_a - t_i)\delta(t_b - t_i) dt_1 \cdots dt_n = \delta(t_b - t_a) \cdot T^{n-1} \cdot n$$

$$\sum_{i \neq j} \int_0^T \cdots \int_0^T \delta(t_a - t_i)\delta(t_b - t_j) dt_1 \cdots dt_n = T^{n-2} \cdot n(n-1)$$

we obtain

$$E[M_P(t_a)M_P(t_b)] = \varrho e^{-\varrho T}\delta(t_b - t_a)\sum_{n=2}^{\infty}\frac{1}{n!}\varrho^n e^{-\varrho T}\left(\delta(t_b - t_a)T^{n-1}n + T^{n-2}n(n-1)\right)$$

$$= \delta(t_b - t_a)e^{-\varrho T}\left(\varrho + \sum_{n=2}^{\infty}\frac{\varrho^n}{(n-1)!}T^{n-1}\right) + \sum_{n=2}^{\infty}\frac{1}{(n-2)!}\varrho^n T^{n-2} = \delta(t_b - t_a)\varrho + \varrho^2.$$

Exercise 5. See `gamma_corr.m`.

Exercise 6. See `rand_fig3.m`.

Exercise 7. According to the results of Exercises 7.13 and 7.14,

$$S(\omega) = S(-\omega) = S(\omega)^*,$$

which completes the proof.

Exercise 8. See `gamma_powersp.m`.

Exercise 9. Starting from Eq. (16.20),

$$P(\text{spike in } (t+\tau, t+\tau+\Delta t)|\text{spike at } t) = E[N(t+\tau+\Delta t, t) - N(t+\tau, t)] + o(\Delta t^2)$$

$$= E[N(t+\tau+\Delta t, t)] - E[N(t+\tau, t)] + o(\Delta t^2).$$

Now divide by Δt on both sides and take the limit $\Delta t \to 0$ to arrive at

$$\chi_c(\tau) = \frac{d}{d\tau}E[N(t+\tau, t)],$$

where a spike is assumed to have occurred at t. Since the process is stationary, the right hand side is independent of t and we arrive at

$$\chi_c(\tau) = \frac{d}{d\tau}E[N(\tau, 0)],$$

where a spike is assumed to have occurred at $t = 0$.

Exercise 10. According to Exercise 9, $\chi_c(\tau) = dm_{N(0,\tau)}/d\tau$, with the notation $m_{N(0,\tau)} = E[N(0,\tau)]$ introduced in §15.3. Since $m_{N(0,0)} = 0$, application of Eq. (3.16) yields $\mathcal{L}(\chi_c)(s) = s\mathcal{L}(m_{N(0,\tau)})(s)$ and the result follows immediately from Exercise 15.9.

Exercise 11. Since $\mathcal{L}(p_n)(s) = \varrho^n/(\varrho+s)^n$,

$$1 - \mathcal{L}(p_n)(s) = 0 \Leftrightarrow (\varrho+s)^n - \varrho^n = 0$$

or

$$(\varrho+s)^n = \varrho^n \Rightarrow \varrho+s = \varrho z_k,$$

where $z_k = \exp(2\pi i k/n)$, $k = 0,\ldots n-1$ is an nth root of unity. This implies $s_k = \varrho(z_k - 1)$.

Exercise 12. The roots of $1 - g(s)$ are clearly simple as may be seen by a geometric drawing. Multiplying the right hand side of Eq. (16.21) by $(s - s_i)$ and letting $s \to s_i$ yields α_i. On the left hand side we obtain

$$\lim_{s \to s_i} \frac{(s - s_i)g(s)}{1 - g(s)} = \frac{0}{0}.$$

According to l'Hôpital's rule,

$$\lim_{s \to s_i} \frac{(s - s_i)g(s)}{1 - g(s)} = \lim_{s \to s_i} \frac{g(s) + (s - s_i)g'(s)}{-g'(s)} = \frac{-1}{g'(s_i)}$$

since $g(s_i) = 1$ and

$$g'(s_i) = \frac{\varrho^n}{(\varrho + s_i)^n} \frac{-n}{\varrho + s_i} = \frac{-n}{\varrho + s_i} \neq 0.$$

Since

$$\alpha_i = \frac{-1}{g'(s_i)} = \frac{1}{n}(\varrho + s_i) = \frac{1}{n}\varrho z_i,$$

plugging this result in Eq. (16.21) completes the exercise.

Exercise 13. According to Exercise 10

$$\mathcal{L}(\chi_t)(s) = \frac{\varrho}{n}\left(\frac{1}{s} + \sum_{i=1}^{n-1} \frac{\varrho z_i}{s - s_i}\right).$$

The result is immediate by applying Eq. (3.14).

Exercise 17. According to Eq. (16.24),

$$x_1 + \cdots + x_l = \int_0^{t_1} \varrho_s(y)\,dy + \cdots + \int_{t_{l-1}}^{t_l} \varrho_s(y)\,dy = \int_0^{t_l} \varrho_s(y)\,dy.$$

This implies that $P(N_s(0,t) \geq l) = P(S_l \leq s(t))$ where $S_l = X_1 + \cdots + X_l$ is the sum of the l successive random thresholds. Just as in Exercise 15.8, this implies

$$P(N_s(0,t) = l) = P(S_l \leq s(t)) - P(S_{l+1} \leq s(t)).$$

From this we obtain $E[N_s(0,t)] = \sum_{l=1}^{\infty} K_l(s(t))$. Taking the time derivative, we obtain

$$\frac{d}{dt}E[N_s(0,t)] = \sum_{l=1}^{\infty}\frac{d}{dt}K_l(s(t)) = \sum_{l=1}^{\infty}\frac{d}{ds}K_l(s(t))\frac{ds}{dt} = \left(\sum_{l=1}^{\infty}k_l(s(t))\right)\frac{ds}{dt} = \chi_c(s(t))\varrho_s(t),$$

which completes the proof.

Exercise 18. With $\lambda_m = 10$ spk/s, we first need to compute

$$s(t)\int_0^t \varrho_s(y)\,dy = \int_0^t \lambda_m\left(\sin(2\pi f_s t - \pi/2) + 1\right)dy$$

$$= \lambda_m t - \frac{1}{2\pi f_s}\cos(2\pi f_s y - \pi/2)\Big|_0^t = \lambda_m\left(t - \frac{1}{2\pi f_s}\cos(2\pi f_s t - \pi/2)\right)$$

since $d\cos(t)/dt = -\sin(t)$. For the numerics, see rand_gamfit.m.

Exercise 19. If the process started in the infinite past, the threshold sequence is a stationary gamma process and consequently its rate is time independent: $\chi_c(t) = \chi$. The result is immediate by plugging this result in Eq. (16.23). Alternatively, the transformed spike times, $s(t_i)$, are distributed as the random threshold sequence, therefore their rate is time independent, since the random threshold sequence is stationary, and given by χ, the random threshold rate. Since $\chi \Delta s = \chi_{sc}(t) \Delta t$ we have $\chi_{sc}(t) = \chi \cdot ds/dt = \chi \varrho_s(t)$.

Exercise 21.

$$E[N(0,t)] = E_\varrho[E[N(0,t)|\varrho(t)]] = E_\varrho\left[\int_0^t \varrho(s)\,ds\right] = \int_0^t E[\varrho(s)]\,ds = \bar{\varrho}t.$$

Since

$$E[(N(0,t) - E[N(0,t)])^2] = E_\varrho[E[N(0,t)^2|\varrho]] - E[N(0,t)]^2$$

we need only compute the first term. Now, just as for a homogeneous Poisson process,

$$E[N(0,t)^2|\varrho] = \sum_{k=0}^\infty k^2 P(N(0,t)=k) = e^{-\kappa}\sum_{k=1}^\infty k^2\frac{\kappa^k}{k!}$$

$$= e^{-\kappa}\sum_{k=1}^\infty\left((k-1)\frac{\kappa}{(k-1)!} + \frac{\kappa^k}{(k-1)!}\right) = e^{-\kappa}\left(\kappa^2 e^\kappa + \kappa e^\kappa\right) = \kappa^2 + \kappa$$

where $\kappa = \int_0^t \varrho(y)\,dy$. This leads to

$$E_\varrho[E[N(0,t)^2|\varrho]] - E[N(0,t)]^2 = E\left[\int_0^t \varrho(y_1)\,dy_1\int_0^t \varrho(y_2)\,dy_2\right] + E\left[\int_0^t \varrho(y)\,dy\right] - (\bar{\varrho}t)^2$$

$$= \int_0^t\int_0^t E[(\varrho(y_1)-\bar{\varrho})(\varrho(y_2)-\bar{\varrho})]\,dy_1dy_2 + \bar{\varrho}t$$

$$= \int_0^t\int_0^t C_\varrho(y_2-y_1)\,dy_1dy_2 + \bar{\varrho}t.$$

The integration variable $y_2 - y_1$ ranges between $-t$ and $+t$. However, since $C_\varrho(-y) = C_\varrho(y)$ we can multiply by a factor two and consider only values between 0 and t. For each fixed value of $u = y_2 - y_1 \in [0,t]$ there are $t - u$ distinct combinations of y_1, y_2 values in $[0,t]$. Hence,

$$\int_0^t\int_0^t C_\varrho(y_2-y_1)\,dy_1dy_2 = \int_0^t (t-u)C_\varrho(u)\,du$$

and

$$E[(N(0,t) - E[N(0,t)])^2] = \int_0^t (t-u)C_\varrho(u)du + \bar{\varrho}t.$$

Exercise 22. Since

$$\sigma^2 = C(0) = \int_{-\infty}^{\infty} S(\omega) \mathbb{1}_{(-f_N, f_N)}(\omega) d\omega = \int_{-f_N}^{f_N} S(\omega) d\omega$$

and $S(\omega)$ is independent of ω we obtain

$$\sigma^2 = 2 f_N S(\omega) \Rightarrow S(\omega) = \frac{\sigma^2}{2 f_N}$$

between $-f_N$ and f_N and zero otherwise. Furthermore,

$$
\begin{aligned}
C(\tau) = \int_{-\infty}^{\infty} S(\omega) e^{2\pi i \omega \tau} d\omega &= \int_{-\infty}^{\infty} \frac{\sigma^2}{2 f_N} \mathbb{1}_{(-f_N, f_N)} e^{2\pi i \omega \tau} d\omega \\
&= \frac{\sigma^2}{2 f_N} \int_{-f_N}^{f_N} e^{2\pi i \omega \tau} d\omega = \frac{\sigma^2}{2 f_N} \int_{-f_N}^{f_N} \frac{1}{2\pi i \tau} \frac{d}{d\omega} e^{2\pi i \omega \tau} d\omega \\
&= \frac{\sigma^2}{2 f_N} \frac{1}{2\pi i \tau} (e^{2\pi i f_N \tau} - e^{-2\pi i f_N \tau}) = \sigma^2 \frac{\sin 2\pi f_N \tau}{2\pi f_N \tau}.
\end{aligned}
$$

Exercise 23. According to §11.10, for a gamma distribution of order 2,

$$p_2(t) = \varrho^2 t \exp(-\varrho t).$$

The corresponding cumulative distribution is

$$F(t) = \varrho^2 \int_0^t x e^{-\varrho x} dx.$$

Integration by parts, with $u = x$, $du/dx = 1$, $dv/dx = \exp(-\varrho x)$, $v = (-1/\varrho) \exp(-\varrho x)$, yields

$$
\begin{aligned}
\int_0^t x e^{-\varrho x} dx &= x \left(-\frac{1}{\varrho} e^{-\varrho x} \right) \Big|_0^t - \int_0^t \left(\frac{-1}{\varrho} \right) e^{-\varrho x} dx \\
&= \frac{-t}{\varrho} e^{-\varrho t} - \frac{1}{\varrho^2} e^{-\varrho t} \Big|_0^t = \frac{1}{\varrho^2} - \frac{1}{\varrho^2} e^{-\varrho t} - \frac{t}{\varrho} e^{-\varrho t}.
\end{aligned}
$$

Therefore $F(t) = 1 - \exp(-\varrho t) - \varrho t \exp(-\varrho t)$. From this we deduce that

$$h(t) = \frac{p_2(t)}{1 - F(t)} = \frac{\varrho^2 t e^{-\varrho t}}{e^{-\varrho t} + \varrho t e^{-\varrho t}} = \frac{\varrho^2 t}{1 + \varrho t}.$$

Exercise 24.

(i) According to Eq. (16.27),

$$s(t_j) = s(t_{j-1}) + \int_{t_{j-1}}^{t_j} \varrho_i(t | t_{j-1}) dt$$

and

$$\int_{t_{j-1}}^{t_j} \varrho_i(t|t_{j-1})\,dt = \int_{t_{j-1}}^{t_j} h(t-t_{j-1})\,dt = \int_{0}^{t_j-t_{j-1}} h(t)\,dt = \int_{0}^{t_j-t_{j-1}} \frac{\varrho^2 t}{1+\varrho t}\,dt.$$

Setting $y = \varrho t$ so that $dy = \varrho\,dt$, we obtain

$$\int_{t_{j-1}}^{t_j} \varrho_i(t|t_{j-1})\,dt = \int_{0}^{\varrho(t_j-t_{j-1})} \frac{y}{1+y}\,dy$$

$$= y - \log(1+y)\Big|_0^{\varrho(t_j-t_{j-1})} = \varrho(t_j - t_{j-1}) - \log\big(1 + \varrho(t_j - t_{j-1})\big).$$

(ii) See `time_rescaling.m`.

28.16 CHAPTER 17

Exercise 1. Since $p'_{11} = -\alpha p_{11} + \beta p_{12}$ and $p_{11} + p_{12} = 1$ we have

$$p'_{11} = -\alpha p_{11} + \beta(1 - p_{11}) = -(\alpha + \beta)p_{11} + \beta \tag{28.8}$$

and steady state, $p'_{11} = 0$, implies $p_{11} = q_\infty$, with $q_\infty = \beta/(\alpha + \beta)$. Now set $\tau = 1/(\alpha + \beta)$ and $p_{11}(t) = q_\infty + C\exp(-t/\tau)$. Plugging this "Ansatz" on both sides of Eq. (28.8) shows that it indeed solves the differential equation:

$$p'_{11} = C \cdot (-(\alpha + \beta))e^{-t/\tau}$$
$$-(\alpha + \beta)p_{11} + \beta = -(\alpha + \beta)Ce^{-t/\tau}.$$

The initial condition $p_{11}(0) = 1$ means that

$$\frac{\beta}{\alpha + \beta} + C = 1 \Rightarrow C = 1 - \frac{\beta}{\alpha + \beta} = \frac{\alpha}{\alpha + \beta}.$$

Define $p_\infty = \alpha/(\alpha + \beta)$. By symmetry,

$$p_{11}(t) = q_\infty + p_\infty e^{-t/\tau}, p_{12}(t) = 1 - p_{11}(t)$$
$$p_{22}(t) = p_\infty + q_\infty e^{-t/\tau}, p_{21}(t) = 1 - p_{22}(t).$$

Exercise 2. First compute

$$\mathbf{I} + \Delta t\mathbf{Q} = \begin{pmatrix} 1 - \alpha\Delta t & \alpha\Delta t \\ \beta\Delta t & 1 - \beta\Delta t \end{pmatrix} = \begin{pmatrix} p_{11}(\Delta t) & p_{12}(\Delta t) \\ p_{21}(\Delta t) & p_{22}(\Delta t) \end{pmatrix}.$$

We conclude from the Markov property that

$$\mathbf{P}(t)(\mathbf{I} + \Delta t\mathbf{Q}) = \mathbf{P}(t + \Delta t)$$

and

$$(\mathbf{I} + \Delta t\mathbf{Q})\mathbf{P}(t) = \mathbf{P}(t + \Delta t).$$

Equating the left hand sides of the last two equations yields

$$\mathbf{P}(t)\mathbf{Q} = \mathbf{Q}\mathbf{P}(t).$$

Exercise 4. See `twostatechan.m`.

Exercise 7. Let $\boldsymbol{\pi}_e$ be the equilibrium state of $\mathbf{Q}$, $\boldsymbol{\pi}_e\mathbf{Q} = 0$, $\sum_{i=1}^{n}\pi_{ei} = 1$ and assume that

$$\pi_{en}q_{nm} = \pi_{em}q_{mn}.$$

Multiplying both sides by $\pi_{en}^{1/2}\pi_{em}^{-1/2}$ we obtain

$$\pi_{en}^{1/2}\pi_{en}q_{nm}\pi_{em}^{-1/2} = \pi_{en}^{-1/2}\pi_{em}q_{mn}\pi_{em}^{-1/2}. \tag{28.9}$$

By definition of $\mathbf{R}$, $R_{ij} = \pi_{ei}^{1/2}q_{ij}\pi_{ej}^{-1/2}$, therefore Eq. (28.9) implies $R_{ij} = R_{ji}$ or $\mathbf{R} = \mathbf{R}^T$. Let $\mathbf{R}\mathbf{v}_i = \lambda_i\mathbf{v}_i$ be the eigenvalues and eigenvectors of $\mathbf{R}$. If we define $\mathbf{w}_i = \mathbf{C}^{-1}\mathbf{v}_i$, then

$$\mathbf{Q}\mathbf{w}_i = \mathbf{C}^{-1}\mathbf{R}\mathbf{C}\mathbf{C}^{-1}\mathbf{v}_i = \lambda_i\mathbf{C}^{-1}\mathbf{v}_i = \lambda_i\mathbf{w}_i.$$

If $\mathbf{V}$ and $\boldsymbol{\Lambda}$ are the corresponding matrices of eigenvectors and eigenvalues of $\mathbf{R}$, then

$$\mathbf{R} = \mathbf{V}\boldsymbol{\Lambda}\mathbf{V}^{-1}, \quad \mathbf{V}^{-1} = \mathbf{V}^T, \quad \text{and} \quad \mathbf{Q} = \mathbf{C}^{-1}\mathbf{V}\boldsymbol{\Lambda}\mathbf{V}^{-1}\mathbf{C}$$

and

$$\exp(t\mathbf{Q}) = \mathbf{C}^{-1}\mathbf{V}\exp(t\boldsymbol{\Lambda})\mathbf{V}^{-1}\mathbf{C}.$$

Exercise 9. See `na_openmax.m`.

Exercise 10. See `na_detbal.m`.

Exercise 11. See `na_detbal.m`.

Exercise 12. If we denote by π_{e1}^m, π_{e2}^m the equilibrium distribution of the m gate and by π_{e1}^h, π_{e2}^h the equilibrium distribution of the h gate, we obtain the equilibrium distribution of the eight state sodium channel model by the same combinatorial argument used to derive Figure 17.3. The corresponding states and equilibrium distributions are as follows. State 1, m_0h_0: $(\pi_{e1}^m)^3\pi_{e1}^h$; State 2, m_1h_0: $3(\pi_{e1}^m)^2\pi_{e2}^m\pi_{e1}^h$; State 3, m_2h_0: $3\pi_{e1}^m(\pi_{e2}^m)^2\pi_{e1}^h$; State 4, m_3h_0: $(\pi_{e2}^m)^3\pi_{e1}^h$; State 5, m_0h_1: $(\pi_{e1}^m)^3\pi_{e2}^h$; State 6, m_1h_1: $3(\pi_{e1}^m)^2\pi_{e2}^m\pi_{e2}^h$; State 7, m_2h_1: $3\pi_{e1}^m(\pi_{e2}^m)^2\pi_{e2}^h$; State 8, m_3h_1: $(\pi_{e2}^m)^3\pi_{e2}^h$. See `na_detbal.m`.

Exercise 13. See `nachan.m`.

Exercise 15. According to Eq. (17.7),

$$X(t+\mathrm{d}t)^2 = X(t)^2 - \frac{1}{\tau}X(t)^2\mathrm{d}t + c^{1/2}X(t)N(t)(\mathrm{d}t)^{1/2} - \frac{1}{\tau}X(t)^2\mathrm{d}t + \frac{1}{\tau^2}X(t)^2(\mathrm{d}t)^2$$
$$+ \frac{c^{1/2}}{\tau}X(t)N(t)(\mathrm{d}t)^{3/2} + c^{1/2}X(t)N(t)(\mathrm{d}t)^{1/2} - \frac{c^{1/2}}{\tau}X(t)N(t)(\mathrm{d}t)^{3/2} + cN(t)^2\mathrm{d}t.$$

To order $(\mathrm{d}t)^1$ and smaller,

$$X(t+\mathrm{d}t)^2 = X(t)^2 - \frac{2}{\tau}X(t)^2\mathrm{d}t + 2c^{1/2}X(t)N(t)(\mathrm{d}t)^{1/2} + cN(t)^2\mathrm{d}t.$$

Averaging,

$$E[X(t+dt)^2] = E[X(t)^2] - \frac{2}{\tau}E[X(t)^2]\,dt + 2c^{1/2}E[X(t)N(t)](dt)^{1/2} + cE[N(t)^2)]\,dt.$$

But $E[N(t)^2] = 1$ and $E[N(t)] = 0$. In addition, $X(t_1)$ and $N(t_2)$ are independent for $t_1 \le t_2$. Therefore, $E[X(t_1)N(t_2)] = 0$ for $t_1 \le t_2$. Hence,

$$E[X(t+dt)^2] = E[X(t)^2] - \frac{2}{\tau}E[X(t)^2]\,dt + c\,dt$$

or

$$\frac{E[X(t+dt)^2] - E[X(t)]^2}{dt} = \frac{-2}{\tau}E[X(t)^2] + c.$$

By taking the limit $dt \to 0$ and with $f(t) = E[X(t)^2]$ we have

$$f'(t) = -\frac{2}{\tau}f(t) + c$$

with the initial condition $f(t_0) = E[X(t_0)^2] = x_0^2$, since $X(t_0) \sim \mathcal{N}(x_0, 0)$. Set $g(t) = f(t) - \tau c/2$ so that $dg/dt = df/dt$ and $g'(t) = -2g(t)/\tau$. This differential equation is solved by the "Ansatz" $g(t) = C\exp(-2t/\tau)$. To determine C we turn to the initial condition:

$$g(t_0) = f(t_0) - \frac{\tau c}{2} = x_0^2 - \frac{\tau c}{2}$$

which implies

$$Ce^{-2t_0/\tau} = x_0^2 - \frac{\tau c}{2}$$

or $C = (x_0^2 - \tau c/2)\exp(2t_0/\tau)$. This in turn means that

$$f(t) = g(t) + \tau c/2 = (x_0^2 - \tau c/2)e^{-2(t-t_0)/\tau} + \tau c/2.$$

From this we conclude that

$$v(t) = f(t) - m(t)^2 = \left(x_0^2 - \frac{\tau c}{2}\right)e^{-2(t-t_0)/\tau} + \frac{\tau c}{2} - x_0^2 e^{-2(t-t_0)/\tau}$$

$$= \frac{\tau c}{2} - \frac{\tau c}{2}e^{-2(t-t_0)/\tau} = \frac{\tau c}{2}(1 - e^{-2(t-t_0)/\tau}).$$

Exercise 16. See `ou_f1.m`.

Exercise 17. With $h(t_1, t_2) = E[X(t_1)X(t_2)]$, $C(t_1, t_2) = h(t_1, t_2) - m(t_1)m(t_2)$. We multiply the stochastic differential equation, Eq. (17.7), for X at $t = t_2$ with $X(t_1)$

$$X(t_1)X(t_2 + dt_2) = X(t_1)X(t_2) - \frac{1}{\tau}X(t_1)X(t_2)\,dt_2 + c^{1/2}X(t_1)N(t_2)\,dt_2^{1/2}$$

and average, taking advantage of the fact that $E[X(t_1)N(t_2)] = 0$ for $t_1 \le t_2$

$$E[X(t_1)X(t_2 + dt_2)] = E[X(t_1)X(t_2)] - \frac{1}{\tau}E[X(t_1)X(t_2)]\,dt_2$$

or

$$\frac{E[X(t_1)X(t_2+dt_2)] - E[X(t_1)X(t_2)]}{dt_2} = -\frac{1}{\tau}E[X(t_1)X(t_2)]$$

and taking the limit $dt \to 0$

$$\frac{d}{dt_2}h(t_1,t_2) = -\frac{1}{\tau}h(t_1,t_2).$$

This differential equation is solved by the "Ansatz" $h(t_1,t_2) = C(t_1)\exp(-t_2/\tau)$ and $C(t_1)$ is determined by the initial condition $h(t_1,t_1) = f(t_1)$ which implies

$$C(t_1)e^{-t_1/\tau} = \left(x_0^2 - \frac{\tau c}{2}\right)e^{-2(t_1-t_0)/\tau} + \frac{\tau c}{2}$$

or

$$C(t_1) = \left(x_0^2 - \frac{\tau c}{2}\right)e^{-2(t_1-t_0)/\tau}e^{t_1/\tau} + \frac{\tau c}{2}e^{t_1/\tau}.$$

This means that

$$h(t_1,t_2) = \left(\left(x_0^2 - \frac{\tau c}{2}\right)e^{(-2t_1+2t_0+t_1)/\tau} + \frac{\tau c}{2}e^{t_1/\tau}\right)e^{-t_2/\tau}$$
$$= \left(x_0^2 - \frac{\tau c}{2}\right)e^{(-t_1+2t_0-t_2)/\tau} + \frac{\tau c}{2}e^{(t_1-t_2)/\tau},$$

which in turn implies that

$$C(t_1,t_2) = h(t_1,t_2) - m(t_1)m(t_2)$$
$$= \left(x_0^2 - \frac{\tau c}{2}\right)e^{(-t_1+2t_0-t_2)/\tau} + \frac{\tau c}{2}e^{(t_1-t_2)/\tau} - x_0e^{(-t_1+t_0)/\tau}x_0e^{(-t_2+t_0)/\tau}$$
$$= x_0^2 e^{(-t_1+2t_0-t_2)/\tau} - \frac{\tau c}{2}e^{(-t_1+2t_0-t_2)/\tau} + \frac{\tau c}{2}e^{(t_1-t_2)/\tau} - x_0^2 e^{(-t_1+2t_0-t_2)/\tau}$$
$$= \frac{c\tau}{2}\left(e^{(t_1-t_2)/\tau} - e^{(-t_1+2t_0-t_2)/\tau}\right) = \frac{c\tau}{2}e^{-(t_2-t_1)/\tau}(1 - e^{-2(t_1-t_0)/\tau}).$$

When $t_0 \to -\infty$, $m(t) \to 0$, $v(t) \to c\tau/2$, and

$$C(t_1,t_2) = \frac{c\tau}{2}e^{-(t_2-t_1)/\tau} \quad \text{for} \quad t_2 \ge t_1.$$

Hence, with $h = t_2 - t_1$, $C(h) = (c\tau/2)\exp(-h/\tau)$ for $h \ge 0$ or $C(h) = (c\tau/2)\exp(-|h|/\tau)$.

Exercise 18. See `ou_f2.m`.

Exercise 19. See `destex_f1.m` and `destex_f2.m`.

28.17 CHAPTER 18

Exercise 1. If $E[(aX(t) + Y(t+\tau))^2] = 0$ then $Y(t+\tau) = -aX(t)$ with probability 1. In this case,

$$C_{XY}(\tau) = E[X(t)Y(t+\tau)] = -aE[X(t)X(t)] = -aC_{XX}(0)$$

so that $|C_{XY}|^2 = a^2 C_{XX}(0)^2$. Similarly, $C_{YY}(0) = E[Y(t)Y(t)] = a^2 C_{XX}(0)$, and therefore $C_{XX}(0)C_{YY}(0) = a^2 C_{XX}(0)^2$, which verifies Eq. (18.10) in this case. When the inequality is strict,

$$0 < E[(aX(t) + Y(t+\tau))^2]$$
$$< E[a^2 X(t)^2 + 2aX(t)Y(t+\tau) + Y(t+\tau)^2]$$
$$< a^2 C_{XX}(0) + 2aC_{XY}(\tau) + C_{YY}(0).$$

This implies $\Delta = 4C_{XY}(\tau) - 4C_{XX}(0)C_{YY}(0) < 0$ since the quadratic equation in a has no real solution.

Exercise 2. This result follows by repeating step by step the proof of the Wiener–Khinchin theorem in §16.5 but replacing

$$\hat{X}_T(\mu,\omega)^* = \int_{-T/2}^{T/2} X_T(\mu,t_1) e^{2\pi i\omega t_1} dt_1, \quad \text{and} \quad \hat{X}_T(\mu,\omega) = \int_{-T/2}^{T/2} X_T(\mu,t_2) e^{-2\pi i\omega t_2} dt_2,$$

by

$$\hat{X}_T(\mu,\omega)^* = \int_{-T/2}^{T/2} X_T(\mu,t_1) e^{2\pi i\omega t_1} dt_1, \quad \text{and} \quad \hat{Y}_T(\mu,\omega) = \int_{-T/2}^{T/2} Y_T(\mu,t_2) e^{-2\pi i\omega t_2} dt_2,$$

respectively.

Exercise 3. When $E[|\hat{X}_T(\omega) + a\hat{Y}_T(\omega)\exp(i\phi)|^2] = 0$ we have $\hat{X}_T(\omega) = -a\hat{Y}_T(\omega)\exp(i\phi)$ with probability 1. Therefore $E[\hat{X}(\omega)^* Y_T(\omega)] = -aE[\hat{Y}_T(\omega)^* \hat{Y}_T(\omega)]\exp(-i\phi)$ and the left hand side of Eq. (18.11) is equal to $a^2 E[|\hat{Y}_T(\omega)|^2]^2$. Since $E[\hat{X}_T(\omega)^* \hat{X}_T(\omega)] = a^2 E[\hat{Y}_T(\omega)^* \hat{Y}_T(\omega)]$ the right hand side has the same value as well. We now compute

$$E[|\hat{X}_T(\omega) + a\hat{Y}_T(\omega)e^{i\phi}|^2] = E[(\hat{X}_T(\omega) + a\hat{Y}_T(\omega)e^{i\phi})(\hat{X}_T(\omega)^* + a\hat{Y}_T(\omega)^* e^{-i\phi})]$$
$$= E[\hat{X}_T(\omega)\hat{X}_T(\omega)^* + a\hat{Y}_T(\omega)e^{i\phi}\hat{X}_T(\omega)^* + a\hat{Y}_T(\omega)^* e^{-i\phi}\hat{X}_T(\omega) + a^2 \hat{Y}_T(\omega)^* \hat{Y}_T(\omega)]$$
$$= E[|\hat{X}_T(\omega)|^2] + a(E[\hat{X}_T(\omega)^* \hat{Y}_T(\omega)]e^{i\phi} + E[\hat{X}_T(\omega)\hat{Y}_T(\omega)^*]e^{-i\phi}) + E[|\hat{Y}_T(\omega)|^2].$$

With $E[\hat{X}_T(\omega)^* \hat{Y}_T(\omega)] = |E[\hat{X}_T(\omega)^* Y_T(\omega)]|e^{i\psi}$ we have

$$0 < E[|\hat{X}_T(\omega)|^2] + 2a|E[\hat{X}_T(\omega)^* \hat{Y}_T(\omega)]|\cos(\psi + \phi) + a^2 E[|\hat{Y}_T(\omega)|^2].$$

This implies

$$\Delta = 4|E[\hat{X}_T(\omega)^* \hat{Y}_T(\omega)]|^2 \cos(\psi + \phi)^2 - 4E[|\hat{Y}_T(\omega)|^2]E[|\hat{X}_T(\omega)|^2] < 0$$

and setting $\psi = -\phi$ we obtain Eq. (18.11).

Exercise 4.

$$E[X(t)Y(t+\tau)] = E[X(t)\int h(t+\tau-t_0)X(t_0)\,dt_0] = \int h(t+\tau-t_0)E[X(t)X(t_0)]\,dt_0.$$

Set $t_0 = t + t_1$ or $t_1 = t_0 - t$ so that

$$C_{XY}(\tau) = \int h(t+\tau-t-t_1)E[X(t)X(t+t_1)]\,dt_1$$

$$= \int h(\tau-t_1)C_{XX}(t_1)\,dt_1 = h \star C_{XX}(\tau).$$

Similarly,

$$C_{YY}(\tau) = E[Y(t)Y(t+\tau)] = E\left[\int h(t-t_0)X(t_0)\,dt_0 \int h(t+\tau-t_1)X(t_1)\,dt_1\right]$$

$$= \iint h(t-t_0)h(t+\tau-t_1)E[X(t_0)X(t_1)]\,dt_0dt_1$$

$$= \iint h(t-t_0)h(t+\tau-t_1)E[X(0)X(t_1-t_0)]\,dt_0dt_1.$$

For t_0 fixed set $y = t_1 - t_0$ so that $-t_1 = -t_0 - y$. Hence,

$$C_{YY}(\tau) = \int h(t-t_0)\int h(t+\tau-y-t_0)E[X(0)X(y)]\,dy dt_0$$

$$= \int h(t-t_0)(h \star C_{XX})(t+\tau-t_0)\,dt_0.$$

Set $\tilde{h}(z) = h(-z)$ so that

$$C_{YY}(\tau) = \int \tilde{h}(t_0-t)(h \star C_{XX})(\tau-(t_0-t))dt_0, \quad \text{set } t = 0$$

$$= \tilde{h} \star (h \star C_{XX})(\tau).$$

We now apply the result of Exercises 7.10 and 7.13 to derive the corresponding Fourier transforms.

Exercise 5. The autocorrelation of the error is, with $t_1 = t_0 + \tau$,

$$E[e(t_0)e(t_1)] = E[(Y(t_0) - h \star X(t_0))(Y(t_1) - h \star X(t_1))]$$

$$= C_{YY}(\tau) - e[h \star X(t_0)Y(t_1)] - E[Y(t_0)h \star X(t_1)] + E[h \star X(t_0)h \star X(t_1)]$$

$$= C_{YY}(\tau) - E\left[\int h(t)X(t_0-t)Y(t_1)\,dt\right] - E\left[Y(t_0)\int h(t)x(t_1-t)\,dt\right] + (h \star \tilde{h}) \star C_{XX}(\tau).$$

But,

$$E[X(t_0-t)Y(t_1)] = E[X(0)Y(t_1-t_0+t)] = C_{XY}(t+\tau)$$

and

$$E[Y(t_0)X(t_1-t)] = E[X(t_1-t)Y(t_0)] = E[X(0)Y(t_0-t_1+t)] = C_{XY}(-\tau+t).$$

Therefore the first term is

$$E\left[\int h(t)X(t_0-t)Y(t_1)\,dt\right] = \int h(t)C_{XY}(t+\tau)\,dt = \int h(-t)C_{XY}(\tau-t)dt = \tilde{h} \star C_{XY}(\tau)$$

and

$$E\left[Y(t_0)\int h(t)x(t_1-t)\,dt\right] = \int h(t)E[Y(t_0)X(t_1-t)]\,dt$$

$$= \int h(t)C_{XY}(-\tau+t)\,dt = \int h(-t)C_{YX}(\tau-t)dt$$

$$= h \star C_{YX}(\tau).$$

Since $C_{XY}(t) = C_{YX}(-t)$. Finally,

$$E[e(t_0)e(t_1)] = C_{YY}(\tau) - \tilde{h} \star C_{XY}(\tau) - h \star C_{YX}(\tau) + (h \star \tilde{h}) \star C_{XX}(\tau).$$

Exercise 8. First,

$$\hat{g}(\omega) = \int_{-\infty}^{\infty} p_{2T}(\tau)(1 - |\tau|/T)e^{-2\pi i\omega\tau}\, d\tau = \int_{-T}^{T} (1 - |\tau|/T)e^{-2\pi i\omega\tau}\, d\tau$$

$$= \int_{-T}^{T} e^{-2\pi i\omega\tau}\, d\tau - \frac{1}{T}\int_{-T}^{T} |\tau|e^{-2\pi i\omega\tau}\, d\tau = A - B/T.$$

(28.10)

We compute A and B separately,

$$A = \int_{-T}^{T} \frac{1}{(-2\pi i\omega)}\frac{d}{d\tau}e^{-2\pi i\omega\tau}\, d\tau = \frac{1}{(-2\pi i\omega)}e^{-2\pi i\omega\tau}\Big|_{-T}^{T} = \frac{1}{2\pi i\omega}(e^{2\pi i\omega T} - e^{-2\pi i\omega T}),$$

and

$$B = \int_{-T}^{T} |\tau|e^{-2\pi i\omega\tau}\, d\tau = \int_{-T}^{0} (-\tau)e^{-2\pi i\omega\tau}\, d\tau + \int_{0}^{T} \tau e^{-2\pi i\omega\tau}\, d\tau = B_1 + B_2.$$

For B_2, we use integration by parts,

$$\int_{a}^{b} u\, dv = uv\big|_{a}^{b} - \int_{a}^{b} v\, du$$

with $u = \tau \Rightarrow du = d\tau$ and

$$\frac{dv}{d\tau} = e^{-2\pi i\omega\tau} \Rightarrow v = \frac{1}{(-2\pi i\omega)}e^{-2\pi i\omega\tau}$$

we obtain

$$B_2 = \int_{0}^{T} \tau e^{-2\pi i\omega\tau}\, d\tau = \frac{\tau}{(-2\pi i\omega)}e^{-2\pi i\omega\tau}\Big|_{0}^{T} - \int_{0}^{T} \frac{1}{(-2\pi i\omega)}e^{-2\pi i\omega\tau}\, d\tau$$

$$= \frac{Te^{-2\pi i\omega T}}{(-2\pi i\omega)} - \frac{1}{(-2\pi i\omega)^2}\int_{0}^{T} \frac{d}{d\tau}e^{-2\pi i\omega\tau}\, d\tau$$

$$= \frac{T}{(-2\pi i\omega)}e^{-2\pi i\omega T} - \frac{1}{(-2\pi i\omega)^2}e^{-2\pi i\omega T}\Big|_{0}^{T} = \frac{-T}{2\pi i\omega}e^{-2\pi i\omega T} + \frac{1}{(2\pi\omega)^2}(e^{-2\pi i\omega T} - 1).$$

After changing the integration variable from τ to $-\tau$ and using integration by parts as above, we obtain

$$B_1 = \int_{-T}^{0} (-\tau) e^{-2\pi i \omega \tau} \, d\tau = \int_{T}^{0} \tau e^{2\pi i \omega \tau} \, d\tau = \int_{0}^{T} \tau e^{2\pi i \omega \tau} \, d\tau$$

$$= \frac{\tau}{2\pi i \omega} e^{2\pi i \omega \tau} \Big|_{0}^{T} - \int_{0}^{T} \frac{1}{2\pi i \omega} e^{2\pi i \omega \tau} \, d\tau$$

$$= \frac{T}{2\pi i \omega} e^{2\pi i \omega T} - \frac{1}{(2\pi i \omega)^2} \int_{0}^{T} \frac{d}{d\tau} e^{2\pi i \omega \tau} \, d\tau$$

$$= \frac{T}{2\pi i \omega} e^{2\pi i \omega T} - \frac{1}{(2\pi i \omega)^2} e^{2\pi i \omega T} \Big|_{0}^{T} = \frac{T}{2\pi i \omega} e^{2\pi i \omega T} + \frac{1}{(2\pi \omega)^2} (e^{2\pi i \omega T} - 1).$$

Plugging the values of A, B_1, and B_2 in Eq. (28.10),

$$\hat{g}(\omega) = \frac{1}{2\pi i \omega} (e^{2\pi i \omega T} - e^{-2\pi i \omega T}) - \left(\frac{e^{2\pi i \omega T}}{2\pi i \omega} + \frac{1}{T(2\pi \omega)^2} (e^{2\pi i \omega T} - 1) \right) - \left(\frac{e^{-2\pi i \omega T}}{-2\pi i \omega} + \frac{1}{T(2\pi \omega)^2} (e^{-2\pi i \omega T} - 1) \right)$$

$$= \frac{1}{T(2\pi \omega)^2} (2 - (e^{2\pi i \omega T} + e^{-2\pi i \omega T})) = \frac{1}{T(2\pi \omega)^2} 2(1 - \cos 2\pi \omega T) = \frac{\sin^2(\pi \omega T)}{T(\pi \omega)^2}$$

since $\sin^2 x/2 = (1 - \cos x)/2$.

Exercise 9. By taking the expectation of Eq. (18.12) and plugging in the definition of the covariance, we obtain

$$E[S_{hx}(\omega)] = \int\int_{-\infty}^{\infty} h(t_1) h(t_2) e^{-2\pi i \omega t_1} e^{2\pi i \omega t_2} C(t_2 - t_1) \, dt_1 \, dt_2.$$

We now use the definition of the Fourier transform of h and C:

$$E[S_{hx}(\omega)] = \int\int\int\int\int_{-\infty}^{\infty} e^{2\pi i (\omega_1 - \omega - \omega_3) t_1} e^{2\pi i (\omega_2 + \omega + \omega_3) t_2} \hat{h}(\omega_1) \hat{h}(\omega_2) S(\omega_3) \, dt_1 \, dt_2 d\omega_1 \, d\omega_2 \, d\omega_3$$

$$= \int\int\int_{-\infty}^{\infty} \delta(\omega_1 - \omega - \omega_3) \delta(\omega_2 + \omega + \omega_3) \hat{h}(\omega_1) \hat{h}(\omega_2) S(\omega_3) \, d\omega_1 \, d\omega_2 \, d\omega_3.$$

The first δ function implies $\omega_1 - \omega - \omega_3 = 0$ or $\omega_3 = \omega_1 - \omega$. The second δ function implies $\omega_2 = -\omega - \omega_3$. Using the first result, $\omega_2 = -\omega - \omega_1 + \omega = -\omega_1$. Plugging this in the last equality yields

$$E[S_{hx}(\omega)] = \int_{-\infty}^{\infty} \hat{h}(\omega_1) \hat{h}(-\omega_1) S(\omega_1 - \omega) \, d\omega_1$$

$$= \int_{-\infty}^{\infty} |\hat{h}(\omega_1)|^2 S(\omega_1 - \omega) \, d\omega_1 = \int_{-\infty}^{\infty} |\hat{h}(\omega_1)|^2 S(\omega - \omega_1) d\omega_1.$$

Exercise 10. See `cross_poiss.m`.

Exercise 11. We have $E[Z(t_1)X(t_2)] = E[X(t_1)X(t_2)]$ since $Z = X + Y$ and X is independent of Y. This implies

$$\gamma(\omega) = \frac{S_{ZX}(\omega)}{\sqrt{S_{XX}(\omega)}\sqrt{S_{ZZ}(\omega)}} = \frac{\sqrt{S_{XX}(\omega)}}{\sqrt{S_{ZZ}(\omega)}}$$

and $S_{ZZ}(\omega) = S_{XX}(\omega) + S_{YY}(\omega)$. With $S_{XX}(\omega) = 2\sigma_{OU}/(1 + (2\pi\tau\omega)^2)$ and $S_{YY}(\omega) = \sigma_w^2/2f_N$ we obtain

$$\gamma(\omega) = \frac{\sqrt{2\sigma_{OU}\tau}}{\sqrt{1 + (2\pi\tau\omega)^2}} \frac{1}{\sqrt{\frac{2\sigma_{OU}\tau}{1 + (2\pi\tau\omega)^2} + \frac{\sigma^2}{2f_N}}}.$$

See `coherence_est.m` for the numerical implementation.

Exercise 12.

(i) Follows immediately from

$$\hat{x}_{-j} = \sum_{k=0}^{N-1} x_k e^{2\pi ijk/N} = \left(\sum_{k=0}^{N-1} x_k e^{-2\pi ijk/N}\right)^* = \hat{x}_j^*.$$

(ii) Since both x_{jr} and x_{ji} are linear combinations of Gaussian random variables they are Gaussian as well, according to §11.9. Furthermore,

$$E[x_{jr}] = \sum_{k=0}^{N-1} E[x_k]\cos 2\pi kj/N = 0, \quad E[x_{ji}] = \sum_{k=0}^{N-1} E[x_k]\sin 2\pi kj/N = 0.$$

(iii)

$$E[\hat{x}_j\hat{x}_l] = \sum_{k,m=0}^{N-1} E[x_k x_m]e^{-2\pi ikj/N}e^{-2\pi iml/N} = \sum_{k,m=0}^{N-1} C_{k-m}e^{-2\pi ikj/N}e^{-2\pi iml/N}$$

$$= \sum_{m,n=0}^{N-1} C_n e^{-2\pi i(m+n)j/N}e^{-2\pi iml/N} = \left(\sum_{n=0}^{N-1} C_n e^{-2\pi inj/N}\right)\left(\sum_{m=0}^{N-1} e^{-2\pi im(j+l)/N}\right) = S_n N\delta_{j-l}.$$

(iv) Applying (iii) to $l = j$, we obtain

$$0 = E[\hat{x}_j\hat{x}_j] = E[\hat{x}_{jr}^2] - E[\hat{x}_{ji}^2] + 2iE[\hat{x}_{ji}\hat{x}_{jr}]$$

which implies $E[\hat{x}_{ji}\hat{x}_{jr}] = 0$ and $E[\hat{x}_{jr}^2] = E[\hat{x}_{ji}^2]$. Setting $l = -j$, we obtain $E[|\hat{x}_j|^2] = E[\hat{x}_{jr}^2] + E[\hat{x}_{ji}^2] = NS_j$.

(v) For $j \neq \pm l$ the result of (iii), $E[\hat{x}_j\hat{x}_l] = 0$, implies

$$E[\hat{x}_{jr}\hat{x}_{lr}] = E[\hat{x}_{ji}\hat{x}_{li}], \quad E[\hat{x}_{jr}\hat{x}_{li}] = -E[\hat{x}_{ji}\hat{x}_{lr}].$$

Similarly, since $\hat{x}_{-l} = \hat{x}_{lr} - i\hat{x}_{li}$, we obtain

$$E[\hat{x}_{jr}\hat{x}_{lr}] = -E[\hat{x}_{ji}\hat{x}_{li}] \quad E[\hat{x}_{ji}\hat{x}_{lr}] = E[\hat{x}_{jr}\hat{x}_{li}].$$

Taken together these equations imply $E[\hat{x}_{jr}\hat{x}_{lr}] = 0$, $E[\hat{x}_{ji}\hat{x}_{li}] = 0$, $E[\hat{x}_{ji}\hat{x}_{lr}] = 0$, and $E[\hat{x}_{jr}\hat{x}_{li}] = 0$.

(vi) For a frequency $\omega_j = j/(N\Delta t) \in [-f_N, f_N]$ we have

$$\frac{\sigma^2}{2f_N} = S(\omega_j) \approx \frac{\Delta t}{N} E[|\hat{x}_j|^2]$$

which implies

$$E[|\hat{x}_j|^2] = \frac{N\sigma^2}{2f_N\Delta t}.$$

(vii) See `coherence_est.m`.

Exercise 13.

(i) Since $g_{\alpha,l} = \alpha g_{1,l}$, it is sufficient to show that $g_{1,l}(x) \in (-1,1)$, which follows from

$$\frac{1}{\sqrt{2\pi}l}\int_0^\infty e^{-t^2/2l^2}\,dt = \frac{1}{2}.$$

If we set $y = t/\sqrt{2}l$, $dy = dt/\sqrt{2}l$, we obtain

$$g_{1,l}(x) = \sqrt{\frac{2}{\pi}}\frac{1}{l}\int_0^{x/\sqrt{2}l} e^{-y^2}\sqrt{2}l\,dy = \frac{2}{\sqrt{\pi}}\int_0^{x/\sqrt{2}l} e^{-y^2}\,dy = \mathrm{erf}\!\left(\frac{y}{\sqrt{2}l}\right).$$

(ii) and (iii) See `coherence_est.m`.

Exercise 15.

(i) Since f_k is real,

$$|\hat{f}(\omega)|^2 = \sum_{j,k=0}^{N-1} f_k f_j e^{2\pi i(j-k)\omega}.$$

Hence,

$$\int_{-W}^{W} |\hat{f}(\omega)|^2\,d\omega = \sum_{j,k=0}^{N-1} f_k f_j \int_{-W}^{W} e^{2\pi i(j-k)\omega}\,d\omega.$$

When $W = 1/2$ the last integral is equal to 1 and otherwise

$$\int_{-W}^{W} e^{2\pi i(j-k)\omega}\,d\omega = \int_{-W}^{W} \frac{1}{2\pi i(j-k)}\frac{d}{d\omega}e^{2\pi i\omega(j-k)}\,d\omega$$

$$= \frac{1}{2\pi i(j-k)} e^{2\pi i(j-k)\omega}\Big|_{-W}^{W}$$

$$= \frac{1}{2\pi i(j-k)}\left(e^{2\pi i(j-k)W} - e^{-2\pi i(j-k)W}\right) = \frac{1}{2\pi i(j-k)}2i\sin(2\pi(j-k)W)$$

$$= \frac{\sin(2\pi(j-k)W)}{\pi(j-k)}.$$

These results immediately lead to Eq. (18.14), with $\mathbf{A} = (A_{jk})$,

$$A_{jk} = \frac{\sin(2\pi(j-k)W)}{\pi(j-k)}, \quad j,k = 1,\dots,N$$

and $\mathbf{f} = (f_0,\dots,f_{N-1})^T$.

(ii) Since the sine function is odd,

$$A_{jk} = \frac{\sin(2\pi(j-k)W)}{\pi(j-k)} = \frac{-\sin(2\pi(k-j)W)}{\pi(j-k)} = \frac{\sin(2\pi(k-j)W)}{\pi(k-j)} = A_{kj}$$

and therefore $\mathbf{A} = \mathbf{A}^T$. Furthermore,

$$\mathbf{f}^T \mathbf{A} \mathbf{f} = \int\limits_{-W}^{W} |\hat{f}(\omega)|^2 \, d\omega \geq 0$$

implying positive semidefiniteness. According to Parseval's identity,

$$\mathbf{f}^T \mathbf{A} \mathbf{f} \leq \int\limits_{-1/2}^{1/2} |\hat{f}(\omega)|^2 \, d\omega = \mathbf{f}^T \mathbf{f}.$$

According to Exercise 6.8, this implies that the highest eigenvalue of $\mathbf{A}$ is ≤ 1.

(iii) We compute

$$\frac{\partial}{\partial f_k} \frac{\mathbf{f}^T \mathbf{A} \mathbf{f}}{\mathbf{f}^T \mathbf{f}} = \frac{1}{\mathbf{f}^T \mathbf{f}} \sum_{i,j=1}^{N} \frac{\partial f_{i-1}}{\partial f_k} \left\{ A_{ij} f_{j-1} + f_{i-1} A_{ij} \frac{\partial f_{j-1}}{\partial f_k} \right\}$$
$$- \frac{\mathbf{f}^T \mathbf{A} \mathbf{f}}{(\mathbf{f}^T \mathbf{f})^2} \sum_{i=1}^{N} 2 f_{i-1} \frac{\partial f_{i-1}}{\partial f_k}.$$

Since the gradient is equal to zero at the maximum, this implies

$$0 = \mathbf{f}^T \mathbf{f} \sum_{i,j=1}^{N} \left\{ \frac{\partial f_{i-1}}{\partial f_k} A_{ij} f_{j-1} + f_{i-1} A_{ij} \frac{\partial f_{j-1}}{\partial f_k} \right\} - \mathbf{f}^T \mathbf{A} \mathbf{f} \sum_{i=1}^{N} 2 f_{i-1} \frac{\partial f_{i-1}}{\partial f_k}$$
$$= \mathbf{f}^T \mathbf{f} \sum_{i,j=1}^{N} \{ \delta_{i-1,k} A_{ij} f_{j-1} + f_{i-1} A_{ij} \delta_{j-1,k} \} - \mathbf{f}^T \mathbf{A} \mathbf{f} \sum_{i=1}^{N} 2 f_{i-1} \delta_{i-1,k}$$
$$= \mathbf{f}^T \mathbf{f} \left(\sum_{j=1}^{N} A_{(k+1)j} f_{j-1} + \sum_{i=1}^{N} f_{i-1} A_{i(k+1)} \right) - \mathbf{f}^T \mathbf{A} \mathbf{f} 2 f_k$$
$$= 2 \mathbf{f}^T \mathbf{f} (\mathbf{A} \mathbf{f})_{k+1} - 2 \mathbf{f}^T \mathbf{A} \mathbf{f} (\mathbf{f})_{k+1}.$$

This implies

$$\mathbf{A} \mathbf{f} = \frac{\mathbf{f}^T \mathbf{A} \mathbf{f}}{\mathbf{f}^T \mathbf{f}} \mathbf{f}$$

or equivalently $\mathbf{f}$ is an eigenvector of $\mathbf{A}$. Clearly an eigenvector to the largest eigenvalue will yield the largest value of $\beta^2(W, \hat{f})$.

28.18 CHAPTER 19

Exercise 1. See `disp_hist.m` and `scene_2d.m`.

Exercise 2. See `disp_im.m` and `scene_2d.m`.

Exercise 3. See disp_ts2.m.

Exercise 4. See disp_ts2.m.

28.19 CHAPTER 20

Exercise 1. Since the receptive field is described by a difference of two Gaussians, we treat first the case of a single Gaussian, corresponding to either the center or the surround of the receptive field,

$$w(x,y) = ke^{-(r/r_0)^2}, \quad \text{with} \quad r = \sqrt{x^2 + y^2}.$$

The one-dimensional receptive field $u(x)$ is obtained from $w(x,y)$ by integrating over y,

$$u(x) = \int ke^{-(x^2+y^2)/r_0^2}\, dy = ke^{-x^2/r_0^2} \int e^{-y^2/r_0^2}\, dy.$$

Using Eq. (20.19), we have

$$\int_{-\infty}^{\infty} e^{-y^2/r_0^2}\, dy = 2\frac{\sqrt{\pi}}{2 \cdot 1/r_0} = r_0\sqrt{\pi}.$$

Therefore,

$$u(x) = kr_0\sqrt{\pi}e^{-x^2/r_0^2}.$$

This result immediately generalizes to Eq. (20.9) by subtracting a second Gaussian corresponding to the receptive field surround.

Exercise 4. If we define $f_n(t) = t^n e^{-\alpha t}\mathbb{1}(t)$ we may write,

$$w_t(t) = f_1(t) - \frac{\alpha}{2}f_2(t).$$

If we define $s = \alpha + 2\pi i\omega_t$, the Fourier transform of f_n can be computed as follows:

$$\hat{f}_n(\omega_t) = \int_0^{\infty} e^{-2\pi i\omega_t t} t^n e^{-\alpha t}\, dt = \int_0^{\infty} t^n e^{-st}\, dt.$$

According to Eq. (3.34),

$$\hat{w}_t(\omega_t) = \frac{1}{(\alpha + 2\pi i\omega_t)^2} - \frac{\alpha}{2}\frac{2}{(\alpha + 2\pi i\omega_t)^3} = \frac{2\pi i\omega_t}{(\alpha + 2\pi i\omega_t)^3}.$$

28.20 CHAPTER 21

Exercise 1. Let $f(x) = f_1(x)f_2(x)$, $h(x) = f_1(x)f_3(x)$ with

$$f_1(x) = \frac{1}{\sqrt{2\pi}\sigma_x}e^{-x^2/2\sigma_x^2}, \quad f_2(x) = \cos\left(2\pi(k_x x - \phi_x)\right), \quad f_3(x) = \sin\left(2\pi(k_x x - \phi_x)\right).$$

Using the results derived in Exercises 7.11 and 7.15 and the convolution theorem, Eq. (7.29), yields,

$$\hat{f}(\omega_x) = \frac{1}{2}e^{-2\pi i\phi_x}\int e^{-\sigma_x^2(2\pi)^2(\omega_x-\eta)^2/2}\delta(k_x-\eta)\,d\eta + \frac{1}{2}e^{2\pi i\phi_x}\int e^{-\sigma_x^2(2\pi)^2(\omega_x-\eta)^2/2}\delta(k_x+\eta)\,d\eta$$

$$= \frac{1}{2}(e^{-2\pi i\phi_x}e^{-\sigma_x^2(2\pi)^2(\omega_x-k_x)^2/2} + e^{i\phi_x}e^{-\sigma_x^2(2\pi)^2(\omega_x+k_x)^2}).$$

(28.11)

Similarly,

$$\hat{h}(\omega_x) = \frac{1}{2i}(e^{-2\pi i\phi_x}e^{-\sigma_x^2(2\pi)^2(\omega_x-k_x)^2/2} - e^{i\phi_x}e^{-\sigma_x^2(2\pi)^2(\omega_x+k_x)^2}).$$

(28.12)

Exercise 3.

$$R_{drift}(t) = \int w(x,y)c_{drift}(x,y,t)\,dxdy$$

$$= \int w(x,y)\cos(2\pi(\eta_x x + \eta_y y - \eta_t t - \eta_0))\,dxdy$$

$$= \Re\left(\int w(x,y)e^{-2\pi i(\eta_x x + \eta_y y - \eta_t t - \eta_0)}\,dxdy\right)$$

$$= \Re\left(e^{2\pi i(\eta_t t + \eta_0)}\int w(x,y)e^{-2\pi i(\eta_x x + \eta_y y)}\,dxdy\right)$$

$$= \Re\left(e^{2\pi i(\eta_t t + \eta_0)}\hat{w}(\eta_x,\eta_y)\right)$$

$$= \Re\left(e^{2\pi i(\eta_t t + \eta_0)}\frac{1}{2}(e^{-2\pi i\phi_x}e^{-\sigma_x^2(2\pi)^2(\eta_x-k_x)^2/2} + e^{2\pi i\phi_x}e^{-\sigma_x^2(2\pi)^2(\eta_x+k_x)^2/2})e^{-\sigma_y^2(2\pi)^2\eta_y^2/2}\right)$$

$$= \frac{1}{2}\cos(2\pi(\eta_t t + \eta_0 - \phi_x)e^{-\sigma_x^2(2\pi)^2(\eta_x-k_x)^2/2}e^{-\sigma_y^2(2\pi)^2\eta_y^2/2} +$$

$$\frac{1}{2}\cos(2\pi(\eta_t t - \eta_0 + \phi_x))e^{-\sigma_x^2(2\pi)^2(\eta_x+k_x)^2/2}e^{-\sigma_y^2(2\pi)^2\eta_y^2/2}.$$

Exercise 4. We are looking for the values of η_x such that,

$$e^{-\sigma_x^2(2\pi)^2(\eta_x-k_x)^2/2} = \frac{1}{2}$$

holds. Taking logarithms on both sides of this equation and rearranging we obtain:

$$\sigma_x^2(2\pi)^2(\eta_x-k_x)^2 = 2\log 2$$

$$\pm\sigma_x(\eta_x-k_x) = \sqrt{2\log 2}/2\pi$$

$$\eta_x = k_x \pm \sqrt{2\log 2}/2\pi\sigma_x.$$

The corresponding bandwidth is $b = \log_2 \eta_h/\eta_l$ with $\eta_h = k_x + \sqrt{2\log 2}/2\pi\sigma_x$ and $\eta_l = k_x - \sqrt{2\log 2}/2\pi\sigma_x$. This gives

$$b = \log_2\frac{2\pi k_x\sigma_x + \sqrt{2\log 2}}{2\pi k_x\sigma_x - \sqrt{2\log 2}}, \quad \text{or} \quad 2\pi k_x\sigma_x = \sqrt{2\log 2}\frac{2^b+1}{2^b-1}.$$

Note that the logarithm in base 2 is obtained from the natural logarithm as follows: $\log_2(x) = \log(x)/\log(2)$.

Exercise 6. By definition,

$$\hat{g}_e^-(\omega_x,\omega_t) = \hat{g}_{se}(\omega_x)\hat{f}_{te}(\omega_t) + \hat{g}_{so}(\omega_x)\hat{f}_{to}(\omega_t),$$

$$\hat{g}_o^-(\omega_x,\omega_t) = \hat{g}_{so}(\omega_x)\hat{f}_{te}(\omega_t) - \hat{g}_{se}(\omega_x)\hat{f}_{to}(\omega_t).$$

The Fourier transform of each component has been derived in Exercise 2. Plugging in this result yields the formula given in the main text for $\hat{g}_e^-$, Eq. (21.9). For $\hat{g}_o^-$ we obtain:

$$\hat{g}_o^- (\omega_x, \omega_t) = \frac{1}{2i} \left(e^{-\sigma_x^2 (2\pi)^2 (\omega_x - k_x)^2 / 2} e^{-\sigma_t^2 (2\pi)^2 (\omega_t + k_t)^2 / 2} - e^{-\sigma_x^2 (2\pi)^2 (\omega_x + k_x)^2 / 2} e^{-\sigma_t^2 (2\pi)^2 (\omega_t - k_t)^2 / 2} \right).$$

Exercise 7. See `temp_space_rfs.m`.

28.21 CHAPTER 22

Exercise 1. First, from $\mathbf{AF} = -\mathbf{B}$ we deduce $\mathbf{F} = -\mathbf{A}^{-1}\mathbf{B}$ and plugging this in $\mathbf{H} = \mathbf{D} - \mathbf{CA}^{-1}\mathbf{B}$ we obtain $\mathbf{H} = \mathbf{D} + \mathbf{CF}$. Second, from $\mathbf{GA} = -\mathbf{C}$ we have $\mathbf{G} = -\mathbf{CA}^{-1}$ and plugging this in $\mathbf{H} = \mathbf{D} - \mathbf{CA}^{-1}\mathbf{B}$ we obtain $\mathbf{H} = \mathbf{D} + \mathbf{GB}$. We can now compute $\mathbf{MM}^{-1}$ and $\mathbf{M}^{-1}\mathbf{M}$:

$$
\begin{aligned}
\mathbf{MM}^{-1} &= \begin{pmatrix} \mathbf{A} & \mathbf{B} \\ \mathbf{C} & \mathbf{D} \end{pmatrix} \left(\begin{pmatrix} \mathbf{A}^{-1} & 0 \\ 0 & 0 \end{pmatrix} + \begin{pmatrix} \mathbf{F} \\ \mathbf{I} \end{pmatrix} \mathbf{H}^{-1} (\mathbf{G} \ \ \mathbf{I}) \right) \\
&= \begin{pmatrix} \mathbf{A} & \mathbf{B} \\ \mathbf{C} & \mathbf{D} \end{pmatrix} \begin{pmatrix} \mathbf{A}^{-1} & 0 \\ 0 & 0 \end{pmatrix} + \begin{pmatrix} \mathbf{A} & \mathbf{B} \\ \mathbf{C} & \mathbf{D} \end{pmatrix} \begin{pmatrix} \mathbf{F} \\ \mathbf{I} \end{pmatrix} \mathbf{H}^{-1} (\mathbf{G} \ \ \mathbf{I}) \\
&= \begin{pmatrix} \mathbf{I} & 0 \\ \mathbf{CA}^{-1} & 0 \end{pmatrix} + \begin{pmatrix} \mathbf{AF} + \mathbf{B} \\ \mathbf{CF} + \mathbf{D} \end{pmatrix} \mathbf{H}^{-1} (\mathbf{G} \ \ \mathbf{I}) \\
&= \begin{pmatrix} \mathbf{I} & 0 \\ \mathbf{CA}^{-1} & 0 \end{pmatrix} + \begin{pmatrix} 0 \\ \mathbf{CF} + \mathbf{D} \end{pmatrix} \mathbf{H}^{-1} (\mathbf{G} \ \ \mathbf{I}) \\
&= \begin{pmatrix} \mathbf{I} & 0 \\ \mathbf{CA}^{-1} & 0 \end{pmatrix} + \begin{pmatrix} 0 \\ (\mathbf{CF} + \mathbf{D})\mathbf{H}^{-1} \end{pmatrix} (\mathbf{G} \ \ \mathbf{I}) \\
&= \begin{pmatrix} \mathbf{I} & 0 \\ \mathbf{CA}^{-1} & 0 \end{pmatrix} + \begin{pmatrix} 0 \\ \mathbf{I} \end{pmatrix} (\mathbf{G} \ \ \mathbf{I}) \\
&= \begin{pmatrix} \mathbf{I} & 0 \\ \mathbf{CA}^{-1} & 0 \end{pmatrix} + \begin{pmatrix} 0 & 0 \\ \mathbf{G} & \mathbf{I} \end{pmatrix} \\
&= \begin{pmatrix} \mathbf{I} & 0 \\ \mathbf{CA}^{-1} + \mathbf{G} & \mathbf{I} \end{pmatrix} \\
&= \begin{pmatrix} \mathbf{I} & 0 \\ 0 & \mathbf{I} \end{pmatrix},
\end{aligned}
$$

$$
\begin{aligned}
\mathbf{M}^{-1}\mathbf{M} &= \left(\begin{pmatrix} \mathbf{A}^{-1} & 0 \\ 0 & 0 \end{pmatrix} + \begin{pmatrix} \mathbf{F} \\ \mathbf{I} \end{pmatrix} \mathbf{H}^{-1} (\mathbf{G} \ \ \mathbf{I}) \right) \begin{pmatrix} \mathbf{A} & \mathbf{B} \\ \mathbf{C} & \mathbf{D} \end{pmatrix} \\
&= \begin{pmatrix} \mathbf{A}^{-1} & 0 \\ 0 & 0 \end{pmatrix} \begin{pmatrix} \mathbf{A} & \mathbf{B} \\ \mathbf{C} & \mathbf{D} \end{pmatrix} + \begin{pmatrix} \mathbf{F} \\ \mathbf{I} \end{pmatrix} \mathbf{H}^{-1} (\mathbf{G} \ \ \mathbf{I}) \begin{pmatrix} \mathbf{A} & \mathbf{B} \\ \mathbf{C} & \mathbf{D} \end{pmatrix} \\
&= \begin{pmatrix} \mathbf{I} & \mathbf{A}^{-1}\mathbf{B} \\ 0 & 0 \end{pmatrix} + \begin{pmatrix} \mathbf{F} \\ \mathbf{I} \end{pmatrix} \mathbf{H}^{-1} (\mathbf{GA} + \mathbf{C} \ \ \mathbf{GB} + \mathbf{D}) \\
&= \begin{pmatrix} \mathbf{I} & \mathbf{A}^{-1}\mathbf{B} \\ 0 & 0 \end{pmatrix} + \begin{pmatrix} \mathbf{F} \\ \mathbf{I} \end{pmatrix} (0 \ \ \mathbf{H}^{-1}(\mathbf{GB} + \mathbf{D})) \\
&= \begin{pmatrix} \mathbf{I} & \mathbf{A}^{-1}\mathbf{B} \\ 0 & 0 \end{pmatrix} + \begin{pmatrix} \mathbf{F} \\ \mathbf{I} \end{pmatrix} (0 \ \ \mathbf{I}) \\
&= \begin{pmatrix} \mathbf{I} & \mathbf{A}^{-1}\mathbf{B} \\ 0 & 0 \end{pmatrix} + \begin{pmatrix} 0 & \mathbf{F} \\ 0 & \mathbf{I} \end{pmatrix} \\
&= \begin{pmatrix} \mathbf{I} & \mathbf{A}^{-1}\mathbf{B} + \mathbf{F} \\ 0 & \mathbf{I} \end{pmatrix} \\
&= \begin{pmatrix} \mathbf{I} & 0 \\ 0 & \mathbf{I} \end{pmatrix}.
\end{aligned}
$$

Exercise 2. For the first identity,

$$\begin{pmatrix} I & 0 \\ H & I \end{pmatrix} \begin{pmatrix} C_{XX} & 0 \\ 0 & Q \end{pmatrix} \begin{pmatrix} I & H^T \\ 0 & I \end{pmatrix} = \begin{pmatrix} C_{XX} & C_{XX}H^T \\ HC_{XX} & HC_{XX}H^T + Q \end{pmatrix}. \tag{28.13}$$

Since $H = C_{YX}C_{XX}^{-1}$, C_{XX} is symmetric, and $C_{YX}^T = C_{XY}$, we have $H^T = C_{XX}^{-1}C_{XY}$. Hence,

$$HC_{XX} = C_{YX}, \quad C_{XX}H^T = C_{XY}, \tag{28.14}$$

and

$$HC_{XX}H^T + Q = C_{YX}C_{XX}^{-1}C_{XX}C_{XX}^{-1}C_{XY} + C_{YY} - C_{YX}C_{XX}^{-1}C_{XY} = C_{YY}.$$

Plugging these results in Eq. (28.13) shows that the right hand side is equal to C_{ZZ}. For the second identity,

$$\begin{pmatrix} I & 0 \\ -H & I \end{pmatrix} \begin{pmatrix} C_{XX} & C_{XY} \\ C_{YX} & C_{YY} \end{pmatrix} \begin{pmatrix} I & -H^T \\ 0 & I \end{pmatrix} = \begin{pmatrix} I & 0 \\ -H & I \end{pmatrix} \begin{pmatrix} C_{XX} & -C_{XX}H^T + C_{XY} \\ C_{YX} & -C_{YX}H^T + C_{YY} \end{pmatrix}$$

$$= \begin{pmatrix} C_{XX} & -C_{XX}H^T + C_{XY} \\ -HC_{XX}C_{YX} & -HC_{XX}H^T - HC_{XY} - C_{YX}H^T + C_{YY} \end{pmatrix}.$$

The off-diagonal terms vanish according to Eq. (28.14) and the lower diagonal term is equal to

$$-HC_{XX}H^T - HC_{XY} - C_{YX}H^T + C_{YY} = C_{YX}C_{XX}^{-1}C_{XY}$$
$$- C_{YX}C_{XX}^{-1}C_{XY} - C_{YX}C_{XX}^{-1}C_{XY} + C_{YY} = Q.$$

Exercise 3.

$$E\left[\begin{pmatrix} v_X \\ v_N \end{pmatrix} (v_X \quad v_N) \right] = E\left[\begin{pmatrix} I & 0 \\ -H & I \end{pmatrix} \begin{pmatrix} v_X \\ v_Y \end{pmatrix} (v_X \quad v_Y) \begin{pmatrix} I & -H^T \\ 0 & I \end{pmatrix} \right]$$

$$= \begin{pmatrix} I & 0 \\ -H & I \end{pmatrix} E\left[\begin{pmatrix} v_X \\ v_Y \end{pmatrix} (v_X \quad v_Y) \right] \begin{pmatrix} I & -H^T \\ 0 & I \end{pmatrix}$$

$$= \begin{pmatrix} I & 0 \\ -H & I \end{pmatrix} C_{ZZ} \begin{pmatrix} I & -H^T \\ 0 & I \end{pmatrix} = \begin{pmatrix} C_{XX} & 0 \\ 0 & Q \end{pmatrix}.$$

Exercise 4.

(i) Since $Y(t)$ is a Gaussian stochastic process,

$$p(y_1, y_2) = (2\pi)^{-1} |\det C_{YY}|^{-1/2} \exp\left(-\frac{1}{2} (y_1 \quad y_2) C_{YY}^{-1} \begin{pmatrix} y_1 \\ y_2 \end{pmatrix} \right) \tag{28.15}$$

with

$$C_{YY} = \begin{pmatrix} \sigma^2 & \sigma^2\rho \\ \sigma^2\rho & \sigma^2 \end{pmatrix} = \sigma^2 \begin{pmatrix} 1 & \rho \\ \rho & 1 \end{pmatrix} = \sigma^2 C_1.$$

Note that the variances of Y_1 and Y_2 (i.e., σ^2) are equal since $Y(t)$ is stationary. Furthermore, $\det C_{YY} = \sigma^4(1 - \rho^2)$. The constant ρ is the correlation coefficient between Y at time t and $t + \tau$. We use the identity derived in Exercise 1 to write

$$C_1^{-1} = \begin{pmatrix} 1 & 0 \\ 0 & 1 \end{pmatrix} + \begin{pmatrix} -\rho \\ 1 \end{pmatrix} \frac{1}{1-\rho^2} \begin{pmatrix} -\rho & 1 \end{pmatrix}$$

$$= \begin{pmatrix} 1 & 0 \\ 0 & 1 \end{pmatrix} + \frac{1}{1-\rho^2} \begin{pmatrix} \rho^2 & -\rho \\ -\rho & 1 \end{pmatrix}.$$

By symmetry between y_1 and y_2 and after multiplying by σ^{-2},

$$C_{YY}^{-1} = \sigma^{-2} \left(\begin{pmatrix} 1 & 0 \\ 0 & 1 \end{pmatrix} + \frac{1}{1-\rho^2} \begin{pmatrix} 1 & -\rho \\ -\rho & \rho^2 \end{pmatrix} \right),$$

so that

$$(y_1 \quad y_2) C_{YY}^{-1} \begin{pmatrix} y_1 \\ y_2 \end{pmatrix} = \sigma^{-2} \left(y_2^2 + \frac{1}{1-\rho^2} (y_1 \quad y_2) \begin{pmatrix} 1 & -\rho \\ -\rho & \rho^2 \end{pmatrix} \begin{pmatrix} y_1 \\ y_2 \end{pmatrix} \right)$$

$$= \sigma^{-2} \left(y_2^2 + (1-\rho^2)^{-1} \left(y_1^2 - 2\rho y_1 y_2 + \rho^2 y_2^2 \right) \right)$$

$$= \sigma^{-2} \left(y_2^2 + (1-\rho^2)^{-1} (y_1 - \rho y_2)^2 \right).$$

Plugging this result in Eq. (28.15) we obtain the desired formula.

(ii)

$$C_{YZ_0}(\tau) = E[Y_1 g(Y_2)] = \int\!\!\!\int_{-\infty}^{\infty} y_1 g(y_2)\, dy_1 dy_2$$

$$= \frac{1}{2\pi\sigma^2\sqrt{1-\rho^2}} \int_{-\infty}^{\infty} g(y_2) e^{-\frac{1}{2\sigma^2} y_2^2} \left(\int_{-\infty}^{\infty} y_1 e^{-\frac{1}{2\sigma^2(1-\rho^2)}(y_1-\rho y_2)^2}\, dy_1 \right).$$

The integral in parenthesis is the mean of the Gaussian density integrand, up to a scaling factor equal to $\sqrt{2\pi}$ times the standard deviation of the Gaussian integrand. Hence, it is equal to $\rho y_2 \sqrt{2\pi}\sigma\sqrt{1-\rho^2}$. Therefore,

$$C_{YZ_0}(\tau) = \rho \frac{1}{\sqrt{2\pi}\sigma} \int_{-\infty}^{\infty} g(y_2) y_2 e^{-\frac{1}{2\sigma^2} y_2^2}$$

$$= \rho E[yg(y)].$$

Since $\sigma^2 \rho = C_{YY}(\tau)$, we obtain the desired result.

Exercise 5. See lgn_est3.m.

Exercise 6. See lgn_est5.m.

Exercise 7. According to Bussgang's theorem,

$$C_{XY}(\tau) = \frac{1}{\sigma_X^2} C_{XX}(\tau) \int_{-\infty}^{\infty} x g_{\alpha,l}(x) p(x)\, dx.$$

We therefore need to evaluate

$$A = \int_{-\infty}^{\infty} x g_{\alpha,l}(x) p(x)\, dx = \int_{-\infty}^{\infty} x \left(\frac{2}{\sqrt{\pi}} \int_{0}^{x/\sqrt{2}l} e^{-z^2}\, dz \right) \frac{1}{\sqrt{2\pi}} e^{-x^2/2}\, dx.$$

We integrate by parts,

$$A = \int_a^b u\,dv = uv\big|_a^b - \int_a^b v\,du$$

with

$$u = g(x) \Rightarrow du = \frac{2}{\sqrt{\pi}} e^{-x^2/2l^2} \frac{1}{\sqrt{2}l} dx = \frac{\sqrt{2}}{\sqrt{\pi}} \frac{1}{l} e^{-x^2/2l^2} dx$$

and

$$dv = x \frac{1}{\sqrt{2\pi}} e^{-x^2/2} dx \Rightarrow v = \frac{-1}{\sqrt{2\pi}} e^{-x^2/2}.$$

This yields

$$A = g(x)\left(\frac{-1}{\sqrt{2\pi}} e^{-x^2/2}\right)\Big|_{-\infty}^{\infty} + \frac{\sqrt{2}}{\sqrt{2\pi}} \frac{1}{l} \int_{-\infty}^{\infty} e^{-x^2(1+1/l^2)/2} dx = \frac{1}{\pi} \frac{1}{l} \int_{-\infty}^{\infty} e^{x^2(1+1/l^2)/2} dx.$$

Set $1/\sigma_1^2 = 1 + 1/l^2$ or $\sigma_1^2 = l^2/(1+l^2)$ and since

$$\frac{1}{\sqrt{2\pi}\sigma_1} \int_{-\infty}^{\infty} e^{-x^2/2\sigma_1^2} dx = 1$$

we obtain

$$C_{XY}(\tau) = \frac{C_{XX}(\tau)}{\sigma_X^2} \sqrt{\frac{2}{\pi}} \sqrt{\frac{l^2}{1+l^2}} \frac{1}{l} = \frac{C_{XX}}{\sigma_X^2} \sqrt{\frac{2}{\pi}} \frac{1}{\sqrt{1+l^2}}.$$

Exercise 8. See `coherence_est.m`.

28.22 CHAPTER 23

Exercise 1. See `lgn_revcor_wn3.m`.

Exercise 2. The optimal filter is given by

$$\hat{h}(\omega) = \frac{S_{YX}(\omega)}{S_{YY}(\omega)}.$$

But since X and N are independent,

$$C_{YX}(\tau) = E[(k \star X(t) + N(t))X(t+\tau)]$$
$$= E[k \star X(t)X(t+\tau)] = \tilde{k} \star C_{XX}(\tau).$$

The last equality follows from

$$E[k \star X(t)X(t+\tau)] = E\left[\int k(t-t_0)X(t_0)\,dt_0\,X(t+\tau)\right]$$

$$= \int k(t-t_0)E[X(t_0)X(t+\tau)]\,dt_0$$

$$= \int k(t-t_0)E[X(t_0)X(t_0+t-t+\tau)]\,dt_0$$

$$= \int k(t-t_0)C_{XX}(t-t_0+\tau)\,dt_0$$

$$= \int \tilde{k}(t_0-t)C_{XX}(t-t_0+\tau)\,dt_0, \quad t_1 = t_0 - t$$

$$= \int \tilde{k}(t_1)C_{XX}(\tau-t_1)\,dt_1 = \tilde{k} \star C_{XX}(\tau).$$

Similarly,

$$C_{YY}(\tau) = (k \star \tilde{k}) \star C_{XX}(\tau) + C_{NN}(\tau).$$

Fourier transforming these two results immediately leads to Eq. (23.6).

Exercise 3. See `rec_wn.8`.

28.23 CHAPTER 24

Exercise 1. See `poiss1.m`.

Exercise 2. From Eq. (24.2) we compute

$$\frac{p(n|s_1)}{p(n|s_0)} = e^{((n-n_0)^2 - (n-n_1)^2)/2\sigma_n^2}$$

$$= e^{(n^2 - 2nn_0 + n_0^2 - n^2 + 2nn_1 - n_1^2)/2\sigma_n^2} = e^{-(n_0-n_1)n/\sigma_n^2}e^{-(n_1^2-n_0^2)/2\sigma_n^2}$$

which implies

$$l(n) = \log\frac{p(n|s_1)}{p(n|s_0)} = (n_1 - n_0)\frac{n}{\sigma_n^2} - \frac{(n_1^2 - n_0^2)}{2\sigma_n^2}$$

$$= \frac{(n_1 - n_0)}{\sigma_n^2}n - \frac{(n_1 - n_0)(n_1 + n_0)}{2\sigma_n^2} = \frac{n_1 - n_0}{\sigma_n^2}\left(n - \frac{n_1 + n_0}{2}\right).$$

Exercise 3. Under hypothesis s_0, $n \sim \mathcal{N}(n_0, \sigma_n^2)$ and

$$l_0 = E[l|s_0] = \frac{(n_1 - n_0)}{\sigma_n^2}\left(n_0 - \frac{n_1 + n_0}{2}\right) = \frac{n_1 - n_0}{\sigma_n^2}\frac{n_0 - n_1}{2}.$$

Define $d^2 = (n_1 - n_0)^2/\sigma_n^2$ so that $l_0 - d^2/2$. Furthermore,

$$E[(l - l_0)^2|s_0] = \frac{(n_1 - n_0)^2}{\sigma_n^4}E[(n - n_0)^2] = \frac{(n_1 - n_0)^2}{\sigma_n^4}\sigma_n^2 = \frac{(n_1 - n_0)^2}{\sigma_n^2} = d^2.$$

The second assertion under s_1 follows in the same manner.

Exercise 4. According to Eq. (24.4),

$$P_{FA} = \int\limits_{\xi}^{\infty} p(l|s_0)\mathrm{d}l = \int\limits_{\xi}^{\infty} \frac{1}{\sqrt{2\pi}d} e^{-(y+d^2/2)^2/2d^2}\mathrm{d}y$$

set $z=(y+d^2/2)/d$, $\mathrm{d}z=\mathrm{d}y/d$ and with $y=\xi$, $z=\xi_0=(\xi+d^2/2)/d$, we obtain

$$P_{FA} = \int\limits_{\xi_0}^{\infty} \frac{1}{\sqrt{2\pi}} e^{-z^2/2}\mathrm{d}z = 1-\Phi(\xi_0).$$

Similarly,

$$P_D = \int\limits_{\xi}^{\infty} \frac{1}{\sqrt{2\pi}d} e^{-(y-d^2/2)^2/2d^2}\mathrm{d}y$$

and with $z=(y-d^2/2)/d$, $\xi_1=(\xi-d^2/2)/d=\xi_0-d$, we obtain

$$P_D = \int\limits_{\xi_1}^{\infty} e^{-z^2/2}\mathrm{d}z = 1-\Phi(\xi_1) = 1-\Phi(\xi_0-d).$$

The error is

$$\varepsilon(\xi_0) = \frac{1}{2}P_{FA} + \frac{1}{2}(1-P_D) = \frac{1}{2}(1-\Phi(\xi_0)+\Phi(\xi_0-d))$$

and its derivative with respect to ξ_0 has to vanish at the minimum, $\xi_{0\,min}$,

$$\left.\frac{\mathrm{d}\varepsilon}{\mathrm{d}\xi_0}\right|_{\xi_0=\xi_{0min}} = -\frac{1}{2}\left.\frac{\mathrm{d}\Phi(\xi_0)}{\mathrm{d}\xi_0}\right|_{\xi_0=\xi_{0min}} + \frac{1}{2}\left.\frac{\mathrm{d}\Phi(\xi_0-d)}{\mathrm{d}\xi_0}\right|_{\xi_0=\xi_{0min}}$$

$$= -\frac{1}{2}\frac{1}{\sqrt{2\pi}}e^{-\xi_0^2/2} + \frac{1}{2}\frac{1}{\sqrt{2\pi}}e^{-(\xi_0-d)^2/2}.$$

This implies

$$\xi_0^2 = (\xi_0-d)^2 \Leftrightarrow \pm\xi_0 = \pm(\xi_0-d).$$

Case 1: $\xi_0=\xi_0-d \Rightarrow d=0$ and ξ_0 is arbitrary, this leads to 100% error.
Case 2: $-\xi_0=-(\xi_0-d) \Rightarrow d=0$, as in Case 1.
Case 3: $\xi_0=-(\xi_0-d) \Rightarrow 2\xi_0=d$ or $\xi_0=d/2$.
Case 4: $-\xi_0=(\xi_0-d) \Rightarrow 2\xi_0=d$ or $\xi_0=d/2$, as in Case 3.

The corresponding value of ξ given $\xi_0=d/2$ is

$$\frac{d}{2} = \left(\xi+\frac{d^2}{2}\right)\Big/ d \Leftrightarrow \frac{d^2}{2} = \xi+\frac{d^2}{2} \Rightarrow \xi=0.$$

This means that the likelihood ratio threshold is $\exp(\xi)=1$. Since $\Phi(d/2)=1-\Phi(-d/2)$,

$$P_C = \frac{P_D}{2} + \frac{1-P_{FA}}{2} = \frac{1}{2}(1-\Phi(-d/2)) + \frac{1}{2}\Phi(d/2)$$

$$= \frac{1}{2}(1-\Phi(-d/2)) + \frac{1}{2}(1-\Phi(-d/2)) = 1-\Phi(-d/2).$$

Exercise 5. According to Eq. (24.10) and Eq. (24.11),

$$P_{FA} = \int_k^\infty q(l_r \mid s_0)\,dl_r, \quad \frac{dP_{FA}}{dk} = -q(k \mid s_0)$$

$$P_D = \int_k^\infty q(l_r \mid s_1)\,dl_r, \quad \frac{P_D}{dk} = -q(k \mid s_1)$$

$$\varepsilon(k) = \frac{1}{2}\left(P_{FA}(k) + 1 - P_D(k)\right)$$

$$\frac{d\varepsilon}{dk} = \frac{1}{2}\left(q(k \mid s_0) + q(k \mid s_1)\right) = \frac{1}{2}\left(-q(k \mid s_0) + kq(k \mid s_0)\right) = \frac{1}{2}q(k \mid s_0)(k-1).$$

Assuming $q(k \mid s_0) \neq 0$ we have $d\varepsilon/dk < 0$ for $k < 1$, $d\varepsilon/dk > 0$ for $k > 1$ and $d\varepsilon/dk = 0$ at $k = 1$ which is therefore the minimum. Maximum errors on each side of this minimum occur at $k = 0$ and $k = \infty$.

Exercise 8.

$$E[(l - l_1)^2 \mid s_1] = E\left[\left(\mathbf{w}^T(\mathbf{x} - \mathbf{x}_0) - \frac{1}{2}\mathbf{w}^T(\mathbf{n}_1 - \mathbf{n}_0)\right)^2\right]$$

$$= E\left[\left(\mathbf{w}^T\left(\mathbf{x} - \frac{1}{2}(\mathbf{n}_0 + \mathbf{n}_1) - \frac{1}{2}(\mathbf{n}_1 - \mathbf{n}_0)\right)\right)^2\right]$$

$$= E\left[\left(\mathbf{w}^T\left(\mathbf{x} - \frac{1}{2}\mathbf{n}_0 - \frac{1}{2}\mathbf{n}_1 - \frac{1}{2}\mathbf{n}_1 + \frac{1}{2}\mathbf{n}_0\right)\right)^2\right]$$

$$= E\left[(\mathbf{w}^T(\mathbf{x} - \mathbf{n}_1))^2\right] = E\left[\mathbf{w}^T(\mathbf{x} - \mathbf{n}_1)(\mathbf{x} - \mathbf{n}_1)^T\mathbf{w}\right]$$

$$= \mathbf{w}^T\mathbf{C}\mathbf{w} = (\mathbf{n}_1 - \mathbf{n}_0)^T\mathbf{C}^{-1}\mathbf{C}\mathbf{C}^{-1}(\mathbf{n}_1 - \mathbf{n}_0)$$

$$= (\mathbf{n}_1 - \mathbf{n}_0)^T\mathbf{C}^{-1}(\mathbf{n}_1 - \mathbf{n}_0) = d^2.$$

Exercise 10. The requirement $\mathbf{C}\mathbf{C}^{-1} = \mathbf{I}$ and $\mathbf{C}^{-1}\mathbf{C} = \mathbf{I}$, where $\mathbf{C}^{-1}$ is defined through Eq. (24.19), is equivalent to:

$$a + (k-1)bc = 1 \quad \text{(diagonal terms)},$$
$$b + (a + (k-2)b)c = 0 \quad \text{(off-diagonal terms)}.$$

To solve this system of equations for a and b we rearrange as follows:

$$ca + (1 + (k-2)c)b = 0$$
$$a + (k-1)cb = 1.$$

The first equation leads to $a = -(1 + (k-2)c)b/c$ and multiplying the second equation by c and subtracting the first one yields

$$(k-1)c^2b - (1 + (k-2)c)b = c \quad \text{or} \quad b((k-1)c^2 - (k-2)c - 1) = c$$

which implies

$$b = \frac{c}{(k-1)c^2 - (k-2)c - 1} \quad \text{and} \quad a = -\frac{(1 + (k-2)c)}{c}b.$$

Note that $b = 0$ when $c = 0$ and $a = 1$.

Exercise 11. Since

$$\sum_{i=1}^{k} v_i \sum_{j=1,j\neq i}^{k} v_j = \left(\sum_{i=1}^{k} v_i\right)^2 - \sum_{i=1}^{k} v_i^2$$

we may rewrite Eq. (24.21) as follows

$$d^2 = \frac{1}{\sigma_n^2}\left(a\sum_{i=1}^{k} v_i^2 + b\left(\sum_{i=1}^{k} v_i\right)^2 - b\sum_{i=1}^{k} v_i^2\right)$$

$$= \frac{1}{\sigma_n^2}\left((a-b)\sum_{i=1}^{k} v_i^2 + b\left(\sum_{i=1}^{k} v_i\right)^2\right)$$

$$= \frac{1}{\sigma_n^2}\left((a-b)k\frac{1}{k}\sum_{i=1}^{k} v_i^2 + bk^2\frac{1}{k^2}\left(\sum_{i=1}^{k} v_i\right)^2\right)$$

$$= \frac{1}{\sigma_n^2}\left((a-b)k\frac{1}{k}\sum_{i=1}^{k} v_i^2 + bk^2\mu_v^2\right).$$

Since

$$\sigma_v^2 = \frac{1}{k}\sum_{i=1}^{k}(v_i - \mu_v)^2 = \frac{1}{k}\sum_{i=1}^{k} v_i^2 - \mu_v^2$$

we have

$$\frac{1}{k}\sum_{i=1}^{k} v_i^2 = \mu_v^2 + \sigma_v^2$$

and

$$d^2 = \frac{1}{\sigma_n^2}\left((a-b)k(\mu_v^2 + \sigma_v^2) + bk^2\mu_v^2\right)$$

$$= \frac{\mu_v^2}{\sigma_v^2}\left((a-b)k + bk^2 + (a-b)k\frac{\sigma_v^2}{\mu_v^2}\right)$$

$$= \frac{\mu_v^2}{\sigma_v^2}\left(k(a+b(k-1)) + (a-b)k\frac{\sigma_v^2}{\mu_v^2}\right).$$

We now compute the two factors

$$
\begin{aligned}
k(a+b(k-1)) &= k\left(\frac{-(1+(k-2)c)}{(k-1)c^2-(k-2)c-1}+\frac{c(k-1)}{(k-1)c^2-(k-2)c-1}\right)\\
&= k\left(\frac{-1-(k-2)c+(k-1)c}{k(c^2-c)-c^2+2c-1}\right)\\
&= k\left(\frac{-1+2c-c}{kc(c-1)-(c-1)^2}\right)\\
&= \frac{k(c-1)}{(c-1)(kc-c+1)}\\
&= \frac{k}{kc-c+1}\to\frac{1}{c}\quad(k\to\infty)
\end{aligned}
$$

and

$$
\begin{aligned}
(a-b)k &= \left(\frac{-(1+(k-2)c)}{(k-1)c^2-(k-2)c-1}-\frac{c}{(k-1)c^2-(k-2)c-1}\right)k\\
&= \frac{(-1-kc+2c-c)}{(c-1)(kc-c+1)}k\\
&= \frac{(-kc+c-1)k}{(c-1)(kc-c+1)}=\frac{-k}{c-1}=\frac{k}{1-c}.
\end{aligned}
$$

Plugging these two results in the last expression for d^2 yields Eq. (24.22).

Exercise 12. Since $\sigma_v^2=\rho\mu_v^2$, we have from Eq. (24.18),

$$
E[d_s^2]=\frac{\mu_v^2}{\sigma_n^2}+\rho\frac{\mu_v^2}{\sigma_n^2}=\frac{\mu_v^2}{\sigma_n^2}(1+\rho)
$$

or $\mu_v^2/\sigma_v^2=E[d_s^2]/(1+\rho)$. Plugging these results in Eq. (24.22)

$$
\begin{aligned}
d^2 &= \frac{E[d_s^2]}{1+\rho}\left(\frac{k}{kc-c+1}+\frac{k}{1-c}\rho\right)\\
&= E[d_s^2]\frac{k}{1+\rho}\left(\frac{1}{kc-c+1}+\frac{1}{1-c}\rho\right).
\end{aligned}
$$

Exercise 13. Clearly,

$$
\mathbf{w}^T\mathbf{S}_C\mathbf{w}=\frac{1}{2}\mathbf{w}^T\mathbf{C}_0\mathbf{w}+\frac{1}{2}\mathbf{w}^T\mathbf{C}_1\mathbf{w}=\frac{1}{2}(\sigma_0^2+\sigma_1^2)>0
$$

and therefore $\mathbf{S}_C$ is positive definite. If $\mathbf{C}=\mathbf{U}^T\mathbf{U}$ and $\mathbf{x}=\mathbf{U}\mathbf{w}$ then

$$
\mathbf{w}^T\mathbf{C}\mathbf{w}=\mathbf{w}^T\mathbf{U}^T\mathbf{U}\mathbf{w}=(\mathbf{U}\mathbf{w})^T\mathbf{x}=\mathbf{x}^T\mathbf{x}
$$

and since $\mathbf{w}=\mathbf{U}^{-1}\mathbf{x}$,

$$
\mathbf{w}^T\mathbf{S}_n\mathbf{w}=(\mathbf{U}^{-1}\mathbf{x})^T\mathbf{S}_n\mathbf{U}^{-1}\mathbf{x}=\mathbf{x}^T(\mathbf{U}^{-1})^T\mathbf{S}_n\mathbf{U}^{-1}\mathbf{x}.
$$

According to Exercise 18.15,

$$(\mathbf{U}^{-1})^T \mathbf{S}_n \mathbf{U}^{-1} \mathbf{x} = \lambda \mathbf{x}$$
$$\mathbf{S}_n \mathbf{w} = \lambda \mathbf{U}^T \mathbf{U} \mathbf{w}$$
$$\mathbf{S}_n \mathbf{w} = \lambda \mathbf{S}_C \mathbf{w}.$$

28.24 CHAPTER 25

Exercise 1. See hsp.m.

Exercise 2. See darknoise.m.

Exercise 3. Call the first presentation interval I_0 and the second presentation I_1. Let s_0 be the hypothesis that the stimulus is presented in interval I_0 and s_1 the hypothesis that the stimulus is presented in interval I_1. Denote by $\mathbf{x}$ the vector $(x_1, x_2)^T$, where x_1 is the value of X in interval I_0 and x_2 the value of X in interval I_1. Let also p_0 be the probability density of X given noise and p_1 the probability of X given the stimulus. Since the random variable X is selected independently in I_0 and I_1 (except that one is selected from the noise and the other from the signal distribution), we have the following expression for the probability densities q_0, q_1 of $\mathbf{x}$ under s_0 and s_1, respectively:

$$s_0 : q_0(\mathbf{x}) = p_0(x_1)p_1(x_2)$$
$$s_1 : q_1(\mathbf{x}) = p_1(x_1)p_0(x_2).$$

The likelihood ratio for $\mathbf{x}$ is

$$l_r(\mathbf{x}) = \frac{q_1(\mathbf{x})}{q_0(\mathbf{x})} = \frac{p_0(x_1)p_1(x_2)}{p_1(x_1)p_0(x_2)} = \frac{l_r(x_2)}{l_r(x_1)}.$$

According to the Neyman–Pearson lemma, the optimal test statistics is

$$l_r(x_2) \gtreqless k l_r(x_1)$$

and the minimum error test compares the likelihood ratios directly with $k = 1$.

Exercise 4. According to Eq. (24.10),

$$P_{FA} = \int_k^\infty q(l_r \mid s_0) dl_r \quad \text{or} \quad \frac{dP_{FA}}{dk} = -q(k \mid s_0).$$

We also have $k = \infty$ when $P_{FA} = 0$ and $k = 0$ when $P_{FA} = 1$. Therefore,

$$P_C = \int_0^1 P_D(P_{FA}) dP_{FA} = \int_0^\infty P_D(k) q(k \mid s_0) dk.$$

Plugging in Eq. (24.11) for $P_D(k)$, we obtain

$$P_C = \int_0^\infty \left(\int_k^\infty q(l_r \mid s_1) dl_r \right) q(k \mid s_0) dk. \tag{28.16}$$

To see that this expression is equal to the probability of correct performance in the 2-AFC task, first note that if the likelihood ratio takes the value k when noise is present (s_0), then correct performance will be achieved only if the value of the likelihood ratio is larger than k for s_1,

$$P_C(k\,|\,s_0) = \int\limits_k^\infty q(l_r\,|\,s_1)\mathrm{d}l_r.$$

The probability of correct performance is obtained by multiplying by the probability density of k given s_0, i.e., $q(k\,|\,s_0)$ and integrating over all possible values of k, which yields Eq. (28.16).

Exercise 5. In the 2-AFC model the decision variable is $l_s - l_n$, where l_s is the log-likelihood ratio in the case the stimulus is present and l_n in the case the noise is present. A correct decision will be made when $l_s - l_n > 0$. Hence $P_C = P(l_s - l_n > 0)$. Since $l_s \sim \mathcal{N}(d^2/2, d^2)$, $l_n \sim \mathcal{N}(-d^2/2, d^2)$, and these two variables are assumed to be independent, we have $\Delta l = l_s - l_n \sim \mathcal{N}(d^2, 2d^2)$ and

$$P_C = \int\limits_0^\infty \frac{1}{\sqrt{2\pi}}\frac{1}{\sqrt{2}d}e^{-(x-d^2)^2/2\cdot 2d^2}\,\mathrm{d}x.$$

With $y = (x - d^2)/\sqrt{2}d$, $x = 0 \Rightarrow y = -d/\sqrt{2}$ and

$$P_C = \int\limits_{-d/\sqrt{2}}^\infty \frac{1}{\sqrt{2\pi}}e^{-y^2/2}\,\mathrm{d}y = 1 - \Phi\left(-\frac{d}{\sqrt{2}}\right).$$

Exercise 6. For notational simplicity, set $m_n = m_{null}$, $m_s = m_{preferred}$, $\sigma_n = \sigma_{null}$, and $\sigma_s = \sigma_{preferred}$ and let x denote the firing rate. Then

$$p_n(x) = \frac{1}{\sqrt{2\pi}\sigma_n}e^{-(x-m_n)^2/2\sigma_n^2} \quad \text{and} \quad p_s(x) = \frac{1}{\sqrt{2\pi}\sigma_s}e^{-(x-m_s)^2/2\sigma_s^2}.$$

With $Y = (X - m_n)/\sigma_n$ we have $Y \sim \mathcal{N}(0,1)$ under n, and $Y \sim \mathcal{N}(\mu_Y, \sigma_Y^2)$ under s, where $\mu_Y = E[Y\,|\,s] = (m_s - m_n)/\sigma_n$ and $\sigma_Y^2 = E[Y^2\,|\,s] - E[Y\,|\,s]^2$. We compute first

$$\begin{aligned}
E[Y^2\,|\,s] &= E\left[\frac{X^2}{\sigma_n^2} - \frac{2X}{\sigma_n^2}m_n + \frac{m_n^2}{\sigma_n^2}\,\Big|\,s\right] \\
&= \frac{1}{\sigma_n^2}E[X^2\,|\,s] - \frac{2}{\sigma_n^2}E[X\,|\,s]m_n + \frac{m_n^2}{\sigma_n^2} \\
&= \frac{1}{\sigma_n^2}(\sigma_s^2 + m_s^2) - \frac{2}{\sigma_n^2}m_s m_n + \frac{m_n^2}{\sigma_n^2} = \frac{\sigma_s^2}{\sigma_n^2} + \frac{(m_s - m_n)^2}{\sigma_n^2},
\end{aligned}$$

which implies

$$E[Y^2\,|\,s] - E[Y\,|\,s]^2 = \frac{\sigma_s^2}{\sigma_n^2} + \frac{(m_s - m_n)^2}{\sigma_n^2} - \frac{m_s - m_n)^2}{\sigma_n^2} = \frac{\sigma_s^2}{\sigma_n^2}.$$

We have $\sigma_Y > 1$ since $\sigma_s > \sigma_n$. Now

$$p(y\,|\,n) = \frac{1}{\sqrt{2\pi}}e^{-y^2/2} \quad \text{and} \quad p(y\,|\,s) = \frac{1}{\sqrt{2\pi}\sigma_y}e^{-(y-\mu_Y)^2/2\sigma_Y^2}$$

so that

$$\log \frac{p(y|s)}{p(y|n)} = \log \frac{\exp(-(y-\mu_Y)^2/2\sigma_Y^2)/\sqrt{2\pi}\,\sigma_Y}{\exp(-y^2/2)/\sqrt{2\pi}}$$

$$= -\log \sigma_Y + \log \exp(-(y-\mu_Y)^2/2\sigma_Y^2 + y^2)$$

$$= -\log \sigma_Y + \left(-\frac{(y-\mu_Y)^2}{2\sigma_Y^2} + \frac{y^2}{2}\right)$$

$$= -\log \sigma_Y + \frac{1}{2\sigma_Y^2}\left((\sigma_Y^2-1)y^2 + 2y\mu_Y - \mu_Y^2\right).$$

We solve this equation for y, given a fixed value, l_{th}, of the log-likelihood ratio. Since

$$l_{th} = -\log \sigma_Y + \frac{1}{2\sigma_Y^2}\left((\sigma_Y^2-1)y^2 + 2y\mu_Y - \mu_Y^2\right)$$

or, equivalently,

$$2\sigma_Y^2(l_{th} + \log \sigma_Y) = \left((\sigma_Y^2-1)y^2 + 2y\mu_Y - \mu_Y^2\right)$$

we define $\rho = 2\sigma_Y^2(l_{th} + \log \sigma_Y)$ which leads to the quadratic equation

$$(\sigma_Y^2-1)y^2 + 2\mu_Y y - \mu_Y^2 - \rho = 0.$$

With $a = \sigma_Y^2 - 1$, $b = 2\mu_Y$, $c = -\mu_Y^2 - \rho$ we have

$$\Delta = 4\mu_Y^2 - 4(\sigma_Y^2 - 1)(-\mu_Y^2 - \rho)$$

$$= 4\mu_Y^2 + 4\sigma_Y^2\mu_Y^2 + 4\sigma_Y^2\rho - 4\mu_Y^2 - 4\rho$$

$$= 4(\sigma_Y^2(\mu_Y^2 + \rho) - \rho) > 0, \text{ since } \sigma_Y > 1.$$

This leads to

$$y_\pm = \frac{-\mu_Y \pm \sqrt{\sigma_Y^2(\mu_Y^2 + \rho) - \rho}}{\sigma_Y^2 - 1}.$$

28.25 CHAPTER 26

Exercise 1. With respect to the standard basis, $\{\mathbf{e}_1\ \mathbf{e}_2\}$, of $\mathbb{R}^2$,

$$\phi_1 = \begin{pmatrix} 1 \\ 0 \end{pmatrix}, \ \phi_2 = \begin{pmatrix} -1/2 \\ \sqrt{3}/2 \end{pmatrix}, \ \phi_3 = \begin{pmatrix} -1/2 \\ -\sqrt{3}/2 \end{pmatrix}, \text{ and } \mathbf{v} = \begin{pmatrix} v_1 \\ v_2 \end{pmatrix}.$$

Furthermore,

$$g_1 = \begin{pmatrix} v_1 & v_2 \end{pmatrix}\begin{pmatrix} 1 \\ 0 \end{pmatrix} = v_1,$$

$$g_2 = \begin{pmatrix} v_1 & v_2 \end{pmatrix}\begin{pmatrix} -1/2 \\ \sqrt{3}/2 \end{pmatrix} = -\frac{1}{2}v_1 + \frac{\sqrt{3}}{2}v_2,$$

$$g_3 = \begin{pmatrix} v_1 & v_2 \end{pmatrix}\begin{pmatrix} -1/2 \\ -\sqrt{3}/2 \end{pmatrix} = -\frac{1}{2}v_1 - \frac{\sqrt{3}}{2}v_2$$

and

$$\sum_{i=1}^{3} g_i \phi_i = v_1 \begin{pmatrix} 1 \\ 0 \end{pmatrix} + \left(-\frac{1}{2} v_1 + \frac{\sqrt{3}}{2} v_2 \right) \begin{pmatrix} -1/2 \\ \sqrt{3}/2 \end{pmatrix} + \left(-\frac{1}{2} v_1 - \frac{\sqrt{3}}{2} v_2 \right) \begin{pmatrix} -1/2 \\ -\sqrt{3}/2 \end{pmatrix}$$

$$= \begin{pmatrix} v_1 + \frac{1}{4} v_1 - \frac{\sqrt{3}}{4} v_2 + \frac{1}{4} v_1 + \frac{\sqrt{3}}{4} v_2 \\ -\frac{\sqrt{3}}{4} v_1 + \frac{3}{4} v_2 + \frac{\sqrt{3}}{4} v_1 + \frac{3}{4} v_2 \end{pmatrix}$$

$$= \frac{3}{2} \begin{pmatrix} v_1 \\ v_2 \end{pmatrix}.$$

Hence,

$$\frac{2}{3} \sum_{i=1}^{3} g_i \phi_i = \begin{pmatrix} v_1 \\ v_2 \end{pmatrix} = \mathbf{v}.$$

To derive the general result, first note that

$$\mathbf{U} = \begin{pmatrix} 1 & 0 \\ \cos \frac{2\pi}{m} & \sin \frac{2\pi}{m} \\ \vdots & \vdots \\ \cos \frac{2\pi(m-1)}{m} & \sin \frac{2\pi(m-1)}{m} \end{pmatrix}$$

which immediately implies that

$$\mathbf{U}^T \mathbf{U} = \begin{pmatrix} \sum_{j=0}^{m-1} \cos^2 \frac{2\pi j}{m} & \sum_{j=0}^{m-1} \cos \frac{2\pi j}{m} \sin \frac{2\pi j}{m} \\ \sum_{j=0}^{m-1} \cos \frac{2\pi j}{m} \sin \frac{2\pi j}{m} & \sum_{j=0}^{m-1} \cos^2 \frac{2\pi j}{m} \end{pmatrix}.$$

Next, we show that

$$\sum_{j=0}^{m-1} z_j^2 = \sum_{j=0}^{m-1} (e^{2\pi i j/m})^2 = \sum_{j=0}^{m-1} e^{4\pi i j/m}$$

$$= \sum_{j=0}^{m-1} w^j, \quad w = e^{4\pi i/m}$$

$$= \frac{1 - w^m}{1 - w} = 0.$$

Taking the real and imaginary part of the left hand side, this implies

$$\sum_{j=0}^{m-1} \cos \frac{4\pi j}{m} = 0 \quad \text{and} \quad \sum_{j=0}^{m-1} \sin \frac{4\pi j}{m} = 0. \tag{28.17}$$

To derive the four identities, we start by computing

$$\cos 2\alpha + i \sin 2\alpha = \exp(2\alpha i) = \exp(\alpha i) \exp(\alpha i)$$

$$= (\cos \alpha + i \sin \alpha)(\cos \alpha + i \sin \alpha)$$

$$= (\cos^2 \alpha - \sin^2 \alpha) + 2i \sin \alpha \cos \alpha$$

from which we immediately deduce the two identities on the left. Furthermore,

$$\cos 2\alpha = \cos^2\alpha - \sin^2\alpha + \cos^2\alpha + \sin^2\alpha - 1 = 2\cos^2\alpha - 1 \tag{28.18}$$

proving the top right identity. The bottom right identity follows from

$$\sin^2\alpha = 1 - \cos^2\alpha = 1 - \frac{1+\cos 2\alpha}{2} = \frac{1-\cos 2\alpha}{2}. \tag{28.19}$$

We may now plug the product formula for $\sin 2\alpha$ in the second equality of Eq. (28.17) to find

$$0 = \sum_{j=0}^{m-1} \sin\frac{4\pi j}{m} = 2\sum_{j=0}^{m-1} \sin\frac{2\pi j}{m}\cos\frac{2\pi j}{m}.$$

Therefore the off-diagonal terms of $\mathbf{U}^T\mathbf{U}$ vanish. To compute the diagonal terms use Eq. (28.18),

$$\sum_{j=0}^{m-1} \cos^2\frac{2\pi j}{m} = \sum_{j=0}^{m-1} \frac{1+\cos 4\pi j/m}{2} = \frac{m}{2} + \frac{1}{2}\sum_{j=0}^{m-1}\cos\frac{4\pi j}{m} = \frac{m}{2},$$

where we used the first equality of Eq. (28.17). Finally, using Eq. (28.19)

$$\sum_{j=0}^{m-1} \sin^2\frac{2\pi j}{m} = \sum_{j=0}^{m-1} \frac{1-\cos 4\pi j/m}{2} = \frac{m}{2} - \frac{1}{2}\sum_{j=0}^{m-1}\cos\frac{4\pi j}{m} = \frac{m}{2}.$$

From this we conclude that the frame determined by $\{\phi_j\}$, $j=1,\dots m$, is tight with $\lambda_1 = \lambda_2 = m/2$. Therefore, according to Eq. (26.8)

$$\mathbf{v} = \frac{2}{m}\sum_{j=1}^{m} g_i\phi_j.$$

Exercise 3.

$$E\left[\left((\check{\mathbf{v}} - E[\check{\mathbf{v}}]) + (E[\check{\mathbf{v}}] - \mathbf{v})\right)\left((\check{\mathbf{v}} - E[\check{\mathbf{v}}]) + (E[\check{\mathbf{v}}] - \mathbf{v})\right)^T\right] = E\left[(\check{\mathbf{v}} - E[\check{\mathbf{v}}])(\check{\mathbf{v}} - E[\check{\mathbf{v}}])^T\right] + (E[\check{\mathbf{v}}] - \mathbf{v})(E[\check{\mathbf{v}}] - \mathbf{v})^T$$
$$+ E\left[(E[\check{\mathbf{v}}] - \mathbf{v})(\check{\mathbf{v}} - E[\check{\mathbf{v}}])^T\right] + E\left[(\check{\mathbf{v}} - E[\check{\mathbf{v}}])(E[\check{\mathbf{v}}] - \mathbf{v})^T\right].$$

However,

$$E[(E[\check{\mathbf{v}}] - \mathbf{v})(\check{\mathbf{v}} - E[\check{\mathbf{v}}])^T] = E[\check{\mathbf{v}}]E[\check{\mathbf{v}}]^T - E[\check{\mathbf{v}}]E[\check{\mathbf{v}}]^T - \mathbf{v}E[\check{\mathbf{v}}]^T + \mathbf{v}E[\check{\mathbf{v}}]^T = 0.$$

The last term can be shown to vanish in the same manner.

Exercise 4. Since $E[\mathbf{n}] = 0$ it follows that $E[\mathbf{g}] = \mathbf{U}\mathbf{v}$. Therefore, we immediately see that

$$E[\check{\mathbf{v}}] = \mathbf{F}E[\mathbf{g}] = (\mathbf{U}^T\mathbf{C}^{-1}\mathbf{U})^{-1}\mathbf{U}^T\mathbf{C}^{-1}\mathbf{U}\mathbf{v} = \mathbf{v}.$$

Exercise 5.

$$E[\mathbf{s}(\mathbf{v},\mathbf{g})] = \int \mathbf{s}(\mathbf{v},\mathbf{g})p(\mathbf{g}|\mathbf{v})\,d\mathbf{g}$$

$$= \int \left(\nabla_{\mathbf{v}}\log(f_{\mathbf{v}}(g))\right)p(\mathbf{g}|\mathbf{v})d\mathbf{g}$$

$$= \int \frac{1}{f_{\mathbf{v}}(\mathbf{g})}\nabla_{\mathbf{v}}(f_{\mathbf{v}}(\mathbf{g}))p(\mathbf{g}|\mathbf{v})\,d\mathbf{g} \quad \text{but} \quad f_{\mathbf{v}}(\mathbf{g}) = p(\mathbf{g}|\mathbf{v}) \quad \text{and so}$$

$$= \nabla_{\mathbf{v}}\int p(\mathbf{g}|\mathbf{v})d\mathbf{g} = \nabla_{\mathbf{v}}1 = 0.$$

Exercise 6.

$$0 = \nabla_{\mathbf{v}}\int f_{\mathbf{v}}(\mathbf{g})(\check{\mathbf{v}}-\mathbf{v})^T d\mathbf{g}$$

$$= \int \nabla_{\mathbf{v}}(f_{\mathbf{v}}(\mathbf{g})(\check{\mathbf{v}}-\mathbf{v})^T)d\mathbf{g}$$

$$= \int (\nabla_{\mathbf{v}}f_{\mathbf{v}}(\mathbf{g}))(\check{\mathbf{v}}-\mathbf{v})^T d\mathbf{g} + \int f_{\mathbf{v}}(\mathbf{g})\nabla_{\mathbf{v}}(\check{\mathbf{v}}-\mathbf{v})^T d\mathbf{g}$$

$$= \int f_{\mathbf{v}}(\mathbf{g})\left(\nabla_{\mathbf{v}}\log(f_{\mathbf{v}}(\mathbf{g}))\right)(\check{\mathbf{v}}-\mathbf{v})^T d\mathbf{g} - \int f_{\mathbf{v}}(\mathbf{g})\mathbf{I}d\mathbf{g}$$

$$= E[\mathbf{s}(\mathbf{v},\mathbf{g})(\check{\mathbf{v}}-\mathbf{v})^T] - \mathbf{I},$$

where we have used $\nabla_{\mathbf{v}}\log(f_{\mathbf{v}}(\mathbf{g})) = \left(\nabla_{\mathbf{v}}f_{\mathbf{v}}(\mathbf{g})\right)/f_{\mathbf{v}}(\mathbf{g})$ to derive the second to last equality.

Exercise 7. By assumption $E[\check{\mathbf{v}}-\mathbf{v}]$ is equal to zero since the estimator $\check{\mathbf{v}}$ is unbiased. In addition, according to Exercise 5, $E[\mathbf{s}(\mathbf{v},\mathbf{g})] = 0$, which implies $E[\mathbf{q}] = 0$. For the covariance,

$$\mathbf{Q} = E[\mathbf{q}\mathbf{q}^T] = E\left[\begin{pmatrix} \check{\mathbf{v}}-\mathbf{v} \\ \mathbf{s}(\mathbf{v},\mathbf{g}) \end{pmatrix}\left((\check{\mathbf{v}}-\mathbf{v})^T \quad \mathbf{s}(\mathbf{v},\mathbf{g})^T\right)\right]$$

$$= \begin{pmatrix} E[(\check{\mathbf{v}}-\mathbf{v})(\check{\mathbf{v}}-\mathbf{v})^T] & E[(\check{\mathbf{v}}-\mathbf{v})\mathbf{s}(\mathbf{v},\mathbf{g})^T] \\ E[\mathbf{s}(\mathbf{v},\mathbf{g})(\check{\mathbf{v}}-\mathbf{v})^T] & E[\mathbf{s}(\mathbf{v},\mathbf{g})\mathbf{s}(\mathbf{v},\mathbf{g})^T] \end{pmatrix}$$

$$= \begin{pmatrix} \mathbf{C} & \mathbf{I} \\ \mathbf{I} & \mathbf{J} \end{pmatrix},$$

where we have used the definition of $\mathbf{J}$ and Eq. (26.16). Straightforward matrix multiplication yields

$$\mathbf{A}^T\mathbf{Q}\mathbf{A} = \begin{pmatrix} \mathbf{I} & -\mathbf{J}^{-1} \\ \mathbf{0} & \mathbf{I} \end{pmatrix}\mathbf{Q} = \begin{pmatrix} \mathbf{C} & \mathbf{I} \\ \mathbf{I} & \mathbf{J} \end{pmatrix}\cdot\begin{pmatrix} \mathbf{I} & \mathbf{0} \\ -\mathbf{J}^{-1} & \mathbf{I} \end{pmatrix}$$

$$= \begin{pmatrix} \mathbf{C}-\mathbf{J}^{-1} & \mathbf{0} \\ \mathbf{0} & \mathbf{J} \end{pmatrix}.$$

With $\mathbf{x} = \begin{pmatrix} \mathbf{x}_1 & \mathbf{0} \end{pmatrix}^T$ we have

$$0 \le \mathbf{x}^T\mathbf{A}^T\mathbf{Q}\mathbf{A}\mathbf{x} = \mathbf{x}_1^T(\mathbf{C}-\mathbf{J}^{-1})\mathbf{x}_1$$

and therefore

$$\mathbf{x}_1^T\mathbf{J}^{-1}\mathbf{x}_1 \le \mathbf{x}_1^T\mathbf{C}\mathbf{x}_1.$$

Exercise 8. First, according to Eq. (26.11),

$$\mathbf{s}(\mathbf{v},\mathbf{g}) = \nabla_{\mathbf{v}} \log f_{\mathbf{v}}(\mathbf{g}) = \nabla_{\mathbf{v}} \left(-\frac{m}{2} \log 2\pi - \frac{1}{2} \log |\det \mathbf{C}| - \frac{1}{2}\left((\mathbf{g}-\mathbf{Uv})^T \mathbf{C}^{-1}(\mathbf{g}-\mathbf{Uv}) \right) \right)$$

$$= -\frac{1}{2} \nabla_{\mathbf{v}} \left((\mathbf{g}-\mathbf{Uv})^T \mathbf{C}^{-1}(\mathbf{g}-\mathbf{Uv}) \right).$$

Second, the matrix $\mathbf{D} = \mathbf{ba}^T$ has elements $D_{ij} = b_i a_j$, $i,j = 1,\ldots,n$. Therefore

$$\mathrm{tr}\,\mathbf{ba}^T = \mathrm{tr}\,\mathbf{D} = \sum_{i=1}^n D_{ii} = \sum_{i=1}^n b_i a_i = \mathbf{a}^T \mathbf{b}.$$

From this we deduce that

$$(\mathbf{g}-\mathbf{Uv})^T \mathbf{C}^{-1}(\mathbf{g}-\mathbf{Uv}) = \mathrm{tr}\,\mathbf{C}^{-1}(\mathbf{g}-\mathbf{Uv})(\mathbf{g}-\mathbf{Uv})^T$$

which immediately implies the third assertion. Next observe that

$$\frac{\partial}{\partial v_i}(\mathbf{g}-\mathbf{Uv})(\mathbf{g}-\mathbf{Uv})^T = -\left((\mathbf{Uf}_i)(\mathbf{g}-\mathbf{Uv})^T + (\mathbf{g}-\mathbf{Uv})(\mathbf{Uf}_i)^T \right)$$

so that

$$-\frac{1}{2}\frac{\partial}{\partial v_i}\mathrm{tr}\,\mathbf{C}^{-1}(\mathbf{g}-\mathbf{Uv})(\mathbf{g}-\mathbf{Uv})^T = \frac{1}{2}\mathrm{tr}\,\mathbf{C}^{-1}\left((\mathbf{Uf}_i)(\mathbf{g}-\mathbf{Uv})^T + (\mathbf{g}-\mathbf{Uv})(\mathbf{Uf}_i)^T \right)$$

$$= \frac{1}{2}\mathrm{tr}\,\mathbf{C}^{-1}\left((\mathbf{Uf}_i)(\mathbf{g}-\mathbf{Uv})^T + \frac{1}{2}\mathrm{tr}\,\mathbf{C}^{-1}(\mathbf{g}-\mathbf{Uv})(\mathbf{Uf}_i)^T \right)$$

$$= \frac{1}{2}(\mathbf{g}-\mathbf{Uv})^T \mathbf{C}^{-1}(\mathbf{Uf}_i) + \frac{1}{2}(\mathbf{Uf}_i)^T \mathbf{C}^{-1}(\mathbf{g}-\mathbf{Uv})$$

$$= (\mathbf{Uf}_i)^T \mathbf{C}^{-1}(\mathbf{g}-\mathbf{Uv}),$$

since $\mathbf{C}^{-1}$ is symmetric. This means that

$$\mathbf{s}(\mathbf{v},\mathbf{g})_i = \mathbf{f}_i^T \mathbf{U}^T \mathbf{C}^{-1}(\mathbf{g}-\mathbf{Uv})$$

and therefore $\mathbf{s}(\mathbf{v},\mathbf{g}) = \mathbf{U}^T \mathbf{C}^{-1}(\mathbf{g}-\mathbf{Uv})$.

28.26 CHAPTER 27

Exercise 1. As there are 2^N distinct $\mathbf{s} \in \{-1,1\}^N$ there are at most 2^N distinct values taken by the action of the ith row of $\mathbf{W}$ onto the admissible $\mathbf{s}$, i.e., by

$$\sum_{j=1}^N W_{ij}s_j.$$

As a result, this set has a smallest strictly positive element. If we denote that number by $2b_i$ and insert the associated $\mathbf{b}$ into Eq. (27.40) then if $(\mathbf{Ws})_i > 0$ then in fact $(\mathbf{Ws})_i > b_i$ and so $\mathrm{Hop}((\mathbf{Ws})_i) = \mathrm{Hop}^\sharp((\mathbf{Ws})_i)_i = 1$. Next, if $(\mathbf{Ws})_i \le 0$ then clearly $(\mathbf{Ws})_i < b_i$ and so $\mathrm{Hop}((\mathbf{Ws})_i) = \mathrm{Hop}^\sharp((\mathbf{Ws})_i)_i = -1$.

Exercise 4. $w = 0.27$.

Exercise 6. See `sotofreq.m`.

Exercise 9. If $u(\theta,t) = U(\theta + \Gamma(t))$ then

$$\begin{aligned}
\tau u_t(\theta,t) &= \tau U'(\theta + \Gamma(t))\Gamma'(t) = U'(\theta + \Gamma(t))\gamma(t)\\
&= W'(\theta + \Gamma(t)) \star f(\theta + \Gamma(t))\gamma(t)\\
&= (w(\theta + \Gamma(t),t) - W(\theta + \Gamma(t))) \star f(\theta + \Gamma(t))\\
&= w(\theta + \Gamma(t),t) \star \sigma(U(\theta + \Gamma(t))) - W(\theta + \Gamma(t)) \star f(\theta + \Gamma(t))\\
&= w(\theta,t) \star \sigma(u(\theta,t)) - u(\theta,t)
\end{aligned}$$

as claimed.

References

L. F. Abbott and P. Dayan. *Theoretical Neuroscience*. MIT Press, 2001.

E. H. Adelson and J. R. Bergen. Spatiotemporal energy models for the perception of motion. *J Opt Soc Am A*, 2(2):284–299, 1985.

R. D. Airan, L. A. Meltzer, M. Roy, Y. Gong, H. Chen, and K. Deisseroth. High-speed imaging reveals neurophysiological links to behavior in an animal model of depression. *Science*, 317(5839):819–823, 2007. doi: 10.1126/science.1144400. URL http://dx.doi.org/10.1126/science.1144400.

D. G. Albrecht and D. B. Hamilton. Striate cortex of monkey and cat: contrast response function. *J Neurophysiol*, 48(1):217–237, 1982.

J. M. Alonso, W. M. Usrey, and R. C. Reid. Rules of connectivity between geniculate cells and simple cells in cat primary visual cortex. *J Neurosci*, 21:4002–4015, 2001.

D. J. Amit. *Modeling Brain Function: The World of Attractor Neural Networks*. Cambridge University Press, 1992.

S. M. Baer and J. Rinzel. Propagation of dendritic spikes mediated by excitable spines: a continuum theory. *J Neurophysiol*, 65(4): 874–890, 1991.

K. G. Baimbridge, M. R. Celio, and J. H. Rogers. Calcium-binding proteins in the nervous system. *Trends Neurosci*, 15(8):303–308, 1992.

H. B. Barlow. Retinal noise and absolute threshold. *J Opt Soc Am*, 46(8):634–639, 1956.

H. B. Barlow, W. R. Levick, and M. Yoon. Responses to single quanta of light in retinal ganglion cells of the cat. *Vision Res*, Suppl 3:87–101, 1971.

D. A. Baylor, T. D. Lamb, and K. W. Yau. Responses of retinal rods to single photons. *J Physiol*, 288:613–634, 1979.

C. C. Bell, V. Z. Han, Y. Sugawara, and K. Grant. Synaptic plasticity in a cerebellum-like structure depends on temporal order. *Nature*, 387(6630):278–281, 1997. doi: 10.1038/387278a0. URL http://dx.doi.org/10.1038/387278a0.

J. S. Bendat. *Nonlinear System Analysis and Identification from Random Data*. John Wiley & Sons, 1990.

J. S. Bendat and A. G. Piersol. *Random Data: Analysis and Measurement Procedures*, 3rd edition. John Wiley & Sons, 2000.

M. J. Berridge. Neuronal calcium signaling. *Neuron*, 21(1):13–26, 1998.

G. Q. Bi and M. M. Poo. Synaptic modifications in cultured hippocampal neurons: dependence on spike timing, synaptic strength, and postsynaptic cell type. *J Neurosci*, 18(24):10464–10472, 1998.

W. Bialek, F. Rieke, R. R. de Ruyter van Steveninck, and D. Warland. Reading a neural code. *Science*, 252(5014):1854–1857, 1991.

P. Billingsley. *Probability and Measure*. Wiley-Interscience, 3rd edition. 1995.

J. A. Blundon and S. S. Zakharenko. Dissecting the components of long-term potentiation. *Neuroscientist*, 14(6):598–608, 2008. doi: 10.1177/1073858408320643. URL http://dx.doi.org/10.1177/1073858408320643.

P. Bonifazi, M. Goldin, M. A. Picardo, I. Jorquera, A. Cattani, G. Bianconi, A. Represa, Y. Ben-Ari, and R. Cossart. Gabaergic hub neurons orchestrate synchrony in developing hippocampal networks. *Science*, 326(5958):1419–1424, 2009. doi: 10.1126/science.1175509. URL http://dx.doi.org/10.1126/science.1175509.

V. Booth and A. Bose. Neural mechanisms for generating rate and temporal codes in model CA3 pyramidal cells. *J Neurophysiol*, 85(6):2432–2445, 2001.

B. G. Borghuis, P. Sterling, and R. G. Smith. Loss of sensitivity in an analog neural circuit. *J Neurosci*, 29(10):3045–3058, 2009. doi: 10.1523/JNEUROSCI.5071-08.2009. URL http://dx.doi.org/10.1523/JNEUROSCI.5071-08.2009.

W. H. Bosking, Y. Zhang, B. Schofield, and D. Fitzpatrick. Orientation selectivity and the arrangement of horizontal connections in tree shrew striate cortex. *J Neurosci*, 17(6):2112–2127, 1997.

J. M. Bower and D. Beeman. *The Book of GENESIS: Exploring Realistic Neural Models with the General Neural Simulation System*. Springer-Verlag, 1998.

I. A. Boyd and A. R. Martin. The end-plate potential in mammalian muscle. *J Physiol*, 132(1):74–91, 1956.

V. Braitenberg and A. Schüz. *Cortex: Statistics and Geometry of Neuronal Connectivity*. Springer-Verlag, 1998.

P. Brémaud. *An Introduction to Probabilistic Modeling*. Springer-Verlag, 1994.

W. L. Briggs and V. E. Henson. *The DFT: An Owners' Manual for the Discrete Fourier Transform*. Society for Industrial and Applied Math, 1987.

E. N. Brown, R. Barbieri, V. Ventura, R. E. Kass, and L. M. Frank. The time-rescaling theorem and its application to neural spike train data analysis. *Neural Comput*, 14(2):325–346, 2002. doi: 10.1162/08997660252741149. URL http://dx.doi.org/10.1162/08997660252741149.

D. A. Butts, C. Weng, J. Jin, C.-I. Yeh, N. A. Lesica, J.-M. Alonso, and G. B. Stanley. Temporal precision in the neural code and the timescales of natural vision. *Nature*, 449(7158):92–95, 2007. doi: 10.1038/nature06105. URL http://dx.doi.org/10.1038/nature06105.

G. Buzsáki. Large-scale recording of neuronal ensembles. *Nat Neurosci*, 7(5):446–451, 2004. doi: 10.1038/nn1233. URL http://dx.doi.org/10.1038/nn1233.

R. C. Cannon, D. A. Turner, G. K. Pyapali, and H. V. Wheal. An on-line archive of reconstructed hippocampal neurons. *J Neurosci Methods*, 84(1–2):49–54, 1998.

T. J. Carew. *Behavioral Neurobiology: The Cellular Organization of Natural Behavior*. Sinauer Associates, 2000.

N. T. Carnevale and M. L. Hines. *The Neuron Book*. Cambridge University Press, 2006.

G. C. Carter. Coherence and time delay estimation. In J. L. Lacoume, T. S. Durrani, and R. Stora, editors, *Traitement du Signal—Signal Processing*, volume II, chapter 9, pages 515–571. North-Holland, 1987.

M. J. Chacron and J. Bastian. Population coding by electrosensory neurons. *J Neurophysiol*, 99(4):1825–1835, 2008. doi: 10.1152/jn.01266.2007. URL http://dx.doi.org/10.1152/jn.01266.2007.

M. J. Chacron, A. Longtin, and L. Maler. Negative interspike interval correlations increase the neuronal capacity for encoding time-dependent stimuli. *J Neurosci*, 21(14):5328–5343, 2001.

E. W. Cheney and D. R. Kincaid. *Numerical Mathematics and Computing*. Brooks/Cole, 2007.

K. L. Chung. *A Course in Probability Theory*. Academic Press, 2000.

CIE. Standard colorimetric observer y2(lambda) data (between 380 nm and 780 nm at 5 nm intervals). Technical report, Commission internationale de l'éclairage, 1931. URL http://www.cie.co.at. (Accessed July 28, 2009).

M. R. Cohen and W. T. Newsome. Estimates of the contribution of single neurons to perception depend on timescale and noise correlation. *J Neurosci*, 29(20):6635–6648, 2009. doi: 10.1523/JNEUROSCI.5179-08.2009. URL http://dx.doi.org/10.1523/JNEUROSCI.5179-08.2009.

D. R. Cox. *Renewal Theory*. Methuen & Co LTD, 1962.

S. J. Cox. A new method for extracting cable parameters from input impedance data. *Math Biosci*, 153(1):1–12, 1998.

S. J. Cox. Estimating the location and time course of synaptic input from multi-site potential recordings. *J Comput Neurosci*, 17(2):225–243, 2004. doi: 10.1023/B:JCNS.0000037684.04521.d8. URL http://dx.doi.org/10.1023/B:JCNS.0000037684.04521.d8.

S. J. Cox and B. E. Griffith. Recovering quasi-active properties of dendritic neurons from dual potential recordings. *J Comput Neurosci*, 11(2):95–110, 2001.

D. R. Cox and V. Isham. *Point Processes*. Chapman & Hall/CRC, 1980.

D. R. Cox and P. A. W. Lewis. *The Statistical Analysis of Series of Events*. Methuen & Co Ltd, 1966.

Y. Dan, J. J. Atick, and R. C. Reid. Efficient coding of natural scenes in the lateral geniculate nucleus: experimental test of a computational theory. *J Neurosci*, 16(10):3351–3362, 1996.

I. Daubechies. *Ten Lectures on Wavelets*. SIAM, 1992.

G. C. DeAngelis, G. M. Ghose, I. Ohzawa, and R. D. Freeman. Functional micro-organization of primary visual cortex: receptive field analysis of nearby neurons. *J Neurosci*, 19(10):4046–4064, 1999.

G. C. DeAngelis, I. Ohzawa, and R. D. Freeman. Receptive-field dynamics in the central visual pathways. *Trends Neurosci*, 18(10):451–458, 1995.

A. E. Desjardins, Y.-X. Li, S. Reinker, R. M. Miura, and R. S. Neuman. The influences of I_h on temporal summation in hippocampal CA1 pyramidal neurons: a modeling study. *J Comput Neurosci*, 15(2):131–142, 2003.

A. Destexhe, Z. F. Mainen, and T. J. Sejnowski. Kinetic models of synaptic transmission. In I. Koch and C. Segev, editors, *Methods in Neuronal Modeling*, pages 1–25. MIT Press, 1998.

A. Destexhe, M. Rudolph, J. M. Fellous, and T. J. Sejnowski. Fluctuating synaptic conductances recreate *in vivo*-like activity in neocortical neurons. *Neuroscience*, 107(1):13–24, 2001.

A. Destexhe, M. Rudolph, and D. Paré. The high-conductance state of neocortical neurons *in vivo*. *Nat Rev Neurosci*, 4(9):739–751, 2003. doi: 10.1038/nrn1198. URL http://dx.doi.org/10.1038/nrn1198.

R. L. DeValois, D. G. Albrecht, and L. G. Thorell. Spatial frequency selectivity of cells in macaque visual cortex. *Vision Res*, 22(5): 545–559, 1982.

R. L. DeValois and K. K. DeValois. *Spatial Vision*. Oxford University Press, 1990.

R. L. DeValois, E. W. Yund, and N. Hepler. The orientation and direction selectivity of cells in macaque visual cortex. *Vision Res*, 22 (5):531–544, 1982.

G. W. De Young and J. Keizer. A single-pool inositol 1,4,5-trisphosphate-receptor-based model for agonist-stimulated oscillations in Ca^{2+} concentration. *Proc Natl Acad Sci U S A*, 89(20):9895–9899, 1992.

B. Doiron, M. J. Chacron, L. Maler, A. Longtin, and J. Bastian. Inhibitory feedback required for network oscillatory responses to communication but not prey stimuli. *Nature*, 421:539–543, 2003.

B. Doiron, A. Longtin, N. Berman, and L. Maler. Subtractive and divisive inhibition: effect of voltage-dependent inhibitory conductances and noise. *Neural Comput*, 13(1):227–248, 2001.

D. W. Dong and J. J. Atick. Statistics of natural time-varying images. *Network: Comput Neural Syst*, 6:345–358, 1995.

D. W. Dong and J. J. Atick. Temporal decorrelation: a theory of lagged and nonlagged responses in the lateral geniculate nucleus. *Network: Comput Neural Syst*, 6:159–178, 1995.

J. L. Doob. *Stochastic Processes*. John Wiley & Sons, 1953.

S. M. Dravid, A. Prakash, and S. F. Traynelis. Activation of recombinant NR1/NR2 NMDA receptors. *J Physiol*, 586(Pt 18):4425–4439, 2008. doi: 10.1113/jphysiol.2008.158634. URL http://dx.doi.org/10.1113/jphysiol.2008.158634.

R. O. Duda, P. E. Hart, and D. G. Stork. *Pattern Classification*, 2nd edition. Wiley & Sons, 2000.

T. Duong and R. D. Freeman. Contrast sensitivity is enhanced by expansive nonlinear processing in the lateral geniculate nucleus. *J Neurophysiol*, 99(1):367–372, 2008. doi: 10.1152/jn.00873.2007. URL http://dx.doi.org/10.1152/jn.00873.2007.

F. A. Edwards, A. Konnerth, and B. Sakmann. Quantal analysis of inhibitory synaptic transmission in the dentate gyrus of rat hippocampal slices: a patch-clamp study. *J Physiol*, 430:213–249, 1990.

J. J. Eggermont, P. M. Johannesma, and A. M. Aertsen. Reverse-correlation methods in auditory research. *Q Rev Biophys*, 16(3): 341–414, 1983.

R. C. Emerson, J. R. Bergen, and E. H. Adelson. Directionally selective complex cells and the computation of motion energy in cat visual cortex. *Vision Res*, 32(2):203–218, 1992.

C. Enroth-Cugell and J. G. Robson. The contrast sensitivity of retinal ganglion cells of the cat. *J Physiol*, 187(3):517–552, 1966.

A. A. Faisal, J. A. White, and S. B. Laughlin. Ion-channel noise places limits on the miniaturization of the brain's wiring. *Curr Biol*, 15(12):1143–1149, 2005. doi: 10.1016/j.cub.2005.05.056. URL http://dx.doi.org/10.1016/j.cub.2005.05.056.

C. Fall, E. Marland, J. Wagner, and J. Tyson, editors. *Computational Cell Biology*. Springer-Verlag, 2005.

P. Fatt and B. Katz. Spontaneous subthreshold activity at motor nerve endings. *J Physiol*, 117(1):109–128, 1952.

D. E. Feldman. Synaptic mechanisms for plasticity in neocortex. *Annu Rev Neurosci*, 32:33–55, 2009. doi: 10.1146/annurev .neuro.051508.135516. URL http://dx.doi.org/10.1146/annurev.neuro.051508.135516.

W. Feller. *An Introduction to Probability Theory and its Applications*, volume I & II, 3rd edition. John Wiley & Sons, 1968.

J.-M. Fellous, M. Rudolph, A. Destexhe, and T. J. Sejnowski. Synaptic background noise controls the input/output characteristics of single cells in an *in vitro* model of *in vivo* activity. *Neuroscience*, 122(3):811–829, 2003.

F. R. Fernandez, W. H. Mehaffey, and R. W. Turner. Dendritic Na^+ current inactivation can increase cell excitability by delaying a somatic depolarizing afterpotential. *J Neurophysiol*, 94(6):3836–3848, 2005. doi: 10.1152/jn.00653.2005. URL http://dx.doi.org/10.1152/jn.00653.2005.

R. P. Feynman, R. B. Leighton, and M. Sands. *The Feynman Lectures on Physics*. AddisonWesley, 1970.

J. C. Fiala, S. Grossberg, and D. Bullock. Metabotropic glutamate receptor activation in cerebellar Purkinje cells as substrate for adaptive timing of the classically conditioned eye-blink response. *J Neurosci*, 16(11):3760–3774, 1996.

R. Fitzhugh. Computation of impulse initiation and saltatory conduction in a myelinated nerve fiber. *Biophys J*, 2:11–21, 1962.

R. Fitzhugh. Mathematical models of threshold phenomena in the nerve membrane. *Bull Math Biophys*, 17:257–278, 1955.

W. J. Freeman and R. Kozma. Scale-free cortical planar networks. In R. Kozmas, B. Bollobas, and D. Miklos, editors, *Handbook of Large-Scale Random Networks*. Springer-Verlag, 2009.

A. S. French and S. Meisner. A new method for wide frequency range dynamic olfactory stimulation and characterization. *Chem Senses*, 32(7):681–688, 2007. doi: 10.1093/chemse/bjm035. URL http://dx.doi.org/10.1093/chemse/bjm035.

F. Gabbiani. Coding of time-varying signals in spike trains of linear and half-wave rectifying neurons. *Network: Comput Neural Syst*, 7:61–85, 1996.

F. Gabbiani and C. Koch. Coding of time-varying signals in spike trains of integrate-and-fire neurons with random threshold. *Neural Comput*, 8:44–66, 1996.

F. Gabbiani and C. Koch. Principles of spike train analysis. In C. Koch and I. Segev, editors, *Methods in Neuronal Modeling*, chapter 9, pages 313–360. MIT Press, 1998.

F. Gabbiani and W. Metzner. Encoding and processing of sensory information in neuronal spike trains. *J Exp Biol*, 202:1267–1279, 1999.

F. Gabbiani, W. Metzner, R. Wessel, and C. Koch. From stimulus encoding to feature extraction in weakly electric fish. *Nature*, 384: 564–567, 1996.

F. Gabbiani and J. Midtgaard. Neural information processing. *Encyclopedia Life Sci*, 2001 doi: 10.1038/npg.els.0000149. URL www.els.net.

A. Gelperin. Olfactory computations and network oscillation. *J Neurosci*, 26(6):1663–1668, 2006. doi: 10.1523/JNEUROSCI.3737-05b.2006. URL http://dx.doi.org/10.1523/JNEUROSCI.3737-05b.2006.

W. Gerstner and W. M. Kistler. *Spiking Neuron Models: Single Neurons, Populations, Plasticity*. Cambridge University Press, 1992.

C. C. A. Gielen, G. H. F. M. Hesselmans, and P. I. M. Johannesma. Sensory interpretation of neural activity patterns. *Math Biosci*, 88:15–35, 1988.

D. T. Gillespie. Exact stochastic simulation of coupled chemical reactions. *J Phys Chem*, 81:2340–2361, 1977.

D. T. Gillespie. The mathematics of Brownian motion and Johnston noise. *Am J Phys*, 64:225–240, 1996.

M. S. Goldman. Memory without feedback in a neural network. *Neuron*, 61(4):621–634, 2009. doi: 10.1016/j.neuron.2008.12.012. URL http://dx.doi.org/10.1016/j.neuron.2008.12.012.

E. Goles-Chacc, F. Fogelman-Soulie, and D. Pellegrin. Decreasing energy functions as a tool for studying threshold networks. *Discrete Appl Math*, 12:261–277, 1985.

G. H. Golub and C. F. van Loan. *Numerical Mathematics and Computing*. The Johns Hopkins University Press, 1996.

A. K. Goodchild, K. K. Ghosh, and P. R. Martin. Comparison of photoreceptor spatial density and ganglion cell morphology in the retina of human, macaque monkey, cat and the marmoset *callithrix jacchus*. *J Comp Neurol*, 366:55–75, 1996.

J. W. Goodman. *Statistical Optics*. John Wiley & Sons, 1985.

R. M. Gray. *Teoplitz and circulant matrices: a review*. Now Publishers, Norwell, Massachusetts, 2006.

C. M. Gray and D. A. McCormick. Chattering cells: superficial pyramidal neurons contributing to the generation of synchronous oscillations in the visual cortex. *Science*, 274:109–113, 1996.

D. M. Green and J. A. Swets. *Signal Detection Theory and Psychophysics*. John Wiley & Sons, 1966.

G. Grynkiewicz, M. Poenie, and R. Y. Tsien. A new generation of Ca^{2+} indicators with greatly improved fluorescence properties. *J Biol Chem*, 260(6):3440–3450, 1985.

Y. Gu, J. Oberwinkler, M. Postma, and R. C. Hardie. Mechanisms of light adaptation in *Drosophila* photoreceptors. *Curr Biol*, 15(13):1228–1234, 2005. doi: 10.1016/j.cub.2005.05.058. URL http://dx.doi.org/10.1016/j.cub.2005.05.058.

D. K. Hartline and D. R. Colman. Rapid conduction and the evolution of giant axons and myelinated fibers. *Curr Biol*, 17(1): R29–R35, 2007. doi: 10.1016/j.cub.2006.11.042. URL http://dx.doi.org/10.1016/j.cub.2006.11.042.

A. G. Hawkes. Stochastic modelling of single ion channels. In J. Feng, editor, *Computational Neuroscience A Comprehensive Approach*, chapter 5, pages 131–157. Chapman & Hall/CRC, 2004.

S. Hecht, S. Shlaer, and M. H. Pirenne. Energy, quanta, and vision. *J Gen Physiol*, 25:819–840, 1942.

W. F. Heiligenberg. *Neural Nets in Electric Fish*. MIT Press, 1991.

B. Hille. *Ion Channels of Excitable Membranes*. Sinauer Associates, 2001.

M. Hines. Efficient computation of branched nerve equations. *Int J Biomed Comput*, 15(1):69–76, 1984.

A. L. Hodgkin and A. F. Huxley. A quantitative description of membrane current and its application to conduction and excitation in nerve. *J Physiol*, 117:500–544, 1952.

G. R. Holt and C. Koch. Shunting inhibition does not have a divisive effect on firing rates. *Neural Comput*, 9(5):1001–1013, 1997.

J. J. Hopfield. Neural networks and physical systems with emergent collective computational abilities. *Proc Natl Acad Sci U S A*, 79 (8):2554–2558, 1982.

A. R. Houweling and M. Brecht. Behavioural report of single neuron stimulation in somatosensory cortex. *Nature*, 451(7174):65–68, 2008. doi: 10.1038/nature06447. URL http://dx.doi.org/10.1038/nature06447.

D. H. Hubel and T. N. Wiesel. Receptive fields, binocular interaction and functional architecture in the cat's visual cortex. *J Physiol*, 160:106–154, 1962.

A. J. Hudspeth and R. S. Lewis. A model for electrical resonance and frequency tuning in saccular hair cells of the bull-frog, *Rana catesbeiana*. *J Physiol*, 400:275–297, 1988.

A. J. Hudspeth and R. S. Lewis. Kinetic analysis of voltage- and ion-dependent conductances in saccular hair cells the bull-frog, *Rana catesbeiana*. *J Physiol*, 400:237–274, 1988.

A. Hyvärinen, J. Hurrk, and P. O. Hoyer. *Natural Image Statistics: A Probabilistic Approach to Early Computational Vision*. Springer, 2009.

E. M. Izhikevich. *Dynamical Systems in Neuroscience: The Geometry of Excitability and Bursting*. MIT Press, 2007.

G. A. Jacobs, J. P. Miller, and Z. Aldworth. Computational mechanisms of mechanosensory processing in the cricket. *J Exp Biol*, 211(Pt 11):1819–1828, 2008. doi: 10.1242/jeb.016402. URL http://dx.doi.org/10.1242/jeb.016402.

D. B. Jaffe and T. H. Brown. Metabotropic glutamate receptor activation induces calcium waves within hippocampal dendrites. *J Neurophysiol*, 72(1):471–474, 1994.

D. B. Jaffe, W. N. Ross, J. E. Lisman, N. Lasser-Ross, H. Miyakawa, and D. Johnston. A model for dendritic Ca^{2+} accumulation in hippocampal pyramidal neurons based on fluorescence imaging measurements. *J Neurophysiol*, 71(3):1065–1077, 1994.

H. Jahnsen and R. Llinàs. Electrophysiological properties of guinea-pig thalamic neurones: an *in vitro* study. *J Physiol*, 349:205–226, 1984.

J. G. Jefferys. Nonsynaptic modulation of neuronal activity in the brain: electric currents and extracellular ions. *Physiol Rev*, 75(4): 689–723, 1995.

D. H. Johnson. Point process models of single-neuron discharges. *J Comput Neurosci*, 3(4):275–299, 1996.

J. P. Jones and L. A. Palmer. The two-dimensional spatial structure of simple receptive fields in cat striate cortex. *J Neurophysiol*, 58(6):1187–1211, 1987.

E. R. Kandel, T. M. Jessell, and J. H. Schwartz. *Principles of Neural Science*. McGraw-Hill, 2008.

B. Katz and O. H. Schmitt. Electric interaction between two adjacent nerve fibres. *J Physiol*, 97(4):471–488, 1940.

M. Kawasaki. Sensory hyperacuity in the jamming avoidance response of weakly electric fish. *Curr Opin Neurobiol*, 7(4):473–479, 1997.

J. Keener and J. Sneyd. *Mathematical Physiology*. Springer-Verlag, 1998.

J. Keizer and L. Levine. Ryanodine receptor adaptation and Ca^{2+}(-)induced Ca^{2+} release-dependent Ca^{2+} oscillations. *Biophys J*, 71(6):3477–3487, 1996. doi: 10.1016/S0006-3495(96)79543-7. URL http://dx.doi.org/10.1016/S0006-3495(96)79543-7.

A. Kellems, D. Roos, N. Xiao, and S. Cox. Low-dimensional, morphologically accurate models of subthreshold membrane potential. *J Comput Neurosci*, 2009. doi: 10.1007/s10827-008-0134-2. URL http://dx.doi.org/10.1007/s10827-008-0134-2.

C. Koch. *Biophysics of Computation*. Oxford University Press, 1999.

T. Kohonen. *Self-Organizing Maps*. Springer-Verlag, 2001.

H. Korn. What central inhibitory pathways tell us about mechanisms of transmitter release. *Exp Brain Res Suppl*, 9:201–224, 1984.

H. Korn and D. S. Faber. The Mauthner cell half a century later: a neurobiological model for decision-making? *Neuron*, 47(1):13–28, 2005. doi: 10.1016/j.neuron.2005.05.019. URL http://dx.doi.org/10.1016/j.neuron.2005.05.019.

H. Korn, A. Mallet, A. Triller, and D. S. Faber. Transmission at a central inhibitory synapse. ii. quantal description of release, with a physical correlate for binomial n. *J Neurophysiol*, 48(3):679–707, 1982.

R. Krahe and F. Gabbiani. Burst firing in sensory systems. *Nat Rev Neurosci*, 5(1):13–23, 2004. doi: 10.1038/nrn1296. URL http://dx.doi.org/10.1038/nrn1296.

H. Kushner and D. Clark. *Stochastic Approximation Methods for Constrained and Unconstrained Systems*. Springer-Verlag, 1978.

C. R. Laing, B. Doiron, A. Longtin, L. Noonan, R. W. Turner, and L. Maler. Type I burst excitability. *J Comput Neurosci*, 14(3):329–342, 2003.

M. F. Land and D. A. Nilsson. *Animal Eyes*. Oxford University Press, 2002.

L. Lapicque. Recherches quantitatives sur l'excitation électrique des nerfs traitée comme une polarisation. *J Physiol Pathol Gen*, 9:620–635, 1907.

S. B. Laughlin. A simple coding procedure enhances a neuron's information capacity. *Z Naturf*, 36c:910–912, 1981.

S. B. Laughlin and R. C. Hardie. Common strategies for light adaptation in the peripheral visual systems of fly and dragonfly. *J Comp Physiol A*, 128:319–340, 1978.

T. S. Lee. Image representation using 2D Gabor wavelets. *IEEE Trans Pattern Anal Mach Intell*, 18:959–971, 1996.

C. Lee, W. H. Rohrer, and D. L. Sparks. Population coding of saccadic eye movements by neurons in the superior colliculus. *Nature*, 332(6162):357–360, 1988. doi: 10.1038/332357a0. URL http://dx.doi.org/10.1038/332357a0.

I. B. Levitan and L. K. Kaczmarek. *The Neuron: Cell and Molecular Biology*. 3rd edition. Oxford University Press, 2001.

W. B. Levy and O. Steward. Temporal contiguity requirements for long-term associative potentiation/depression in the hippocampus. *Neuroscience*, 8(4):791–797, 1983.

M. S. Lewicki. A review of methods for spike sorting: the detection and classification of neural action potentials. *Network*, 9(4): R53–R78, 1998.

J. E. Lewis and W. B. Kristan. A neuronal network for computing population vectors in the leech. *Nature*, 391(6662):76–79, 1998. doi: 10.1038/34172. URL `http://dx.doi.org/10.1038/34172`.

M. S. Livingstone, D. C. Freeman, and D. H. Hubel. Visual responses of V1 of freely viewing monkeys. *Cold Spring Harb Symp Quant Biol*, 61:27–37, 1996.

S. B. Lowen, S. S. Cash, M. Poo, and M. C. Teich. Quantal neurotransmitter secretion rate exhibits fractal behavior. *J Neurosci*, 17(15):5666–5677, 1997.

L. Maffei. Inhibitory and facilitatory spatial interactions in retinal receptive fields. *Vision Res*, 8(9):1187–1194, 1968.

Z. F. Mainen and T. J. Sejnowski. Influence of dendritic structure on firing pattern in model neocortical neurons. *Nature*, 382:363–366, 1996.

R. Malinow and R. C. Malenka. AMPA receptor trafficking and synaptic plasticity. *Annu Rev Neurosci*, 25:103–126, 2002. doi: 10.1146/annurev.neuro.25.112701.142758. URL `http://dx.doi.org/10.1146/annurev.neuro.25.112701.142758`.

R. Malinow and R. W. Tsien. Presynaptic enhancement shown by whole-cell recordings of long-term potentiation in hippocampal slices. *Nature*, 346(6280):177–180, 1990. doi: 10.1038/346177a0. URL `http://dx.doi.org/10.1038/346177a0`.

S. Mallat. *A Wavelet Tour of Signal Processing*. Academic Press, 2008.

J. G. Mancilla, T. J. Lewis, D. J. Pinto, J. Rinzel, and B. W. Connors. Synchronization of electrically coupled pairs of inhibitory interneurons in neocortex. *J Neurosci*, 27(8):2058–2073, 2007. doi: 10.1523/JNEUROSCI.2715-06.2007. URL `http://dx.doi.org/10.1523/JNEUROSCI.2715-06.2007`.

V. Mante, R. A. Frazor, V. Bonin, W. S. Geisler, and M. Carandini. Independence of luminance and contrast in natural scenes and in the early visual system. *Nat Neurosci*, 8(12):1690–1697, 2005. doi: 10.1038/nn1556. URL `http://dx.doi.org/10.1038/nn1556`.

H. Markram, Y. Wang, and M. Tsodyks. Differential signaling via the same axon of neocortical pyramidal neurons. *Proc Natl Acad Sci U S A*, 95:5323–5328, 1998.

P. Z. Marmarelis and V. Z. Marmarelis. *Analysis of Physiological Systems*. Plenum Press, 1978.

G. Marsat, R. D. Proville, and L. Maler. Transient signals trigger synchronous bursts in an identified population of neurons. *J Neurophysiol*, 102(2):714–723, 2009. doi: 10.1152/jn.91366.2008. URL `http://dx.doi.org/10.1152/jn.91366.2008`.

J. H. Maunsell and D. C. VanEssen. Functional properties of neurons in middle temporal visual area of the macaque monkey. I. selectivity for stimulus direction, speed, and orientation. *J Neurophysiol*, 49(5):1127–1147, 1983.

D. A. McCormick and T. Bal. Sleep and arousal: thalamocortical mechanisms. *Annu Rev Neurosci*, 20:185–215, 1997. doi: 10.1146/annurev.neuro.20.1.185. URL `http://dx.doi.org/10.1146/annurev.neuro.20.1.185`.

T. McLaughlin and D. D. M. O'Leary. Molecular gradients and development of retinotopic maps. *Annu Rev Neurosci*, 28:327–355, 2005. doi: 10.1146/annurev.neuro.28.061604.135714. URL `http://dx.doi.org/10.1146/annurev.neuro.28.061604.135714`.

D. L. McLean, J. Fan, S. Higashijima, M. E. Hale, and J. R. Fetcho. A topographic map of recruitment in spinal cord. *Nature*, 446 (7131):71–75, 2007. doi: 10.1038/nature05588. URL `http://dx.doi.org/10.1038/nature05588`.

M. R. Mehta, C. A. Barnes, and B. L. McNaughton. Experience-dependent, asymmetric expansion of hippocampal place fields. *Proc Natl Acad Sci U S A*, 94(16):8918–8921, 1997.

B. W. Mel, D. L. Ruderman, and K. A. Archie. Translation-invariant orientation tuning in visual "complex" cells could derive from intradendritic computations. *J Neurosci*, 18(11):4325–4334, 1998.

R. Menzel and M. Giurfa. Cognitive architecture of a mini-brain: the honeybee. *Trends Cogn Sci*, 5(2):62–71, 2001.

M. Migliore and G. M. Shepherd. Emerging rules for the distributions of active dendritic conductances. *Nat Rev Neurosci*, 3(5): 362–370, 2002. doi: 10.1038/nrn810. URL `http://dx.doi.org/10.1038/nrn810`.

J. P. Miller, G. A. Jacobs, and F. E. Theunissen. Representation of sensory information in the cricket cercal sensory system. I. Response properties of the primary interneurons. *J Neurophysiol*, 66(5):1680–1689, 1991.

M. L. Molineux, F. R. Fernandez, W. H. Mehaffey, and R. W. Turner. A-type and T-type currents interact to produce a novel spike latency-voltage relationship in cerebellar stellate cells. *J Neurosci*, 25:10863–10873, 2005.

B. C. Moore. Principal component analysis in linear systems: controllability, observability, and model reduction. *IEEE Trans Automat Contr*, 26:17–32, 1981.

C. Morris and H. Lecar. Voltage oscillations in the barnacle giant muscle fiber. *Biophys J*, 35(1):193–213, 1981. doi: 10.1016/S0006-3495(81)84782-0. URL `http://dx.doi.org/10.1016/S0006-3495(81)84782-0`.

V. N. Murthy, T. J. Sejnowski, and C. F. Stevens. Heterogeneous release properties of visualized individual hippocampal synapses. *Neuron*, 18(4):599–612, 1997.

E. Neher. A comparison between exocytic control mechanisms in adrenal chromaffin cells and a glutamatergic synapse. *Pflugers Arch*, 453(3):261–268, 2006. doi: 10.1007/s00424-006-0143-9. URL `http://dx.doi.org/10.1007/s00424-006-0143-9`.

W. T. Newsome and E. B. Paré. A selective impairment of motion perception following lesions of the middle temporal visual area (mt). *J Neurosci*, 8(6):2201–2211, 1988.

S. Nicaise. Approche spectrale des problemes de diffusion sur les réseaux. In *Lecture Notes in Math. 1235*, pages 120–140. Springer-Verlag, 1987.

D. G. Nicholls. *Proteins, Transmitters and Synapses*. Blackwell Science Ltd, 1994.

H. Nienborg and B. G. Cumming. Decision-related activity in sensory neurons reflects more than a neuron's causal effect. *Nature*, 459(7243):89–92, 2009. doi: 10.1038/nature07821. URL http://dx.doi.org/10.1038/nature07821.

G. North and R. J. Greenspan, editors. *Invertebrate Neurobiology*. Cold Spring Harbor Laboratory Press, 2007.

D. C. O'Carroll, N. J. Bidwell, S. B. Laughlin, and E. J. Warrant. Insect motion detectors matched to visual ecology. *Nature*, 382: 63–66, 1996.

K. Ohki, S. Chung, P. Kara, M. Hÿbener, T. Bonhoeffer, and R. C. Reid. Highly ordered arrangement of single neurons in orientation pinwheels. *Nature*, 442(7105):925–928, 2006. doi: 10.1038/nature05019. URL http://dx.doi.org/10.1038/nature05019.

E. Oja. A simplified neuron model as a principal component analyzer. *J Math Biol*, 15:267–273, 1982.

A.-M. M. Oswald, M. J. Chacron, B. Doiron, J. Bastian, and L. Maler. Parallel processing of sensory input by bursts and isolated spikes. *J Neurosci*, 24(18):4351–4362, 2004. doi: 10.1523/JNEUROSCI.0459-04.2004. URL http://dx.doi.org/10.1523/JNEUROSCI.0459-04.2004.

L. Paninski. Maximum likelihood estimation of cascade point-process neural encoding models. *Network*, 15(4):243–262, 2004.

A. Papoulis and S. U. Pillai. *Probability, Random Variables and Stochastic Processes*, 4th edition. McGraw-Hill, 2002.

B. E. Peercy. Initiation and propagation of a neuronal intracellular calcium wave. *J Comput Neurosci*, 25(2):334–348, 2008. doi: 10.1007/s10827-008-0082-x. URL http://dx.doi.org/10.1007/s10827-008-0082-x.

D. B. Percival and A. T. Walden. *Spectral Analysis for Physical Applications*. Cambridge University Press, 1993.

J. Perez-Orive, O. Mazor, G. C. Turner, S. Cassenaer, R. I. Wilson, and G. Laurent. Oscillations and sparsening of odor representations in the mushroom body. *Science*, 297(5580):359–365, 2002. doi: 10.1126/science.1070502. URL http://dx.doi.org/10.1126/science.1070502.

A. Pikovsky, M. Rosenblum, and J. Kurths. *Synchronization: A Universal Concept in Nonlinear Sciences*. Cambridge University Press, 2003.

M. A. Pinsky. *Introduction to Fourier Analysis and Wavelets*. Brooks/Cole, 2002.

P. F. Pinsky and J. Rinzel. Intrinsic and network rhythmogenesis in a reduced Traub model for CA3 neurons. *J Comput Neurosci*, 1(1-2):39–60, 1994.

R. Price. A useful theorem for nonlinear devices having Gaussian inputs. *IRE Trans Inf Th*, 4:69–72, 1958.

M .B. Priestley. *Spectral Analysis and Time Series*, volume 1. Academic Press, 1981.

W. Rall. Theoretical significance of dendritic trees for neuronal input-output relations. In R. F. Reiss, editor, *Neural Theory and Modeling*, pages 73–91. Stanford University Press, Palo Alto, CA, 1964. URL senselab.med.yale.edu/modeldb/ShowModel.asp?model=116981.

W. Rall and H. Agmon-Snir. Cable theory for dendritic neurons. In C. Koch and I. Segev, editors, *Methods in Neuronal Modeling*, chapter 2, pages 27–92. MIT Press, 1998.

R. Ratnam and M. E. Nelson. Nonrenewal statistics of electrosensory afferent spike trains: implications for the detection of weak sensory signals. *J Neurosci*, 20(17):6672–6683, 2000.

R. Redheffer and D. Port. *Introduction to Differential Equations*. Jones & Bartlett, 1992.

D. L. Ringach. Mapping receptive fields in primary visual cortex. *J Physiol*, 558(Pt 3):717–728, 2004. doi: 10.1113/jphysiol.2004.065771. URL http://dx.doi.org/10.1113/jphysiol.2004.065771.

H. Ritter, T. Martinetz, and K. Schulten. *Neural Computation and Self-Organizing Maps: An Introduction*. Addison-Wesley, 1992.

J. Rizo and C. Rosenmund. Synaptic vesicle fusion. *Nat Struct Mol Biol*, 15(7):665–674, 2008.

R. W. Rodieck, N. Y. Kiang, and G. L. Gerstein. Some quantitative methods for the study of spontaneous activity of single neurons. *Biophys J*, 2:351–368, 1962.

C. Rosenmund, J. D. Clements, and G. L. Westbrook. Nonuniform probability of glutamate release at a hippocampal synapse. *Science*, 262(5134):754–757, 1993.

W. Rudin. *Functional Analysis*. McGraw-Hill, 1991.

N. C. Rust and J. A. Movshon. In praise of artifice. *Nat Neurosci*, 8(12):1647–1650, 2005. doi: 10.1038/nn1606. URL http://dx.doi.org/10.1038/nn1606.

B. E. A. Saleh and M. C. Teich. Multiplication and refractoriness in the cat's retinal-ganglion-cell discharge at low light levels. *Biol Cybern*, 52:101–107, 1985.

T. D. Sanger. Neural population codes. *Curr Opin Neurobiol* 13(2):238–249, 2003.

L. L. Scharf. *Statistical Signal Processing Detection*. Addison-Wesley, 1991.

V. Scheuss, R. Schneggenburger, and E. Neher. Separation of presynaptic and postsynaptic contributions to depression by covariance analysis of successive EPSCs at the calyx of Held synapse. *J Neurosci*, 22(3):728–739, 2002.

E. Schrödinger. *Science and Humanism*. Cambridge University Press, 1961.

L. Schwartz. *Theorie des distributions*. Hermann, 1966.

E. L. Schwartz. *Computational Neuroscience*. MIT Press, 1990.

O. Schwartz, J. W. Pillow, N. C. Rust, and E. P. Simoncelli. Spike-triggered neural characterization. *J Vis*, 6(4):484–507, 2006. doi: 10.1167/6.4.13. URL http://dx.doi.org/10.1167/6.4.13.

A. Scott. *Neuroscience: A Mathematical Primer*. Springer-Verlag, 2002.

I. Segev. Sound grounds for computing dendrites. *Nature*, 393(6682):207–208, 1998. doi: 10.1038/30340. URL http://dx.doi.org/10.1038/30340.

I. Segev, J. Rinzel, and G. M. Shepherd, editors. *The Theoretical Foundations of Dendritic Function: The Selected Papers of Wilfrid Rall with Commentaries*. MIT Press, 1994.

M. N. Shadlen and W. T. Newsome. The variable discharge of cortical neurons: implications for connectivity, computation, and information coding. *J Neurosci*, 18(10):3870–3896, 1998.

R. D. Shah and M. C. Crair. Mechanisms of response homeostasis during retinocollicular map formation. *J Physiol*, 586(Pt 18):4363–4369, 2008. doi: 10.1113/jphysiol.2008.157222. URL http://dx.doi.org/10.1113/jphysiol.2008.157222.

O. Shriki, D. Hansel, and H. Sompolinsky. Rate models for conductance-based cortical neuronal networks. *Neural Comput*, 15(8):1809–1841, 2003. doi: 10.1162/08997660360675053. URL http://dx.doi.org/10.1162/08997660360675053.

R. A. Silver, J. Lubke, B. Sakmann, and D. Feldmeyer. High-probability uniquantal transmission at excitatory synapses in barrel cortex. *Science*, 302(5652):1981–1984, 2003. doi: 10.1126/science.1087160. URL http://dx.doi.org/10.1126/science.1087160.

R. A. Silver, A. Momiyama, and S. G. Cull-Candy. Locus of frequency-dependent depression identified with multiple-probability fluctuation analysis at rat climbing fibre-Purkinje cell synapses. *J Physiol*, 510 (Pt 3):881–902, 1998.

F. K. Skinner, N. Kopell, and E. Marder. Mechanisms for oscillation and frequency control in reciprocally inhibitory model neural networks. *J Comput Neurosci*, 1(1–2):69–87, 1994.

W. R. Softky and C. Koch. The highly irregular firing of cortical cells is inconsistent with temporal integration of random EPSPs. *J Neurosci*, 13(1):334–350, 1993.

H. Sompolinsky, H. Yoon, K. Kang, and M. Shamir. Population coding in neuronal systems with correlated noise. *Phys Rev E Stat Nonlin Soft Matter Phys*, 64(5 Pt 1):051904, 2001.

S. Song, K. D. Miller, and L. F. Abbott. Competitive Hebbian learning through spike-timing-dependent synaptic plasticity. *Nat Neurosci*, 3(9):919–926, 2000. doi: 10.1038/78829. URL http://dx.doi.org/10.1038/78829.

J. B. Sørensen, R. Fernández-Chacón, T. C. Südhof, and E. Neher. Examining synaptotagmin 1 function in dense core vesicle exocytosis under direct control of Ca^{2+}. *J Gen Physiol*, 122(3):265–276, 2003. doi: 10.1085/jgp.200308855. URL http://dx.doi.org/10.1085/jgp.200308855.

C. Soto-Treviño, K. A. Thoroughman, E. Marder, and L. F. Abbott. Activity-dependent modification of inhibitory synapses in models of rhythmic neural networks. *Nat Neurosci*, 4(3):297–303, 2001. doi: 10.1038/85147. URL http://dx.doi.org/10.1038/85147.

D. L. Sparks. The brainstem control of saccadic eye movements. *Nat Rev Neurosci*, 3(12):952–964, 2002. doi: 10.1038/nrn986. URL http://dx.doi.org/10.1038/nrn986.

D. L. Sparks and I. S. Nelson. Sensory and motor maps in the mammalian superior colliculus. *TINS*, 10:312–317, 1987.

M. Spiegel, S. Lipschutz, J. Schiller, and D. Spellman. *Schaum's Outline of Complex Variables*. McGraw-Hill, 2009.

L. R. Squire, D. Berg, F. Bloom, S. duLac, and A. Ghosh, editors. *Fundamental Neuroscience*. Academic Press, 2008.

M. V. Srinivasan, S. B. Laughlin, and A. Dubs. Predictive coding: a fresh view of inhibition in the retina. *Proc R Soc Lond B Biol Sci*, 216(1205):427–459, 1982.

P. N. Steinmetz, A. Manwani, C. Koch, M. London, and I. Segev. Subthreshold voltage noise due to channel fluctuations in active neuronal membranes. *J Comput Neurosci*, 9(2):133–148, 2000.

W. Strauss. *Partial Differential Equations: An Introduction*. Wiley, 2007.

G. Stuart, N. Spruston, B. Sakmann, and M. Häusser. Action potential initiation and backpropagation in neurons of the mammalian CNS. *Trends Neurosci*, 20(3):125–131, 1997.

N. V. Swindale and H.-B. Bauer. Application of Kohonen's self-organizing feature map algorithm to cortical maps of orientation and direction preference. *Proc R Soc Lond B*, 265:827–838, 1998.

J. S. Taube. The head direction signal: Origins and sensory-motor integration. *Ann Rev Neurosci*, 30:181–207, 2007. URL doi:10.1146/annurev.neuro.29.051605.112854.

M. C. Teich, R. G. Turcott, and R. M. Siegel. Temporal correlation in cat striate-cortex neural spike trains. *IEEE Eng Med Biol Mag*, 15:79–87, 1996.

D. Terman, S. Ahn, X. Wang, and W. Just. Reducing neuronal networks to discrete dynamics. *Physica D*, 237(3):324–338, 2008. doi: 10.1016/j.physd.2007.09.011. URL http://dx.doi.org/10.1016/j.physd.2007.09.011.

D. J. Tolhurst, J. A. Movshon, and A. F. Dean. The statistical reliability of signals in single neurons in cat and monkey visual cortex. *Vision Res*, 23(8):775–785, 1983.

K. Toth, G. Suares, J. J. Lawrence, E. Philips-Tansey, and C. J. McBain. Differential mechanisms of transmission at three types of mossy fiber synapse. *J Neurosci*, 20(22):8279–8289, 2000.

R. D. Traub and R. Miles. *Neuronal networks of the hippocampus*. Cambridge University Press, 1991.

M. V. Tsodyks and H. Markram. The neural code between neocortical pyramidal neurons depends on neurotransmitter release probability. *Proc Natl Acad Sci U S A*, 94(2):719–723, 1997.

H. C. Tuckwell. *Introduction to Theoretical Neurobiology*, volume 2. Cambridge University Press, 1988.

H. C. Tuckwell. *Introduction to Theoretical Neurobiology: Volume 1, Linear Cable Theory and Dendritic Structure*. Cambridge University Press, 1988.

R. W. Turner, L. Maler, T. Deerinck, S. R. Levinson, and M. H. Ellisman. TTX-sensitive dendritic sodium channels underlie oscillatory discharge in a vertebrate sensory neuron. *J Neurosci*, 14(11 Pt 1):6453–6471, 1994.

D. C. Van Essen. Corticocortical and thalamocortical information flow in the primate visual cortex. *Prog Brain Res*, 149:173–185, 2005.

J. H. van Hateren. Processing of natural time series of intensities by the visual system of the blowfly. *Vision Res*, 37:3407–3416, 1997. URL http://hlab.phys.rug.nl/tslib/. (Accessed July 27, 2009).

J. H. van Hateren and H. P. Snippe. Information theoretical evaluation of parametric models of gain control in blowfly photoreceptor cells. *Vision Res*, 41(14):1851–1865, 2001.

J. H. van Hateren and H. P. Snippe. Phototransduction in primate cones and blowfly photoreceptors: different mechanisms, different algorithms, similar response. *J Comp Physiol A Neuroethol Sens Neural Behav Physiol*, 192(2):187–197, 2006. doi: 10.1007/s00359-005-0060-y. URL http://dx.doi.org/10.1007/s00359-005-0060-y.

J. H. van Hateren and A. van der Schaaf. Independent component filters of natural images compared with simple cells in primary visual cortex. *Proc R Soc Lond B*, 265:359–366, 1998. URL http://hlab.phys.rug.nl/imlib. (Accessed July 27, 2009).

G. Von Bekesy. *Experiments in Hearing*. McGraw Hill, 1960.

J. Von Below. Sturm-Liouville eigenvalue problems on networks. *Math Methods Appl Sci*, 10:383–395, 1988.

E. T. Vu and F. B. Krasne. Evidence for a computational distinction between proximal and distal neuronal inhibition. *Science*, 255 (5052):1710–1712, 1992.

J. Wagner and J. Keizer. Effects of rapid buffers on Ca^{2+} diffusion and Ca^{2+} oscillations. *Biophys J*, 67(1):447–456, 1994. doi: 10.1016/S0006-3495(94)80500-4. URL http://dx.doi.org/10.1016/S0006-3495(94)80500-4.

B. A. Wandell. *Foundations of Vision*. Sinauer Associates, 1995.

P. Wallisch, M. Lusignan, M. Benayoun, T. I. Baker, A.S. Dickey, and N. Hatsopoulos. *Matlab for Neuroscientists: An Introduction to Scientific Computing in Matlab*. Academic Press, 2008.

X. J. Wang. Multiple dynamical modes of thalamic relay neurons: rhythmic bursting and intermittent phase-locking. *Neuroscience*, 59(1):21–31, 1994.

M. A. Webster and R. L. DeValois. Relationship between spatial-frequency and orientation tuning of striate-cortex cells. *J Opt Soc Am A*, 2(7):1124–1132, 1985.

R. Wessel, C. Koch, and F. Gabbiani. Coding of time-varying electric field amplitude modulations in a wave-type electric fish. *J Neurophysiol*, 75(6):2280–2293, 1996.

J. A. White, J. T. Rubinstein, and A. R. Kay. Channel noise in neurons. *Trends Neurosci*, 23(3):131–137, 2000.

T. D. Wickens. *Elementary Signal Detection Theory*. Oxford University Press, 2001.

R. W. Williams and K. Herrup. The control of neuron number. *Annu Rev Neurosci*, 11:423–453, 1988. doi: 10.1146/annurev .ne.11.030188.002231. URL http://dx.doi.org/10.1146/annurev.ne.11.030188.002231.

A. R. Willms, D. J. Baro, R. M. Harris-Warrick, and J. Guckenheimer. An improved parameter estimation method for Hodgkin–Huxley models. *J Comput Neurosci*, 6:145–168, 1999.

A. M. Zhabotinsky. Bistability in the $Ca^{(2+)}$/calmodulin-dependent protein kinase-phosphatase system. *Biophys J*, 79(5):2211–2221, 2000. doi: 10.1016/S0006-3495(00)76469-1. URL http://dx.doi.org/10.1016/S0006-3495(00)76469-1.

K. Zhang. Representation of spatial orientation by the intrinsic dynamics of the head-direction cell ensemble: a theory. *J Neurosci*, 16(6):2112–2126, 1996.

K. Zhang and T. J. Sejnowski. Accuracy and learning in neuronal populations. *Prog Brain Res*, 130:333–342, 2001.

M. Zochowski, L. B. Cohen, G. Fuhrmann, and D. Kleinfeld. Distributed and partially separate pools of neurons are correlated with two different components of the gill-withdrawal reflex in aplysia. *J Neurosci*, 20(22):8485–8492, 2000.

A. Zygmund. *Trigonometric Series*. Cambridge University Press, 1959.

Index

2-AFC experiment, 359, 361

A

affinity, 221
aliasing phenomenon, 91
alpha synapse, 14, 97, 108
autocorrelation function, 251
autocovariance function, 251
  and power spectrum, 259
  Gaussian process, 252
  point process, 256
  white noise, 253
  Wiener process, 254
Avogadro's number, 7, 195

B

back-propagating action potential, 119, 130
bandwidth
  frequency, 315
  orientation, 316
Bayes formula, 161
Boltzmann's constant, 11
burst, 146, 238, 354
Bussgang's theorem, 331–333

C

Ca Green, 221
calcium/calmodulin dependent protein kinase II, 209
Channel
  calcium, 146, 148
  calcium, L, N and T-type, 196
  hyperpolarization activated, 59, 147, 148
  potassium, A-type, 40
  potassium, calcium activated, 151, 200
  potassium, delayed rectifier, 34
  sodium, 36
  sodium, persistent, 58, 148
Cholesky factorization, 172
chromaffin cells, 213, 215
coefficient of variation, 159, 180, 181, 246
  and Fano factor, 242, 246
  and refractory period, 239
  gamma distribution, 168
coherence function, 279

command neuron, 363
complex cell, 320, 321, 325
  and frequency doubling, 320
  and motion energy, 321
conditional
  mean, 328, 374
  probability, 161
contrast, 293, 295, 298, 301
  constancy, 293
  sensitivity, 306, 309
convolution, 6, 25, 280, 300, 319, 328, 399
  formula, 162
Convolution Theorem, 26, 89, 93, 95
correlation coefficient, 166, 167, 243, 279, 373
covariance
  matrix, 165
  matrix, empirical, 226
  matrix, noise, 372
  matrix, score, 374
  matrix, uniform, 350
  stochastic process, 251, 279
Cramer–Rao bound, 375
cricket cercal system, 367
CV method, 181

D

De Vries–Rose law, 296
deconvolution, 399
detailed balance, 275, 276
Dirac delta, 23, 100, 179
discrete prolate spheroidal sequence, 284, 286
dissociation constant, 221

E

eigenfunction
  branched, 113, 115
  calcium, 222
  equivalent cylinder, 111
  passive cable, 75, 132
endoplasmic reticulum, 201
Ephaptic, 122
epileptic rhythmic activity, 395
Equivalent Cylinder, 111
error function, 161
estimator bias and variance, 280
exocytosis, 175, 213, 217

F

false-alarm, 344, 357
Fano factor, 240, 242, 244, 246, 264, 265, 358, 365
Faraday's constant, 199
Fick's Law, 11, 198
Fisher information matrix, 374
Fisher linear discriminant, 352
FitzHugh model, 43, 46, 47, 64
forward recurrence time, 247–249
Fourier, 87
  coefficient, 399
  transform, 259, 270, 279, 304, 313, 328, 338
fovea, 301
Fura-2, 221

G

Gabor filter, 312, 318
Gamma function, 171
Gillespie algorithm, 271, 275, 276
Goldman–Hodgkin–Katz equation, 195
graded synapse, 392

H

hazard function, 265, 266
head direction cells, 399
Heaviside function, 6, 101
Hebbian learning, 228
Hill
  dissociation constant, 210
  function, 199, 203
Hopfield network, 382
Hubel and Wiesel model, 322, 323

I

input resistance, 23, 74, 77, 133, 187, 273
integrate and fire neuron, 144
  with random threshold, 259, 264
isopotential, 10

K

kinase, 176, 193, 209, 212
Kirchhoff's Current Law, 13
Kronecker delta, 5

L

Laplace transform, 25, 65, 248, 263
law of mass action, 14

Mathematics for Neuroscientists. DOI: 10.1016/B978-0-12-374882-9.00030-7

leaky integrate-and-fire neuron, 143, 152, 187, 245, 383
leech, 367
LGN, 300, 301, 307–309, 336
Linear Algebra
  concepts
    determinant, 62
    eigenvalue, 55
    eigenvector, 55
    frame, 371, 372
    Gauss–Jordan, 61
    Gaussian Elimination, 51
    Gramian, 230
    invertible matrix, 52
    linear dependence, 54
    linear independence, 56
    Lyapunov equation, 231, 232, 235
    matrix exponential, 58, 230
    noninvertible matrix, 54
    orthonormal, 69
    outer product, 225
    pivot, 52
    principal component, 226, 229
    pseudo–inverse, 233, 371, 372
    score, 226
    unitary matrix, 235
  factorizations
    Cholesky, 82
    LU, 61
    Schur decomposition, 233, 235
    singular value decomposition, 225, 371
  matrices
    circulant matrix, 92, 93, 98, 332
    Hines matrix, 105, 106, 113, 116, 135, 276
    permutation matrix, 52
    second difference matrix, 69, 78, 81, 82, 120, 124
    Toeplitz matrix, 332
LN model, 331
Lorentzian, 270, 272
LTD, 184, 228
LTP, 183–185, 209, 228
luminance, 293

M

MAP estimator, 373
Markov process, 267, 271, 275
matched filter, 229, 234, 351, 352, 354
MATLAB
  contributed
    aliascombined.m, 91
    alphafit.m, 31
    ascconverter.m, 135
    be_vs_trap.m, 30
    beps.m, 28
    bepswI.m, 13
    bevec.m, 106, 107

bkwshift.m, 405
boyd_martin2.m, 179
camk2ss.m, 213
chol_gauss.m, 173
clamp.m, 43
cndrive.m, 73
cnpfib.m, 73
codpm.m, 402, 403
coherence_est.m, 281
Comp2syn.m, 18, 19
convex.m, 26
cross_poiss.m, 287
curvssyn.m, 31
cv_ref_ex.m, 247
darknoise.m, 357
demyelin.m, 139
destex_f1.m, 274
destex_f2.m, 274
disp_hist.m, 294
disp_im.m, 294
disp_ts2.m, 295
distort.m, 63
drfsenoper.m, 140
eigcab.m, 71
evecS.m, 70
EInet.m, 388
EInetComp.m, 392
EInetH.m, 403
Enet.m, 387
exocytosis.m, 216
exp_rand.m, 172
feps.m, 27
ffreq.m, 24
fftexcoarse2.m, 90
fftexfine.m, 92
fhpp.m, 47
fi_curves.m, 144, 172
fisher_fig.m, 353
fleak.m, 283
fourcell.m, 391
fourierex2.m, 88
gab3dresp.m, 324
gabor3dex.m, 324
gamma2_ex1.m, 247
gamma_corr.m, 257
gamma_distr.m, 168
gamma_frect.m, 248
gamma_powersp.m, 260
gamma_spks.m, 242
gauss_fig.m, 165
getVrJac.m, 61
ghk.m, 196
gKCa.m, 201
haircell1.m, 219
haircell2.m, 219
hdnet.m, 401
hhfuncs.m., 35, 36, 37
hhsym.m, 51
hop.m, 382, 383
hsp.m, 356

htrack.m, 60
hyEcabCa1.m, 196, 197
hyEcabCa2drive.m, 200, 201
hyEcabCa3.m, 200, 201, 217
hyEcabCa3Ldrive.m, 218
hyEcabCa3traindrive.m, 217
hyEcabCa4.m, 204, 205
hyEcabCa5.m, 208, 209
hyEprnet.m, 396
hyEprnetdemo.m, 396
hyprEInet.m, 407
INaP.m, 59
ip3fundrive.m, 207
ip3gen.m, 206
lgn_est3.m, 328
lgn_est5.m, 330
lgn_revcor_wn3.m, 337
lif_rand_inp.m, 145
LNTcurves.m, 197
makeH.m, 135
makemd.m, 135
matched.m, 352
ml1.m, 393
ml2.m, 393, 394
moliA.m, 41
molifreq.m, 45
molisynss.m, 42
mt_mod12.m, 189
mt_mod6.m, 188
mt_perf.m, 138
myelins.m, 139
myelinsdriver.m, 362
NaPtrack.m, 59
neg_corr.m, 245
ojasim.m, 230
ou_f1.m, 272
ou_f2.m, 273
over_rep.m, 370
pfibexact.m, 85
photoreceptor_model.m, 297
plot_pp.m, 169
poiss1.m, 344
pop_corr.m, 373
power_auto_g2_g10.m, 289
power_spec.m, 285
pr_complex.m, 152
pr_modes.m, 151
pr_sodca_spike.m, 151
prob_pdfs.m, 158
Qcabnon.m, 133
quasicabspec.m, 132
rand_fig2.m, 254
rand_fig3.m, 255
rec_wn8.m, 339
ref_period2.m, 239
rgc_rf1.m, 310
Rinxs.m, 77
scene_2d.m, 294
sdpop.m, 351
soto.m, 397, 398, 405

sotofreq.m, 406
spikepca.m, 227, 228
ss2e.m, 17
sse.m, 16
ssEI.m, 17
stdobs_plot.m, 292
stE.m, 38, 44–46
stE2cab.m, 124, 125, 136
stE2cabthresh.m, 137
stE2d.m, 46
steady.m, 71
stEcab.m, 137
stEcabgNadriver.m, 124, 136
stEcabnon.m, 127
stEcabQandA.m, 131
stEcabResdrive.m, 134
stEcabsdriver.m, 137
stEcabspine.m, 130
stEcabthreshloc.m, 121
stEdemo.m, 38, 39, 43
stEdemo2.m, 39
stEerr.m, 40
stEfork.m, 134
stEforksyn.m, 135
stEforksyndrive.m, 135
stEforksyngain.m, 135
stEfreq.m, 44
stEKstimdrive.m, 45
stEperdrive.m, 54
stEqa.m, 53, 65
stEqafreq.m, 53
stEqah.m, 60
stEQcab.m, 131
stEQcabBT.m, 232, 235
stEQcabBT2.m, 235
stErefracdrive.m, 44
stEtreesyn.m, 135, 136
stmolidemo.m, 41, 44
stmolierr.m, 42
stmolisyn.m, 42
swcconverter.m, 135
temp_space_rfs.m, 319
threecell.m, 385, 387, 404
threecellI.m, 387
threecellIrast.m, 387
threecellrast.m, 387
thresh_fatigue.m, 146
thvsvth.m, 78
trapcab.m, 72
trapcabspine.m, 81
trapcabsyn.m, 79
trapcabsyninv.m, 97
trapfork.m, 108, 117
trapforkd.m, 117
trapforksyn.m, 108, 116
trapforksynclamp.m, 116
trapforksyngain.m, 109
trapsyn.m, 29, 30
trapsyndrive.m, 15
treeplot.m, 135, 139

ts_rfs.m, 325
tuning_rec.m, 369
twocell.m, 385
twostatechan.m, 269
wang_mod.m, 150
wang_ss.m, 150
function
    chol, 172
    circshift, 90
    colormap, 326
    conv, 324, 333
    cpsd, 287
    cumsum, 173
    diag, 86
    eig, 56, 70
    fft, 90
    fftfilt, 341
    fftshift, 91
    fsolve, 37, 61, 126
    gamrnd, 266
    hist, 266
    ifft, 91, 333, 340
    lsqcurvefit, 31
    lu, 61, 72
    lyapchol, 232
    mesh, 85
    meshc, 326
    meshgrid, 85
    mscohere, 288
    pinv, 234
    pwelch, 288, 298, 341
    round, 72
    speye, 72
    spline, 298
    sprand, 387
    svd, 225
    tfestimate, 333, 340
    view, 326
maximum likelihood, 372, 374
mean squared coherence, 280, 297
method of failures, 180
Mexican hat, 303–305
Michaelis constant, 211
minimum error, 346, 348, 360, 363
miss, 344
mod, 31
moment, 23, 65, 82, 354
Morris Lecar model, 64, 397
motion energy model, 321
MT, 301, 321, 362–364
multi-taper method, 286
myelin, 136

N

Naka–Rushton non-linearity, 309
Nernst Potential, 11
Nernst–Planck equation, 11, 195
neuromuscular junction, 159, 175–178,
    180–183, 190

Newton's Method, 61
Neyman–Pearson test, 346, 360, 363
nodes of Ranvier, 137, 138
nullcline, 46
Nyquist
    frequency, 90, 95
    rate, 91

O

octave, 315
Ohm's Law, 11
Oja's Rule, 233
Ornstein–Uhlenbeck process, 271, 272,
    277, 280, 285, 287
oscillations, 149
overcomplete representation, 369

P

Parseval's Identity, 282
parvalbumin, 198, 221
patch–clamp technique, 181, 267, 275
periodogram, 282
phase plane, 46
phosphatase, 211, 212, 220
phosphorylation, 209
point process, 254
Poisson process
    doubly stochastic, 265
    homogeneous, 168, 240, 246, 256, 260
    inhomogeneous, 257
posterior probability, 161
power spectrum, 259, 279, 328, 338
    natural scenes, 293, 308
    numerical estimate, 282
psychometric function, 360
Purkinje cell, 3, 104, 125, 182, 186

Q

quadrature pair, 320, 323
quantal content, 178, 180, 181
quasi–active
    cable, 130, 230
    cell, 50

R

radiance, 293
random variable
    binomial, 157, 178
    definition, 156
    degenerate, 165
    exponential, 167, 169, 172
    gamma, 167, 241
    Gaussian, 159, 178
    independence, 157
    Poisson, 159, 178
randomized decision rule, 345, 348
rapid buffer approximation, 222

receptive field, 149, 301, 335, 337
  non-separable, 318
  separable, 307
Receptor
  AMPA, 14, 127
  GABA, 14
  IP$_3$, 204
  metabotropic glutamate, 176, 204, 217
  NMDA, 127
  ryanodine, 202
refractory period, 44
Reichardt correlation model, 321
releasable pool
  rapid, 187, 214–216
  slow, 187, 215
renewal process, 240, 246–248, 257, 263, 265
resonance, 53, 57, 131
resonant, 219
retinal ganglion cell, 300, 301, 311, 312, 358, 364, 365
reverse–correlation, 335
ROC curve, 345, 348, 359, 360

S

sample
  mean, 281
  variance, 287
sarco-endoplasmic reticulum calcium ATPase, 203
Schwarz inequality, 5, 234

score
  function, 374
second difference matrix, 200
signal-to-noise ratio, 338, 340, 346, 349, 350
simple cell, 311, 318, 320–323, 325, 336, 337
siz, spike initiation zone, 126
SNARE, 213
space clamp, 34, 132
space constant, 68, 71
spike time-dependent plasticity, 389, 403
spine, 79
standard error of the mean, 281
stationarity, 246, 247, 252, 253, 256, 259, 262, 327, 331
superior colliculus, 367, 375
synaptic
  depression, 184
  facilitation, 183, 185, 188, 190
  plasticity, 209
  potentiation, 183
synaptotagmin, 213

T

tapered cable equation, 86
thalamic relay neuron, 147, 152, 300, 307–309, 311, 322
threshold fatigue, 145, 245, 246
time constant
  channel, 270

effective, 16
  exponential filter, 339
  membrane, 13, 21, 70
Time Marching Scheme
  Backward Euler, 28
  Forward Euler, 27
  Hybrid Euler, 41
  Staggered Euler, 38
  Trapezoid, 28
time rescaling, 262, 266
topographic map, 438

V

V1, 301, 312, 323, 362
voltage clamp, 34, 116

W

wavelets, 322
weakly electric fish, 3, 149, 246, 338–340, 352, 353
Weber's law, 296
Weierstrass M-test, 84
white noise, 253, 288, 333, 336
Wiener process, 252, 259, 263
Wiener–Khinchin theorem, 260, 262, 282
Wiener–Kolmogorov filter, 340
window
  data, 284
  spectral, 285
wrap-around order, 91, 309

Printed in the United States
By Bookmasters